SECTIONAL ANATOMY
by MRI and CT

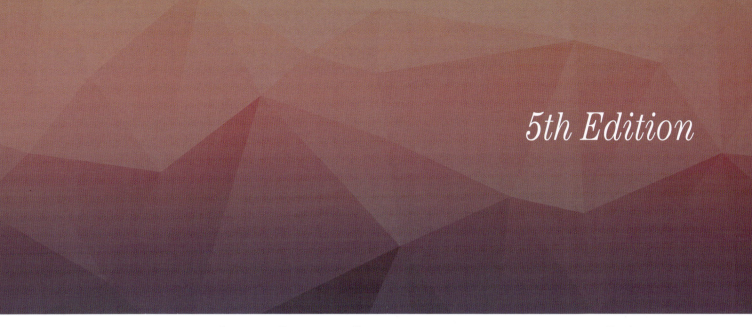

5th Edition

SECTIONAL ANATOMY
by MRI and CT

MARK W. ANDERSON, MD
Harrison Distinguished Teaching Professor of Radiology
Chief of the Division of Musculoskeletal Radiology
Department of Radiology
University of Virginia Health Sciences Center
Charlottesville, Virginia

MICHAEL G. FOX, MD
Musculoskeletal Division Chair
Associate Professor of Radiology
Department of Radiology
Mayo Clinic College of Medicine
Phoenix, Arizona

NICHOLAS C. NACEY, MD
Associate Professor
Department of Radiology and Medical Imaging
University of Virginia Health Science Center
Charlottesville, Virginia

ELSEVIER

Elsevier
1600 John F. Kennedy Blvd.
Ste 1800
Philadelphia, PA 19103-2899

SECTIONAL ANATOMY BY MRI AND CT, FIFTH EDITION   ISBN: 978-0-323-93448-0

Notice

Practitioners and researchers must always rely on their own experience and knowledge in evaluating and using any information, methods, compounds or experiments described herein. Because of rapid advances in the medical sciences, in particular, independent verification of diagnoses and drug dosages should be made. To the fullest extent of the law, no responsibility is assumed by Elsevier, authors, editors or contributors for any injury and/or damage to persons or property as a matter of products liability, negligence or otherwise, or from any use or operation of any methods, products, instructions, or ideas contained in the material herein.

Previous editions copyrighted 2017, 2007, 1995 and 1990.

Senior Content Strategist: Melanie Tucker
Senior Content Development Specialist: Rishabh Gupta
Content Development Manager: Ranjana Sharma
Publishing Services Manager: Shereen Jameel
Project Manager: Haritha Dharmarajan
Design Direction: Brian Salisbury

Printed in India

Last digit is the print number: 9 8 7 6 5 4 3 2 1

Working together
to grow libraries in
developing countries

www.elsevier.com • www.bookaid.org

Preface

With the explosion of cross-sectional imaging, the accessibility of a high-quality anatomic atlas has become essential, and it is with great pleasure that we introduce the fifth edition of this classic atlas.

Since it was first published in 1990, it has become a standard anatomic reference source. The first three editions were masterfully edited by Drs. Georges El-Khoury, Ronald Bergman, and William Montgomery, and we are honored to be able to continue the tradition of excellence that they established.

This new fifth edition includes additional chapters on head CT, brain MRI, and cervical spine MRI. The corresponding online version also allows for easy access anytime/anywhere and provides scroll and zoom functions that should further enhance the user's experience.

We hope that you will find this new edition to be an integral and valuable addition to your practice.

Mark W. Anderson, MD
Michael G. Fox, MD
Nicholas C. Nacey, MD

Acknowledgments

We are indebted to Drs. Georges El-Khoury and Ronald Bergman for their prior efforts in producing and improving this text and for allowing us to continue along the path of excellence they established. We also would like to thank Rishabh Gupta and Melanie Tucker from Elsevier for helping to bring this project to fruition. Thanks as well to our fellow Matthew Schmidt for his assistance. Dr. Anderson would like to thank all the residents and fellows who have made him a better radiologist, and his wife Amy whose sacrifice and support have made it all possible. Dr. Nacey would like to thank his wife Mary as well as his children Ollie, Annie, Emmie, and Zach for all their support. Dr. Fox would like to thank his family (Katherine, Marie, Elizabeth, Michael Jr., and Jonathan) for their love and encouragement. Without their invaluable assistance, it would not have happened!

Mark W. Anderson, MD
Michael G. Fox, MD
Nicholas C. Nacey, MD

Contents

Preface, v
Acknowledgments, vi

SECTION I BRAIN, 1
Chapter 1 CT of the Brain, 3
Chapter 2 MRI of the Brain, 18

SECTION II THORAX, 33
Chapter 3 CT of the Thorax, 35
Chapter 4 MRI of the Heart, 53

SECTION III UPPER EXTREMITY, 65
Chapter 5 MRI of the Pectoral Girdle and Chest Wall, 67
Chapter 6 MRI of the Shoulder, 98
Chapter 7 MR Arthrography of the Shoulder, 130
Chapter 8 MRI of the Arm, 154
Chapter 9 MRI of the Elbow, 178
Chapter 10 MRI of the Forearm, 208
Chapter 11 MRI of the Wrist, 235
Chapter 12 MRI of the Hand, 261

SECTION IV SPINE AND BACK, 285
Chapter 13 MRI of the Cervical Spine, 287
Chapter 14 MRI of the Thoracic Spine, 296
Chapter 15 MRI of the Lumbar Spine, 309

SECTION V ABDOMEN, 323
Chapter 16 CT of the Abdomen, 325
Chapter 17 MRI of the Abdomen, 345

SECTION VI LOWER EXTREMITY, 371
Chapter 18 MRI of the Hip, 373
Chapter 19 MR Arthrography of the Hip, 402
Chapter 20 MRI of the Thigh, 419
Chapter 21 MRI of the Knee, 446
Chapter 22 MRI of the Leg, 473
Chapter 23 MRI of the Ankle, 500
Chapter 24 MRI of the foot, 534

SECTION VII PELVIS, 561
Chapter 25 CT of the Male Pelvis, 563
Chapter 26 CT of the Female Pelvis, 579
Chapter 27 MRI of the Male Pelvis, 594
Chapter 28 MRI of the Female Pelvis, 613

Index, 627

Section

I

Brain

Chapter

1

CT of the Brain

AXIAL
Figure 1.1.1

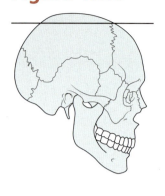

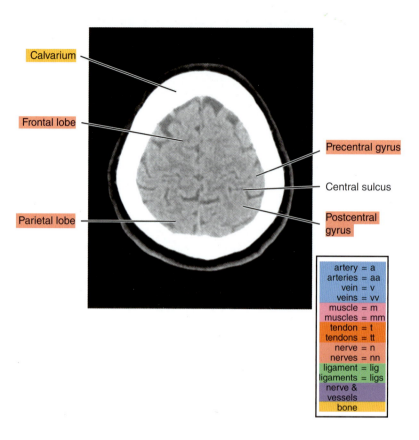

Calvarium

Frontal lobe

Precentral gyrus

Central sulcus

Parietal lobe

Postcentral gyrus

artery = a	
arteries = aa	
vein = v	
veins = vv	
muscle = m	
muscles = mm	
tendon = t	
tendons = tt	
nerve = n	
nerves = nn	
ligament = lig	
ligaments = ligs	
nerve & vessels	
bone	

Figure 1.1.2

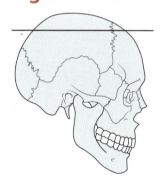

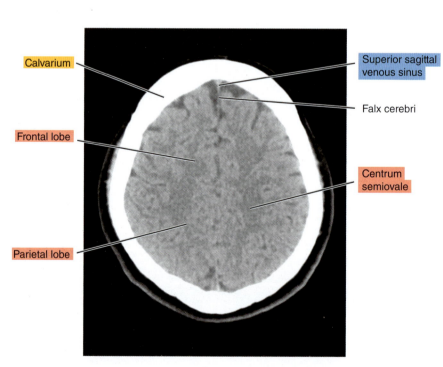

Calvarium

Superior sagittal venous sinus

Falx cerebri

Frontal lobe

Centrum semiovale

Parietal lobe

Figure 1.1.3

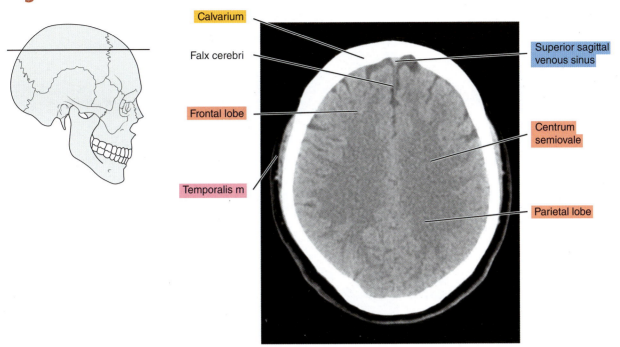

Calvarium

Falx cerebri

Frontal lobe

Temporalis m

Superior sagittal venous sinus

Centrum semiovale

Parietal lobe

Figure 1.1.4

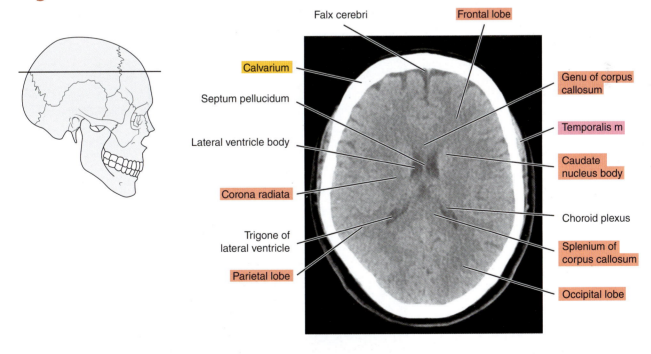

Falx cerebri

Frontal lobe

Calvarium

Septum pellucidum

Lateral ventricle body

Corona radiata

Trigone of lateral ventricle

Parietal lobe

Genu of corpus callosum

Temporalis m

Caudate nucleus body

Choroid plexus

Splenium of corpus callosum

Occipital lobe

Figure 1.1.5

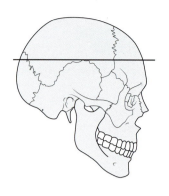

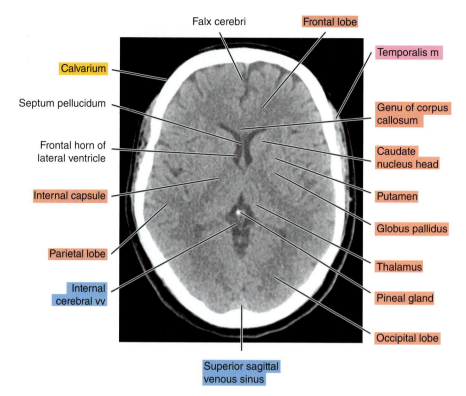

Falx cerebri   Frontal lobe

Temporalis m

Calvarium

Septum pellucidum

Genu of corpus callosum

Frontal horn of lateral ventricle

Caudate nucleus head

Internal capsule

Putamen

Globus pallidus

Parietal lobe

Thalamus

Internal cerebral vv

Pineal gland

Occipital lobe

Superior sagittal venous sinus

Figure 1.1.6

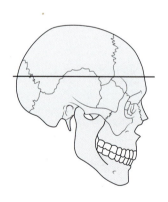

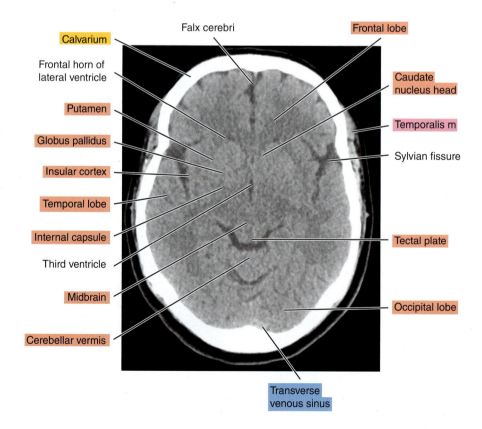

Falx cerebri   Frontal lobe

Calvarium

Frontal horn of lateral ventricle

Caudate nucleus head

Putamen

Temporalis m

Globus pallidus

Sylvian fissure

Insular cortex

Temporal lobe

Internal capsule

Third ventricle

Tectal plate

Midbrain

Occipital lobe

Cerebellar vermis

Transverse venous sinus

Figure 1.1.7

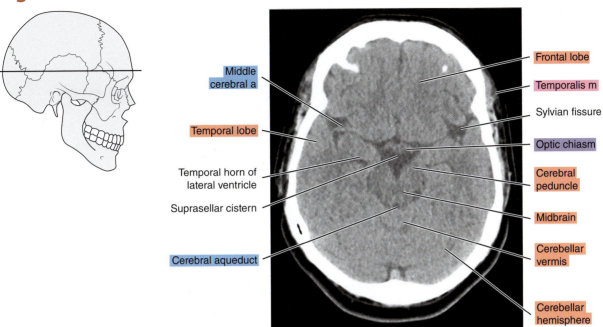

Middle cerebral a

Temporal lobe

Temporal horn of lateral ventricle

Suprasellar cistern

Cerebral aqueduct

Frontal lobe

Temporalis m

Sylvian fissure

Optic chiasm

Cerebral peduncle

Midbrain

Cerebellar vermis

Cerebellar hemisphere

Figure 1.1.8

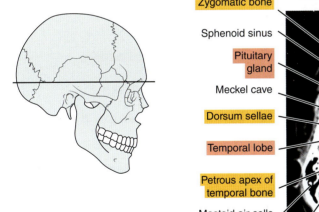

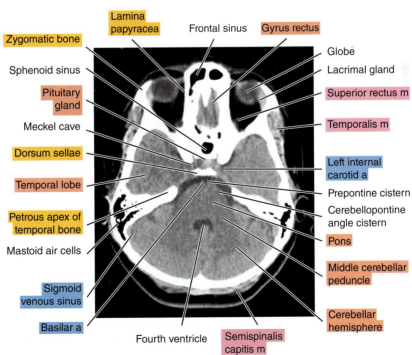

Lamina papyracea

Frontal sinus

Gyrus rectus

Zygomatic bone

Sphenoid sinus

Pituitary gland

Meckel cave

Dorsum sellae

Temporal lobe

Petrous apex of temporal bone

Mastoid air cells

Sigmoid venous sinus

Basilar a

Fourth ventricle

Semispinalis capitis m

Globe

Lacrimal gland

Superior rectus m

Temporalis m

Left internal carotid a

Prepontine cistern

Cerebellopontine angle cistern

Pons

Middle cerebellar peduncle

Cerebellar hemisphere

Figure 1.1.9

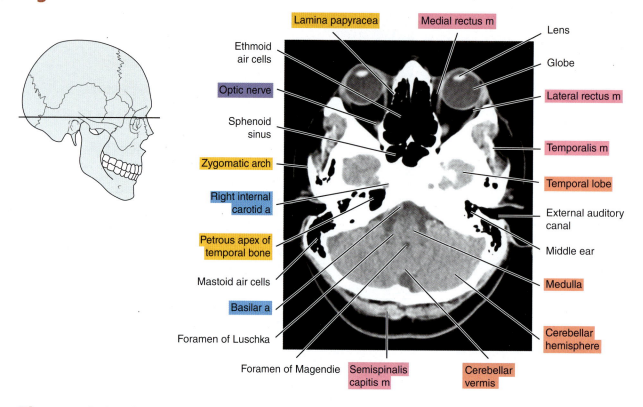

Lamina papyracea
Medial rectus m
Lens
Ethmoid air cells
Globe
Optic nerve
Lateral rectus m
Sphenoid sinus
Temporalis m
Zygomatic arch
Temporal lobe
Right internal carotid a
External auditory canal
Petrous apex of temporal bone
Middle ear
Mastoid air cells
Medulla
Basilar a
Foramen of Luschka
Cerebellar hemisphere
Foramen of Magendie
Semispinalis capitis m
Cerebellar vermis

Figure 1.1.10

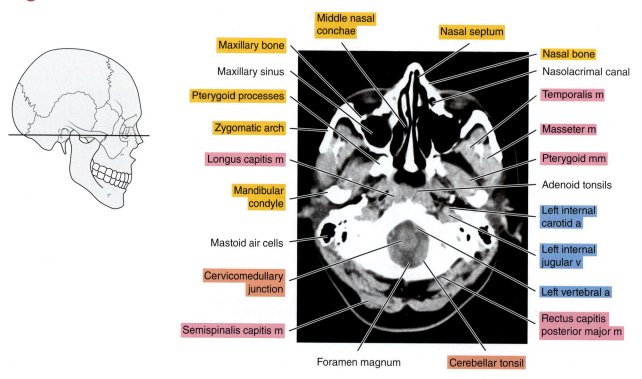

Middle nasal conchae
Nasal septum
Maxillary bone
Nasal bone
Maxillary sinus
Nasolacrimal canal
Pterygoid processes
Temporalis m
Zygomatic arch
Masseter m
Longus capitis m
Pterygoid mm
Mandibular condyle
Adenoid tonsils
Mastoid air cells
Left internal carotid a
Left internal jugular v
Cervicomedullary junction
Left vertebral a
Semispinalis capitis m
Rectus capitis posterior major m
Foramen magnum
Cerebellar tonsil

Figure 1.1.11

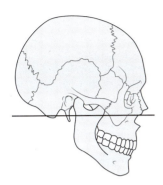

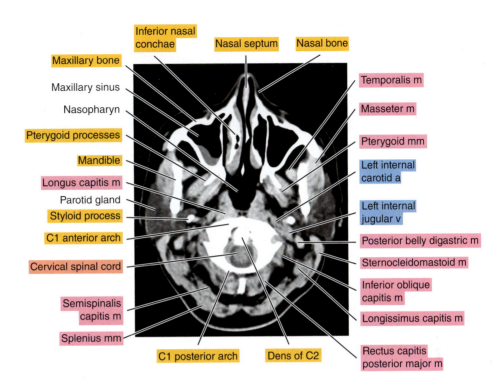

Inferior nasal conchae

Maxillary bone

Maxillary sinus

Nasopharyn

Pterygoid processes

Mandible

Longus capitis m

Parotid gland

Styloid process

C1 anterior arch

Cervical spinal cord

Semispinalis capitis m

Splenius mm

Nasal septum

Nasal bone

Temporalis m

Masseter m

Pterygoid mm

Left internal carotid a

Left internal jugular v

Posterior belly digastric m

Sternocleidomastoid m

Inferior oblique capitis m

Longissimus capitis m

Rectus capitis posterior major m

C1 posterior arch

Dens of C2

SAGITTAL
Figure 1.2.1

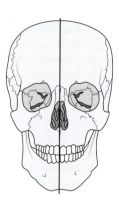

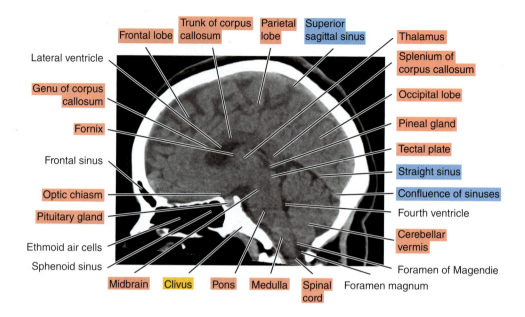

Frontal lobe | Trunk of corpus callosum | Parietal lobe | Superior sagittal sinus | Thalamus

Lateral ventricle

Splenium of corpus callosum

Genu of corpus callosum

Occipital lobe

Fornix

Pineal gland

Frontal sinus

Tectal plate

Optic chiasm

Straight sinus

Pituitary gland

Confluence of sinuses

Ethmoid air cells

Fourth ventricle

Sphenoid sinus

Cerebellar vermis

Foramen of Magendie

Midbrain | Clivus | Pons | Medulla | Spinal cord | Foramen magnum

Figure 1.2.2

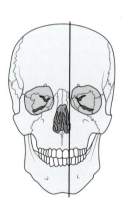

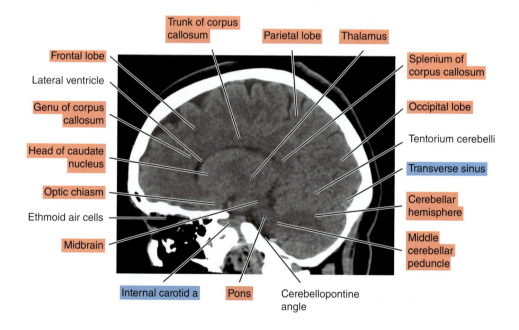

Trunk of corpus callosum | Parietal lobe | Thalamus

Frontal lobe

Splenium of corpus callosum

Lateral ventricle

Occipital lobe

Genu of corpus callosum

Tentorium cerebelli

Head of caudate nucleus

Transverse sinus

Optic chiasm

Cerebellar hemisphere

Ethmoid air cells

Midbrain

Middle cerebellar peduncle

Internal carotid a | Pons | Cerebellopontine angle

Figure 1.2.3

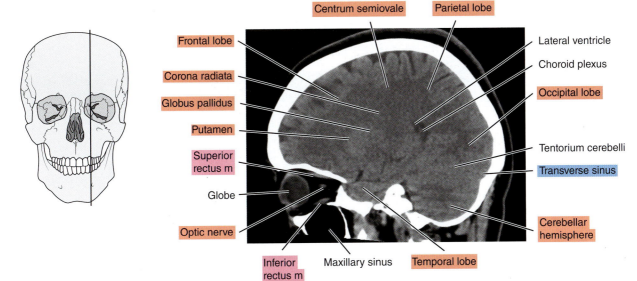

Centrum semiovale

Parietal lobe

Frontal lobe

Corona radiata

Globus pallidus

Putamen

Superior rectus m

Globe

Optic nerve

Inferior rectus m

Maxillary sinus

Temporal lobe

Lateral ventricle

Choroid plexus

Occipital lobe

Tentorium cerebelli

Transverse sinus

Cerebellar hemisphere

Figure 1.2.4

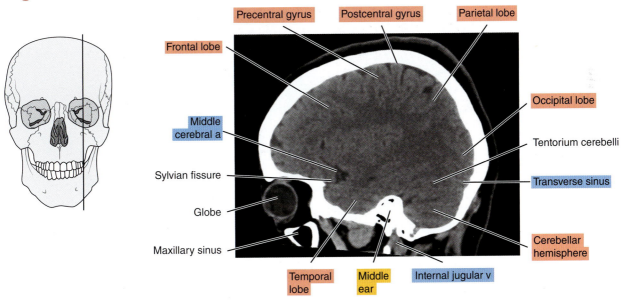

Precentral gyrus

Postcentral gyrus

Parietal lobe

Frontal lobe

Middle cerebral a

Sylvian fissure

Globe

Maxillary sinus

Temporal lobe

Middle ear

Internal jugular v

Occipital lobe

Tentorium cerebelli

Transverse sinus

Cerebellar hemisphere

Figure 1.2.5

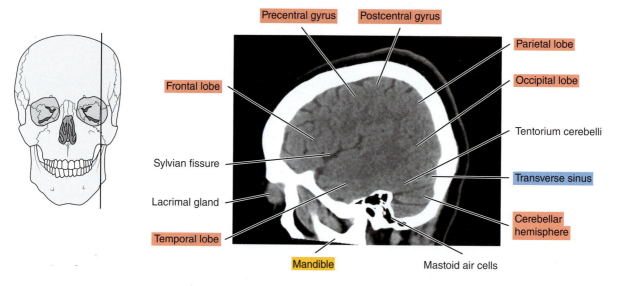

Precentral gyrus

Postcentral gyrus

Parietal lobe

Frontal lobe

Occipital lobe

Tentorium cerebelli

Sylvian fissure

Transverse sinus

Lacrimal gland

Cerebellar hemisphere

Temporal lobe

Mandible

Mastoid air cells

Figure 1.2.6

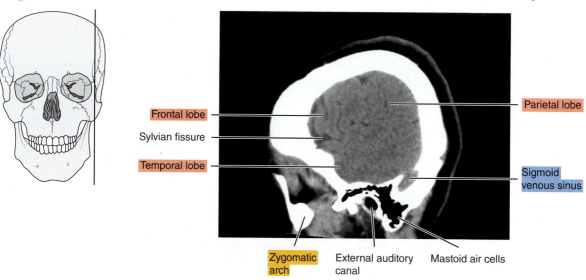

Frontal lobe

Sylvian fissure

Temporal lobe

Parietal lobe

Sigmoid venous sinus

Zygomatic arch

External auditory canal

Mastoid air cells

CORONAL
Figure 1.3.1

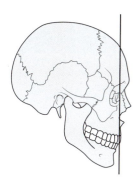

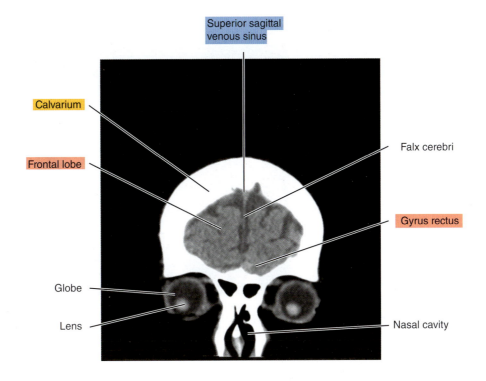

Superior sagittal venous sinus

Calvarium

Frontal lobe

Falx cerebri

Gyrus rectus

Globe

Lens

Nasal cavity

Figure 1.3.2

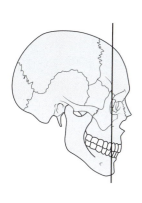

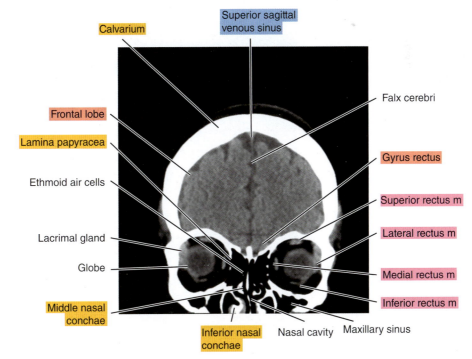

Calvarium

Superior sagittal venous sinus

Frontal lobe

Lamina papyracea

Ethmoid air cells

Lacrimal gland

Globe

Middle nasal conchae

Falx cerebri

Gyrus rectus

Superior rectus m

Lateral rectus m

Medial rectus m

Inferior rectus m

Inferior nasal conchae

Nasal cavity

Maxillary sinus

Figure 1.3.3

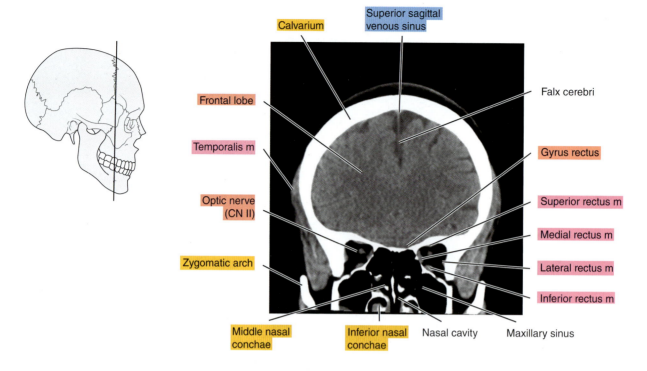

Calvarium
Superior sagittal venous sinus
Falx cerebri
Frontal lobe
Temporalis m
Gyrus rectus
Superior rectus m
Optic nerve (CN II)
Medial rectus m
Lateral rectus m
Zygomatic arch
Inferior rectus m
Middle nasal conchae
Inferior nasal conchae
Nasal cavity
Maxillary sinus

Figure 1.3.4

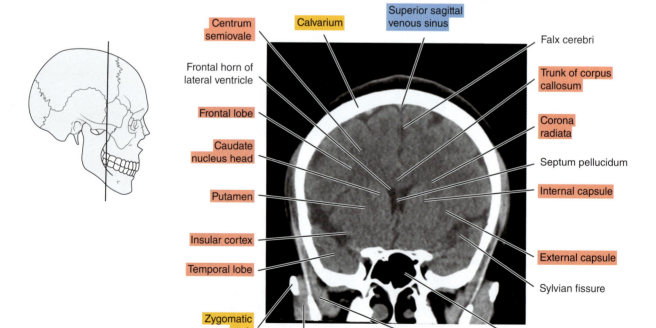

Centrum semiovale
Calvarium
Superior sagittal venous sinus
Falx cerebri
Frontal horn of lateral ventricle
Trunk of corpus callosum
Frontal lobe
Corona radiata
Caudate nucleus head
Septum pellucidum
Putamen
Internal capsule
Insular cortex
External capsule
Temporal lobe
Sylvian fissure
Zygomatic arch
Sphenoid sinus
Masseter m
Temporalis m

Figure 1.3.5

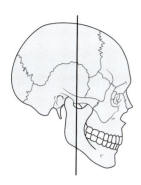

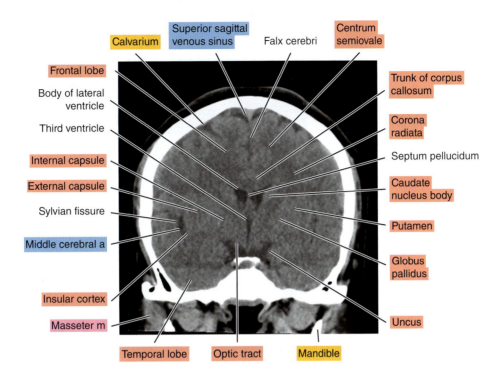

Calvarium — Superior sagittal venous sinus — Falx cerebri — Centrum semiovale

Frontal lobe
Body of lateral ventricle
Third ventricle
Internal capsule
External capsule
Sylvian fissure
Middle cerebral a
Insular cortex
Masseter m

Trunk of corpus callosum
Corona radiata
Septum pellucidum
Caudate nucleus body
Putamen
Globus pallidus
Uncus

Temporal lobe   Optic tract   Mandible

Figure 1.3.6

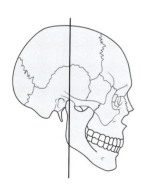

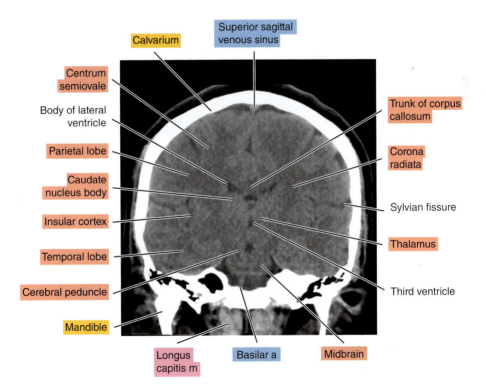

Calvarium — Superior sagittal venous sinus

Centrum semiovale
Body of lateral ventricle
Parietal lobe
Caudate nucleus body
Insular cortex
Temporal lobe
Cerebral peduncle
Mandible

Trunk of corpus callosum
Corona radiata
Sylvian fissure
Thalamus
Third ventricle

Longus capitis m   Basilar a   Midbrain

Figure 1.3.7

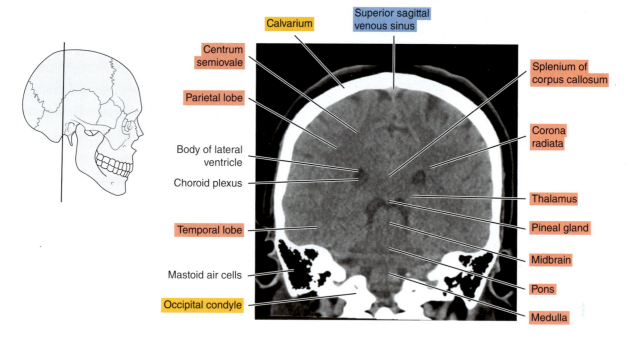

Calvarium
Superior sagittal venous sinus
Centrum semiovale
Splenium of corpus callosum
Parietal lobe
Corona radiata
Body of lateral ventricle
Choroid plexus
Thalamus
Pineal gland
Temporal lobe
Midbrain
Mastoid air cells
Pons
Occipital condyle
Medulla

Figure 1.3.8

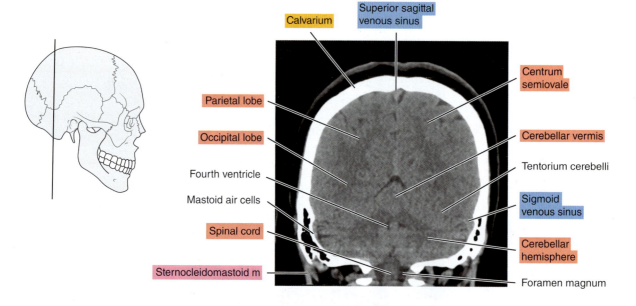

Calvarium
Superior sagittal venous sinus
Centrum semiovale
Parietal lobe
Cerebellar vermis
Occipital lobe
Tentorium cerebelli
Fourth ventricle
Sigmoid venous sinus
Mastoid air cells
Spinal cord
Cerebellar hemisphere
Sternocleidomastoid m
Foramen magnum

Figure 1.3.9

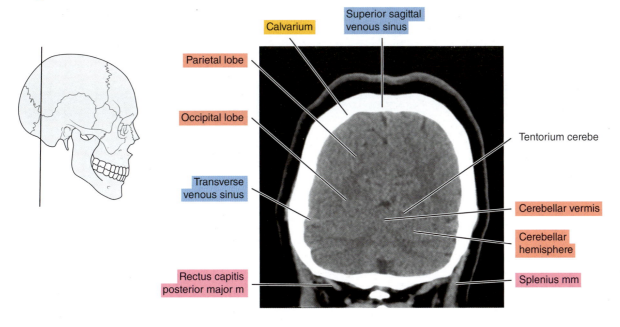

Figure 1.3.10

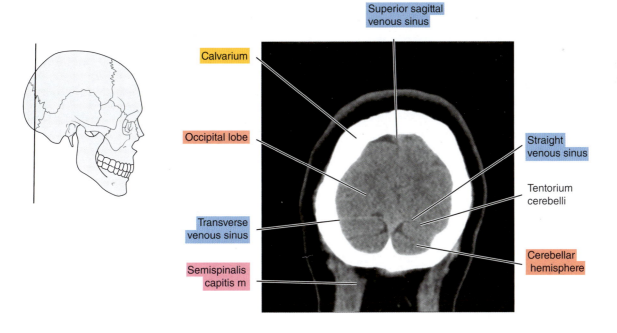

Chapter

2

MRI of the Brain

AXIAL
Figure 2.1.1

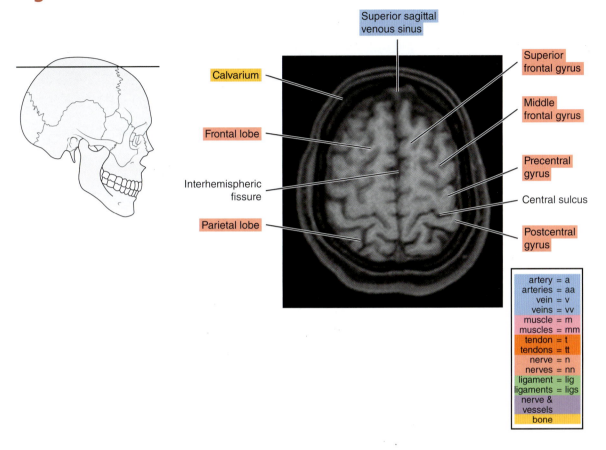

Superior sagittal venous sinus

Calvarium

Frontal lobe

Interhemispheric fissure

Parietal lobe

Superior frontal gyrus

Middle frontal gyrus

Precentral gyrus

Central sulcus

Postcentral gyrus

artery =	a
arteries =	aa
vein =	v
veins =	vv
muscle =	m
muscles =	mm
tendon =	t
tendons =	tt
nerve =	n
nerves =	nn
ligament =	lig
ligaments =	ligs
nerve & vessels	
bone	

Figure 2.1.2

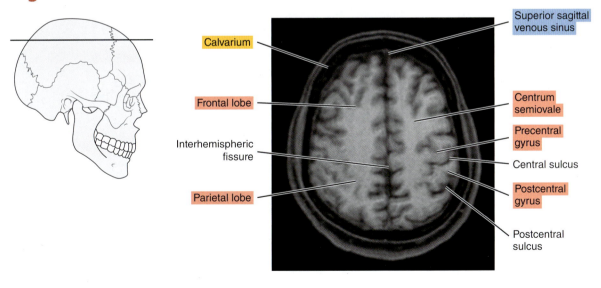

Superior sagittal venous sinus

Calvarium

Frontal lobe

Interhemispheric fissure

Parietal lobe

Centrum semiovale

Precentral gyrus

Central sulcus

Postcentral gyrus

Postcentral sulcus

Figure 2.1.3

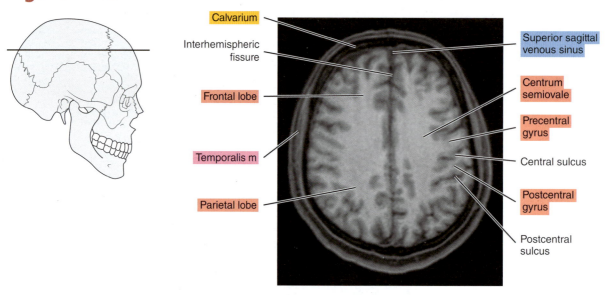

Calvarium

Interhemispheric fissure

Frontal lobe

Temporalis m

Parietal lobe

Superior sagittal venous sinus

Centrum semiovale

Precentral gyrus

Central sulcus

Postcentral gyrus

Postcentral sulcus

Figure 2.1.4

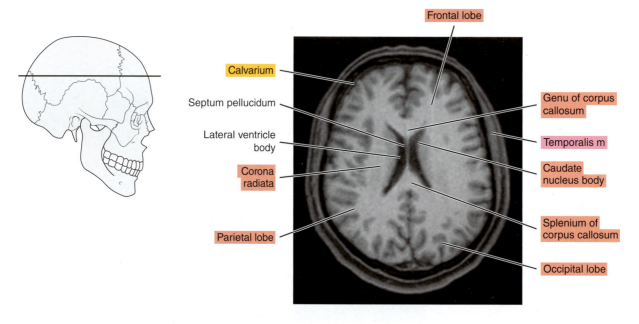

Frontal lobe

Calvarium

Septum pellucidum

Lateral ventricle body

Corona radiata

Parietal lobe

Genu of corpus callosum

Temporalis m

Caudate nucleus body

Splenium of corpus callosum

Occipital lobe

Figure 2.1.5

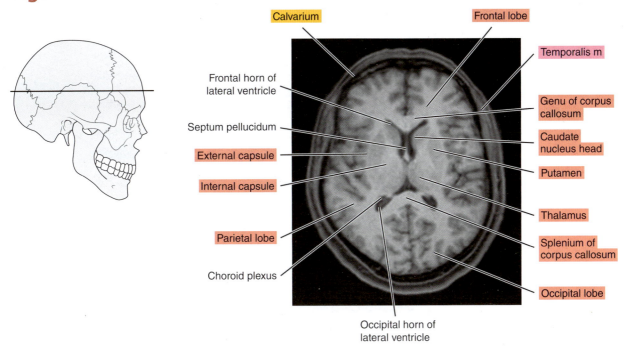

Calvarium

Frontal lobe

Temporalis m

Frontal horn of
lateral ventricle

Genu of corpus
callosum

Septum pellucidum

Caudate
nucleus head

External capsule

Putamen

Internal capsule

Thalamus

Parietal lobe

Splenium of
corpus callosum

Choroid plexus

Occipital lobe

Occipital horn of
lateral ventricle

Figure 2.1.6

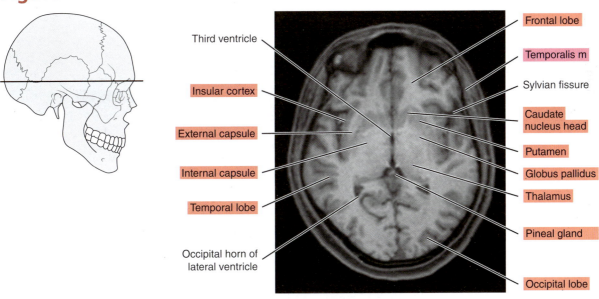

Third ventricle

Frontal lobe

Temporalis m

Insular cortex

Sylvian fissure

External capsule

Caudate
nucleus head

Internal capsule

Putamen

Globus pallidus

Temporal lobe

Thalamus

Occipital horn of
lateral ventricle

Pineal gland

Occipital lobe

Figure 2.1.7

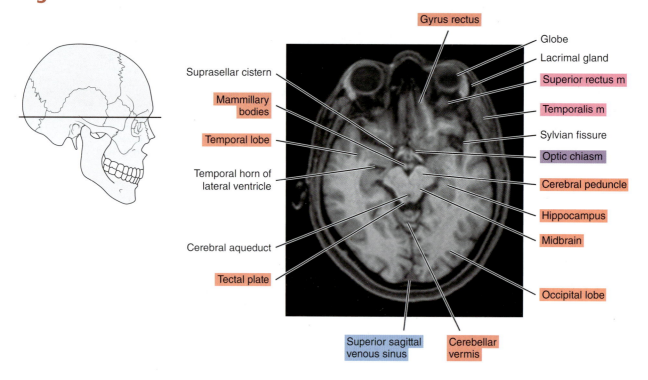

Gyrus rectus

Globe

Lacrimal gland

Superior rectus m

Temporalis m

Sylvian fissure

Optic chiasm

Cerebral peduncle

Hippocampus

Midbrain

Occipital lobe

Suprasellar cistern

Mammillary bodies

Temporal lobe

Temporal horn of lateral ventricle

Cerebral aqueduct

Tectal plate

Superior sagittal venous sinus

Cerebellar vermis

Figure 2.1.8

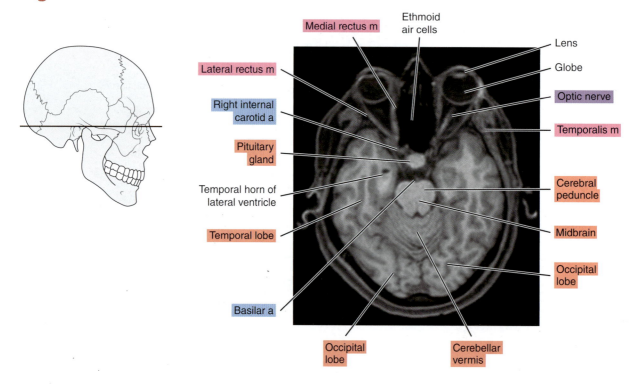

Medial rectus m

Ethmoid air cells

Lens

Globe

Optic nerve

Temporalis m

Lateral rectus m

Right internal carotid a

Pituitary gland

Temporal horn of lateral ventricle

Temporal lobe

Basilar a

Cerebral peduncle

Midbrain

Occipital lobe

Occipital lobe

Cerebellar vermis

Figure 2.1.9

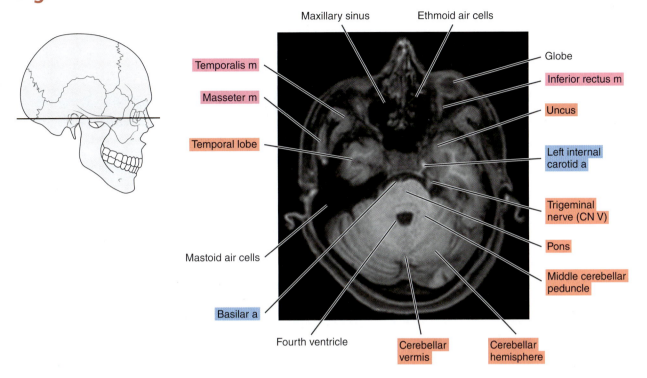

Maxillary sinus

Ethmoid air cells

Temporalis m

Masseter m

Temporal lobe

Mastoid air cells

Basilar a

Fourth ventricle

Cerebellar vermis

Cerebellar hemisphere

Globe

Inferior rectus m

Uncus

Left internal carotid a

Trigeminal nerve (CN V)

Pons

Middle cerebellar peduncle

Figure 2.1.10

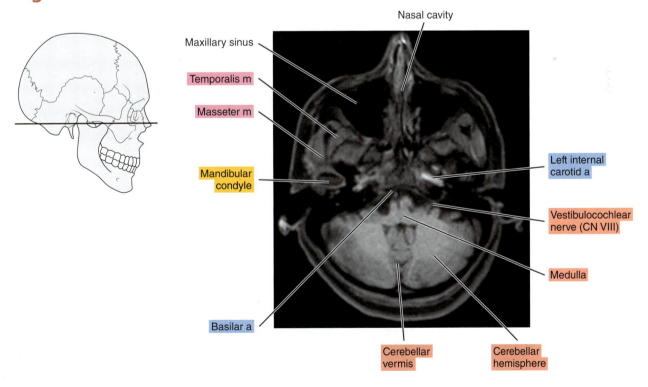

Nasal cavity

Maxillary sinus

Temporalis m

Masseter m

Mandibular condyle

Basilar a

Cerebellar vermis

Cerebellar hemisphere

Left internal carotid a

Vestibulocochlear nerve (CN VIII)

Medulla

Figure 2.1.11

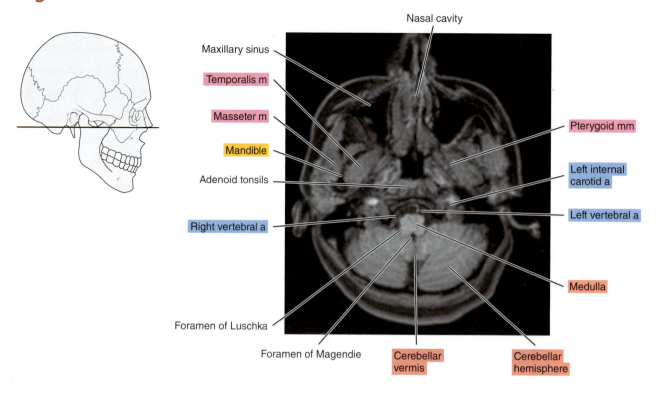

Nasal cavity

Maxillary sinus

Temporalis m

Masseter m

Mandible

Adenoid tonsils

Right vertebral a

Pterygoid mm

Left internal carotid a

Left vertebral a

Medulla

Foramen of Luschka

Foramen of Magendie

Cerebellar vermis

Cerebellar hemisphere

Figure 2.1.12

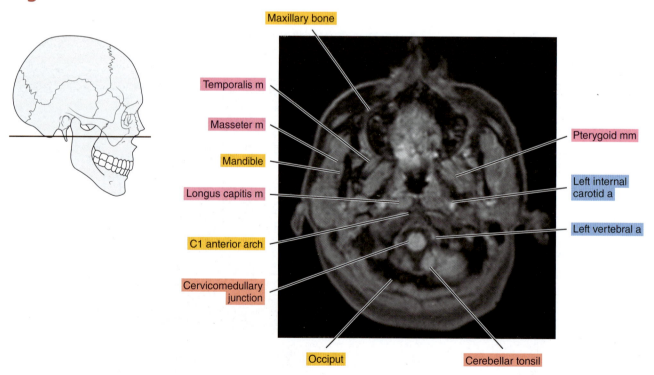

Maxillary bone

Temporalis m

Masseter m

Mandible

Longus capitis m

C1 anterior arch

Cervicomedullary junction

Pterygoid mm

Left internal carotid a

Left vertebral a

Occiput

Cerebellar tonsil

SAGITTAL
Figure 2.2.1

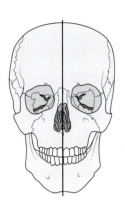

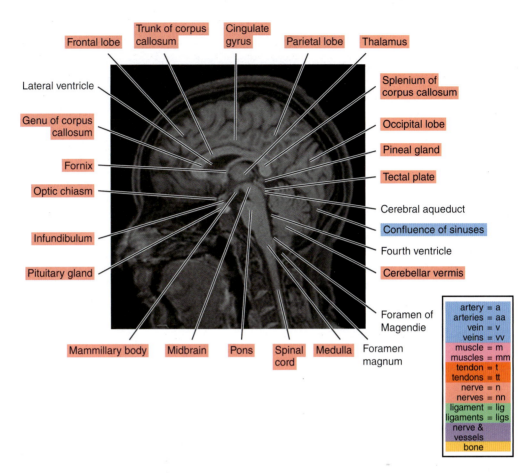

Frontal lobe

Trunk of corpus callosum

Cingulate gyrus

Parietal lobe

Thalamus

Lateral ventricle

Splenium of corpus callosum

Genu of corpus callosum

Occipital lobe

Fornix

Pineal gland

Optic chiasm

Tectal plate

Cerebral aqueduct

Confluence of sinuses

Infundibulum

Fourth ventricle

Cerebellar vermis

Pituitary gland

Foramen of Magendie

Mammillary body

Midbrain

Pons

Spinal cord

Medulla

Foramen magnum

artery	= a
arteries	= aa
vein	= v
veins	= vv
muscle	= m
muscles	= mm
tendon	= t
tendons	= tt
nerve	= n
nerves	= nn
ligament	= lig
ligaments	= ligs
nerve & vessels	
bone	

Figure 2.2.2

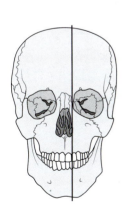

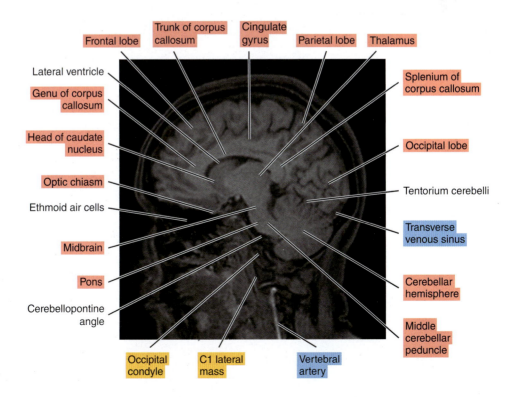

Frontal lobe

Trunk of corpus callosum

Cingulate gyrus

Parietal lobe

Thalamus

Lateral ventricle

Splenium of corpus callosum

Genu of corpus callosum

Head of caudate nucleus

Occipital lobe

Optic chiasm

Tentorium cerebelli

Ethmoid air cells

Transverse venous sinus

Midbrain

Pons

Cerebellar hemisphere

Cerebellopontine angle

Middle cerebellar peduncle

Occipital condyle

C1 lateral mass

Vertebral artery

Figure 2.2.3

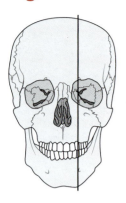

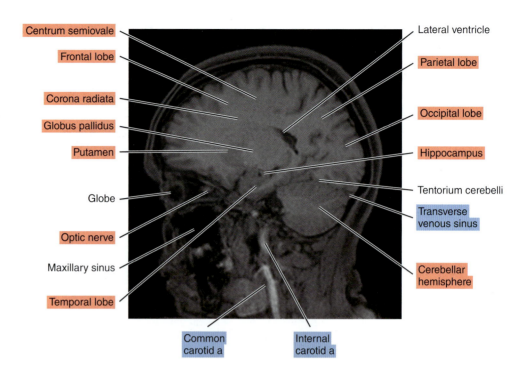

Centrum semiovale

Frontal lobe

Corona radiata

Globus pallidus

Putamen

Globe

Optic nerve

Maxillary sinus

Temporal lobe

Lateral ventricle

Parietal lobe

Occipital lobe

Hippocampus

Tentorium cerebelli

Transverse venous sinus

Cerebellar hemisphere

Common carotid a

Internal carotid a

Figure 2.2.4

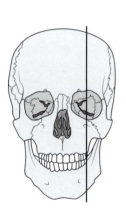

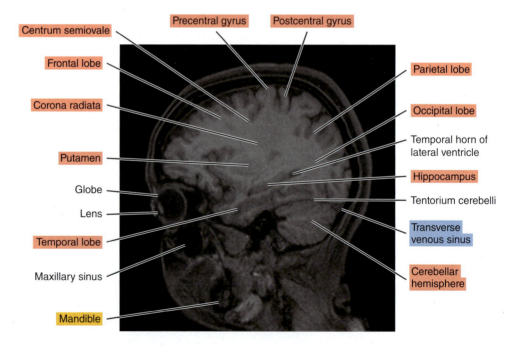

Centrum semiovale

Frontal lobe

Corona radiata

Putamen

Globe

Lens

Temporal lobe

Maxillary sinus

Mandible

Precentral gyrus

Postcentral gyrus

Parietal lobe

Occipital lobe

Temporal horn of lateral ventricle

Hippocampus

Tentorium cerebelli

Transverse venous sinus

Cerebellar hemisphere

Figure 2.2.5

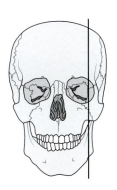
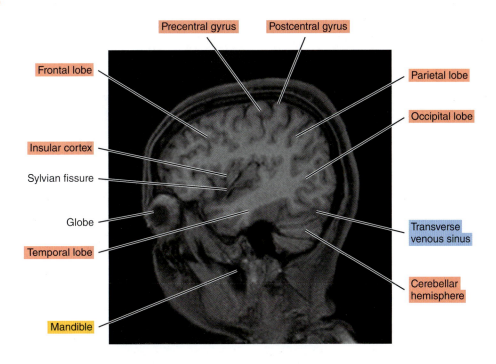

Precentral gyrus

Postcentral gyrus

Frontal lobe

Parietal lobe

Occipital lobe

Insular cortex

Sylvian fissure

Globe

Transverse venous sinus

Temporal lobe

Cerebellar hemisphere

Mandible

Figure 2.2.6

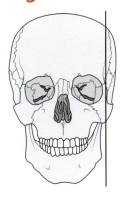
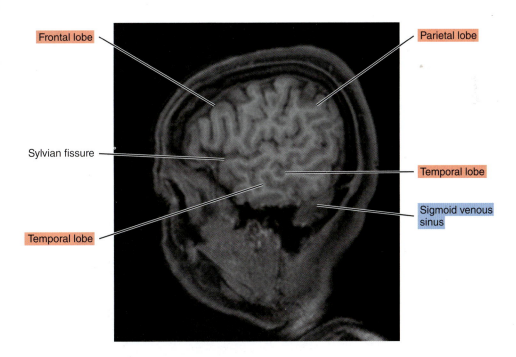

Frontal lobe

Parietal lobe

Sylvian fissure

Temporal lobe

Sigmoid venous sinus

Temporal lobe

SAGITTAL
Figure 2.3.1

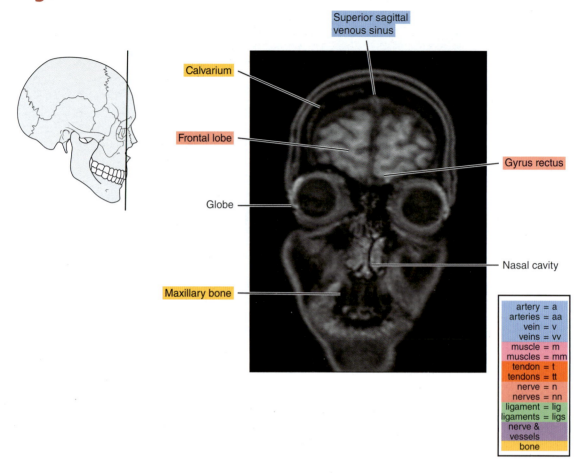

Superior sagittal venous sinus

Calvarium

Frontal lobe

Globe

Maxillary bone

Gyrus rectus

Nasal cavity

artery = a	
arteries = aa	
vein = v	
veins = vv	
muscle = m	
muscles = mm	
tendon = t	
tendons = tt	
nerve = n	
nerves = nn	
ligament = lig	
ligaments = ligs	
nerve & vessels	
bone	

Figure 2.3.2

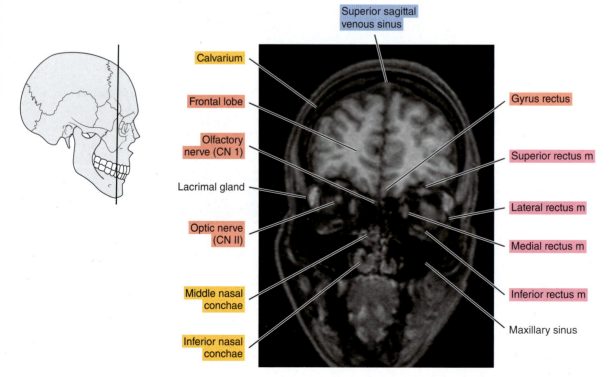

Superior sagittal venous sinus

Calvarium

Frontal lobe

Olfactory nerve (CN 1)

Lacrimal gland

Optic nerve (CN II)

Middle nasal conchae

Inferior nasal conchae

Gyrus rectus

Superior rectus m

Lateral rectus m

Medial rectus m

Inferior rectus m

Maxillary sinus

Figure 2.3.3

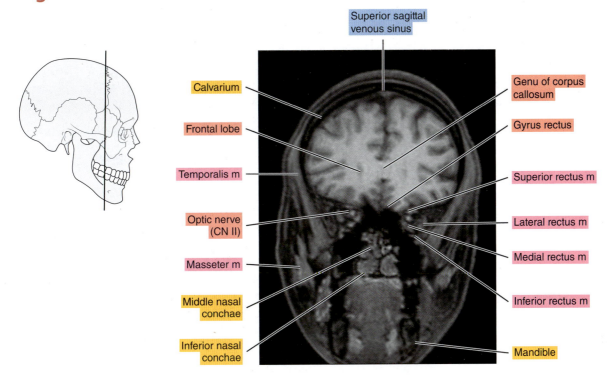

Superior sagittal venous sinus

Calvarium

Frontal lobe

Temporalis m

Optic nerve (CN II)

Masseter m

Middle nasal conchae

Inferior nasal conchae

Genu of corpus callosum

Gyrus rectus

Superior rectus m

Lateral rectus m

Medial rectus m

Inferior rectus m

Mandible

Figure 2.3.4

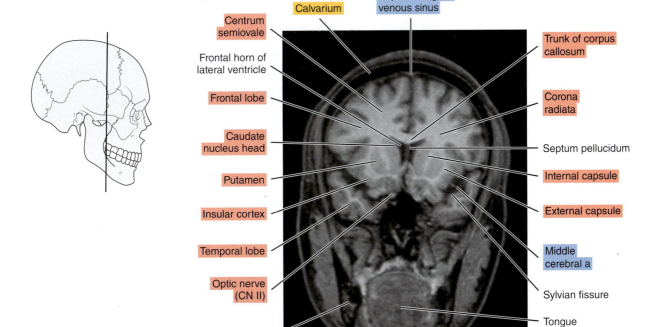

Calvarium

Superior sagittal venous sinus

Centrum semiovale

Frontal horn of lateral ventricle

Frontal lobe

Caudate nucleus head

Putamen

Insular cortex

Temporal lobe

Optic nerve (CN II)

Mandible

Trunk of corpus callosum

Corona radiata

Septum pellucidum

Internal capsule

External capsule

Middle cerebral a

Sylvian fissure

Tongue

Figure 2.3.5

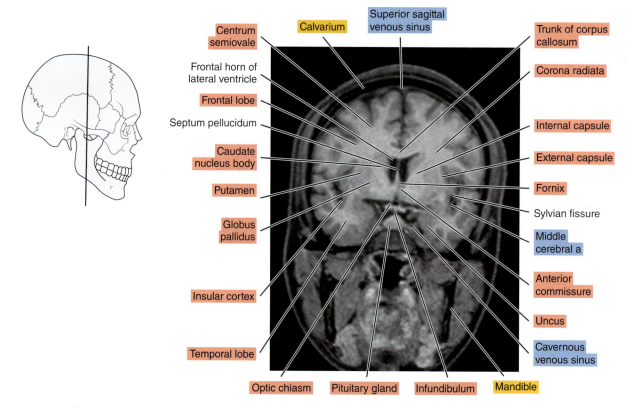

Calvarium · Superior sagittal venous sinus · Centrum semiovale · Trunk of corpus callosum · Frontal horn of lateral ventricle · Corona radiata · Frontal lobe · Septum pellucidum · Internal capsule · Caudate nucleus body · External capsule · Putamen · Fornix · Sylvian fissure · Globus pallidus · Middle cerebral a · Anterior commissure · Insular cortex · Uncus · Cavernous venous sinus · Temporal lobe · Optic chiasm · Pituitary gland · Infundibulum · Mandible

Figure 2.3.6

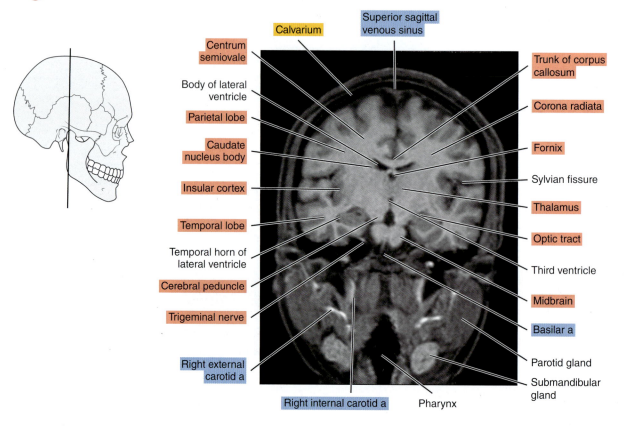

Calvarium · Superior sagittal venous sinus · Centrum semiovale · Trunk of corpus callosum · Body of lateral ventricle · Corona radiata · Parietal lobe · Fornix · Caudate nucleus body · Sylvian fissure · Insular cortex · Thalamus · Temporal lobe · Optic tract · Temporal horn of lateral ventricle · Third ventricle · Cerebral peduncle · Midbrain · Trigeminal nerve · Basilar a · Right external carotid a · Parotid gland · Submandibular gland · Right internal carotid a · Pharynx

Figure 2.3.7

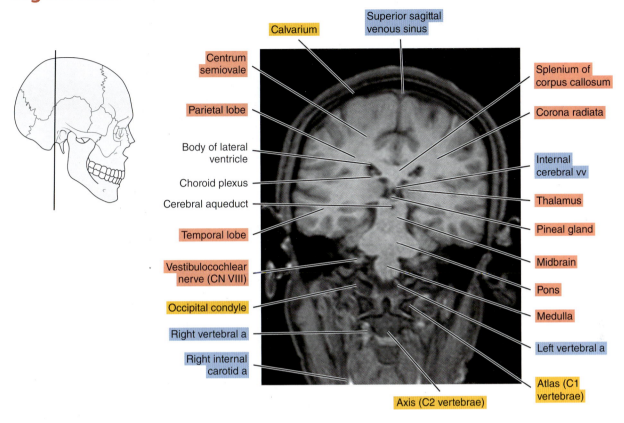

Calvarium
Superior sagittal venous sinus
Centrum semiovale
Splenium of corpus callosum
Parietal lobe
Corona radiata
Body of lateral ventricle
Internal cerebral vv
Choroid plexus
Thalamus
Cerebral aqueduct
Pineal gland
Temporal lobe
Midbrain
Vestibulocochlear nerve (CN VIII)
Pons
Occipital condyle
Medulla
Right vertebral a
Left vertebral a
Right internal carotid a
Atlas (C1 vertebrae)
Axis (C2 vertebrae)

Figure 2.3.8

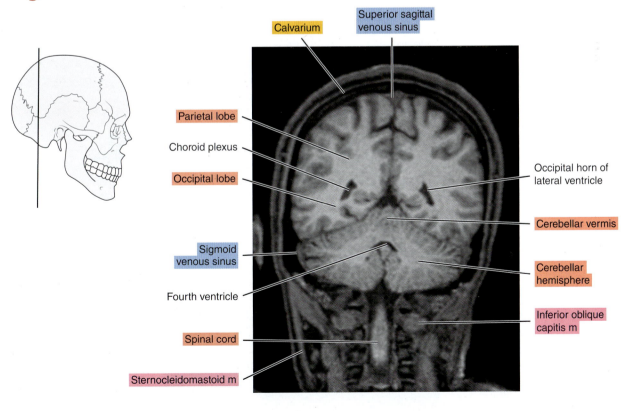

Calvarium
Superior sagittal venous sinus
Parietal lobe
Choroid plexus
Occipital horn of lateral ventricle
Occipital lobe
Cerebellar vermis
Sigmoid venous sinus
Cerebellar hemisphere
Fourth ventricle
Inferior oblique capitis m
Spinal cord
Sternocleidomastoid m

Figure 2.3.9

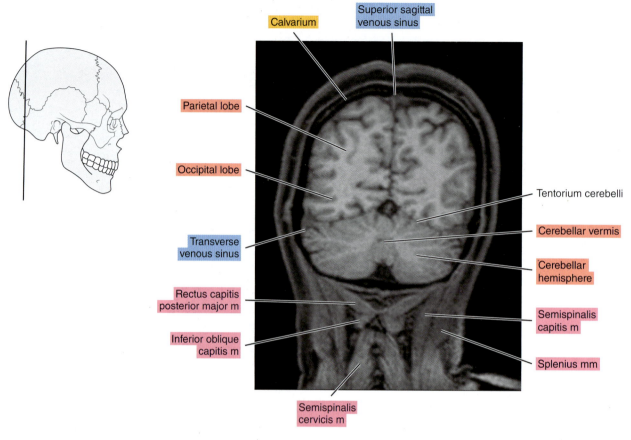

Calvarium

Superior sagittal venous sinus

Parietal lobe

Occipital lobe

Transverse venous sinus

Rectus capitis posterior major m

Inferior oblique capitis m

Tentorium cerebelli

Cerebellar vermis

Cerebellar hemisphere

Semispinalis capitis m

Splenius mm

Semispinalis cervicis m

Figure 2.3.10

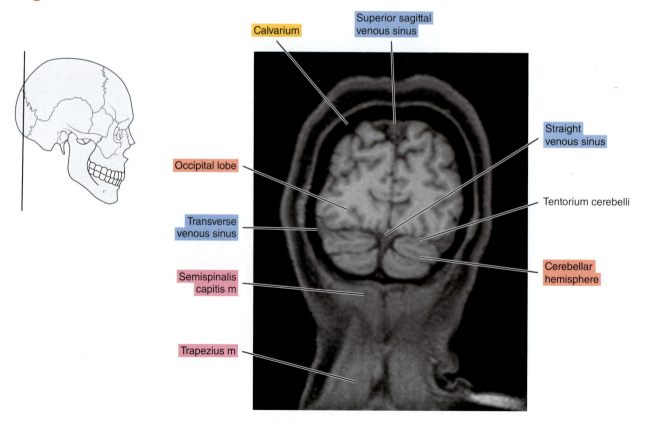

Calvarium

Superior sagittal venous sinus

Occipital lobe

Transverse venous sinus

Semispinalis capitis m

Trapezius m

Straight venous sinus

Tentorium cerebelli

Cerebellar hemisphere

Section II

Thorax

Chapter 3

CT of the Thorax

AXIAL
Figure 3.1.1

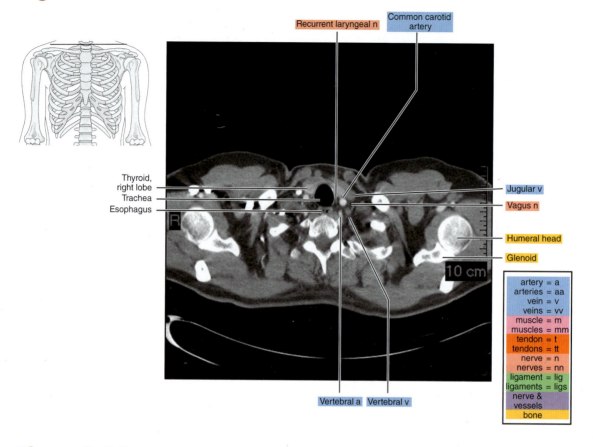

Recurrent laryngeal n

Common carotid artery

Thyroid, right lobe
Trachea
Esophagus

Jugular v

Vagus n

Humeral head

Glenoid

artery = a	
arteries = aa	
vein = v	
veins = vv	
muscle = m	
muscles = mm	
tendon = t	
tendons = tt	
nerve = n	
nerves = nn	
ligament = lig	
ligaments = ligs	
nerve & vessels	
bone	

Vertebral a   Vertebral v

Figure 3.1.2

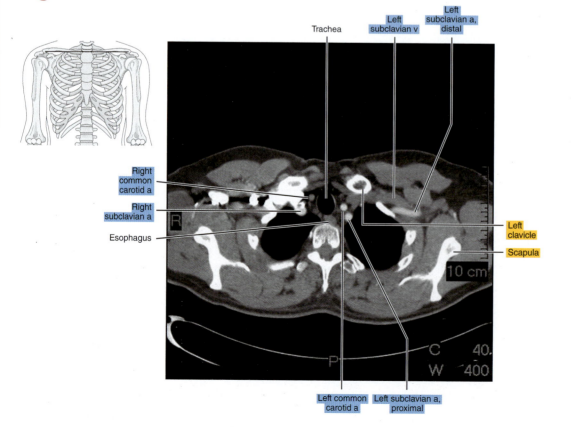

Trachea

Left subclavian v

Left subclavian a, distal

Right common carotid a

Right subclavian a

Esophagus

Left clavicle

Scapula

10 cm

C 40.
W 400

Left common carotid a   Left subclavian a, proximal

Figure 3.1.3

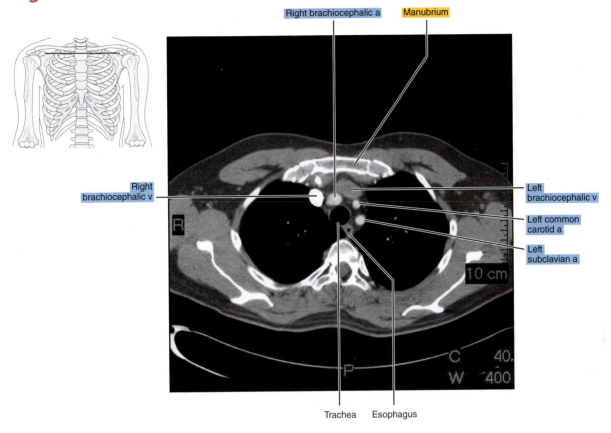

Right brachiocephalic a

Manubrium

Right brachiocephalic v

Left brachiocephalic v

Left common carotid a

Left subclavian a

10 cm

Trachea   Esophagus

Figure 3.1.4

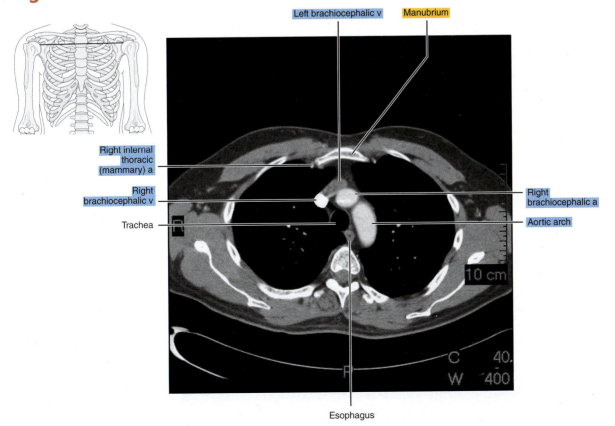

Left brachiocephalic v

Manubrium

Right internal thoracic (mammary) a

Right brachiocephalic v

Right brachiocephalic a

Trachea

Aortic arch

10 cm

Esophagus

Figure 3.1.5

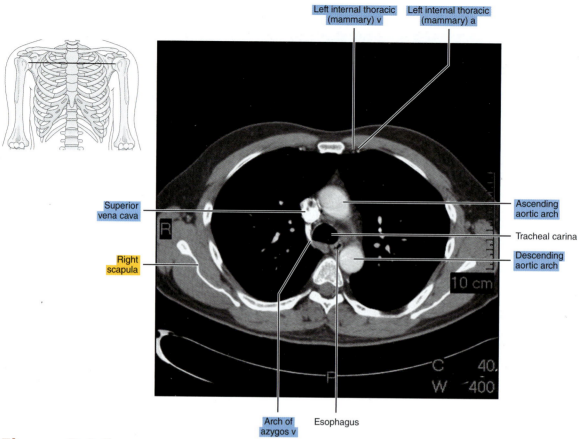

Left internal thoracic (mammary) v

Left internal thoracic (mammary) a

Superior vena cava

Ascending aortic arch

Tracheal carina

Right scapula

Descending aortic arch

10 cm

Arch of azygos v

Esophagus

C 40.
W 400

Figure 3.1.6

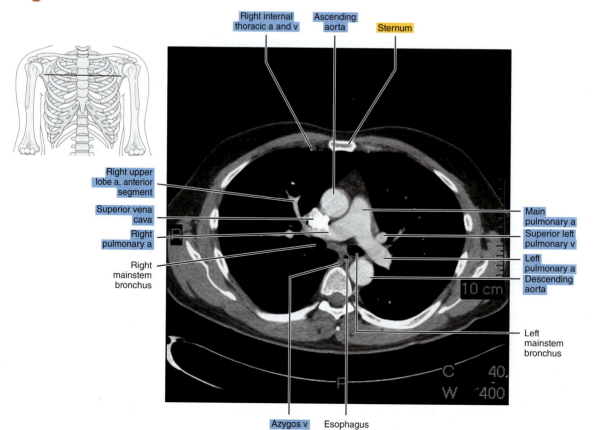

Right internal thoracic a and v

Ascending aorta

Sternum

Right upper lobe a, anterior segment

Superior vena cava

Right pulmonary a

Right mainstem bronchus

Main pulmonary a

Superior left pulmonary v

Left pulmonary a

Descending aorta

Left mainstem bronchus

10 cm

Azygos v

Esophagus

C 40.
W 400

Figure 3.1.7

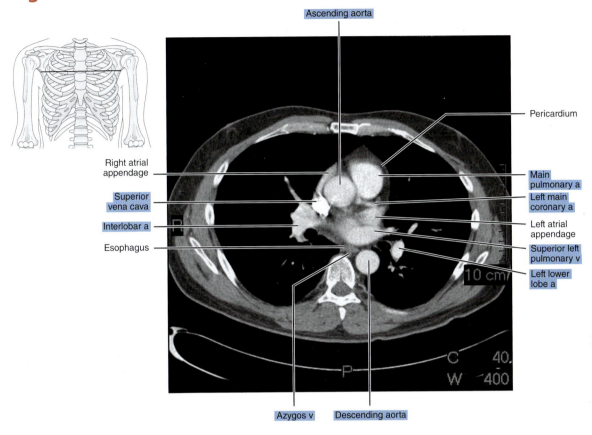

Ascending aorta

Pericardium

Right atrial appendage

Main pulmonary a

Superior vena cava

Left main coronary a

Interlobar a

Left atrial appendage

Esophagus

Superior left pulmonary v

Left lower lobe a

10 cm

C 40.
W 400

Azygos v

Descending aorta

Figure 3.1.8

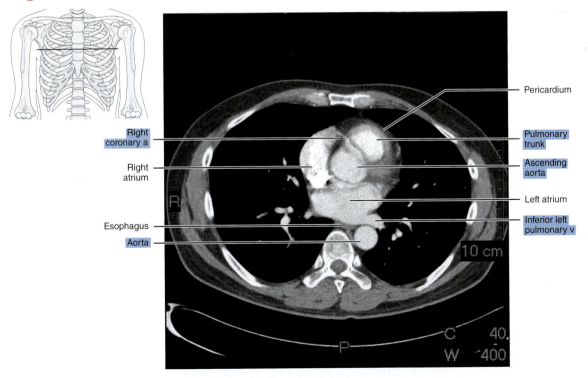

Pericardium

Right coronary a

Pulmonary trunk

Right atrium

Ascending aorta

Left atrium

Esophagus

Inferior left pulmonary v

Aorta

10 cm

C 40.
W 400

Figure 3.1.9

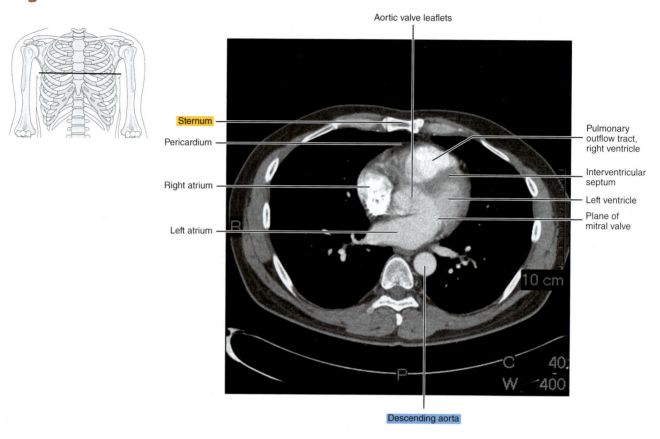

Aortic valve leaflets

Sternum

Pericardium

Right atrium

Left atrium

Pulmonary outflow tract, right ventricle

Interventricular septum

Left ventricle

Plane of mitral valve

10 cm

Descending aorta

Figure 3.1.10

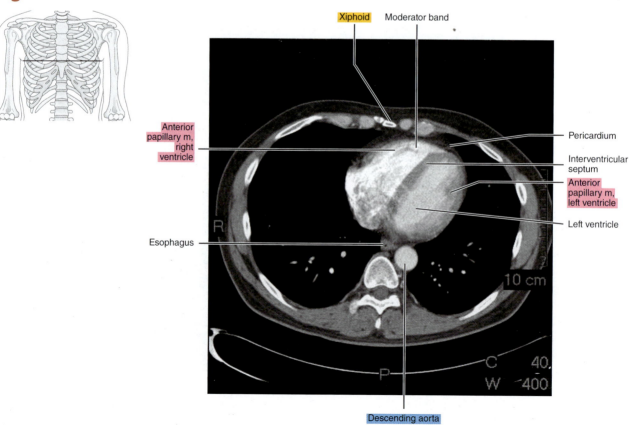

Xiphoid   Moderator band

Anterior papillary m, right ventricle

Esophagus

Pericardium

Interventricular septum

Anterior papillary m, left ventricle

Left ventricle

10 cm

Descending aorta

Figure 3.1.11

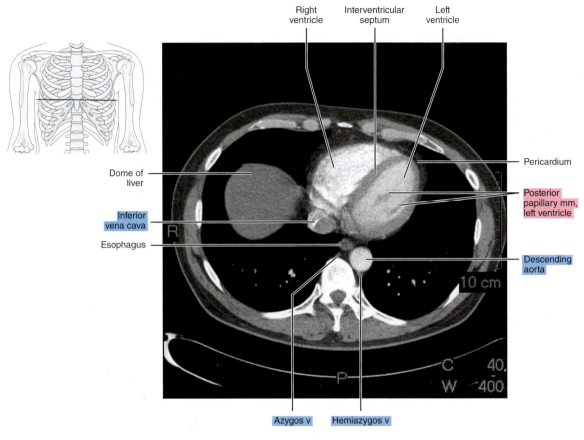

Right ventricle

Interventricular septum

Left ventricle

Pericardium

Dome of liver

Posterior papillary mm, left ventricle

Inferior vena cava

Esophagus

Descending aorta

Azygos v

Hemiazygos v

Figure 3.1.12

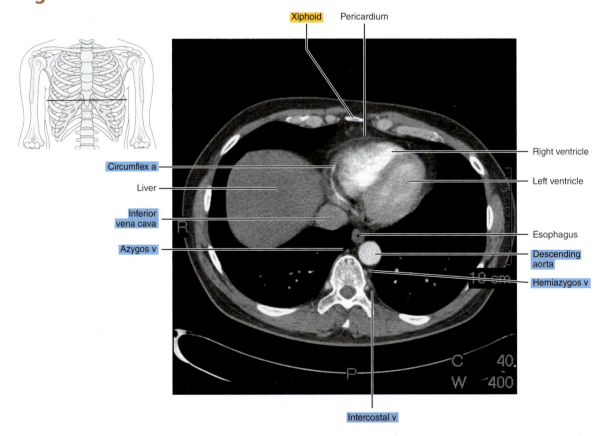

Xiphoid

Pericardium

Circumflex a

Right ventricle

Liver

Left ventricle

Inferior vena cava

Esophagus

Azygos v

Descending aorta

Hemiazygos v

Intercostal v

Figure 3.1.13

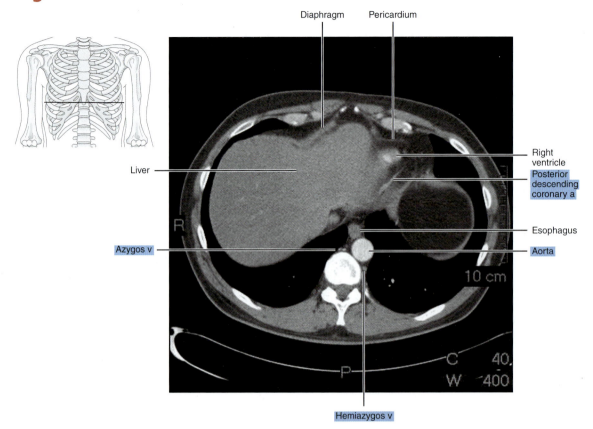

Diaphragm

Pericardium

Liver

R

Azygos v

Right ventricle

Posterior descending coronary a

Esophagus

Aorta

10 cm

P

C 40.
W 400

Hemiazygos v

SAGITTAL
Figure 3.2.1A

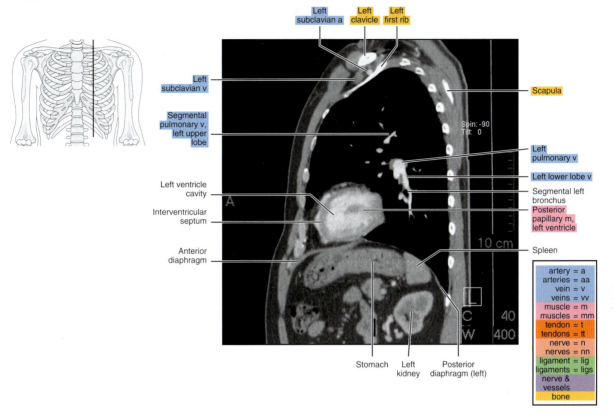

Left subclavian a
Left clavicle
Left first rib
Left subclavian v
Scapula
Segmental pulmonary v, left upper lobe
Spin: -90
Tilt: 0
Left pulmonary v
Left lower lobe v
Left ventricle cavity
Interventricular septum
Segmental left bronchus
Posterior papillary m, left ventricle
10 cm
Anterior diaphragm
Spleen
A
C W
40
400
Stomach
Left kidney
Posterior diaphragm (left)

artery = a	
arteries = aa	
vein = v	
veins = vv	
muscle = m	
muscles = mm	
tendon = t	
tendons = tt	
nerve = n	
nerves = nn	
ligament = lig	
ligaments = ligs	
nerve & vessels	
bone	

Figure 3.2.1B

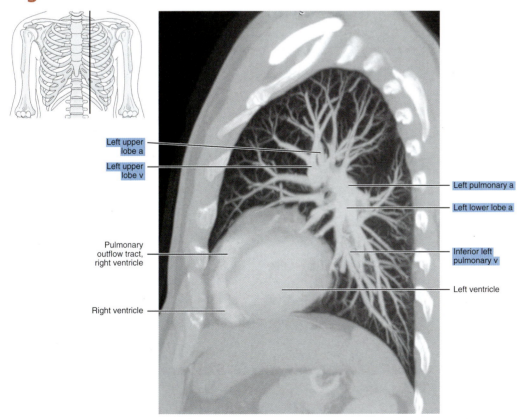

Left upper lobe a
Left upper lobe v
Left pulmonary a
Left lower lobe a
Pulmonary outflow tract, right ventricle
Inferior left pulmonary v
Left ventricle
Right ventricle

Figure 3.2.2

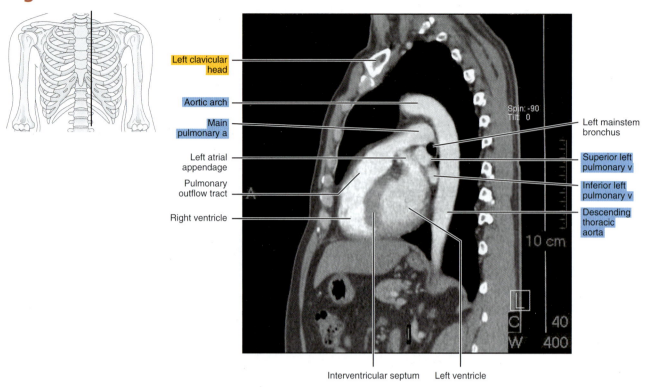

Left clavicular head

Aortic arch

Main pulmonary a

Left atrial appendage

Pulmonary outflow tract

Right ventricle

Left mainstem bronchus

Superior left pulmonary v

Inferior left pulmonary v

Descending thoracic aorta

Spin: -90
Tilt: 0

10 cm

L
C
W

40
400

Interventricular septum   Left ventricle

Figure 3.2.3

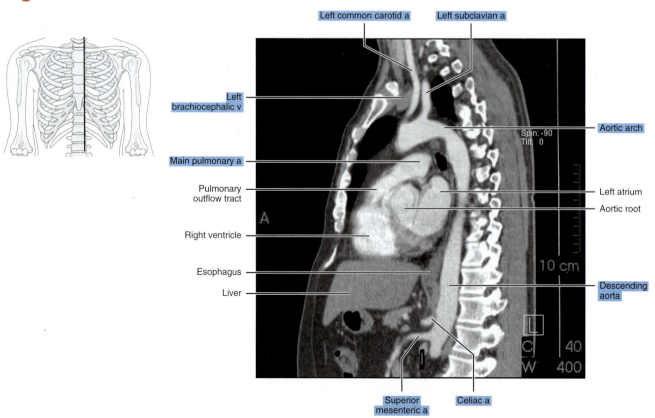

Left common carotid a   Left subclavian a

Left brachiocephalic v

Main pulmonary a

Pulmonary outflow tract

Right ventricle

Esophagus

Liver

Aortic arch

Left atrium

Aortic root

Descending aorta

Spin: -90
Tilt: 0

10 cm

L
C
W

40
400

Superior mesenteric a   Celiac a

Figure 3.2.4

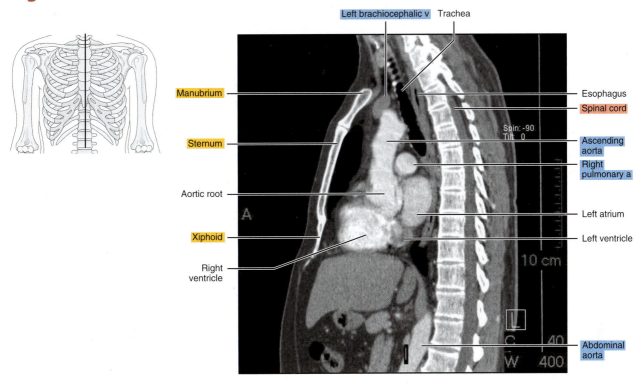

Left brachiocephalic v   Trachea

Manubrium

Esophagus

Spinal cord

Sternum

Ascending aorta

Right pulmonary a

Aortic root

Left atrium

Xiphoid

Left ventricle

Right ventricle

Abdominal aorta

Figure 3.2.5

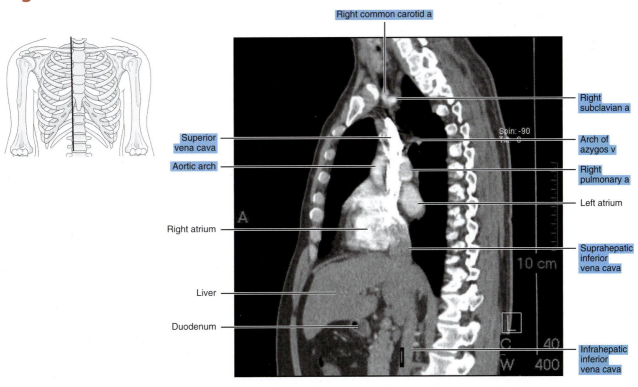

Right common carotid a

Right subclavian a

Superior vena cava

Arch of azygos v

Aortic arch

Right pulmonary a

Left atrium

Right atrium

Suprahepatic inferior vena cava

Liver

Duodenum

Infrahepatic inferior vena cava

Figure 3.2.6

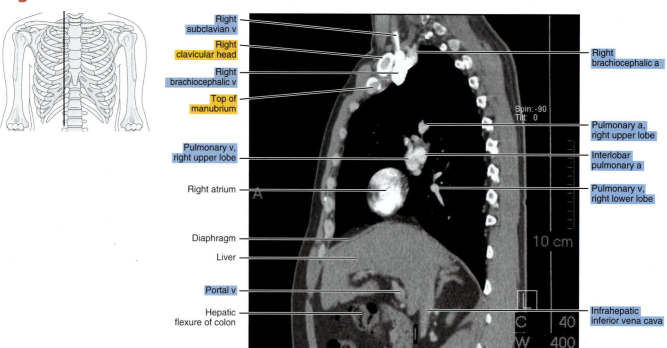

Right subclavian v

Right clavicular head

Right brachiocephalic v

Top of manubrium

Pulmonary v, right upper lobe

Right atrium

Diaphragm

Liver

Portal v

Hepatic flexure of colon

Right brachiocephalic a

Pulmonary a, right upper lobe

Interlobar pulmonary a

Pulmonary v, right lower lobe

Infrahepatic inferior vena cava

Spin: -90
Tilt: 0

10 cm

C   40
W   400

CORONAL
Figure 3.3.1

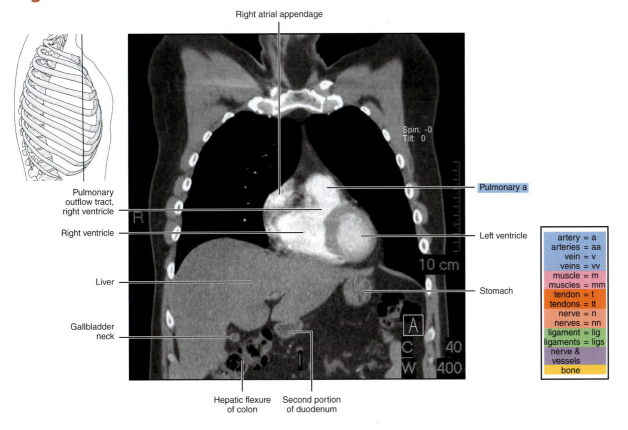

Right atrial appendage

Pulmonary outflow tract, right ventricle

Right ventricle

Liver

Gallbladder neck

Pulmonary a

Left ventricle

Stomach

Hepatic flexure of colon

Second portion of duodenum

Spin: -0
Tilt: 0

10 cm

A

C 40
W 400

artery = a	
arteries = aa	
vein = v	
veins = vv	
muscle = m	
muscles = mm	
tendon = t	
tendons = tt	
nerve = n	
nerves = nn	
ligament = lig	
ligaments = ligs	
nerve & vessels	
bone	

Figure 3.3.2

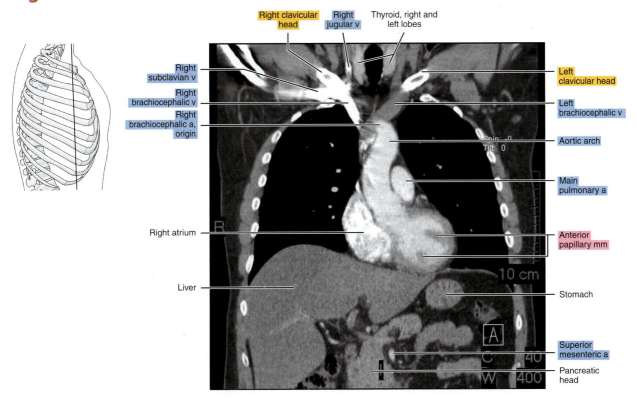

Right clavicular head

Right jugular v

Thyroid, right and left lobes

Right subclavian v

Right brachiocephalic v

Right brachiocephalic a, origin

Left clavicular head

Left brachiocephalic v

Aortic arch

Main pulmonary a

Right atrium

Anterior papillary mm

Liver

Stomach

Superior mesenteric a

Pancreatic head

10 cm

A

C 40
W 400

Figure 3.3.3A

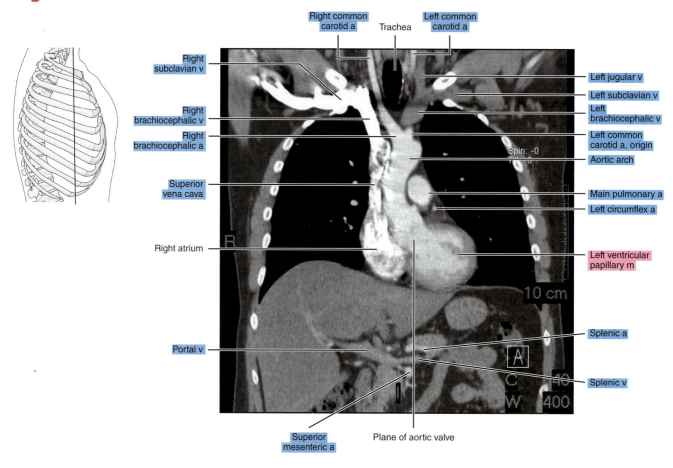

Right common carotid a
Trachea
Left common carotid a
Right subclavian v
Left jugular v
Left subclavian v
Right brachiocephalic v
Left brachiocephalic v
Right brachiocephalic a
Left common carotid a, origin
Aortic arch
Superior vena cava
Main pulmonary a
Left circumflex a
Right atrium
Left ventricular papillary m
Portal v
Splenic a
Splenic v
Superior mesenteric a
Plane of aortic valve

Figure 3.3.3B

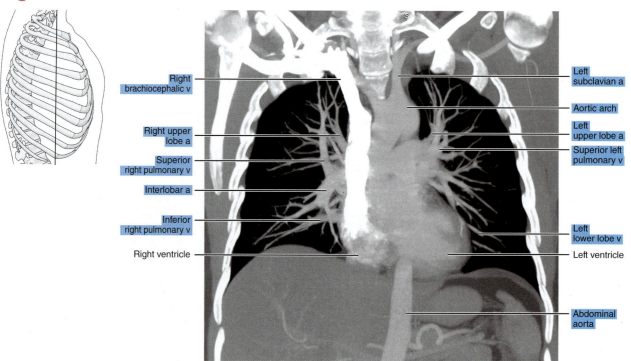

Right brachiocephalic v
Left subclavian a
Aortic arch
Right upper lobe a
Left upper lobe a
Superior right pulmonary v
Superior left pulmonary v
Interlobar a
Inferior right pulmonary v
Left lower lobe v
Right ventricle
Left ventricle
Abdominal aorta

Figure 3.3.4

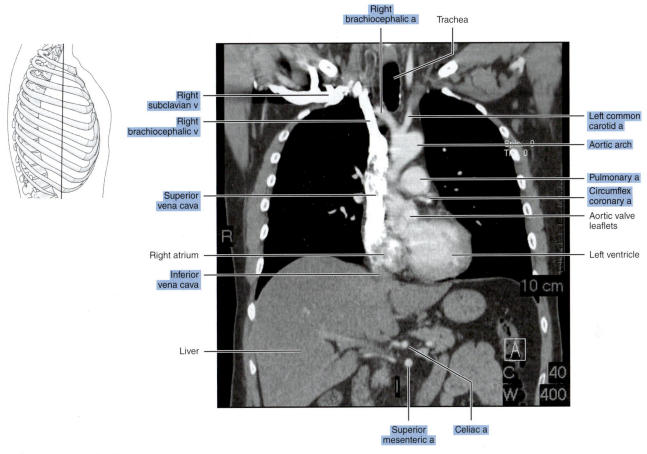

Right brachiocephalic a

Trachea

Right subclavian v

Right brachiocephalic v

Left common carotid a

Aortic arch

Pulmonary a

Circumflex coronary a

Superior vena cava

Aortic valve leaflets

Right atrium

Left ventricle

Inferior vena cava

Liver

Superior mesenteric a

Celiac a

Figure 3.3.5

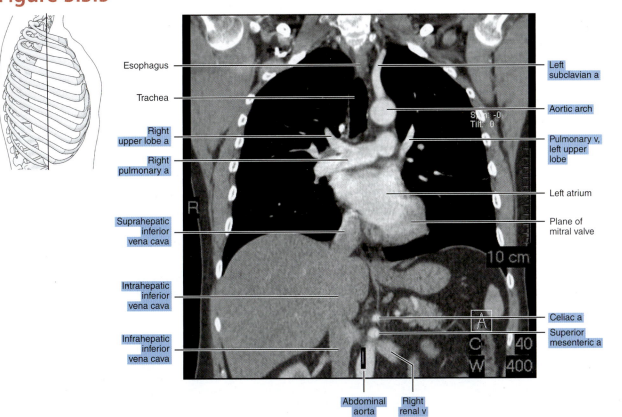

Esophagus

Left subclavian a

Trachea

Aortic arch

Right upper lobe a

Pulmonary v, left upper lobe

Right pulmonary a

Left atrium

Suprahepatic inferior vena cava

Plane of mitral valve

Intrahepatic inferior vena cava

Celiac a

Superior mesenteric a

Infrahepatic inferior vena cava

Abdominal aorta

Right renal v

Figure 3.3.6A

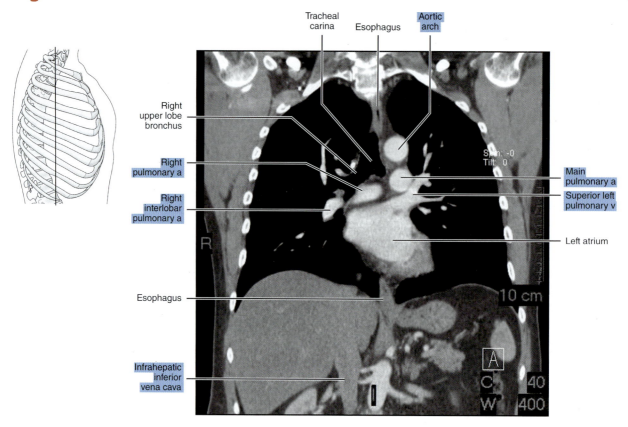

Tracheal carina

Esophagus

Aortic arch

Right upper lobe bronchus

Right pulmonary a

Right interlobar pulmonary a

Esophagus

Infrahepatic inferior vena cava

Main pulmonary a

Superior left pulmonary v

Left atrium

Figure 3.3.6B

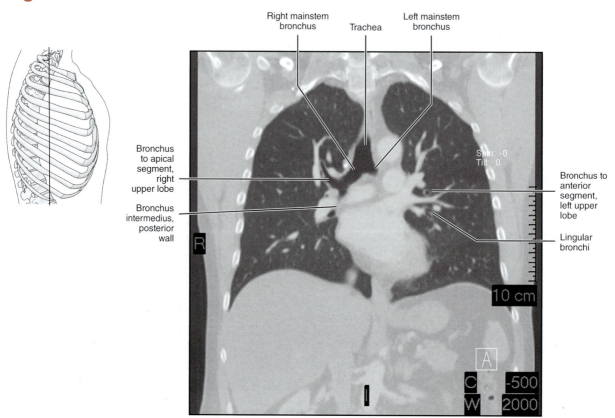

Right mainstem bronchus

Trachea

Left mainstem bronchus

Bronchus to apical segment, right upper lobe

Bronchus intermedius, posterior wall

Bronchus to anterior segment, left upper lobe

Lingular bronchi

Figure 3.3.7A

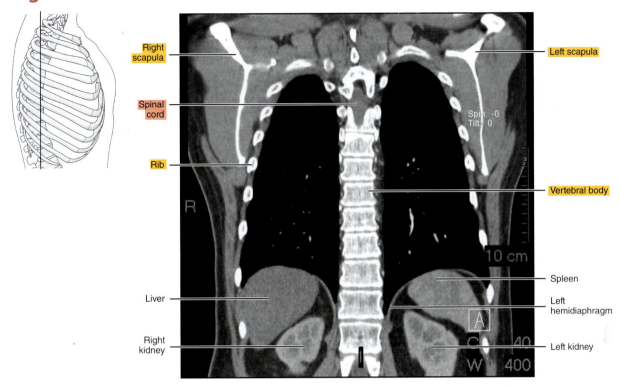

Right scapula
Left scapula
Spinal cord
Rib
Vertebral body
Spleen
Liver
Left hemidiaphragm
Right kidney
Left kidney

Figure 3.3.7B

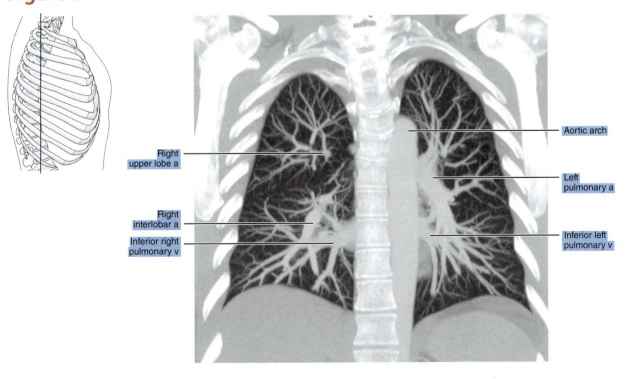

Aortic arch
Right upper lobe a
Left pulmonary a
Right interlobar a
Inferior right pulmonary v
Inferior left pulmonary v

Figure 3.3.8

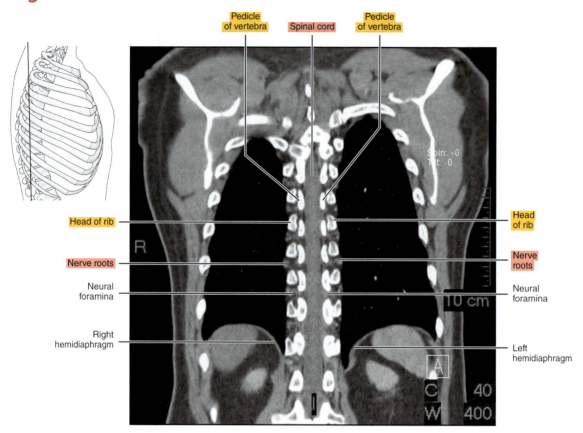

Pedicle of vertebra

Spinal cord

Pedicle of vertebra

Head of rib

Head of rib

Nerve roots

Nerve roots

Neural foramina

Neural foramina

Right hemidiaphragm

Left hemidiaphragm

Spin: -0
Tilt: 0

10 cm

A
C   40
W   400

R

MRI of the Heart

AXIAL
Figure 4.1.1

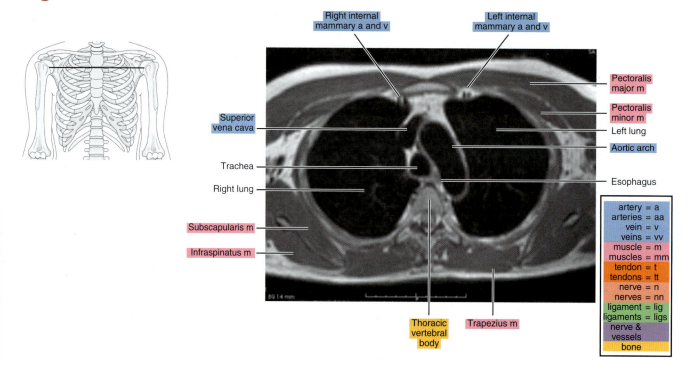

Right internal mammary a and v

Left internal mammary a and v

Pectoralis major m

Pectoralis minor m

Superior vena cava

Left lung

Aortic arch

Trachea

Esophagus

Right lung

Subscapularis m

Infraspinatus m

artery =	a
arteries =	aa
vein =	v
veins =	vv
muscle =	m
muscles =	mm
tendon =	t
tendons =	tt
nerve =	n
nerves =	nn
ligament =	lig
ligaments =	ligs
nerve & vessels	
bone	

Thoracic vertebral body

Trapezius m

Figure 4.1.2

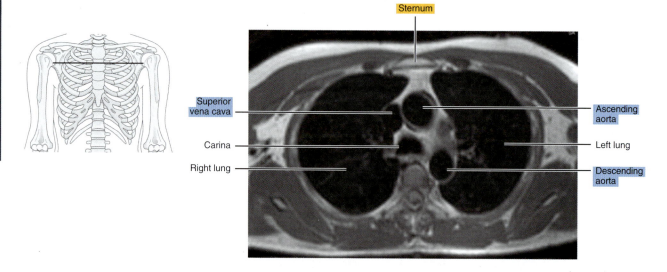

Sternum

Superior vena cava

Ascending aorta

Carina

Left lung

Right lung

Descending aorta

Figure 4.1.3

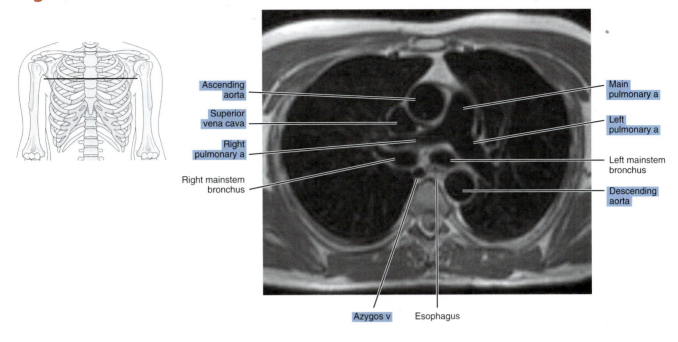

Ascending aorta

Superior vena cava

Right pulmonary a

Right mainstem bronchus

Main pulmonary a

Left pulmonary a

Left mainstem bronchus

Descending aorta

Azygos v

Esophagus

Figure 4.1.4

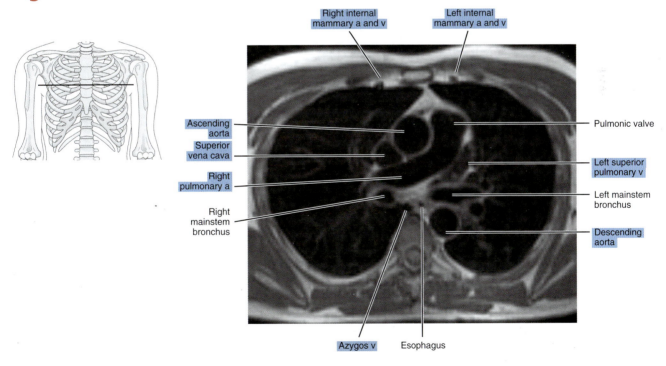

Right internal mammary a and v

Left internal mammary a and v

Ascending aorta

Superior vena cava

Right pulmonary a

Right mainstem bronchus

Pulmonic valve

Left superior pulmonary v

Left mainstem bronchus

Descending aorta

Azygos v

Esophagus

Figure 4.1.5

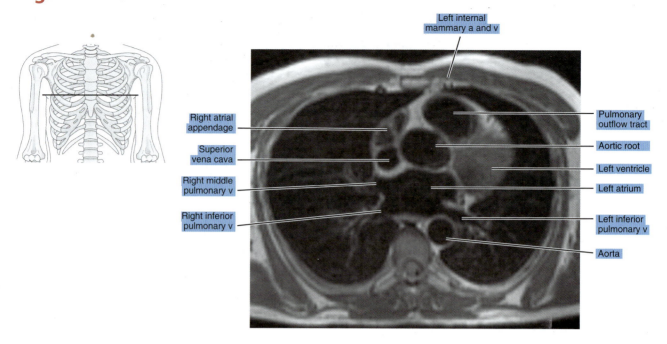

Left internal mammary a and v

Right atrial appendage

Superior vena cava

Right middle pulmonary v

Right inferior pulmonary v

Pulmonary outflow tract

Aortic root

Left ventricle

Left atrium

Left inferior pulmonary v

Aorta

Figure 4.1.6

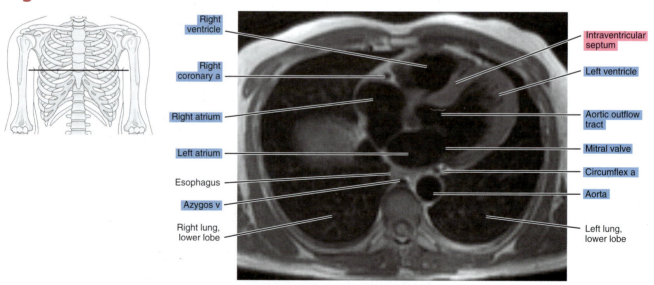

Right ventricle

Right coronary a

Right atrium

Left atrium

Esophagus

Azygos v

Right lung, lower lobe

Intraventricular septum

Left ventricle

Aortic outflow tract

Mitral valve

Circumflex a

Aorta

Left lung, lower lobe

Figure 4.1.7

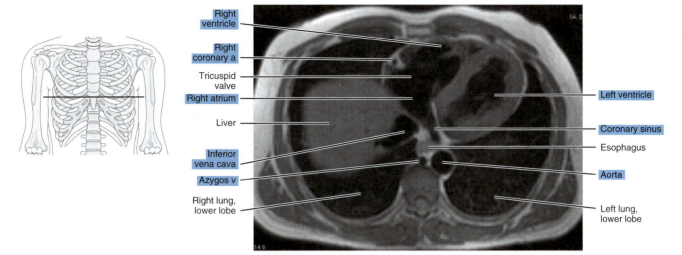

Right ventricle

Right coronary a

Tricuspid valve

Right atrium

Liver

Inferior vena cava

Azygos v

Right lung, lower lobe

Left ventricle

Coronary sinus

Esophagus

Aorta

Left lung, lower lobe

SAGITTAL
Figure 4.2.1

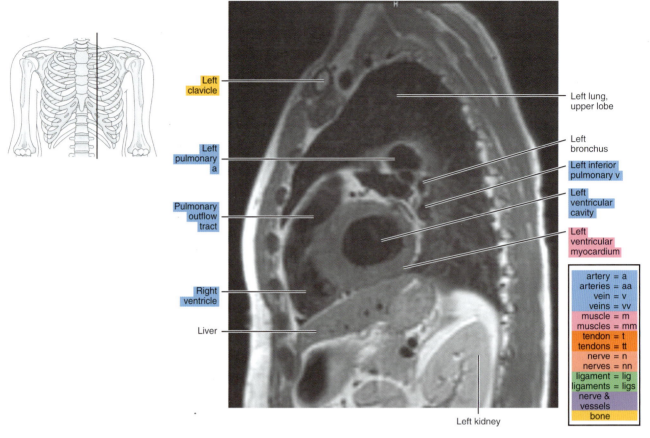

Left clavicle

Left pulmonary a

Pulmonary outflow tract

Right ventricle

Liver

Left lung, upper lobe

Left bronchus

Left inferior pulmonary v

Left ventricular cavity

Left ventricular myocardium

Left kidney

artery = a	
arteries = aa	
vein = v	
veins = vv	
muscle = m	
muscles = mm	
tendon = t	
tendons = tt	
nerve = n	
nerves = nn	
ligament = lig	
ligaments = ligs	
nerve & vessels	
bone	

Figure 4.2.2

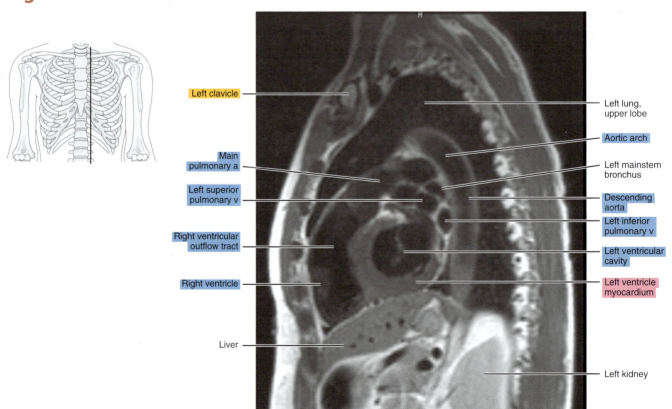

Left clavicle

Main pulmonary a

Left superior pulmonary v

Right ventricular outflow tract

Right ventricle

Liver

Left lung, upper lobe

Aortic arch

Left mainstem bronchus

Descending aorta

Left inferior pulmonary v

Left ventricular cavity

Left ventricle myocardium

Left kidney

Figure 4.2.3

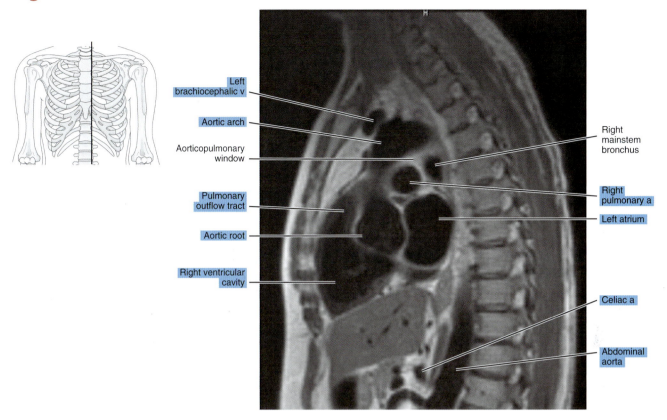

Left brachiocephalic v
Aortic arch
Aorticopulmonary window
Pulmonary outflow tract
Aortic root
Right ventricular cavity
Right mainstem bronchus
Right pulmonary a
Left atrium
Celiac a
Abdominal aorta

Figure 4.2.4

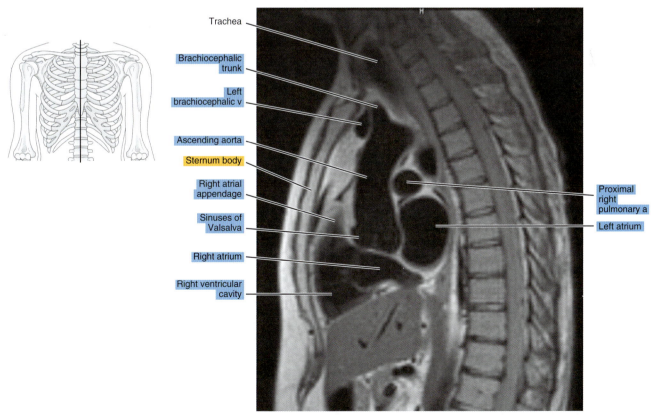

Trachea
Brachiocephalic trunk
Left brachiocephalic v
Ascending aorta
Sternum body
Right atrial appendage
Sinuses of Valsalva
Right atrium
Right ventricular cavity
Proximal right pulmonary a
Left atrium

Figure 4.2.5

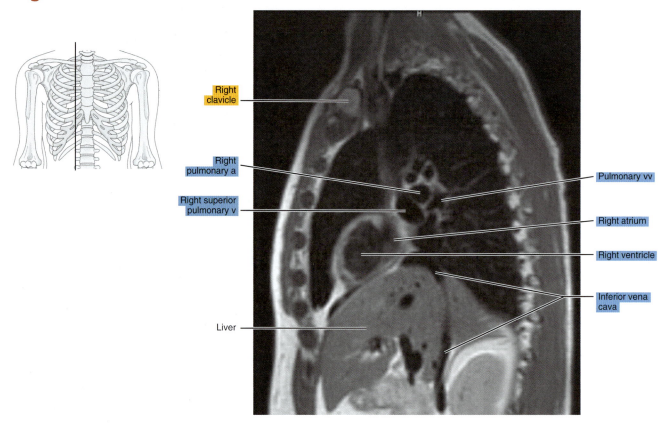

Right clavicle

Right pulmonary a

Right superior pulmonary v

Liver

Pulmonary vv

Right atrium

Right ventricle

Inferior vena cava

CORONAL
Figure 4.3.1

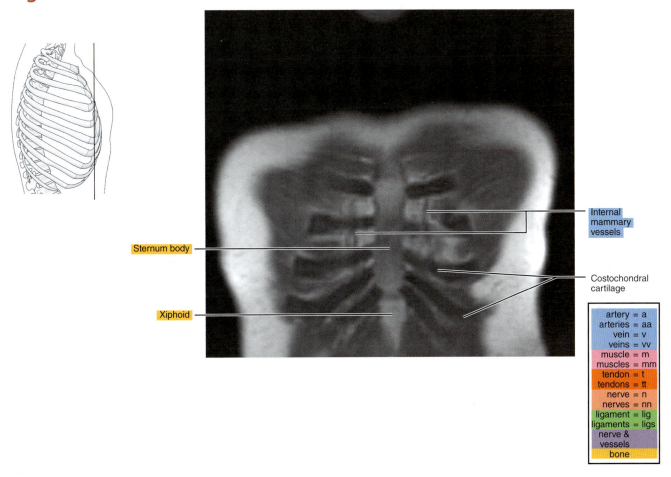

Internal mammary vessels

Sternum body

Costochondral cartilage

Xiphoid

artery = a	
arteries = aa	
vein = v	
veins = vv	
muscle = m	
muscles = mm	
tendon = t	
tendons = tt	
nerve = n	
nerves = nn	
ligament = lig	
ligaments = ligs	
nerve & vessels	
bone	

Figure 4.3.2

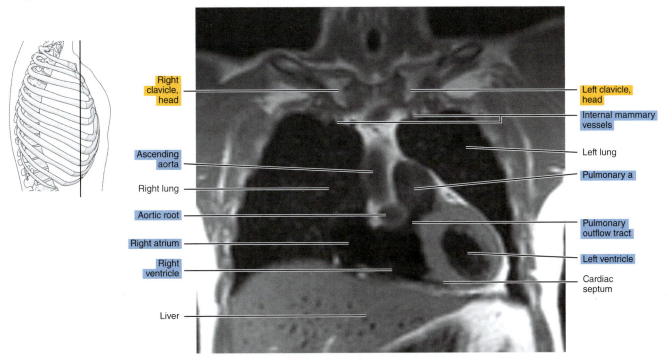

Right clavicle, head

Left clavicle, head

Internal mammary vessels

Ascending aorta

Left lung

Right lung

Pulmonary a

Aortic root

Pulmonary outflow tract

Right atrium

Left ventricle

Right ventricle

Cardiac septum

Liver

Figure 4.3.3

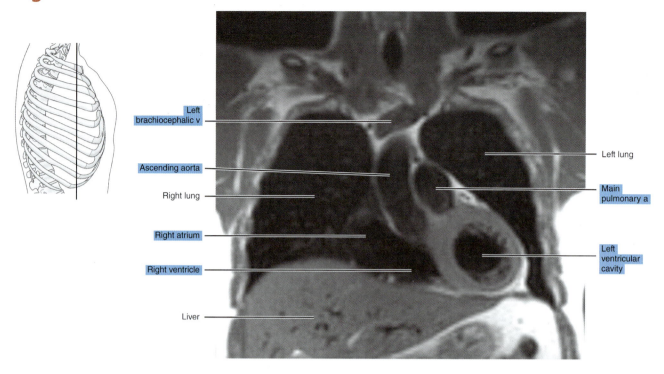

Left brachiocephalic v

Ascending aorta

Right lung

Right atrium

Right ventricle

Liver

Left lung

Main pulmonary a

Left ventricular cavity

Figure 4.3.4

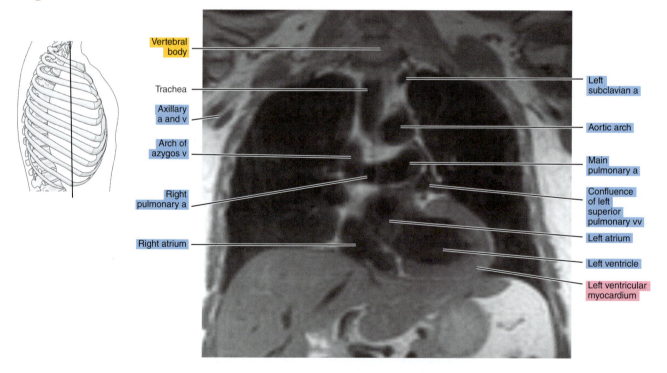

Vertebral body

Trachea

Axillary a and v

Arch of azygos v

Right pulmonary a

Right atrium

Left subclavian a

Aortic arch

Main pulmonary a

Confluence of left superior pulmonary vv

Left atrium

Left ventricle

Left ventricular myocardium

Figure 4.3.5

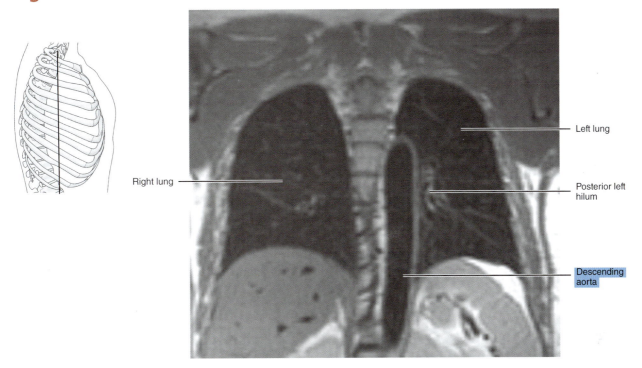

Right lung

Left lung

Posterior left hilum

Descending aorta

III
Section

Upper Extremity

Chapter

5

MRI of the Pectoral Girdle and Chest Wall

AXIAL
Figure 5.1.1

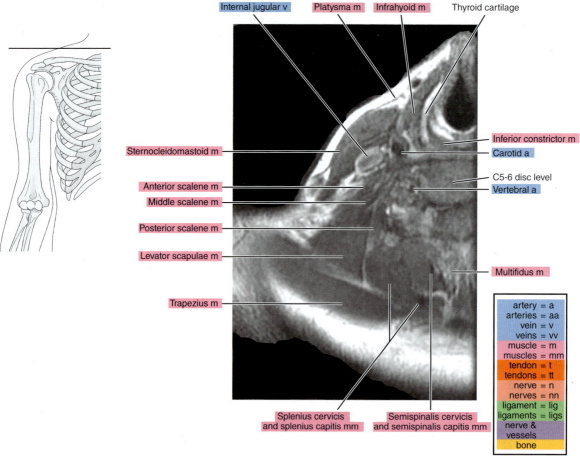

Internal jugular v | Platysma m | Infrahyoid m | Thyroid cartilage

Sternocleidomastoid m

Anterior scalene m

Middle scalene m

Posterior scalene m

Levator scapulae m

Trapezius m

Inferior constrictor m

Carotid a

C5-6 disc level

Vertebral a

Multifidus m

Splenius cervicis and splenius capitis mm | Semispinalis cervicis and semispinalis capitis mm

artery	= a
arteries	= aa
vein	= v
veins	= vv
muscle	= m
muscles	= mm
tendon	= t
tendons	= tt
nerve	= n
nerves	= nn
ligament	= lig
ligaments	= ligs
nerve & vessels	
bone	

Figure 5.1.2

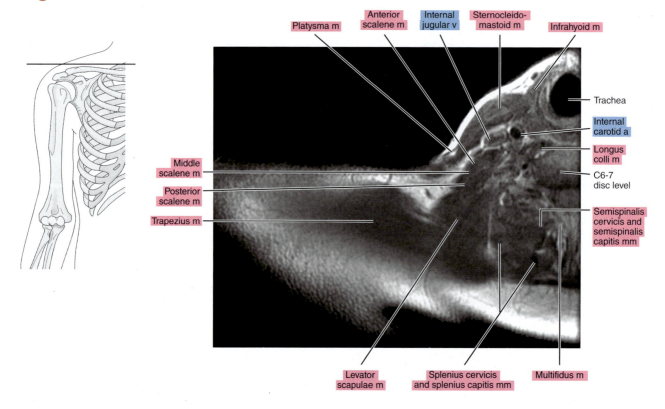

Platysma m | Anterior scalene m | Internal jugular v | Sternocleido-mastoid m | Infrahyoid m

Trachea

Internal carotid a

Longus colli m

C6-7 disc level

Semispinalis cervicis and semispinalis capitis mm

Middle scalene m

Posterior scalene m

Trapezius m

Levator scapulae m | Splenius cervicis and splenius capitis mm | Multifidus m

Figure 5.1.3

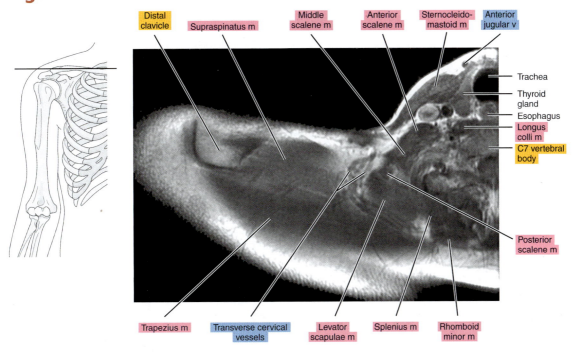

Distal clavicle · Supraspinatus m · Middle scalene m · Anterior scalene m · Sternocleido-mastoid m · Anterior jugular v · Trachea · Thyroid gland · Esophagus · Longus colli m · C7 vertebral body · Posterior scalene m · Trapezius m · Transverse cervical vessels · Levator scapulae m · Splenius m · Rhomboid minor m

Figure 5.1.4

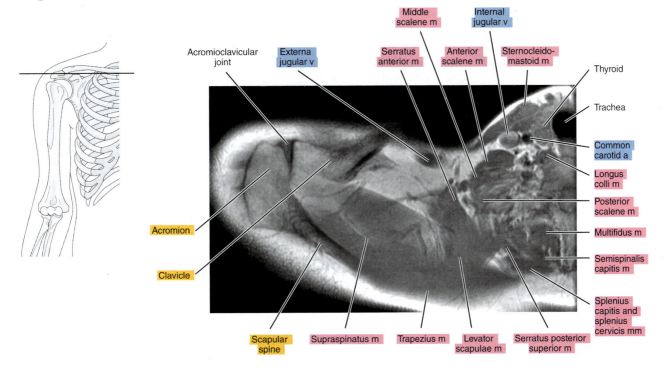

Acromioclavicular joint · Externa jugular v · Middle scalene m · Serratus anterior m · Anterior scalene m · Internal jugular v · Sternocleido-mastoid m · Thyroid · Trachea · Common carotid a · Longus colli m · Posterior scalene m · Multifidus m · Semispinalis capitis m · Splenius capitis and splenius cervicis mm · Acromion · Clavicle · Scapular spine · Supraspinatus m · Trapezius m · Levator scapulae m · Serratus posterior superior m

Figure 5.1.5

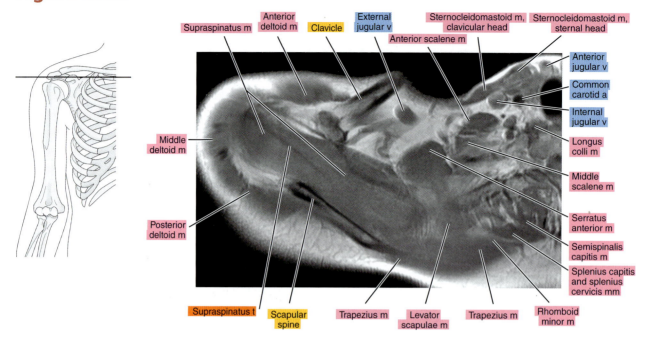

Figure 5.1.6

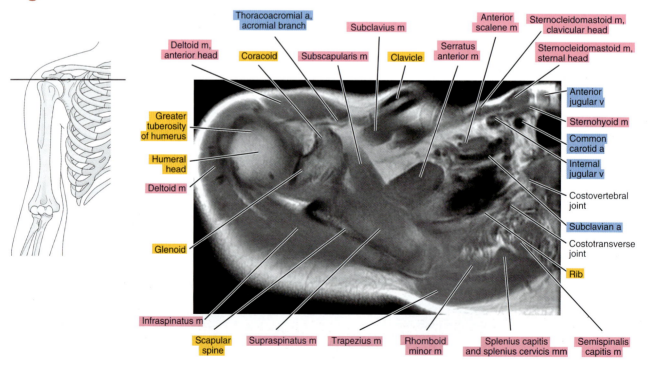

Figure 5.1.7

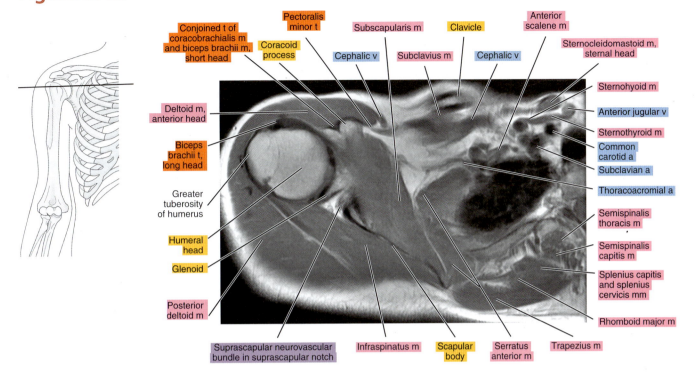

Conjoined t of coracobrachialis m and biceps brachii m, short head

Coracoid process

Pectoralis minor t

Subscapularis m

Clavicle

Anterior scalene m

Cephalic v

Subclavius m

Cephalic v

Sternocleidomastoid m, sternal head

Sternohyoid m

Deltoid m, anterior head

Anterior jugular v

Sternothyroid m

Biceps brachii t, long head

Common carotid a

Subclavian a

Greater tuberosity of humerus

Thoracoacromial a

Semispinalis thoracis m

Humeral head

Semispinalis capitis m

Glenoid

Splenius capitis and splenius cervicis mm

Posterior deltoid m

Rhomboid major m

Suprascapular neurovascular bundle in suprascapular notch

Infraspinatus m

Scapular body

Serratus anterior m

Trapezius m

Figure 5.1.8

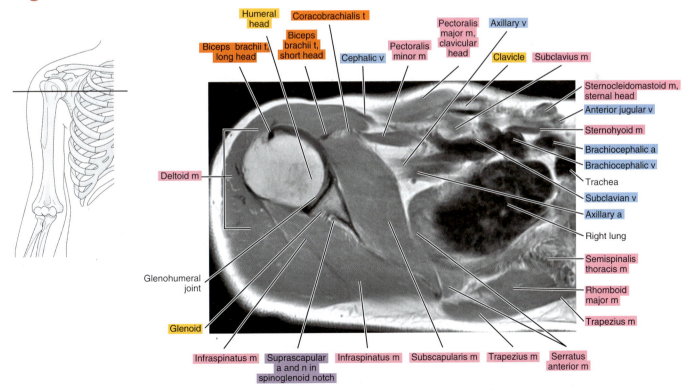

Humeral head

Coracobrachialis t

Pectoralis major m, clavicular head

Axillary v

Biceps brachii t, long head

Biceps brachii t, short head

Cephalic v

Pectoralis minor m

Clavicle

Subclavius m

Sternocleidomastoid m, sternal head

Anterior jugular v

Sternohyoid m

Deltoid m

Brachiocephalic a

Brachiocephalic v

Trachea

Subclavian v

Axillary a

Glenohumeral joint

Right lung

Semispinalis thoracis m

Glenoid

Rhomboid major m

Trapezius m

Infraspinatus m

Suprascapular a and n in spinoglenoid notch

Infraspinatus m

Subscapularis m

Trapezius m

Serratus anterior m

Figure 5.1.9

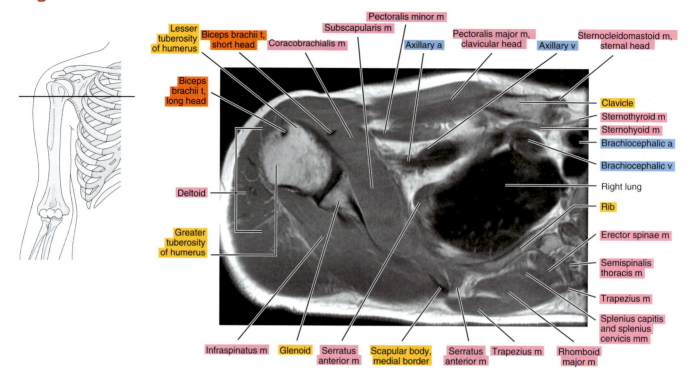

Lesser tuberosity of humerus
Biceps brachii t, short head
Coracobrachialis m
Subscapularis m
Pectoralis minor m
Axillary a
Pectoralis major m, clavicular head
Axillary v
Sternocleidomastoid m, sternal head

Biceps brachii t, long head

Clavicle
Sternothyroid m
Sternohyoid m
Brachiocephalic a
Brachiocephalic v
Right lung
Rib
Erector spinae m
Semispinalis thoracis m
Trapezius m
Splenius capitis and splenius cervicis mm

Deltoid

Greater tuberosity of humerus

Infraspinatus m   Glenoid   Serratus anterior m   Scapular body, medial border   Serratus anterior m   Trapezius m   Rhomboid major m

Figure 5.1.10

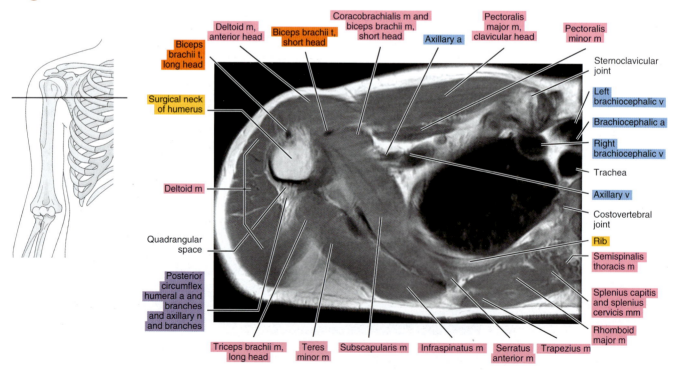

Deltoid m, anterior head
Coracobrachialis m and biceps brachii m, short head
Biceps brachii t, short head
Axillary a
Pectoralis major m, clavicular head
Pectoralis minor m

Biceps brachii t, long head

Surgical neck of humerus

Sternoclavicular joint
Left brachiocephalic v
Brachiocephalic a
Right brachiocephalic v
Trachea
Axillary v
Costovertebral joint
Rib
Semispinalis thoracis m
Splenius capitis and splenius cervicis mm
Rhomboid major m

Deltoid m

Quadrangular space

Posterior circumflex humeral a and branches and axillary n and branches

Triceps brachii m, long head   Teres minor m   Subscapularis m   Infraspinatus m   Serratus anterior m   Trapezius m

Figure 5.1.11

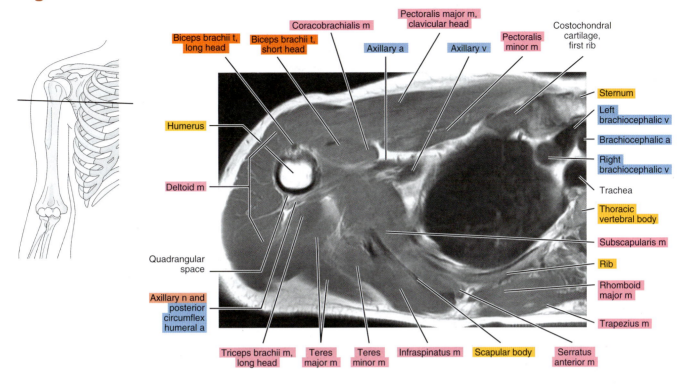

Biceps brachii t, long head
Biceps brachii t, short head
Coracobrachialis m
Pectoralis major m, clavicular head
Axillary a
Axillary v
Pectoralis minor m
Costochondral cartilage, first rib
Humerus
Deltoid m
Sternum
Left brachiocephalic v
Brachiocephalic a
Right brachiocephalic v
Trachea
Thoracic vertebral body
Subscapularis m
Rib
Rhomboid major m
Trapezius m
Quadrangular space
Axillary n and posterior circumflex humeral a
Triceps brachii m, long head
Teres major m
Teres minor m
Infraspinatus m
Scapular body
Serratus anterior m

Figure 5.1.12

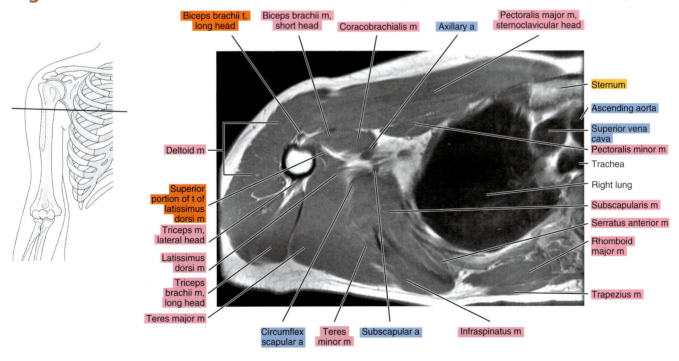

Biceps brachii t, long head
Biceps brachii m, short head
Coracobrachialis m
Axillary a
Pectoralis major m, sternoclavicular head
Deltoid m
Sternum
Ascending aorta
Superior vena cava
Pectoralis minor m
Trachea
Right lung
Subscapularis m
Serratus anterior m
Rhomboid major m
Trapezius m
Superior portion of t of latissimus dorsi m
Triceps m, lateral head
Latissimus dorsi m
Triceps brachii m, long head
Teres major m
Circumflex scapular a
Teres minor m
Subscapular a
Infraspinatus m

Figure 5.1.13

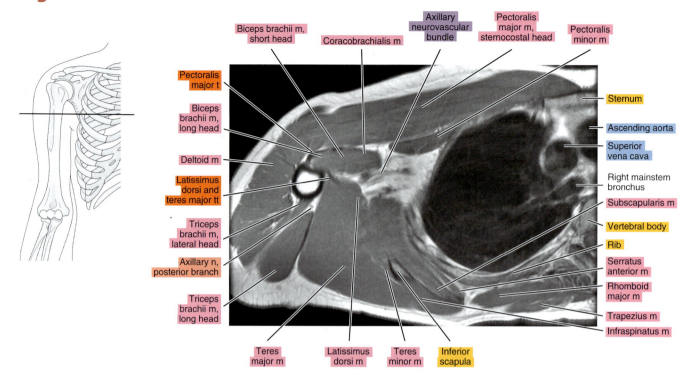

Biceps brachii m, short head
Coracobrachialis m
Axillary neurovascular bundle
Pectoralis major m, sternocostal head
Pectoralis minor m
Pectoralis major t
Biceps brachii m, long head
Deltoid m
Latissimus dorsi and teres major tt
Triceps brachii m, lateral head
Axillary n, posterior branch
Triceps brachii m, long head
Sternum
Ascending aorta
Superior vena cava
Right mainstem bronchus
Subscapularis m
Vertebral body
Rib
Serratus anterior m
Rhomboid major m
Trapezius m
Infraspinatus m
Teres major m
Latissimus dorsi m
Teres minor m
Inferior scapula

Figure 5.1.14

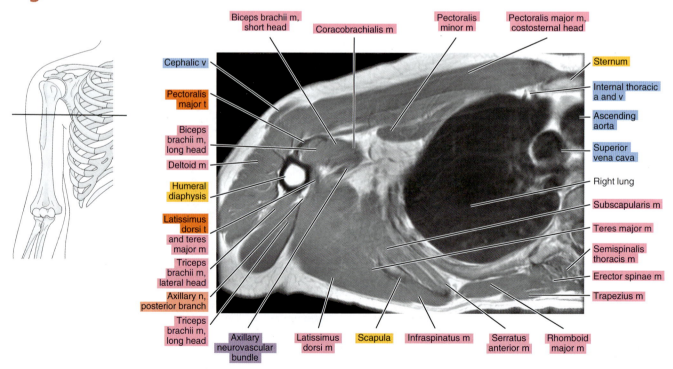

Biceps brachii m, short head
Coracobrachialis m
Pectoralis minor m
Pectoralis major m, costosternal head
Cephalic v
Pectoralis major t
Biceps brachii m, long head
Deltoid m
Humeral diaphysis
Latissimus dorsi t and teres major m
Triceps brachii m, lateral head
Axillary n, posterior branch
Triceps brachii m, long head
Sternum
Internal thoracic a and v
Ascending aorta
Superior vena cava
Right lung
Subscapularis m
Teres major m
Semispinalis thoracis m
Erector spinae m
Trapezius m
Axillary neurovascular bundle
Latissimus dorsi m
Scapula
Infraspinatus m
Serratus anterior m
Rhomboid major m

Figure 5.1.15

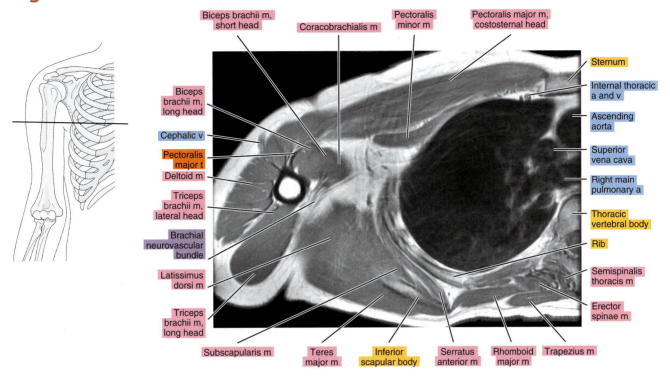

Biceps brachii m, short head
Coracobrachialis m
Pectoralis minor m
Pectoralis major m, costosternal head
Sternum
Internal thoracic a and v
Ascending aorta
Superior vena cava
Right main pulmonary a
Thoracic vertebral body
Rib
Semispinalis thoracis m
Erector spinae m
Biceps brachii m, long head
Cephalic v
Pectoralis major t
Deltoid m
Triceps brachii m, lateral head
Brachial neurovascular bundle
Latissimus dorsi m
Triceps brachii m, long head
Subscapularis m
Teres major m
Inferior scapular body
Serratus anterior m
Rhomboid major m
Trapezius m

Figure 5.1.16

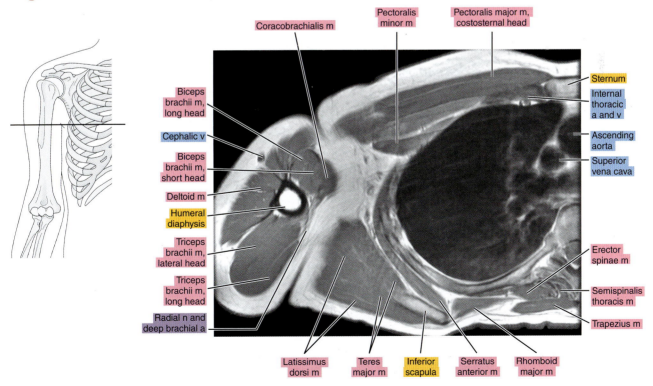

Coracobrachialis m
Pectoralis minor m
Pectoralis major m, costosternal head
Sternum
Internal thoracic a and v
Ascending aorta
Superior vena cava
Erector spinae m
Semispinalis thoracis m
Trapezius m
Biceps brachii m, long head
Cephalic v
Biceps brachii m, short head
Deltoid m
Humeral diaphysis
Triceps brachii m, lateral head
Triceps brachii m, long head
Radial n and deep brachial a
Latissimus dorsi m
Teres major m
Inferior scapula
Serratus anterior m
Rhomboid major m

Figure 5.1.17

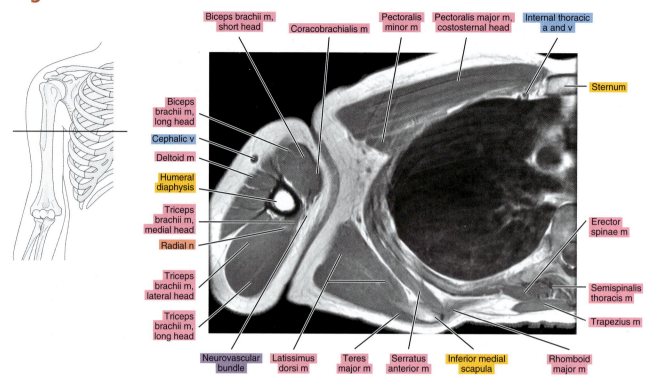

Figure 5.1.18

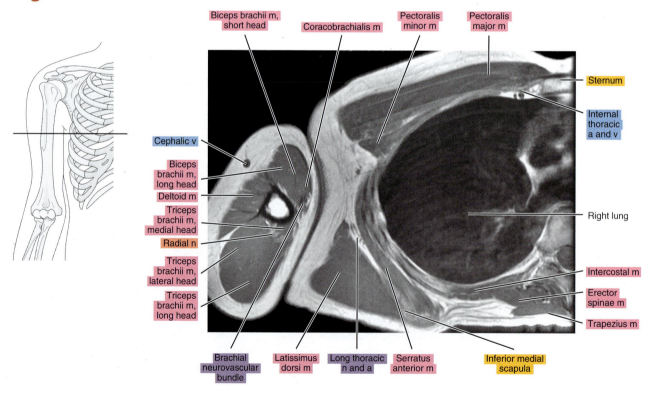

Figure 5.1.19

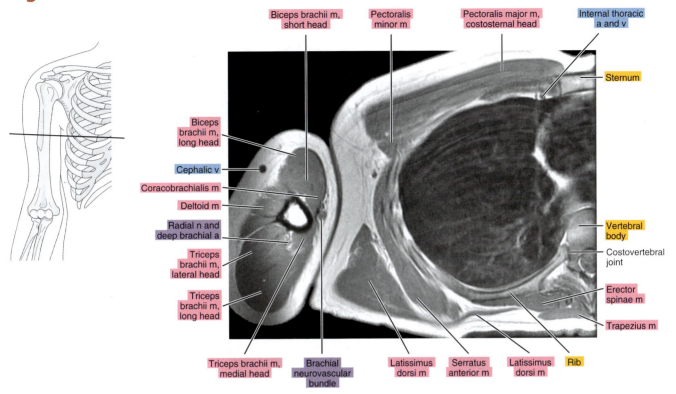

Biceps brachii m, short head

Pectoralis minor m

Pectoralis major m, costosternal head

Internal thoracic a and v

Sternum

Biceps brachii m, long head

Cephalic v

Coracobrachialis m

Deltoid m

Radial n and deep brachial a

Triceps brachii m, lateral head

Triceps brachii m, long head

Vertebral body

Costovertebral joint

Erector spinae m

Trapezius m

Triceps brachii m, medial head

Brachial neurovascular bundle

Latissimus dorsi m

Serratus anterior m

Latissimus dorsi m

Rib

SAGITTAL
Figure 5.2.1

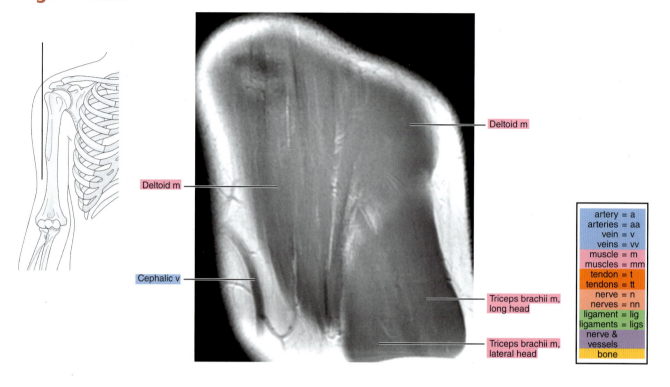

Deltoid m

Deltoid m

Cephalic v

Triceps brachii m, long head

Triceps brachii m, lateral head

artery =	a
arteries =	aa
vein =	v
veins =	vv
muscle =	m
muscles =	mm
tendon =	t
tendons =	tt
nerve =	n
nerves =	nn
ligament =	lig
ligaments =	ligs
nerve & vessels	
bone	

Figure 5.2.2

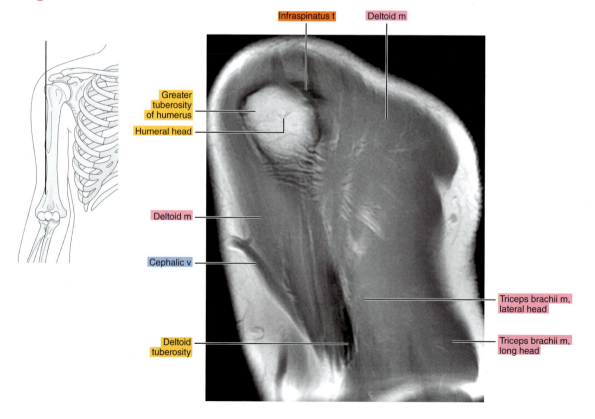

Infraspinatus t

Deltoid m

Greater tuberosity of humerus

Humeral head

Deltoid m

Cephalic v

Deltoid tuberosity

Triceps brachii m, lateral head

Triceps brachii m, long head

Figure 5.2.3

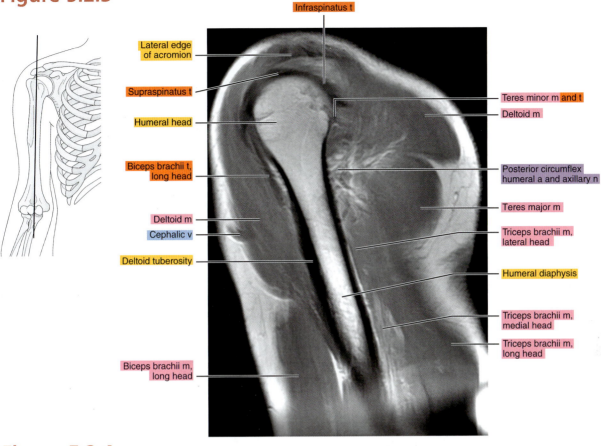

Infraspinatus t

Lateral edge of acromion

Supraspinatus t

Humeral head

Biceps brachii t, long head

Deltoid m

Cephalic v

Deltoid tuberosity

Biceps brachii m, long head

Teres minor m and t

Deltoid m

Posterior circumflex humeral a and axillary n

Teres major m

Triceps brachii m, lateral head

Humeral diaphysis

Triceps brachii m, medial head

Triceps brachii m, long head

Figure 5.2.4

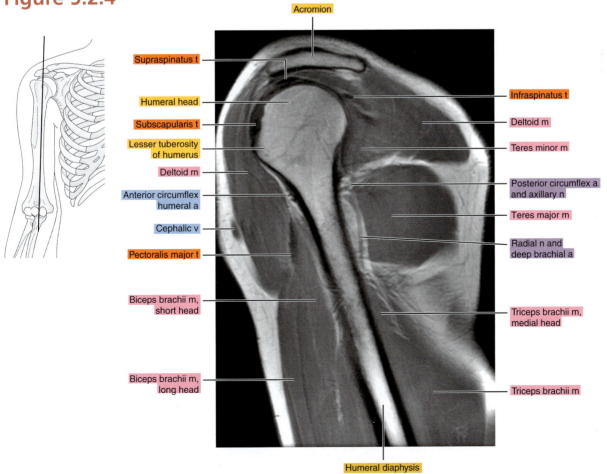

Acromion

Supraspinatus t

Humeral head

Subscapularis t

Lesser tuberosity of humerus

Deltoid m

Anterior circumflex humeral a

Cephalic v

Pectoralis major t

Biceps brachii m, short head

Biceps brachii m, long head

Infraspinatus t

Deltoid m

Teres minor m

Posterior circumflex a and axillary n

Teres major m

Radial n and deep brachial a

Triceps brachii m, medial head

Triceps brachii m

Humeral diaphysis

Figure 5.2.5

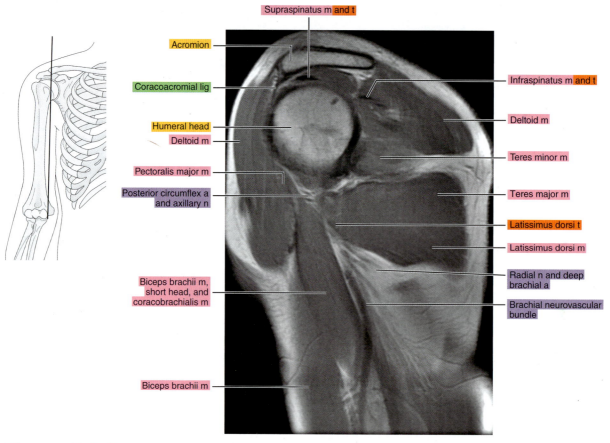

Supraspinatus m and t
Acromion
Coracoacromial lig
Humeral head
Deltoid m
Pectoralis major m
Posterior circumflex a and axillary n
Biceps brachii m, short head, and coracobrachialis m
Biceps brachii m

Infraspinatus m and t
Deltoid m
Teres minor m
Teres major m
Latissimus dorsi t
Latissimus dorsi m
Radial n and deep brachial a
Brachial neurovascular bundle

Figure 5.2.6

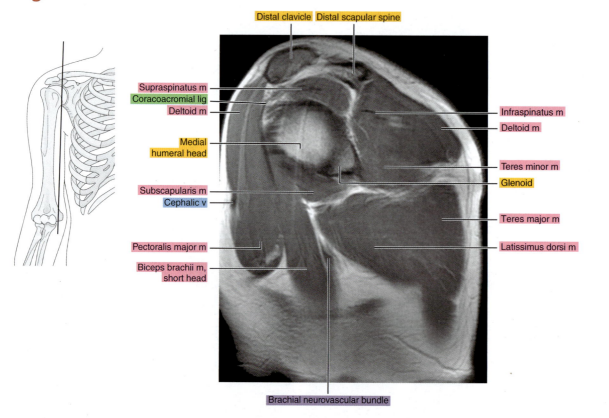

Distal clavicle   Distal scapular spine
Supraspinatus m
Coracoacromial lig
Deltoid m
Medial humeral head
Subscapularis m
Cephalic v
Pectoralis major m
Biceps brachii m, short head

Infraspinatus m
Deltoid m
Teres minor m
Glenoid
Teres major m
Latissimus dorsi m

Brachial neurovascular bundle

Figure 5.2.7

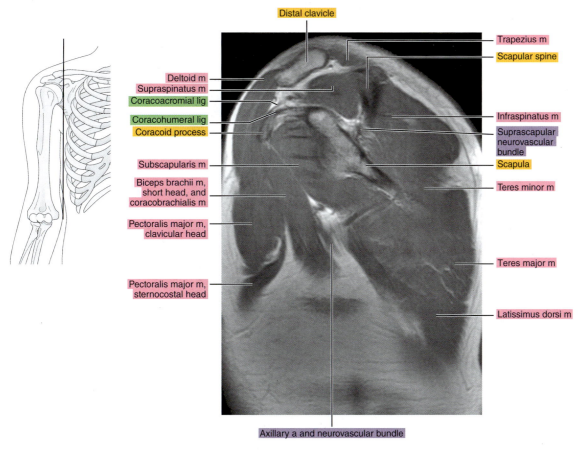

Distal clavicle

Trapezius m

Scapular spine

Deltoid m

Supraspinatus m

Coracoacromial lig

Coracohumeral lig

Coracoid process

Infraspinatus m

Suprascapular neurovascular bundle

Subscapularis m

Scapula

Biceps brachii m, short head, and coracobrachialis m

Teres minor m

Pectoralis major m, clavicular head

Pectoralis major m, sternocostal head

Teres major m

Latissimus dorsi m

Axillary a and neurovascular bundle

Figure 5.2.8

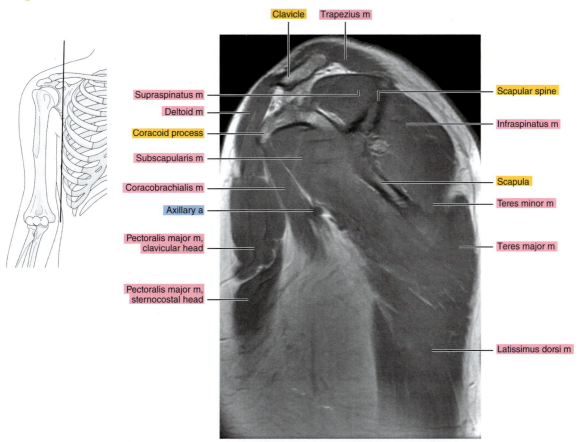

Clavicle

Trapezius m

Supraspinatus m

Scapular spine

Deltoid m

Infraspinatus m

Coracoid process

Subscapularis m

Coracobrachialis m

Scapula

Axillary a

Teres minor m

Pectoralis major m, clavicular head

Teres major m

Pectoralis major m, sternocostal head

Latissimus dorsi m

Figure 5.2.9

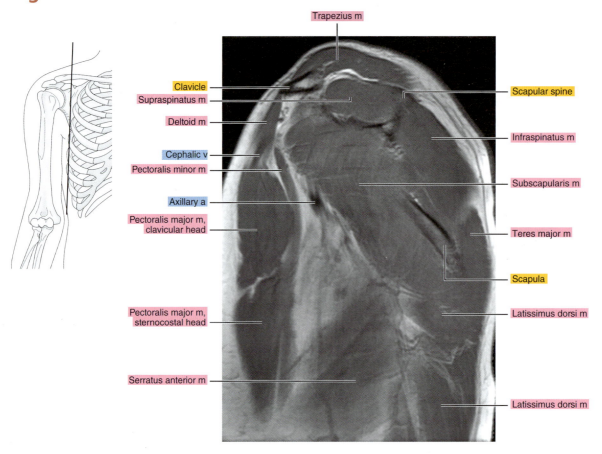

Trapezius m

Clavicle

Supraspinatus m

Deltoid m

Cephalic v

Pectoralis minor m

Axillary a

Pectoralis major m, clavicular head

Pectoralis major m, sternocostal head

Serratus anterior m

Scapular spine

Infraspinatus m

Subscapularis m

Teres major m

Scapula

Latissimus dorsi m

Latissimus dorsi m

Figure 5.2.10

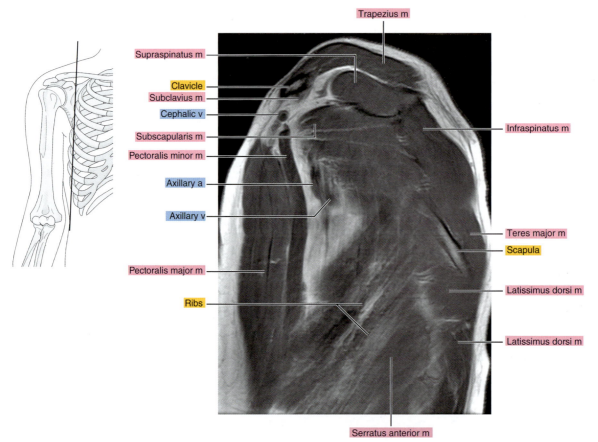

Trapezius m

Supraspinatus m

Clavicle

Subclavius m

Cephalic v

Subscapularis m

Pectoralis minor m

Axillary a

Axillary v

Pectoralis major m

Ribs

Serratus anterior m

Infraspinatus m

Teres major m

Scapula

Latissimus dorsi m

Latissimus dorsi m

Figure 5.2.11

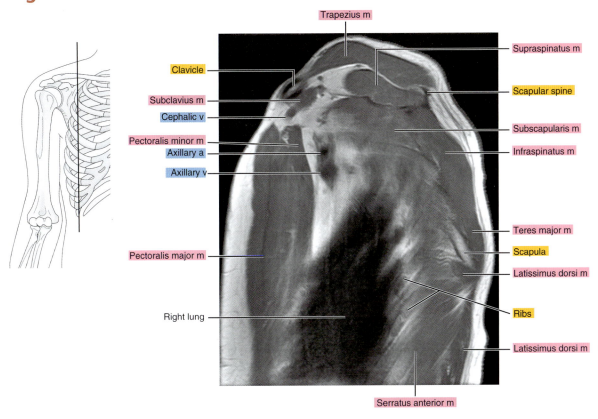

- Trapezius m
- Clavicle
- Subclavius m
- Cephalic v
- Pectoralis minor m
- Axillary a
- Axillary v
- Pectoralis major m
- Right lung
- Supraspinatus m
- Scapular spine
- Subscapularis m
- Infraspinatus m
- Teres major m
- Scapula
- Latissimus dorsi m
- Ribs
- Latissimus dorsi m
- Serratus anterior m

Figure 5.2.12

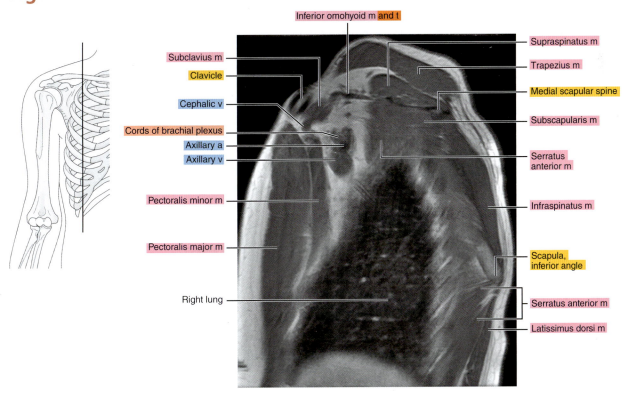

- Inferior omohyoid m and t
- Subclavius m
- Clavicle
- Cephalic v
- Cords of brachial plexus
- Axillary a
- Axillary v
- Pectoralis minor m
- Pectoralis major m
- Right lung
- Supraspinatus m
- Trapezius m
- Medial scapular spine
- Subscapularis m
- Serratus anterior m
- Infraspinatus m
- Scapula, inferior angle
- Serratus anterior m
- Latissimus dorsi m

Figure 5.2.13

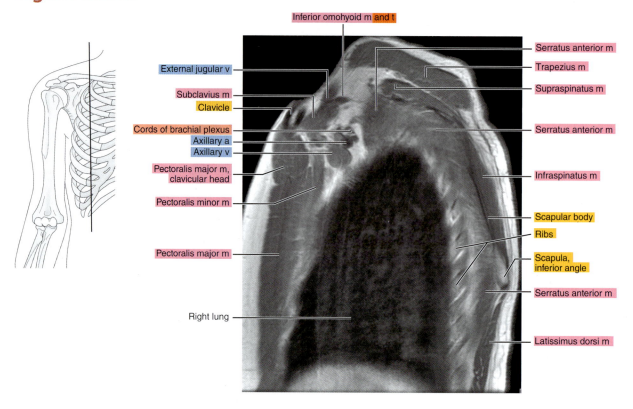

Inferior omohyoid m and t

External jugular v

Subclavius m

Clavicle

Cords of brachial plexus

Axillary a

Axillary v

Pectoralis major m, clavicular head

Pectoralis minor m

Pectoralis major m

Right lung

Serratus anterior m

Trapezius m

Supraspinatus m

Serratus anterior m

Infraspinatus m

Scapular body

Ribs

Scapula, inferior angle

Serratus anterior m

Latissimus dorsi m

Figure 5.2.14

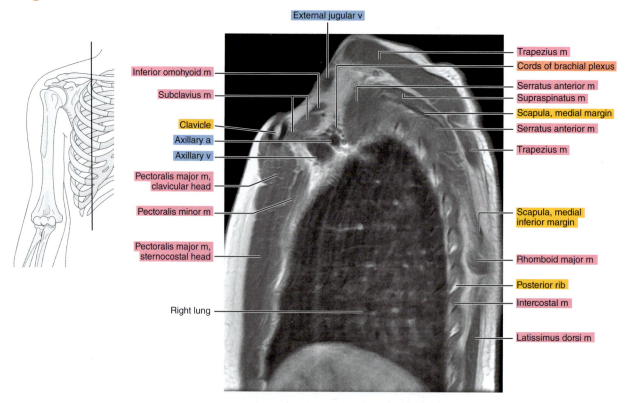

External jugular v

Inferior omohyoid m

Subclavius m

Clavicle

Axillary a

Axillary v

Pectoralis major m, clavicular head

Pectoralis minor m

Pectoralis major m, sternocostal head

Right lung

Trapezius m

Cords of brachial plexus

Serratus anterior m

Supraspinatus m

Scapula, medial margin

Serratus anterior m

Trapezius m

Scapula, medial inferior margin

Rhomboid major m

Posterior rib

Intercostal m

Latissimus dorsi m

Figure 5.2.15

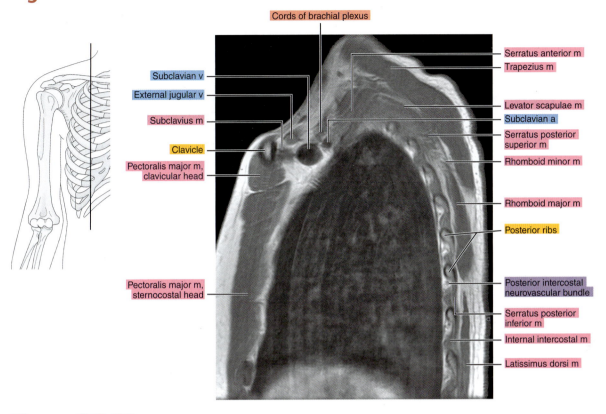

Cords of brachial plexus

Subclavian v

External jugular v

Subclavius m

Clavicle

Pectoralis major m, clavicular head

Pectoralis major m, sternocostal head

Serratus anterior m

Trapezius m

Levator scapulae m

Subclavian a

Serratus posterior superior m

Rhomboid minor m

Rhomboid major m

Posterior ribs

Posterior intercostal neurovascular bundle

Serratus posterior inferior m

Internal intercostal m

Latissimus dorsi m

Figure 5.2.16

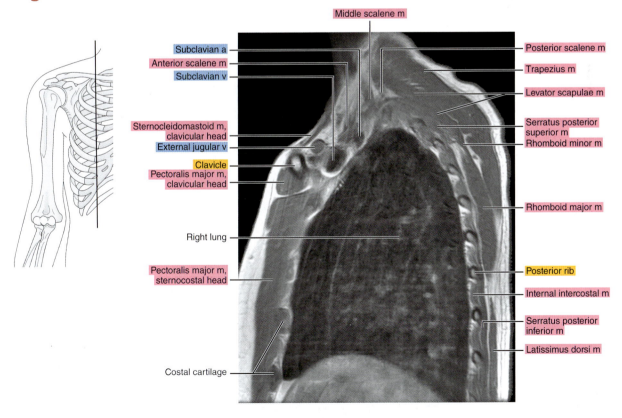

Middle scalene m

Subclavian a

Anterior scalene m

Subclavian v

Sternocleidomastoid m, clavicular head

External jugular v

Clavicle

Pectoralis major m, clavicular head

Right lung

Pectoralis major m, sternocostal head

Costal cartilage

Posterior scalene m

Trapezius m

Levator scapulae m

Serratus posterior superior m

Rhomboid minor m

Rhomboid major m

Posterior rib

Internal intercostal m

Serratus posterior inferior m

Latissimus dorsi m

Figure 5.2.17

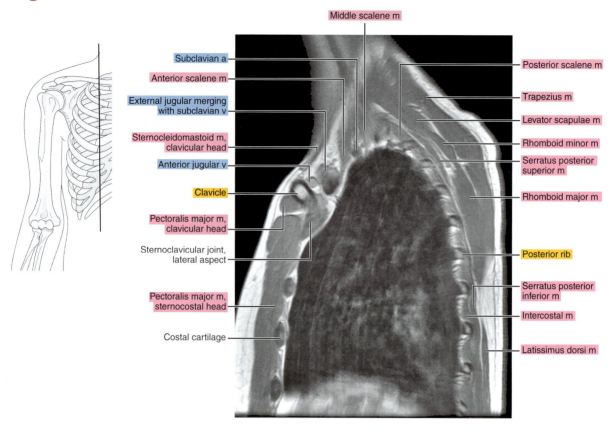

Middle scalene m

Subclavian a

Anterior scalene m

External jugular merging with subclavian v

Sternocleidomastoid m, clavicular head

Anterior jugular v

Clavicle

Pectoralis major m, clavicular head

Sternoclavicular joint, lateral aspect

Pectoralis major m, sternocostal head

Costal cartilage

Posterior scalene m

Trapezius m

Levator scapulae m

Rhomboid minor m

Serratus posterior superior m

Rhomboid major m

Posterior rib

Serratus posterior inferior m

Intercostal m

Latissimus dorsi m

Figure 5.2.18

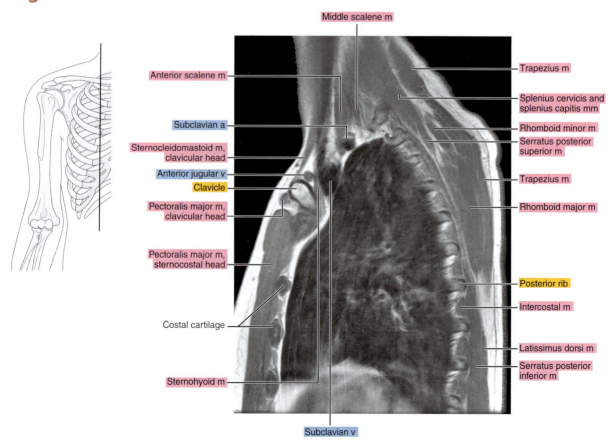

Middle scalene m

Anterior scalene m

Subclavian a

Sternocleidomastoid m, clavicular head

Anterior jugular v

Clavicle

Pectoralis major m, clavicular head

Pectoralis major m, sternocostal head

Costal cartilage

Sternohyoid m

Subclavian v

Trapezius m

Splenius cervicis and splenius capitis mm

Rhomboid minor m

Serratus posterior superior m

Trapezius m

Rhomboid major m

Posterior rib

Intercostal m

Latissimus dorsi m

Serratus posterior inferior m

Figure 5.2.19

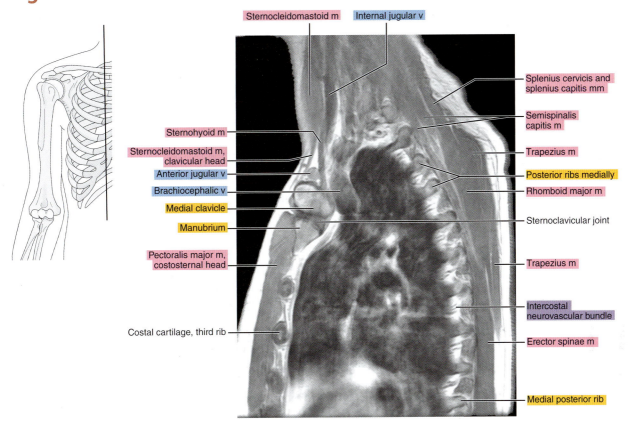

Sternocleidomastoid m

Internal jugular v

Splenius cervicis and splenius capitis mm

Semispinalis capitis m

Sternohyoid m

Sternocleidomastoid m, clavicular head

Trapezius m

Anterior jugular v

Posterior ribs medially

Brachiocephalic v

Rhomboid major m

Medial clavicle

Manubrium

Sternoclavicular joint

Pectoralis major m, costosternal head

Trapezius m

Intercostal neurovascular bundle

Erector spinae m

Costal cartilage, third rib

Medial posterior rib

CORONAL
Figure 5.3.1

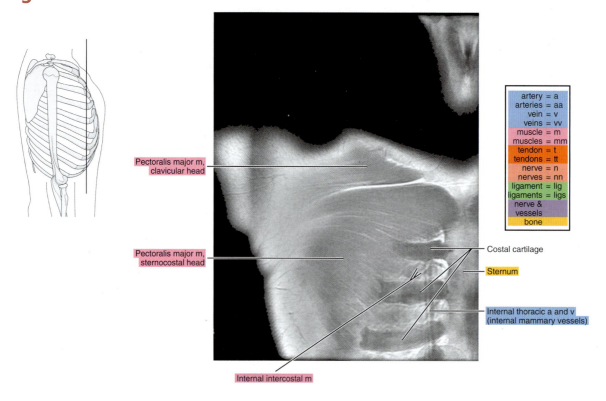

Pectoralis major m, clavicular head

Pectoralis major m, sternocostal head

Internal intercostal m

Costal cartilage

Sternum

Internal thoracic a and v (internal mammary vessels)

artery = a	
arteries = aa	
vein = v	
veins = vv	
muscle = m	
muscles = mm	
tendon = t	
tendons = tt	
nerve = n	
nerves = nn	
ligament = lig	
ligaments = ligs	
nerve & vessels	
bone	

Figure 5.3.2

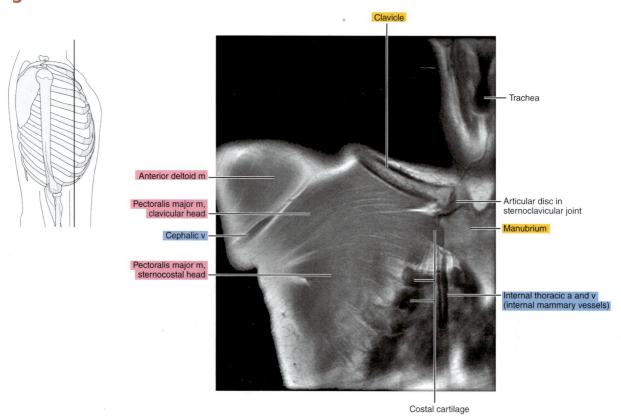

Clavicle

Trachea

Anterior deltoid m

Pectoralis major m, clavicular head

Cephalic v

Pectoralis major m, sternocostal head

Articular disc in sternoclavicular joint

Manubrium

Internal thoracic a and v (internal mammary vessels)

Costal cartilage

Figure 5.3.3

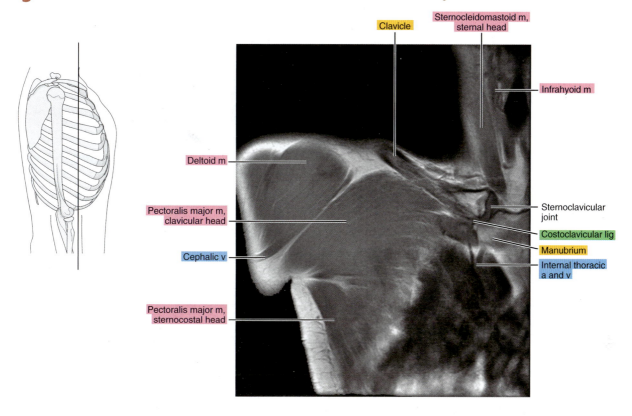

Clavicle

Sternocleidomastoid m, sternal head

Infrahyoid m

Deltoid m

Pectoralis major m, clavicular head

Cephalic v

Pectoralis major m, sternocostal head

Sternoclavicular joint

Costoclavicular lig

Manubrium

Internal thoracic a and v

Figure 5.3.4

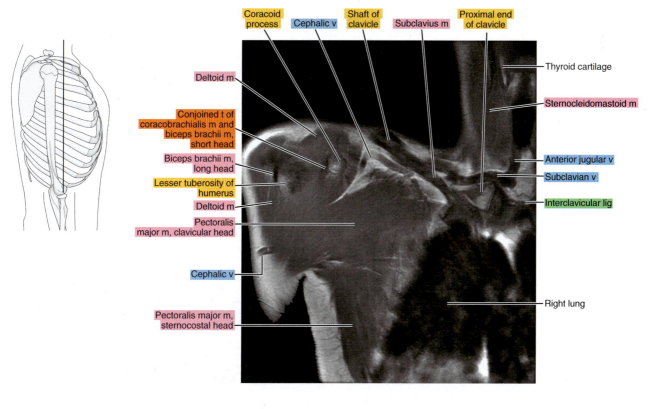

Coracoid process

Cephalic v

Shaft of clavicle

Subclavius m

Proximal end of clavicle

Deltoid m

Conjoined t of coracobrachialis m and biceps brachii m, short head

Biceps brachii m, long head

Lesser tuberosity of humerus

Deltoid m

Pectoralis major m, clavicular head

Cephalic v

Pectoralis major m, sternocostal head

Thyroid cartilage

Sternocleidomastoid m

Anterior jugular v

Subclavian v

Interclavicular lig

Right lung

Figure 5.3.5

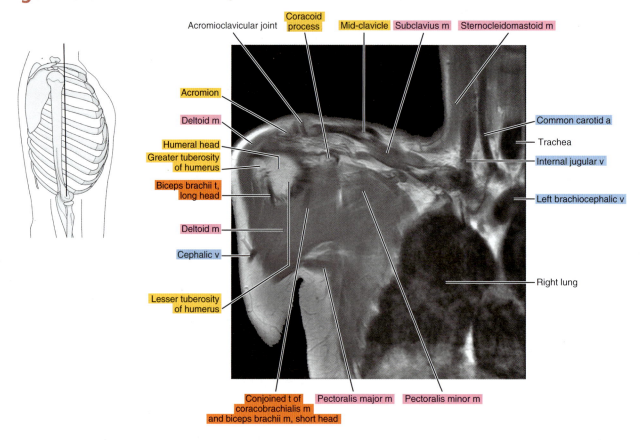

Acromioclavicular joint

Coracoid process

Mid-clavicle

Subclavius m

Sternocleidomastoid m

Acromion

Deltoid m

Humeral head

Greater tuberosity of humerus

Biceps brachii t, long head

Deltoid m

Cephalic v

Lesser tuberosity of humerus

Common carotid a

Trachea

Internal jugular v

Left brachiocephalic v

Right lung

Conjoined t of coracobrachialis m and biceps brachii m, short head

Pectoralis major m

Pectoralis minor m

Figure 5.3.6

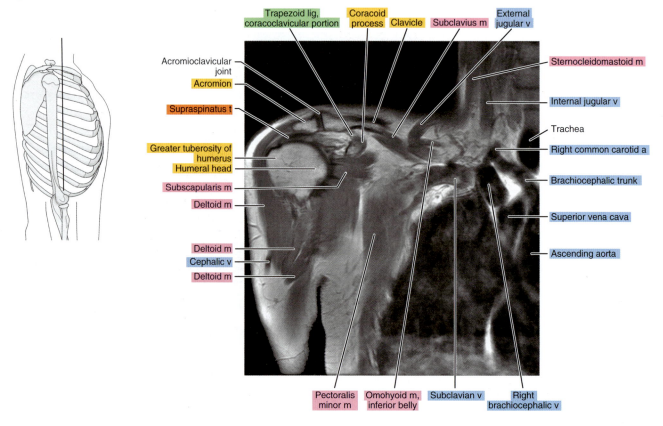

Trapezoid lig, coracoclavicular portion

Coracoid process

Clavicle

Subclavius m

External jugular v

Acromioclavicular joint

Acromion

Supraspinatus t

Greater tuberosity of humerus

Humeral head

Subscapularis m

Deltoid m

Deltoid m

Cephalic v

Deltoid m

Sternocleidomastoid m

Internal jugular v

Trachea

Right common carotid a

Brachiocephalic trunk

Superior vena cava

Ascending aorta

Pectoralis minor m

Omohyoid m, inferior belly

Subclavian v

Right brachiocephalic v

Figure 5.3.7

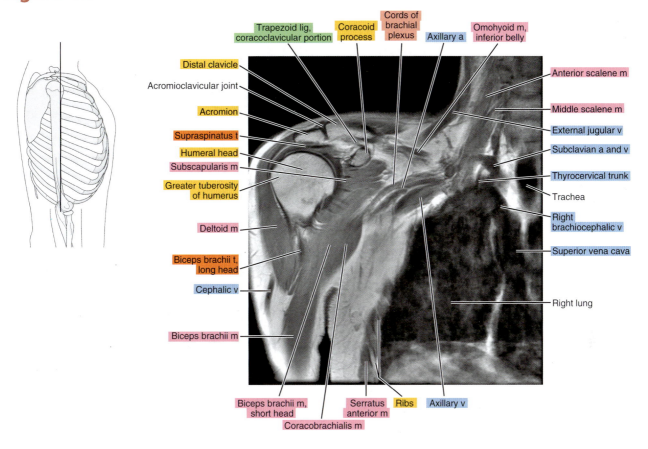

Trapezoid lig, coracoclavicular portion — Coracoid process — Cords of brachial plexus — Axillary a — Omohyoid m, inferior belly

Distal clavicle
Acromioclavicular joint
Acromion
Supraspinatus t
Humeral head
Subscapularis m
Greater tuberosity of humerus
Deltoid m
Biceps brachii t, long head
Cephalic v
Biceps brachii m

Anterior scalene m
Middle scalene m
External jugular v
Subclavian a and v
Thyrocervical trunk
Trachea
Right brachiocephalic v
Superior vena cava
Right lung

Biceps brachii m, short head — Serratus anterior m — Ribs — Axillary v
Coracobrachialis m

Figure 5.3.8

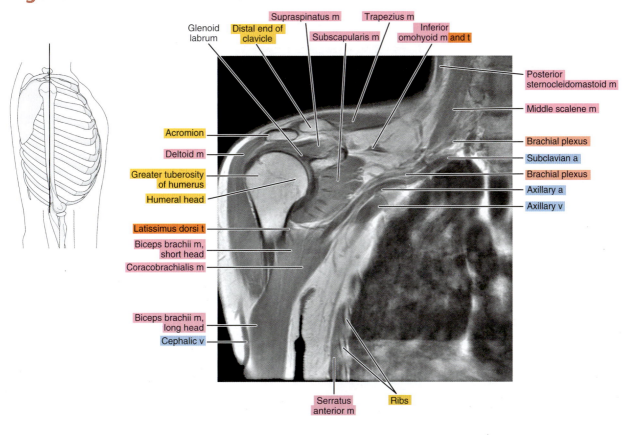

Supraspinatus m — Trapezius m
Glenoid labrum — Distal end of clavicle — Subscapularis m — Inferior omohyoid m and t

Acromion
Deltoid m
Greater tuberosity of humerus
Humeral head
Latissimus dorsi t
Biceps brachii m, short head
Coracobrachialis m
Biceps brachii m, long head
Cephalic v

Posterior sternocleidomastoid m
Middle scalene m
Brachial plexus
Subclavian a
Brachial plexus
Axillary a
Axillary v

Serratus anterior m — Ribs

Figure 5.3.9

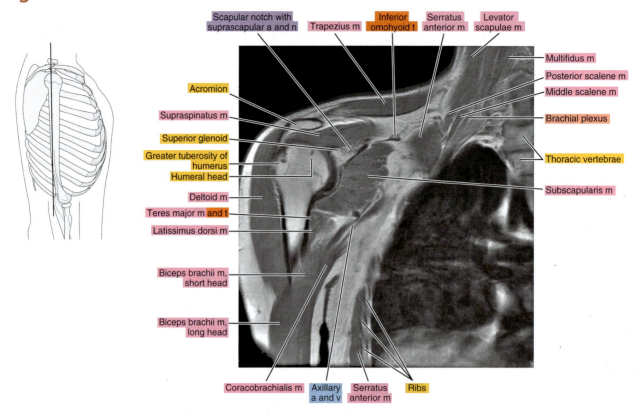

Scapular notch with suprascapular a and n · Trapezius m · Inferior omohyoid t · Serratus anterior m · Levator scapulae m · Multifidus m · Posterior scalene m · Middle scalene m · Brachial plexus · Thoracic vertebrae · Subscapularis m · Acromion · Supraspinatus m · Superior glenoid · Greater tuberosity of humerus · Humeral head · Deltoid m · Teres major m and t · Latissimus dorsi m · Biceps brachii m, short head · Biceps brachii m, long head · Coracobrachialis m · Axillary a and v · Serratus anterior m · Ribs

Figure 5.3.10

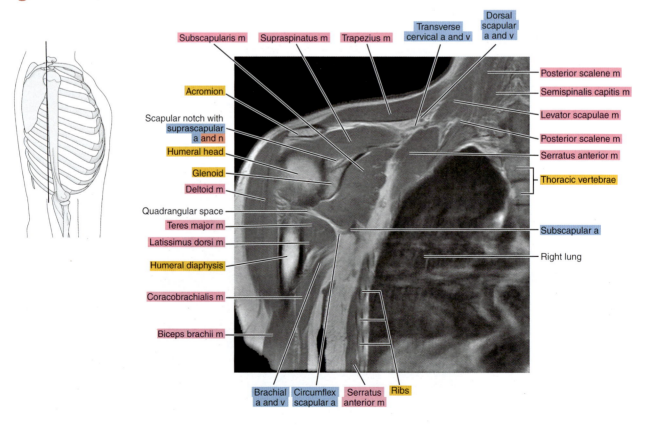

Subscapularis m · Supraspinatus m · Trapezius m · Transverse cervical a and v · Dorsal scapular a and v · Posterior scalene m · Semispinalis capitis m · Levator scapulae m · Posterior scalene m · Serratus anterior m · Thoracic vertebrae · Acromion · Scapular notch with suprascapular a and n · Humeral head · Glenoid · Deltoid m · Quadrangular space · Teres major m · Latissimus dorsi m · Humeral diaphysis · Coracobrachialis m · Biceps brachii m · Subscapular a · Right lung · Brachial a and v · Circumflex scapular a · Serratus anterior m · Ribs

Figure 5.3.11

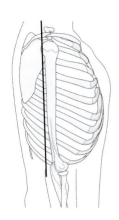
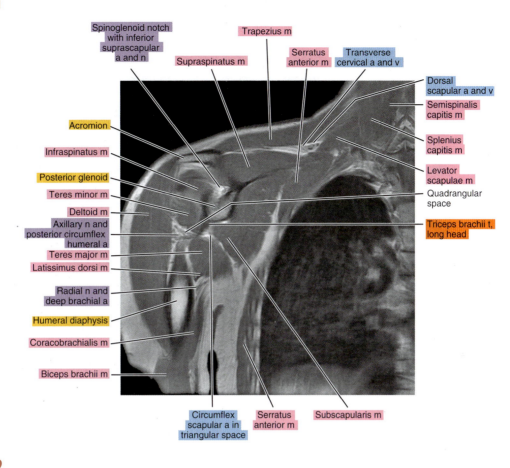

Figure 5.3.12

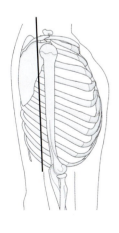
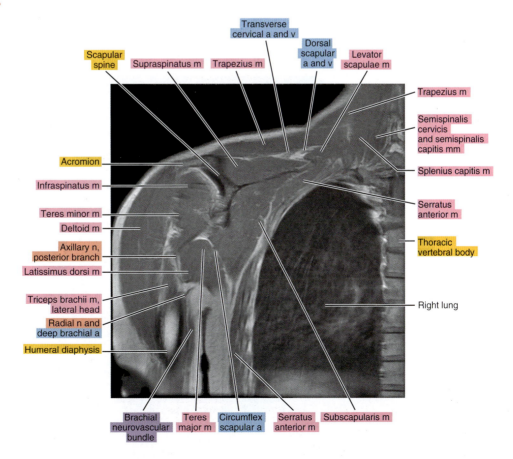

Figure 5.3.13

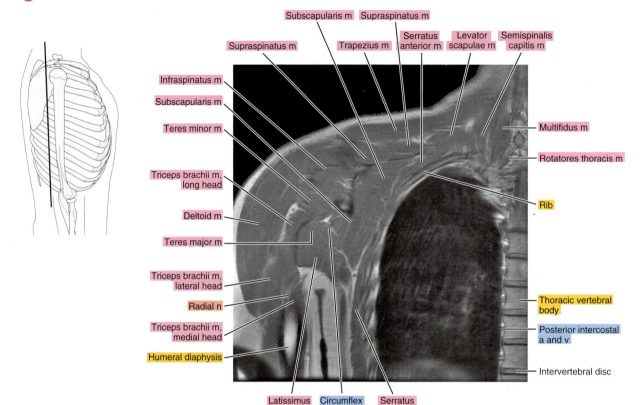

Subscapularis m   Supraspinatus m

Supraspinatus m   Trapezius m   Serratus anterior m   Levator scapulae m   Semispinalis capitis m

Infraspinatus m

Subscapularis m

Teres minor m

Triceps brachii m, long head

Deltoid m

Teres major m

Triceps brachii m, lateral head

Radial n

Triceps brachii m, medial head

Humeral diaphysis

Multifidus m

Rotatores thoracis m

Rib

Thoracic vertebral body

Posterior intercostal a and v

Intervertebral disc

Latissimus dorsi m   Circumflex scapular a   Serratus anterior m

Figure 5.3.14

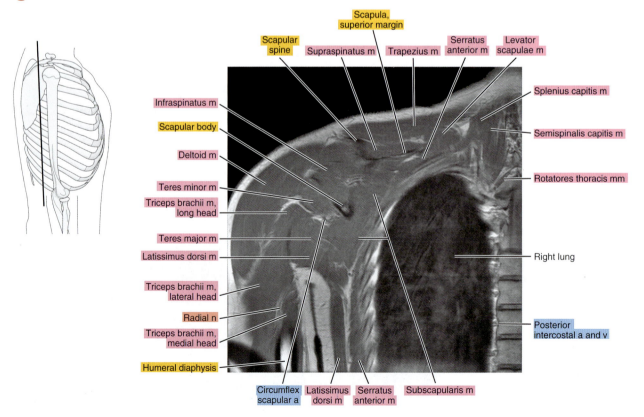

Scapula, superior margin

Scapular spine   Supraspinatus m   Trapezius m   Serratus anterior m   Levator scapulae m

Infraspinatus m

Scapular body

Deltoid m

Teres minor m

Triceps brachii m, long head

Teres major m

Latissimus dorsi m

Triceps brachii m, lateral head

Radial n

Triceps brachii m, medial head

Humeral diaphysis

Splenius capitis m

Semispinalis capitis m

Rotatores thoracis mm

Right lung

Posterior intercostal a and v

Circumflex scapular a   Latissimus dorsi m   Serratus anterior m   Subscapularis m

Figure 5.3.15

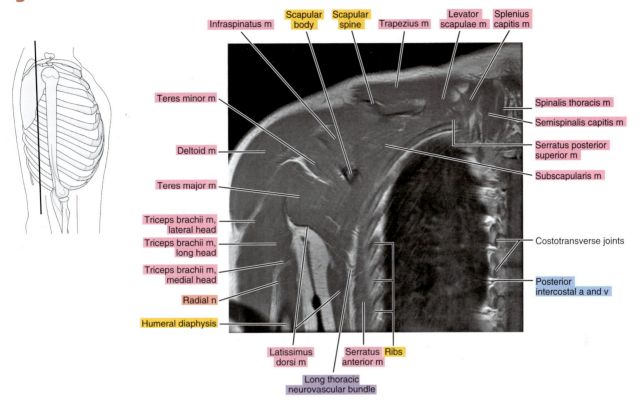

Figure 5.3.16

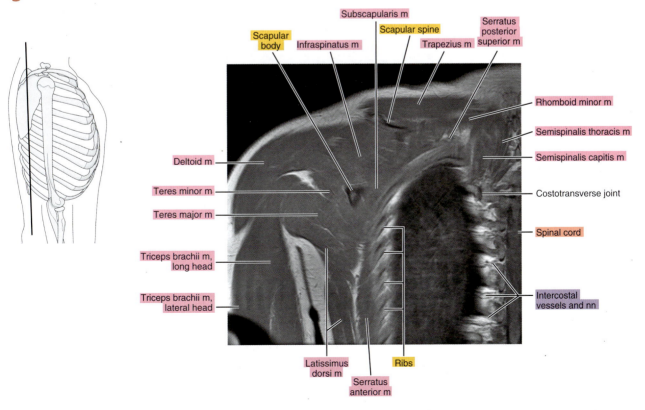

Figure 5.3.17

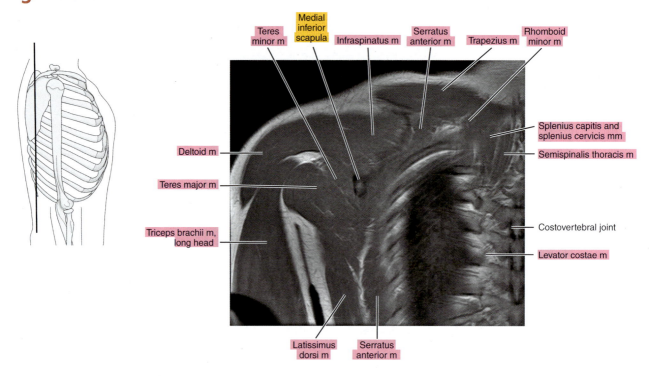

Figure 5.3.18

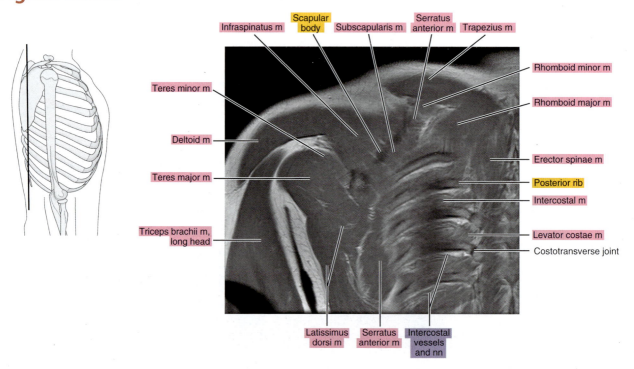

Figure 5.3.19

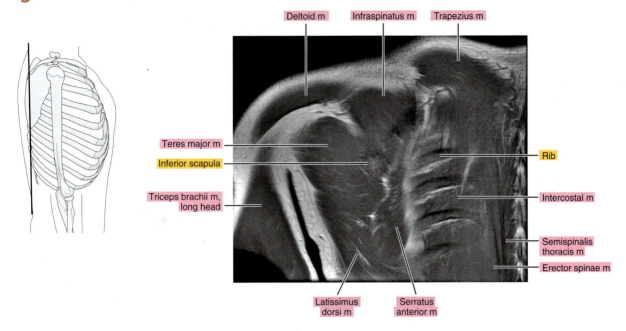

Deltoid m

Infraspinatus m

Trapezius m

Teres major m

Inferior scapula

Rib

Triceps brachii m, long head

Intercostal m

Semispinalis thoracis m

Erector spinae m

Latissimus dorsi m

Serratus anterior m

Figure 5.3.20

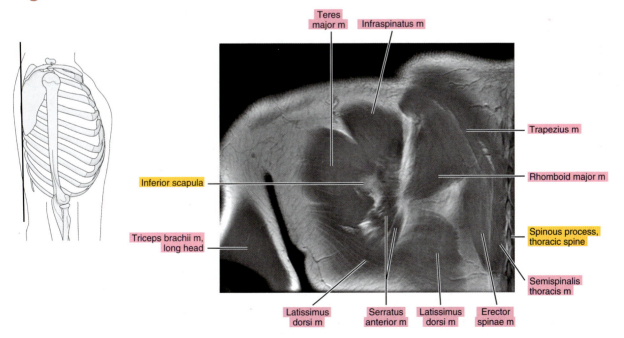

Teres major m

Infraspinatus m

Trapezius m

Inferior scapula

Rhomboid major m

Triceps brachii m, long head

Spinous process, thoracic spine

Semispinalis thoracis m

Latissimus dorsi m

Serratus anterior m

Latissimus dorsi m

Erector spinae m

Chapter

6

MRI of the Shoulder

AXIAL
Figure 6.1.1

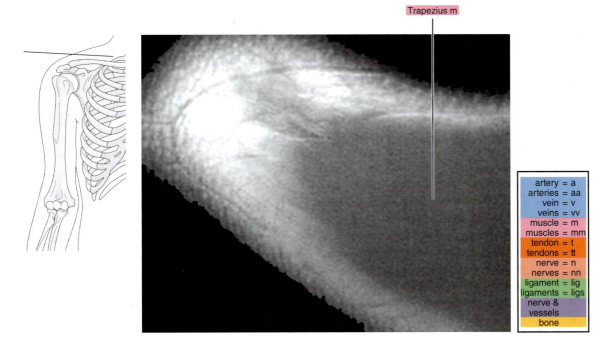

Trapezius m

artery	= a
arteries	= aa
vein	= v
veins	= vv
muscle	= m
muscles	= mm
tendon	= t
tendons	= tt
nerve	= n
nerves	= nn
ligament	= lig
ligaments	= ligs
nerve & vessels	
bone	

Figure 6.1.2

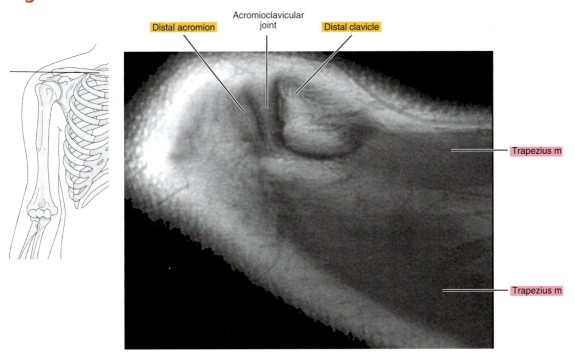

Distal acromion

Acromioclavicular joint

Distal clavicle

Trapezius m

Trapezius m

Figure 6.1.3

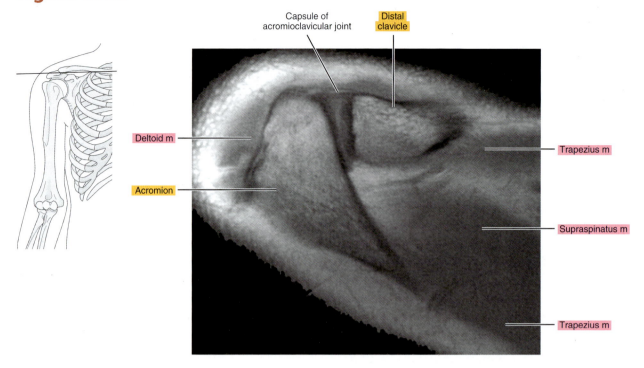

Capsule of acromioclavicular joint

Distal clavicle

Deltoid m

Acromion

Trapezius m

Supraspinatus m

Trapezius m

Figure 6.1.4

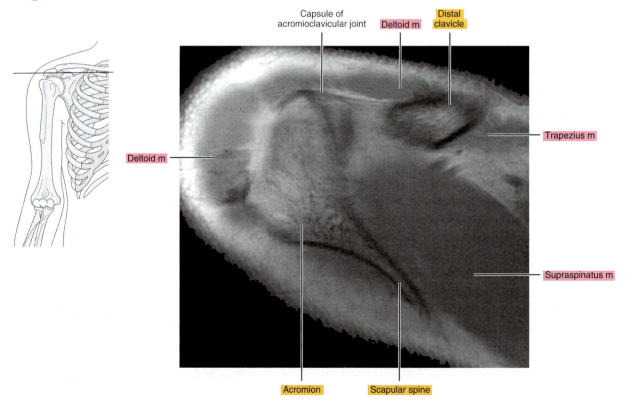

Capsule of acromioclavicular joint

Deltoid m

Distal clavicle

Deltoid m

Trapezius m

Supraspinatus m

Acromion

Scapular spine

Figure 6.1.5

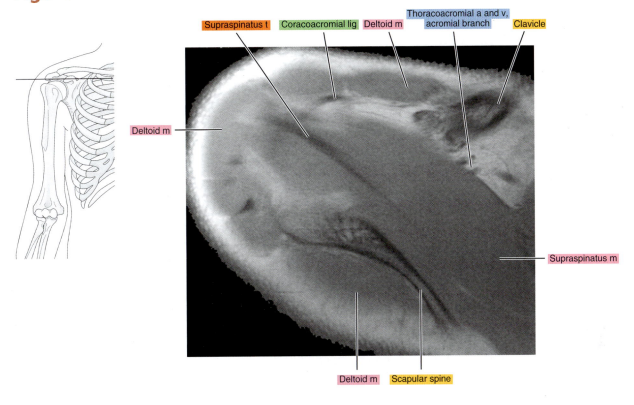

Supraspinatus t | Coracoacromial lig | Deltoid m | Thoracoacromial a and v, acromial branch | Clavicle

Deltoid m

Supraspinatus m

Deltoid m | Scapular spine

Figure 6.1.6

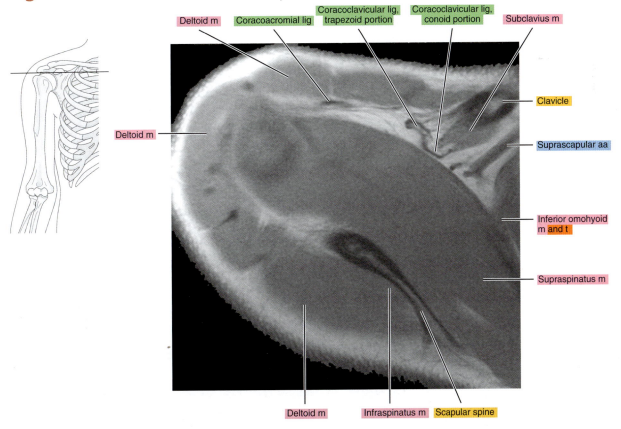

Deltoid m | Coracoacromial lig | Coracoclavicular lig, trapezoid portion | Coracoclavicular lig, conoid portion | Subclavius m

Deltoid m

Clavicle

Suprascapular aa

Inferior omohyoid m and t

Supraspinatus m

Deltoid m | Infraspinatus m | Scapular spine

Figure 6.1.7

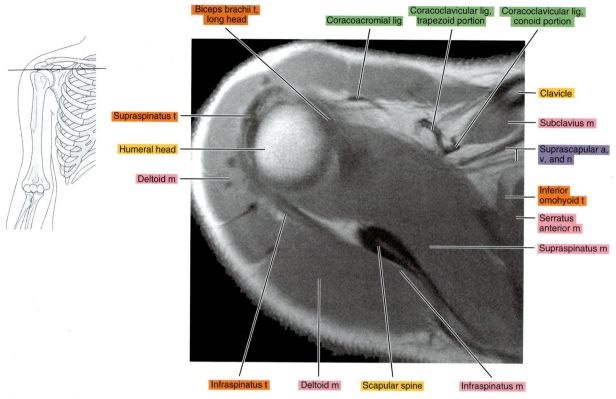

Figure 6.1.8

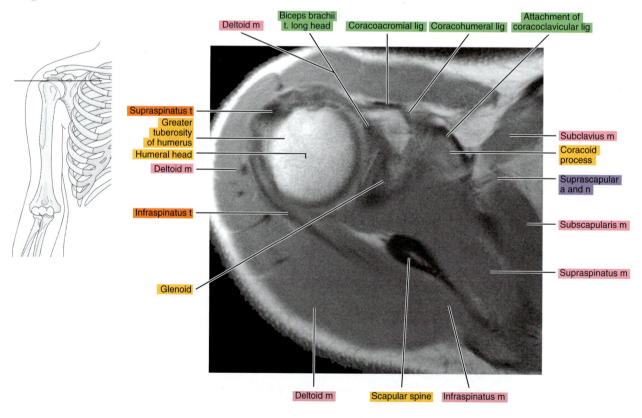

Figure 6.1.9

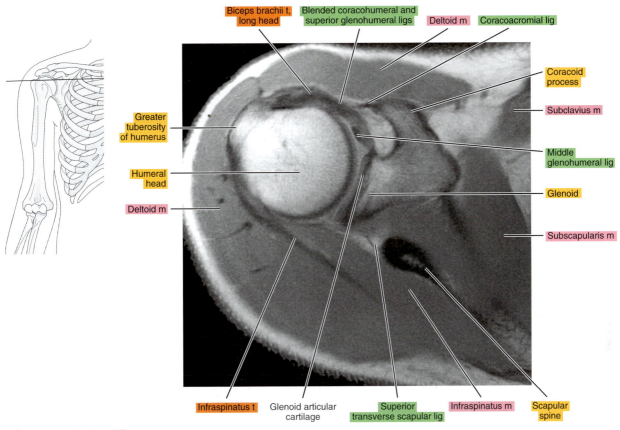

Biceps brachii t, long head — Blended coracohumeral and superior glenohumeral ligs — Deltoid m — Coracoacromial lig

Greater tuberosity of humerus

Humeral head

Deltoid m

Coracoid process

Subclavius m

Middle glenohumeral lig

Glenoid

Subscapularis m

Infraspinatus t — Glenoid articular cartilage — Superior transverse scapular lig — Infraspinatus m — Scapular spine

Figure 6.1.10

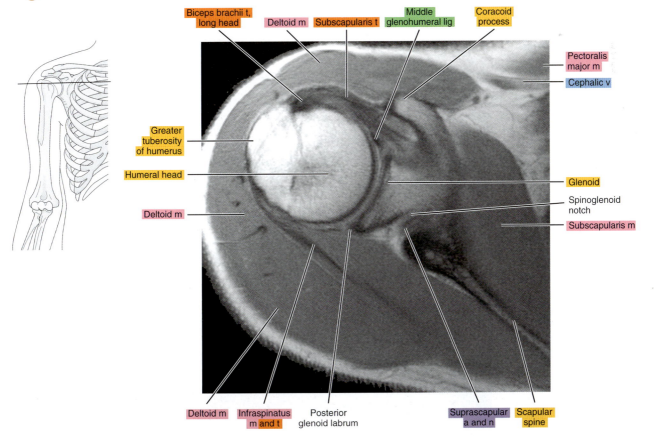

Biceps brachii t, long head — Deltoid m — Subscapularis t — Middle glenohumeral lig — Coracoid process

Pectoralis major m

Cephalic v

Greater tuberosity of humerus

Humeral head

Deltoid m

Glenoid

Spinoglenoid notch

Subscapularis m

Deltoid m — Infraspinatus m and t — Posterior glenoid labrum — Suprascapular a and n — Scapular spine

Figure 6.1.11

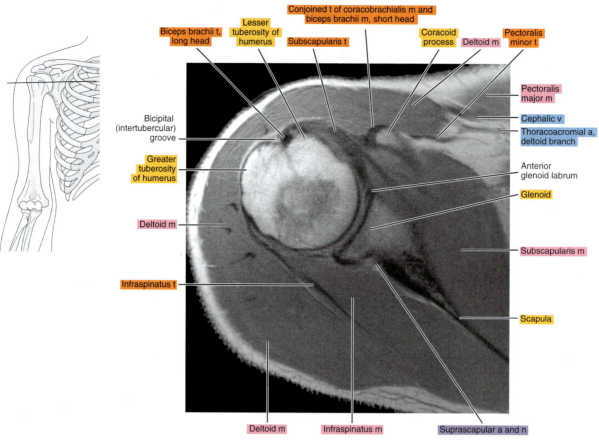

Biceps brachii t, long head

Lesser tuberosity of humerus

Conjoined t of coracobrachialis m and biceps brachii m, short head

Subscapularis t

Coracoid process

Deltoid m

Pectoralis minor t

Pectoralis major m

Cephalic v

Thoracoacromial a, deltoid branch

Bicipital (intertubercular) groove

Greater tuberosity of humerus

Anterior glenoid labrum

Glenoid

Deltoid m

Subscapularis m

Infraspinatus t

Scapula

Deltoid m

Infraspinatus m

Suprascapular a and n

Figure 6.1.12

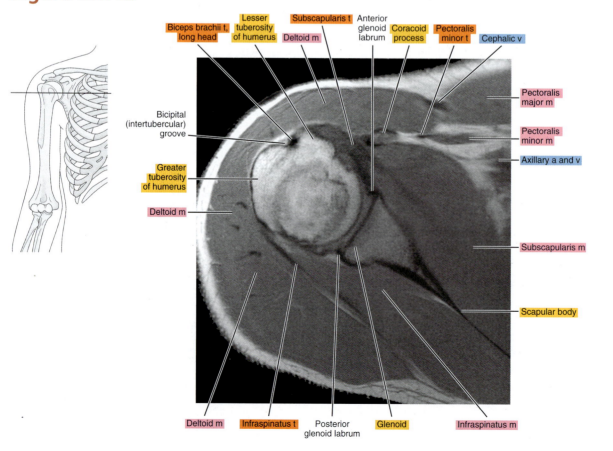

Biceps brachii t, long head

Lesser tuberosity of humerus

Subscapularis t

Deltoid m

Anterior glenoid labrum

Coracoid process

Pectoralis minor t

Cephalic v

Pectoralis major m

Bicipital (intertubercular) groove

Greater tuberosity of humerus

Pectoralis minor m

Axillary a and v

Deltoid m

Subscapularis m

Scapular body

Deltoid m

Infraspinatus t

Posterior glenoid labrum

Glenoid

Infraspinatus m

Figure 6.1.13

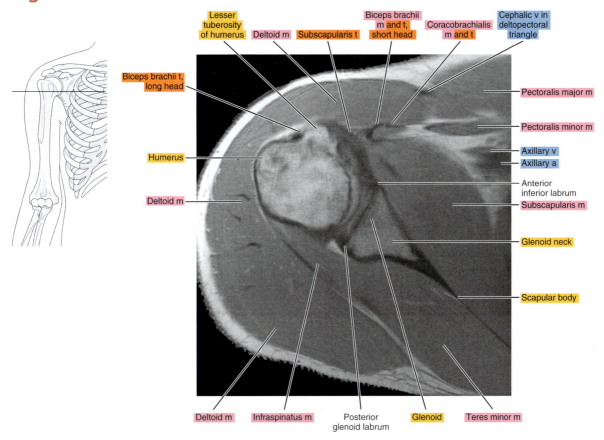

Lesser tuberosity of humerus

Deltoid m

Subscapularis t

Biceps brachii m and t, short head

Coracobrachialis m and t

Cephalic v in deltopectoral triangle

Biceps brachii t, long head

Humerus

Deltoid m

Pectoralis major m

Pectoralis minor m

Axillary v

Axillary a

Anterior inferior labrum

Subscapularis m

Glenoid neck

Scapular body

Deltoid m

Infraspinatus m

Posterior glenoid labrum

Glenoid

Teres minor m

Figure 6.1.14

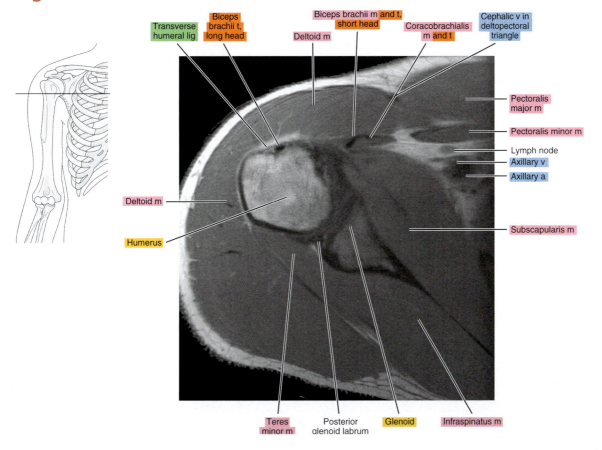

Transverse humeral lig

Biceps brachii t, long head

Biceps brachii m and t, short head

Deltoid m

Coracobrachialis m and t

Cephalic v in deltopectoral triangle

Pectoralis major m

Pectoralis minor m

Lymph node

Axillary v

Axillary a

Deltoid m

Humerus

Subscapularis m

Teres minor m

Posterior glenoid labrum

Glenoid

Infraspinatus m

Figure 6.1.15

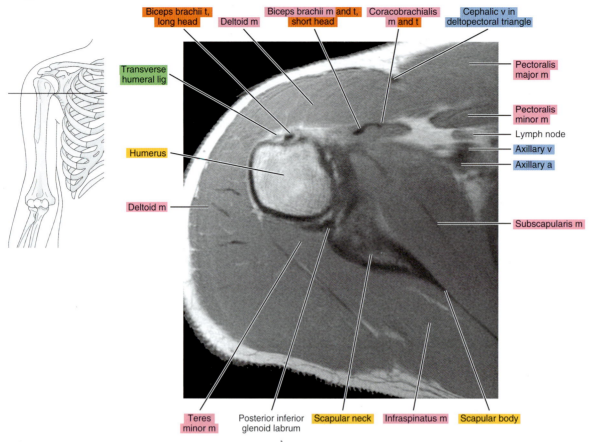

Biceps brachii t, long head — Deltoid m — Biceps brachii m and t, short head — Coracobrachialis m and t — Cephalic v in deltopectoral triangle

Transverse humeral lig

Pectoralis major m

Pectoralis minor m

Lymph node

Axillary v

Axillary a

Humerus

Deltoid m

Subscapularis m

Teres minor m — Posterior inferior glenoid labrum — Scapular neck — Infraspinatus m — Scapular body

Figure 6.1.16

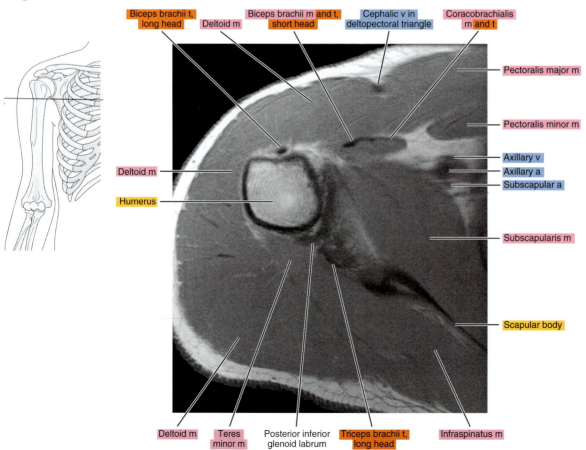

Biceps brachii t, long head — Deltoid m — Biceps brachii m and t, short head — Cephalic v in deltopectoral triangle — Coracobrachialis m and t

Pectoralis major m

Pectoralis minor m

Deltoid m

Axillary v

Axillary a

Subscapular a

Humerus

Subscapularis m

Scapular body

Deltoid m — Teres minor m — Posterior inferior glenoid labrum — Triceps brachii t, long head — Infraspinatus m

Figure 6.1.17

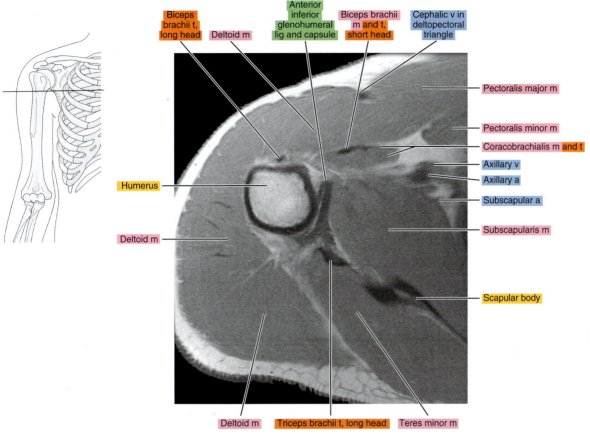

Biceps brachii t, long head
Deltoid m
Anterior inferior glenohumeral lig and capsule
Biceps brachii m and t, short head
Cephalic v in deltopectoral triangle
Pectoralis major m
Pectoralis minor m
Coracobrachialis m and t
Axillary v
Axillary a
Subscapular a
Subscapularis m
Scapular body
Humerus
Deltoid m
Deltoid m
Triceps brachii t, long head
Teres minor m

Figure 6.1.18

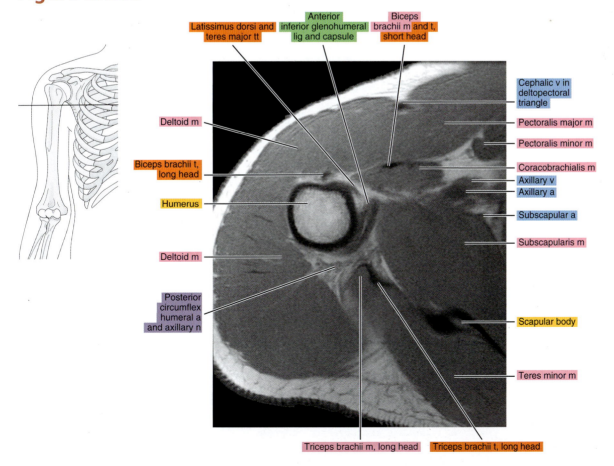

Latissimus dorsi and teres major tt
Anterior inferior glenohumeral lig and capsule
Biceps brachii m and t, short head
Cephalic v in deltopectoral triangle
Pectoralis major m
Pectoralis minor m
Coracobrachialis m
Axillary v
Axillary a
Subscapular a
Subscapularis m
Scapular body
Teres minor m
Deltoid m
Biceps brachii t, long head
Humerus
Deltoid m
Posterior circumflex humeral a and axillary n
Triceps brachii m, long head
Triceps brachii t, long head

Figure 6.1.19

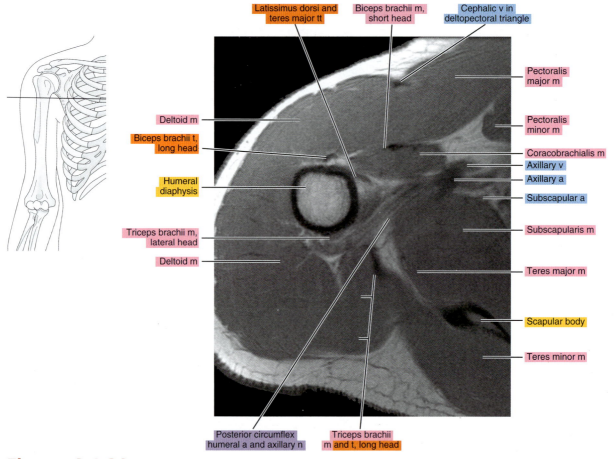

Latissimus dorsi and teres major tt

Biceps brachii m, short head

Cephalic v in deltopectoral triangle

Pectoralis major m

Deltoid m

Pectoralis minor m

Biceps brachii t, long head

Coracobrachialis m

Axillary v

Humeral diaphysis

Axillary a

Subscapular a

Triceps brachii m, lateral head

Subscapularis m

Deltoid m

Teres major m

Scapular body

Teres minor m

Posterior circumflex humeral a and axillary n

Triceps brachii m and t, long head

Figure 6.1.20

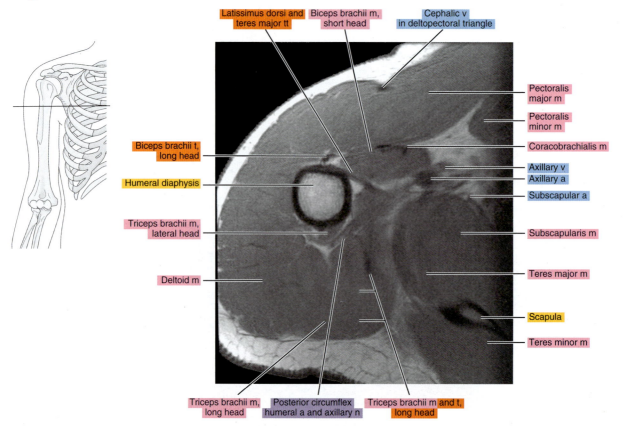

Latissimus dorsi and teres major tt

Biceps brachii m, short head

Cephalic v in deltopectoral triangle

Pectoralis major m

Pectoralis minor m

Biceps brachii t, long head

Coracobrachialis m

Humeral diaphysis

Axillary v

Axillary a

Subscapular a

Triceps brachii m, lateral head

Subscapularis m

Deltoid m

Teres major m

Scapula

Teres minor m

Triceps brachii m, long head

Posterior circumflex humeral a and axillary n

Triceps brachii m and t, long head

OBLIQUE SAGITTAL
Figure 6.2.1

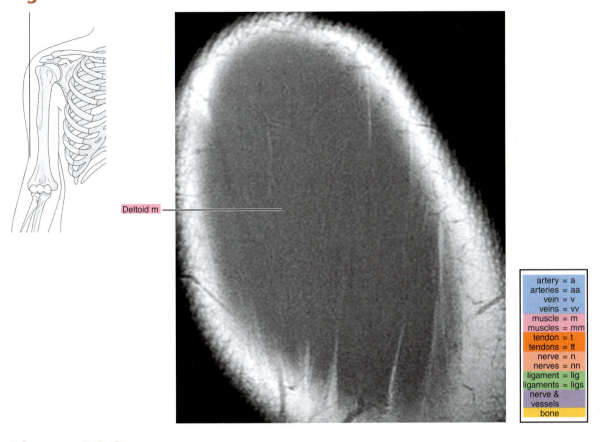

Deltoid m

artery = a	
arteries = aa	
vein = v	
veins = vv	
muscle = m	
muscles = mm	
tendon = t	
tendons = tt	
nerve = n	
nerves = nn	
ligament = lig	
ligaments = ligs	
nerve & vessels	
bone	

Figure 6.2.2

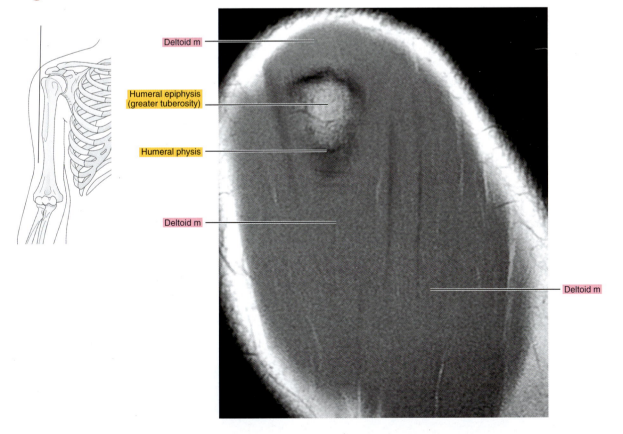

Deltoid m

Humeral epiphysis
(greater tuberosity)

Humeral physis

Deltoid m

Deltoid m

Figure 6.2.3

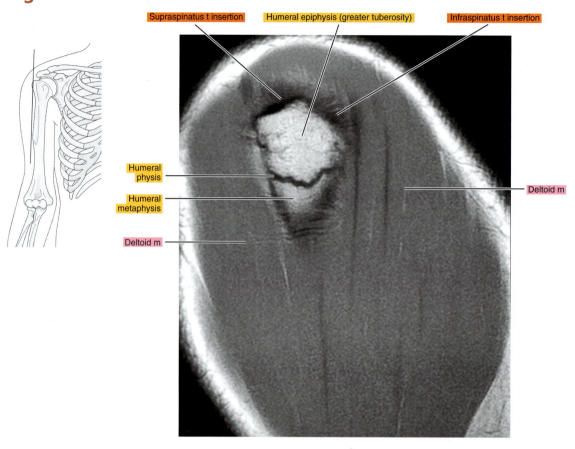

Supraspinatus t insertion | Humeral epiphysis (greater tuberosity) | Infraspinatus t insertion

Humeral physis

Humeral metaphysis

Deltoid m

Deltoid m

Figure 6.2.4

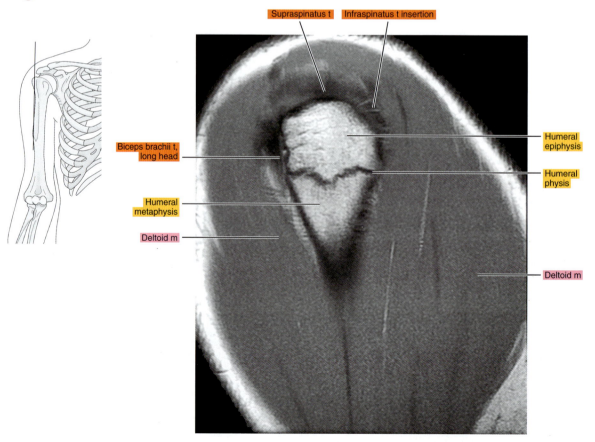

Supraspinatus t | Infraspinatus t insertion

Biceps brachii t, long head

Humeral metaphysis

Deltoid m

Humeral epiphysis

Humeral physis

Deltoid m

Figure 6.2.5

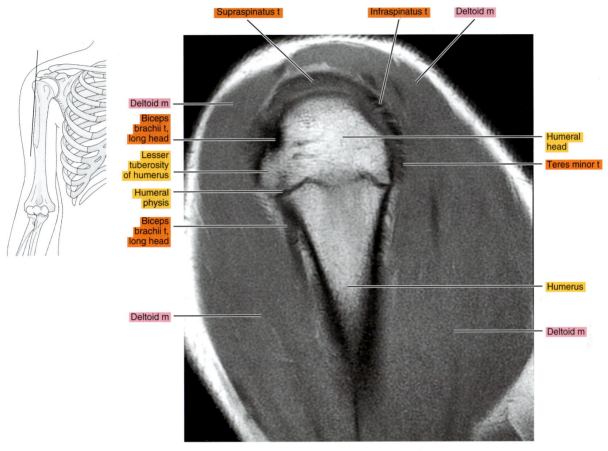

Supraspinatus t — Infraspinatus t — Deltoid m

Deltoid m

Biceps brachii t, long head

Lesser tuberosity of humerus

Humeral physis

Biceps brachii t, long head

Deltoid m

Humeral head

Teres minor t

Humerus

Deltoid m

Figure 6.2.6

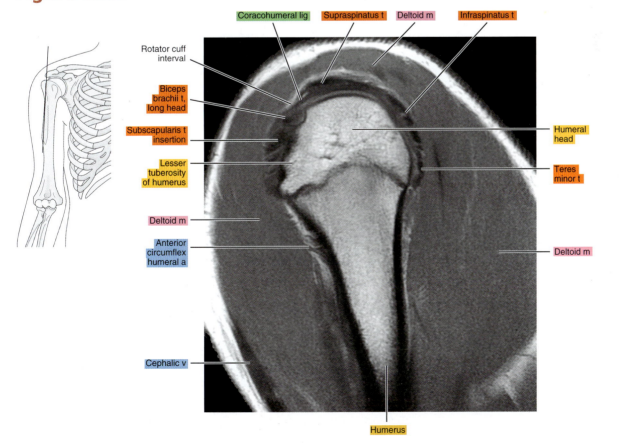

Coracohumeral lig — Supraspinatus t — Deltoid m — Infraspinatus t

Rotator cuff interval

Biceps brachii t, long head

Subscapularis t insertion

Lesser tuberosity of humerus

Deltoid m

Anterior circumflex humeral a

Cephalic v

Humeral head

Teres minor t

Deltoid m

Humerus

Figure 6.2.7

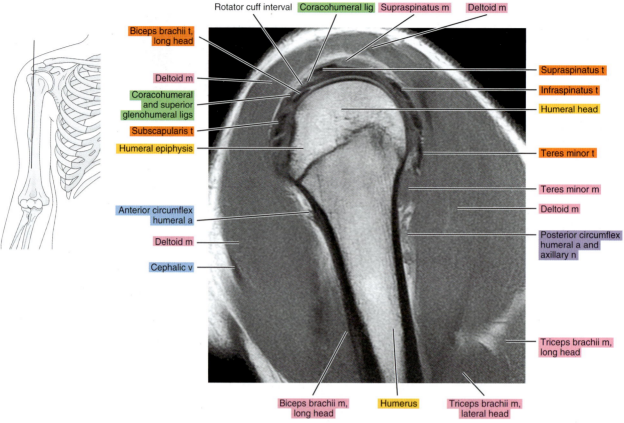

Rotator cuff interval — Coracohumeral lig — Supraspinatus m — Deltoid m

Biceps brachii t, long head

Deltoid m

Coracohumeral and superior glenohumeral ligs

Subscapularis t

Humeral epiphysis

Anterior circumflex humeral a

Deltoid m

Cephalic v

Supraspinatus t

Infraspinatus t

Humeral head

Teres minor t

Teres minor m

Deltoid m

Posterior circumflex humeral a and axillary n

Triceps brachii m, long head

Biceps brachii m, long head — Humerus — Triceps brachii m, lateral head

Figure 6.2.8

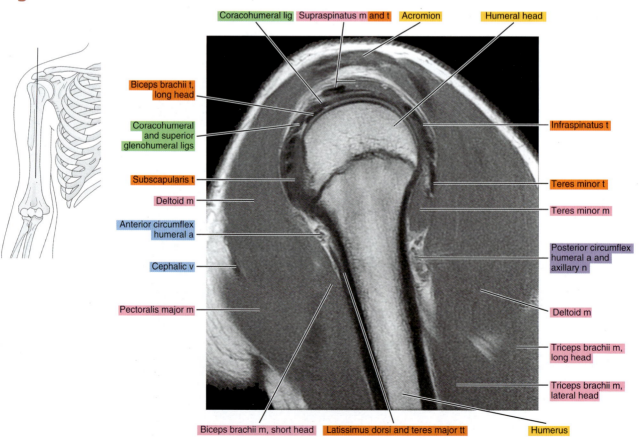

Coracohumeral lig — Supraspinatus m and t — Acromion — Humeral head

Biceps brachii t, long head

Coracohumeral and superior glenohumeral ligs

Subscapularis t

Deltoid m

Anterior circumflex humeral a

Cephalic v

Pectoralis major m

Infraspinatus t

Teres minor t

Teres minor m

Posterior circumflex humeral a and axillary n

Deltoid m

Triceps brachii m, long head

Triceps brachii m, lateral head

Biceps brachii m, short head — Latissimus dorsi and teres major tt — Humerus

Figure 6.2.9

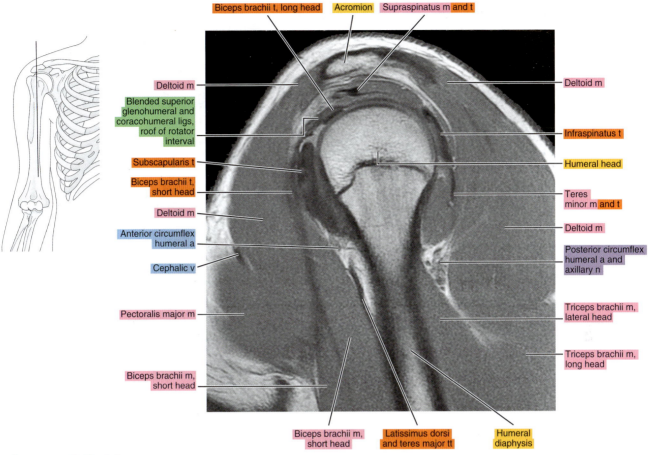

Biceps brachii t, long head — Acromion — Supraspinatus m and t

Deltoid m — Deltoid m

Blended superior glenohumeral and coracohumeral ligs, roof of rotator interval

Infraspinatus t

Subscapularis t — Humeral head

Biceps brachii t, short head — Teres minor m and t

Deltoid m — Deltoid m

Anterior circumflex humeral a — Posterior circumflex humeral a and axillary n

Cephalic v

Pectoralis major m — Triceps brachii m, lateral head

Triceps brachii m, long head

Biceps brachii m, short head

Biceps brachii m, short head — Latissimus dorsi and teres major tt — Humeral diaphysis

Figure 6.2.10

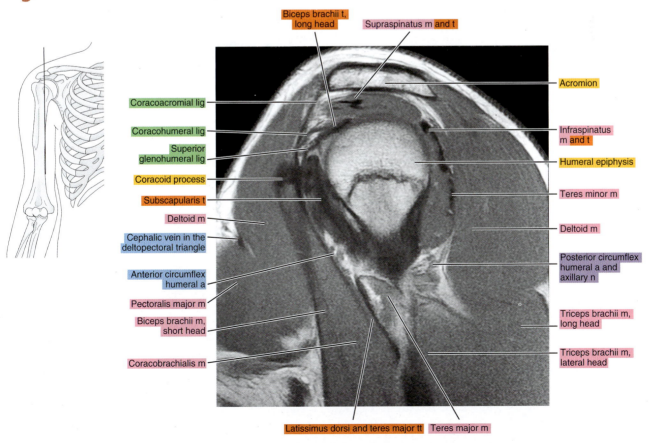

Biceps brachii t, long head — Supraspinatus m and t

Coracoacromial lig — Acromion

Coracohumeral lig — Infraspinatus m and t

Superior glenohumeral lig — Humeral epiphysis

Coracoid process

Subscapularis t — Teres minor m

Deltoid m — Deltoid m

Cephalic vein in the deltopectoral triangle — Posterior circumflex humeral a and axillary n

Anterior circumflex humeral a

Pectoralis major m — Triceps brachii m, long head

Biceps brachii m, short head — Triceps brachii m, lateral head

Coracobrachialis m

Latissimus dorsi and teres major tt — Teres major m

Figure 6.2.11

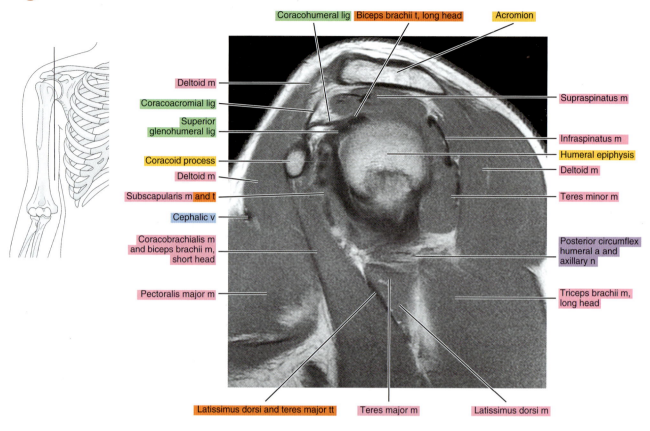

Coracohumeral lig | Biceps brachii t, long head | Acromion

Deltoid m
Coracoacromial lig
Superior glenohumeral lig
Coracoid process
Deltoid m
Subscapularis m and t
Cephalic v
Coracobrachialis m and biceps brachii m, short head
Pectoralis major m

Supraspinatus m
Infraspinatus m
Humeral epiphysis
Deltoid m
Teres minor m
Posterior circumflex humeral a and axillary n
Triceps brachii m, long head

Latissimus dorsi and teres major tt | Teres major m | Latissimus dorsi m

Figure 6.2.12

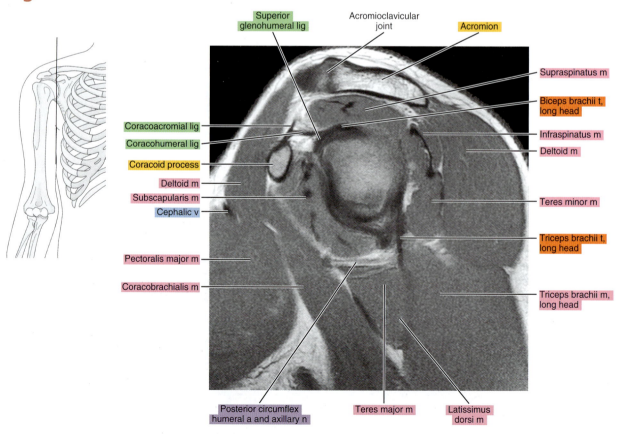

Superior glenohumeral lig | Acromioclavicular joint | Acromion

Coracoacromial lig
Coracohumeral lig
Coracoid process
Deltoid m
Subscapularis m
Cephalic v
Pectoralis major m
Coracobrachialis m

Supraspinatus m
Biceps brachii t, long head
Infraspinatus m
Deltoid m
Teres minor m
Triceps brachii t, long head
Triceps brachii m, long head

Posterior circumflex humeral a and axillary n | Teres major m | Latissimus dorsi m

Figure 6.2.13

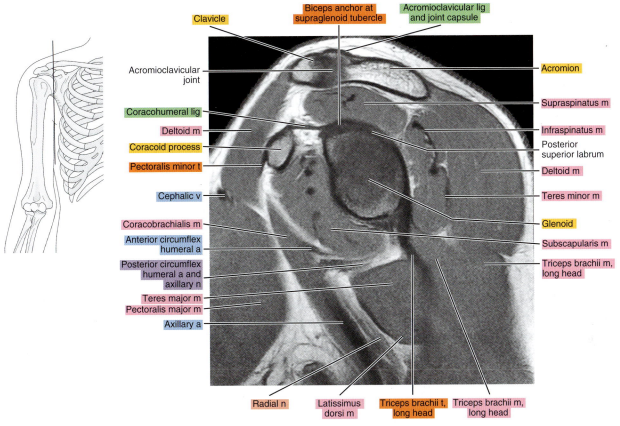

Clavicle
Biceps anchor at supraglenoid tubercle
Acromioclavicular lig and joint capsule
Acromioclavicular joint
Acromion
Coracohumeral lig
Supraspinatus m
Deltoid m
Infraspinatus m
Coracoid process
Posterior superior labrum
Pectoralis minor t
Deltoid m
Cephalic v
Teres minor m
Coracobrachialis m
Glenoid
Anterior circumflex humeral a
Subscapularis m
Posterior circumflex humeral a and axillary n
Triceps brachii m, long head
Teres major m
Pectoralis major m
Axillary a
Radial n
Latissimus dorsi m
Triceps brachii t, long head
Triceps brachii m, long head

Figure 6.2.14

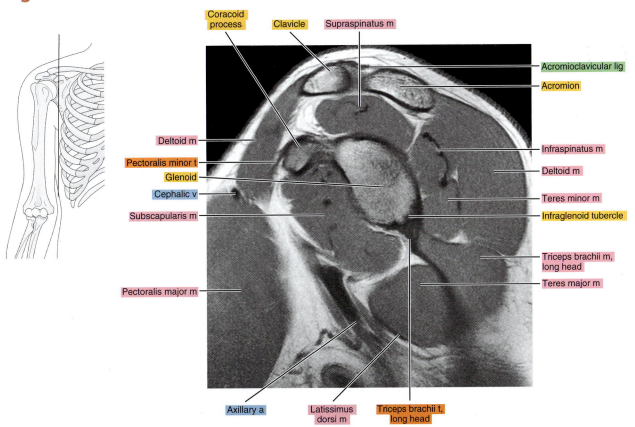

Coracoid process
Clavicle
Supraspinatus m
Acromioclavicular lig
Acromion
Deltoid m
Infraspinatus m
Pectoralis minor t
Deltoid m
Glenoid
Cephalic v
Teres minor m
Subscapularis m
Infraglenoid tubercle
Triceps brachii m, long head
Teres major m
Pectoralis major m
Axillary a
Latissimus dorsi m
Triceps brachii t, long head

Figure 6.2.15

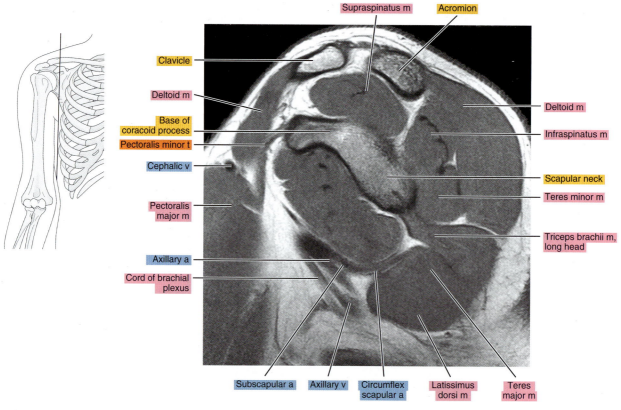

Supraspinatus m
Acromion
Clavicle
Deltoid m
Base of coracoid process
Pectoralis minor t
Cephalic v
Pectoralis major m
Axillary a
Cord of brachial plexus
Deltoid m
Infraspinatus m
Scapular neck
Teres minor m
Triceps brachii m, long head
Subscapular a
Axillary v
Circumflex scapular a
Latissimus dorsi m
Teres major m

Figure 6.2.16

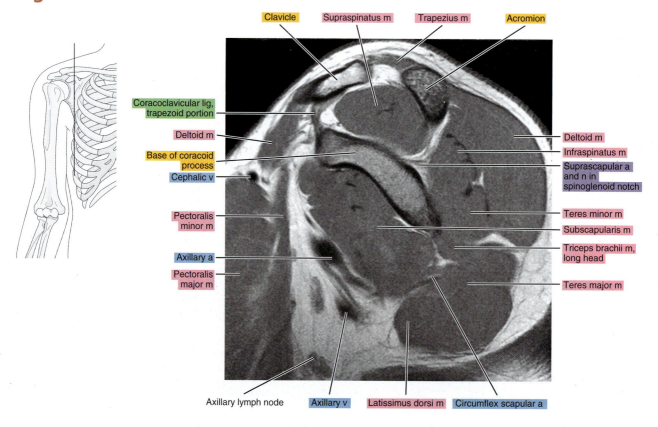

Clavicle
Supraspinatus m
Trapezius m
Acromion
Coracoclavicular lig, trapezoid portion
Deltoid m
Base of coracoid process
Cephalic v
Pectoralis minor m
Axillary a
Pectoralis major m
Deltoid m
Infraspinatus m
Suprascapular a and n in spinoglenoid notch
Teres minor m
Subscapularis m
Triceps brachii m, long head
Teres major m
Axillary lymph node
Axillary v
Latissimus dorsi m
Circumflex scapular a

Figure 6.2.17

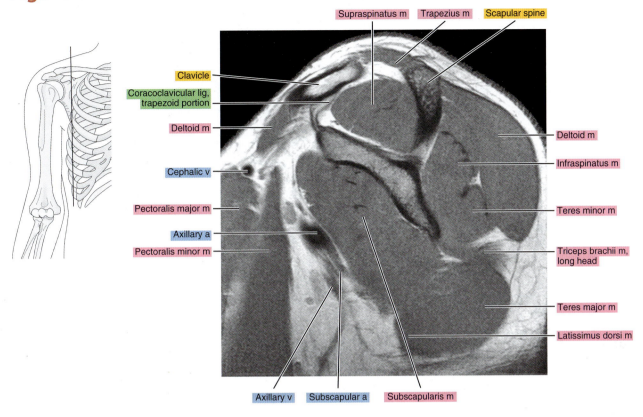

Supraspinatus m   Trapezius m   Scapular spine

Clavicle

Coracoclavicular lig, trapezoid portion

Deltoid m

Cephalic v

Pectoralis major m

Axillary a

Pectoralis minor m

Deltoid m

Infraspinatus m

Teres minor m

Triceps brachii m, long head

Teres major m

Latissimus dorsi m

Axillary v   Subscapular a   Subscapularis m

Figure 6.2.18

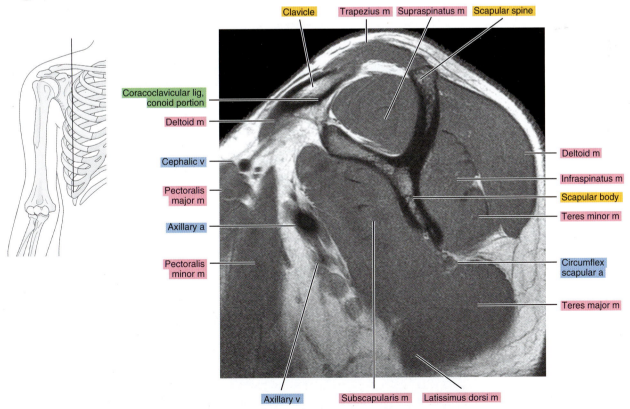

Clavicle   Trapezius m   Supraspinatus m   Scapular spine

Coracoclavicular lig, conoid portion

Deltoid m

Cephalic v

Pectoralis major m

Axillary a

Pectoralis minor m

Deltoid m

Infraspinatus m

Scapular body

Teres minor m

Circumflex scapular a

Teres major m

Axillary v   Subscapularis m   Latissimus dorsi m

Figure 6.2.19

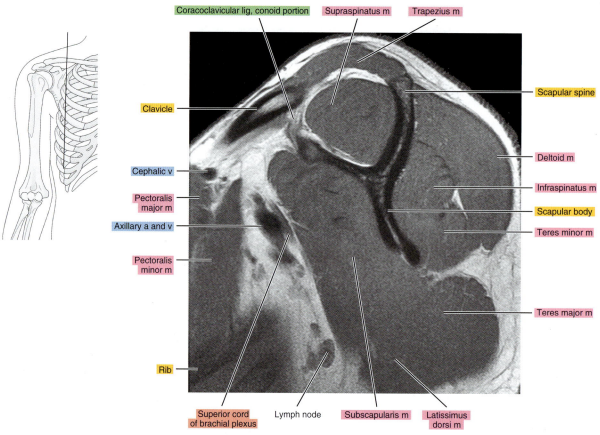

Coracoclavicular lig, conoid portion
Supraspinatus m
Trapezius m
Scapular spine
Clavicle
Deltoid m
Cephalic v
Infraspinatus m
Pectoralis major m
Scapular body
Axillary a and v
Teres minor m
Pectoralis minor m
Teres major m
Rib
Superior cord of brachial plexus
Lymph node
Subscapularis m
Latissimus dorsi m

Figure 6.2.20

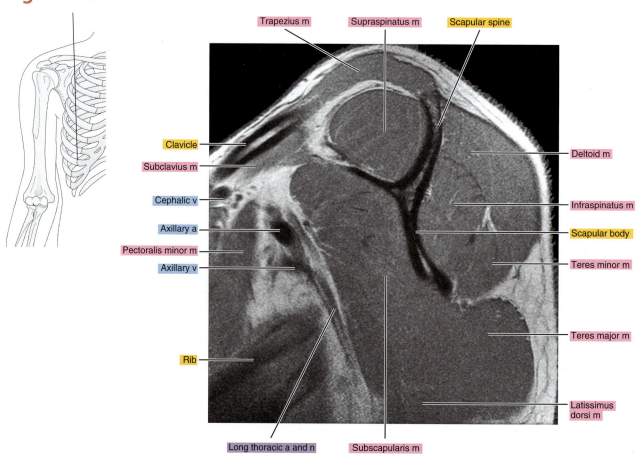

Trapezius m
Supraspinatus m
Scapular spine
Clavicle
Deltoid m
Subclavius m
Cephalic v
Infraspinatus m
Axillary a
Scapular body
Pectoralis minor m
Teres minor m
Axillary v
Rib
Teres major m
Latissimus dorsi m
Long thoracic a and n
Subscapularis m

OBLIQUE CORONAL
Figure 6.3.1

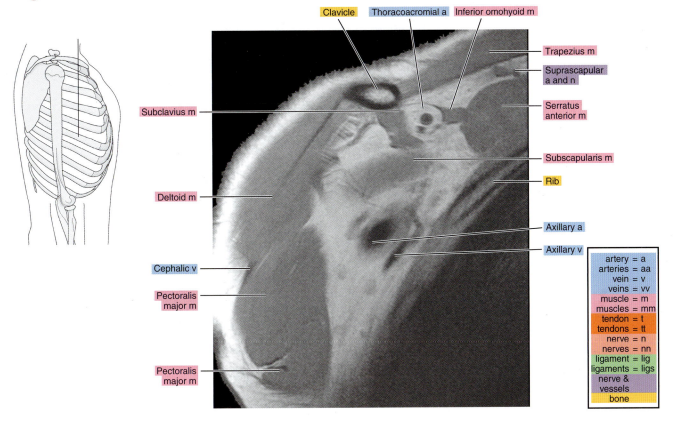

Clavicle — Thoracoacromial a — Inferior omohyoid m

Trapezius m

Suprascapular a and n

Serratus anterior m

Subclavius m

Subscapularis m

Rib

Deltoid m

Axillary a

Axillary v

Cephalic v

Pectoralis major m

Pectoralis major m

| artery = a |
| arteries = aa |
| vein = v |
| veins = vv |
| muscle = m |
| muscles = mm |
| tendon = t |
| tendons = tt |
| nerve = n |
| nerves = nn |
| ligament = lig |
| ligaments = ligs |
| nerve & vessels |
| bone |

Figure 6.3.2

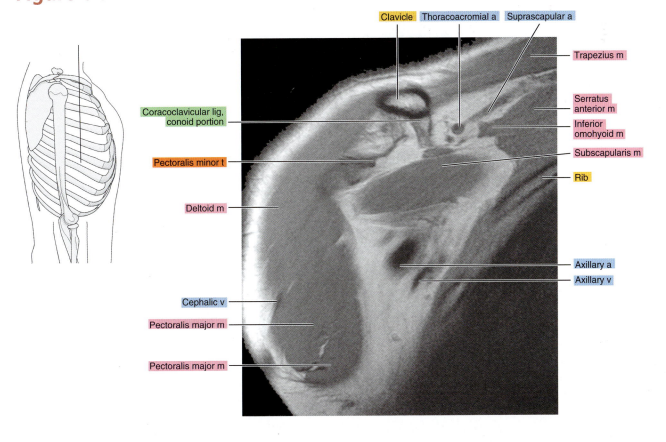

Clavicle — Thoracoacromial a — Suprascapular a

Trapezius m

Serratus anterior m

Inferior omohyoid m

Coracoclavicular lig, conoid portion

Subscapularis m

Pectoralis minor t

Rib

Deltoid m

Axillary a

Axillary v

Cephalic v

Pectoralis major m

Pectoralis major m

Figure 6.3.3

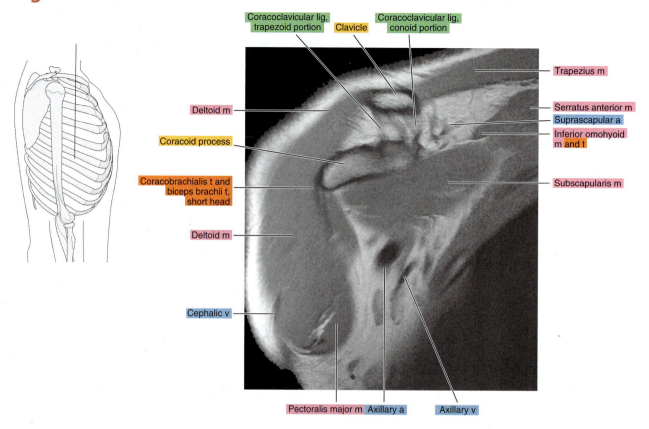

Coracoclavicular lig, trapezoid portion
Clavicle
Coracoclavicular lig, conoid portion
Trapezius m
Deltoid m
Serratus anterior m
Suprascapular a
Coracoid process
Inferior omohyoid m and t
Coracobrachialis t and biceps brachii t, short head
Subscapularis m
Deltoid m
Cephalic v
Pectoralis major m
Axillary a
Axillary v

Figure 6.3.4

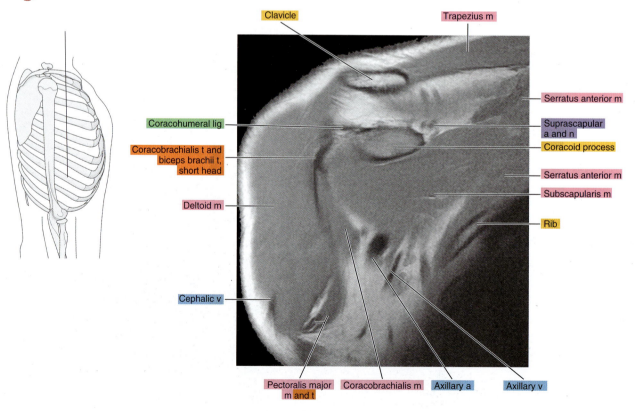

Clavicle
Trapezius m
Serratus anterior m
Coracohumeral lig
Suprascapular a and n
Coracobrachialis t and biceps brachii t, short head
Coracoid process
Serratus anterior m
Subscapularis m
Deltoid m
Rib
Cephalic v
Pectoralis major m and t
Coracobrachialis m
Axillary a
Axillary v

Figure 6.3.5

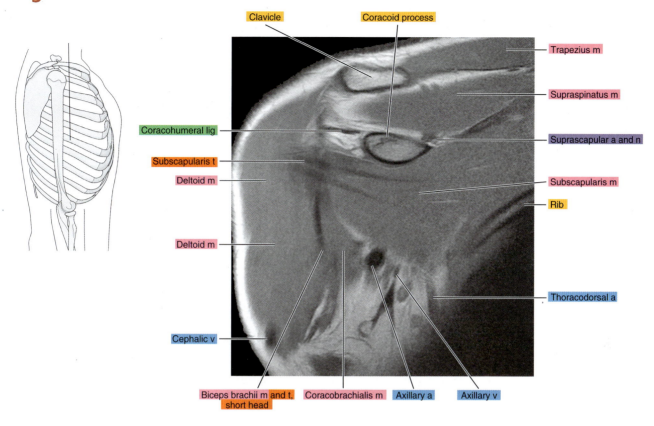

Clavicle

Coracoid process

Trapezius m

Supraspinatus m

Coracohumeral lig

Suprascapular a and n

Subscapularis t

Subscapularis m

Deltoid m

Rib

Deltoid m

Thoracodorsal a

Cephalic v

Biceps brachii m and t, short head

Coracobrachialis m

Axillary a

Axillary v

Figure 6.3.6

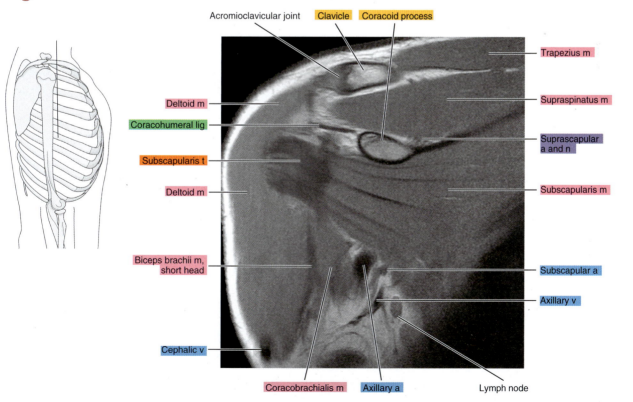

Acromioclavicular joint

Clavicle

Coracoid process

Trapezius m

Deltoid m

Supraspinatus m

Coracohumeral lig

Suprascapular a and n

Subscapularis t

Subscapularis m

Deltoid m

Biceps brachii m, short head

Subscapular a

Axillary v

Cephalic v

Coracobrachialis m

Axillary a

Lymph node

Figure 6.3.7

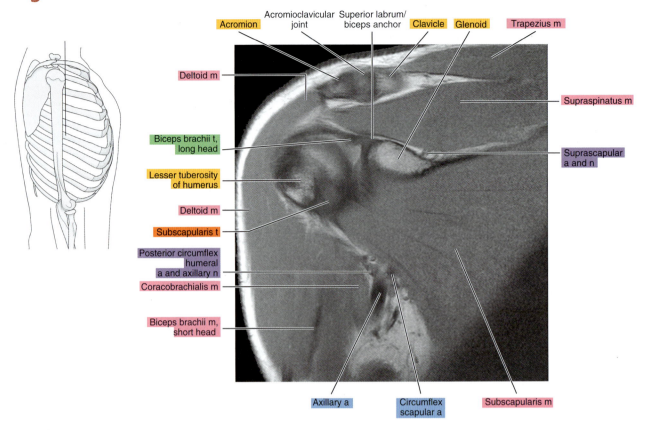

Acromion · Acromioclavicular joint · Superior labrum/biceps anchor · Clavicle · Glenoid · Trapezius m · Deltoid m · Supraspinatus m · Biceps brachii t, long head · Suprascapular a and n · Lesser tuberosity of humerus · Deltoid m · Subscapularis t · Posterior circumflex humeral a and axillary n · Coracobrachialis m · Biceps brachii m, short head · Axillary a · Circumflex scapular a · Subscapularis m

Figure 6.3.8

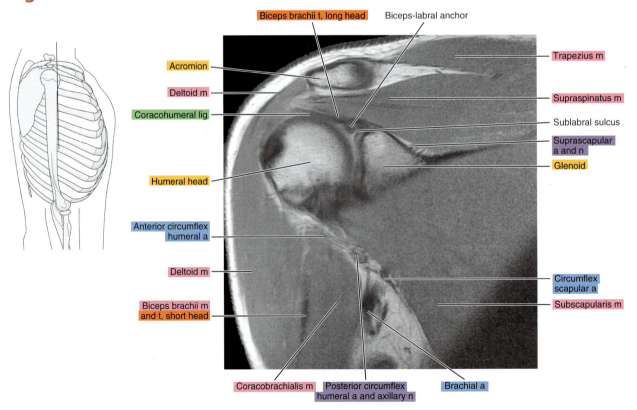

Biceps brachii t, long head · Biceps-labral anchor · Acromion · Trapezius m · Deltoid m · Supraspinatus m · Coracohumeral lig · Sublabral sulcus · Suprascapular a and n · Humeral head · Glenoid · Anterior circumflex humeral a · Deltoid m · Circumflex scapular a · Biceps brachii m and t, short head · Subscapularis m · Coracobrachialis m · Posterior circumflex humeral a and axillary n · Brachial a

Figure 6.3.9

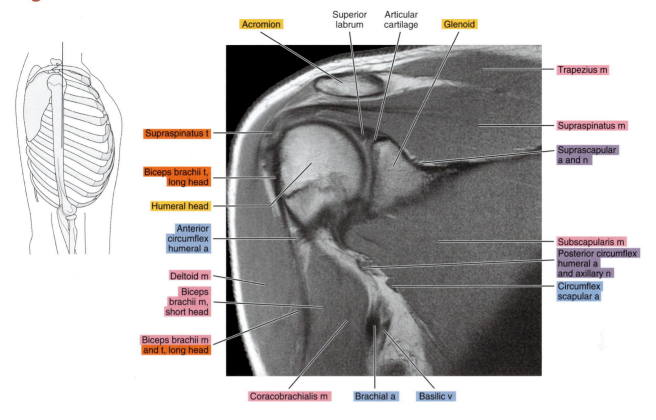

Figure 6.3.10

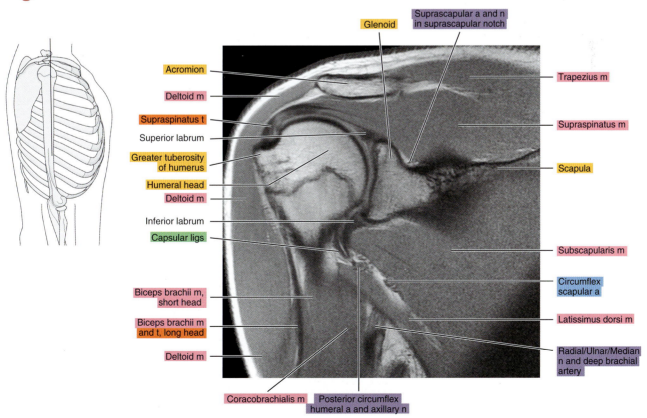

Figure 6.3.11

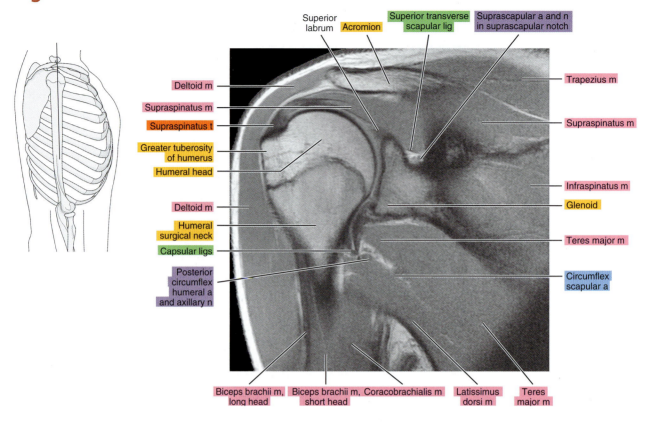

Superior labrum | Acromion | Superior transverse scapular lig | Suprascapular a and n in suprascapular notch

Deltoid m
Supraspinatus m
Supraspinatus t
Greater tuberosity of humerus
Humeral head
Deltoid m
Humeral surgical neck
Capsular ligs
Posterior circumflex humeral a and axillary n

Trapezius m
Supraspinatus m
Infraspinatus m
Glenoid
Teres major m
Circumflex scapular a

Biceps brachii m, long head | Biceps brachii m, short head | Coracobrachialis m | Latissimus dorsi m | Teres major m

Figure 6.3.12

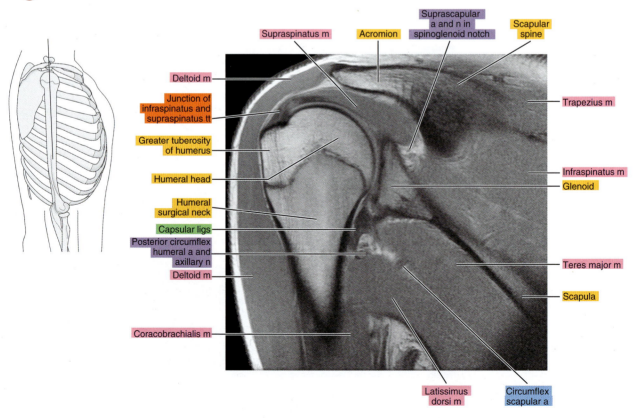

Supraspinatus m | Acromion | Suprascapular a and n in spinoglenoid notch | Scapular spine

Deltoid m
Junction of infraspinatus and supraspinatus tt
Greater tuberosity of humerus
Humeral head
Humeral surgical neck
Capsular ligs
Posterior circumflex humeral a and axillary n
Deltoid m
Coracobrachialis m

Trapezius m
Infraspinatus m
Glenoid
Teres major m
Scapula

Latissimus dorsi m | Circumflex scapular a

Figure 6.3.13

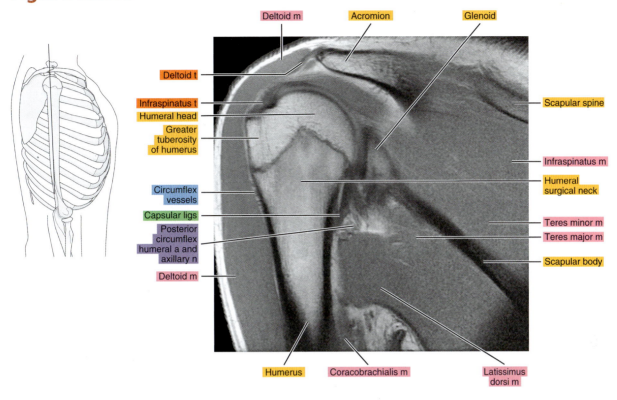

Figure 6.3.14

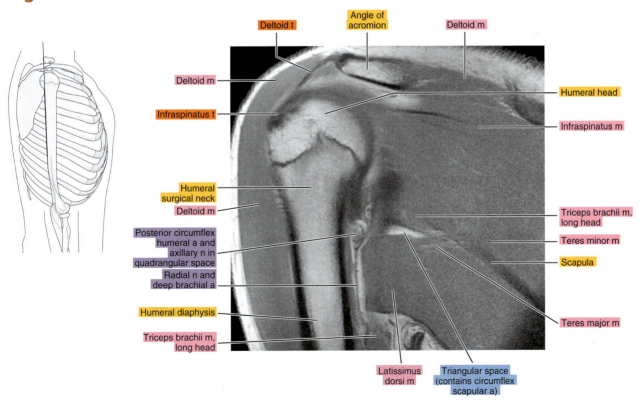

Figure 6.3.15

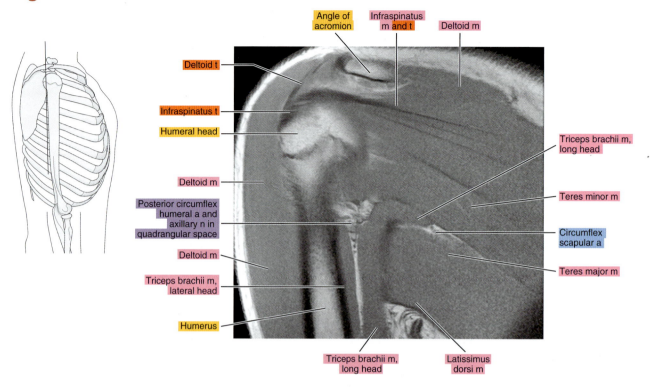

Angle of acromion
Infraspinatus m and t
Deltoid m
Deltoid t
Infraspinatus t
Humeral head
Triceps brachii m, long head
Teres minor m
Deltoid m
Posterior circumflex humeral a and axillary n in quadrangular space
Circumflex scapular a
Deltoid m
Teres major m
Triceps brachii m, lateral head
Humerus
Triceps brachii m, long head
Latissimus dorsi m

Figure 6.3.16

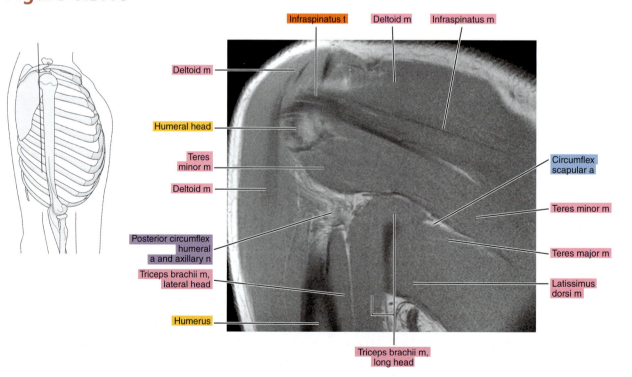

Infraspinatus t
Deltoid m
Infraspinatus m
Deltoid m
Humeral head
Teres minor m
Circumflex scapular a
Deltoid m
Teres minor m
Posterior circumflex humeral a and axillary n
Teres major m
Triceps brachii m, lateral head
Latissimus dorsi m
Humerus
Triceps brachii m, long head

Figure 6.3.17

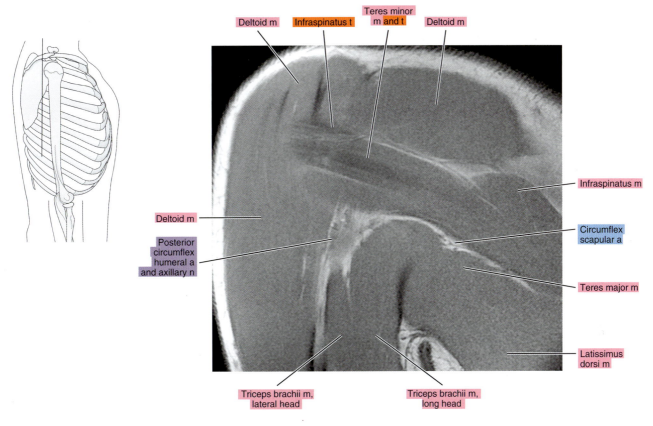

Deltoid m

Infraspinatus t

Teres minor m and t

Deltoid m

Infraspinatus m

Deltoid m

Circumflex scapular a

Posterior circumflex humeral a and axillary n

Teres major m

Latissimus dorsi m

Triceps brachii m, lateral head

Triceps brachii m, long head

Figure 6.3.18

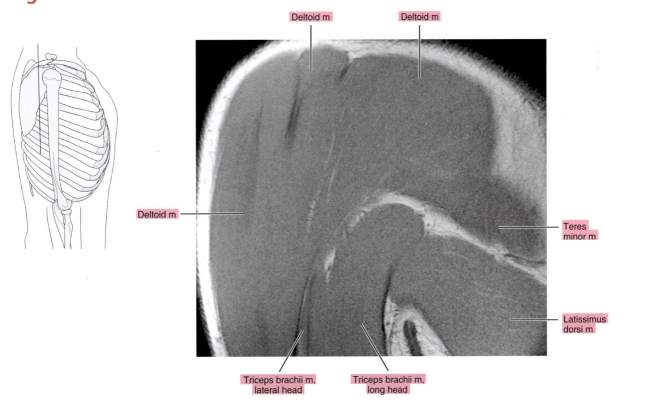

Deltoid m

Deltoid m

Deltoid m

Teres minor m

Latissimus dorsi m

Triceps brachii m, lateral head

Triceps brachii m, long head

Figure 6.3.19

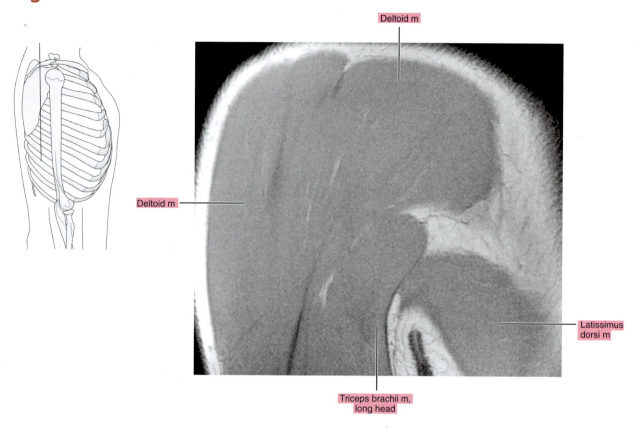

Deltoid m

Deltoid m

Latissimus dorsi m

Triceps brachii m, long head

Figure 6.3.20

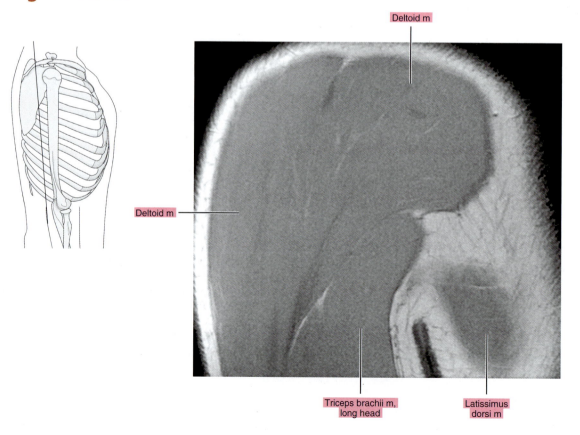

Deltoid m

Deltoid m

Triceps brachii m, long head

Latissimus dorsi m

Table 6-1. Muscles of the Shoulder

MUSCLE	ORIGIN	INSERTION	NERVE SUPPLY
Pectoralis major	Medial half of the anterior surface of the clavicle, side and front of the sternum as far as the sixth costal cartilage, front and surfaces of the cartilage of the second through sixth ribs, osseous ends of the sixth and seventh ribs, and aponeurosis of external abdominal oblique	Crest of the greater tubercle of the humerus, lateral lip of the intertubercular groove, deltoid tubercle, and fibrous periosteum of the intertubercular sulcus.	Lateral and medial pectoral (C5 and C6 for the clavicular part and C7, C8, and T1 for the sternocostal part)
Pectoralis minor	Aponeurotic slips from the second through fifth ribs, near costal cartilages	Anterior half of the medial border and upper surface of the coracoid process of the scapula.	Medial and lateral pectoral (C6, C7, and C8)
Subclavius	First rib and its cartilage	Inferior surface of the clavicle between the costal and coracoid tuberosities.	Nerve to subclavian (C5 or C5 and C6)
Deltoid	Lateral border and upper surface of the lateral third of the clavicle, the acromion, and the scapular spine	Deltoid tuberosity of the humerus.	Axillary (C5, C6)
Supraspinatus	Supraspinous fossa and investing fascia	Shoulder capsule and superior facet of the greater tubercle of the humerus.	Suprascapular (C4, C5, and C6)
Infraspinatus	Infraspinous fossa, scapular spine, investing (deep) fascia, and adjacent aponeurotic septa	Shoulder capsule and middle facet of the greater tubercle of the humerus.	Suprascapular (C4, C5, and C6)
Teres minor	Upper two-thirds of the axillary border of the scapula	Shoulder capsule and inferior facet of the greater tubercle of the humerus.	Axillary (C4, C5, and C6)
Subscapularis	Subscapularis fossa	Shoulder capsule and lesser tubercle of the humerus and its shaft immediately below the tubercle.	Two or three subscapular branches from the posterior cord and upper and lower subscapular (C5, C6, and C7)
Teres major	Inferior angle of the scapula	Medial lip of the intertubercular groove of the humerus.	Lower subscapular (C6 and C7)
Latissimus dorsi	Spine and interspinous ligaments of the lower five or six thoracic vertebrae, upper lumbar vertebrae, thoracodorsal fascia, posterior third of the crest of the ilium, and the lateral surface and upper edge of the lower three or four ribs	Muscle tendon inserts onto the ventral side of the lesser tubercle of the humerus and onto the floor of the intertubercular groove ventral to the tendon of the teres major. The tendon may extend to the greater tubercle of the humerus.	Thoracodorsal (C6, C7, and C8)

MR Arthrography of the Shoulder

AXIAL
Figure 7.1.1

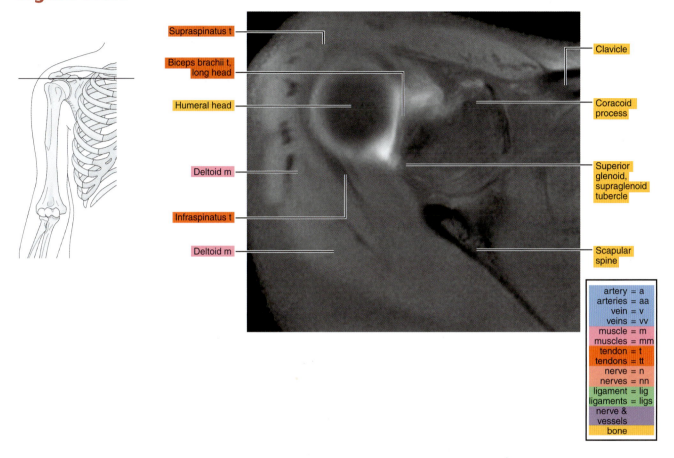

- Supraspinatus t
- Biceps brachii t, long head
- Humeral head
- Deltoid m
- Infraspinatus t
- Deltoid m
- Clavicle
- Coracoid process
- Superior glenoid, supraglenoid tubercle
- Scapular spine

artery = a	
arteries = aa	
vein = v	
veins = vv	
muscle = m	
muscles = mm	
tendon = t	
tendons = tt	
nerve = n	
nerves = nn	
ligament = lig	
ligaments = ligs	
nerve & vessels	
bone	

Figure 7.1.2

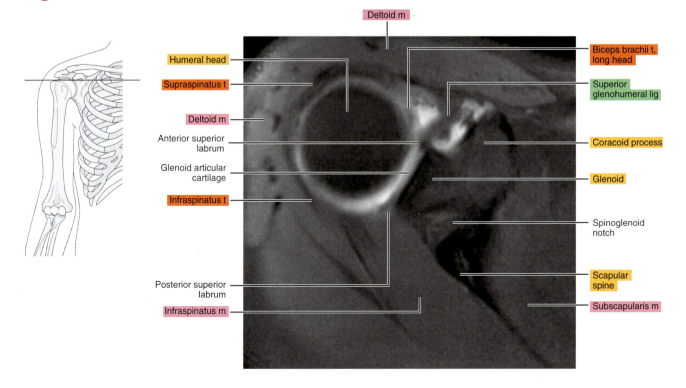

- Deltoid m
- Humeral head
- Supraspinatus t
- Deltoid m
- Anterior superior labrum
- Glenoid articular cartilage
- Infraspinatus t
- Posterior superior labrum
- Infraspinatus m
- Biceps brachii t, long head
- Superior glenohumeral lig
- Coracoid process
- Glenoid
- Spinoglenoid notch
- Scapular spine
- Subscapularis m

Figure 7.1.3

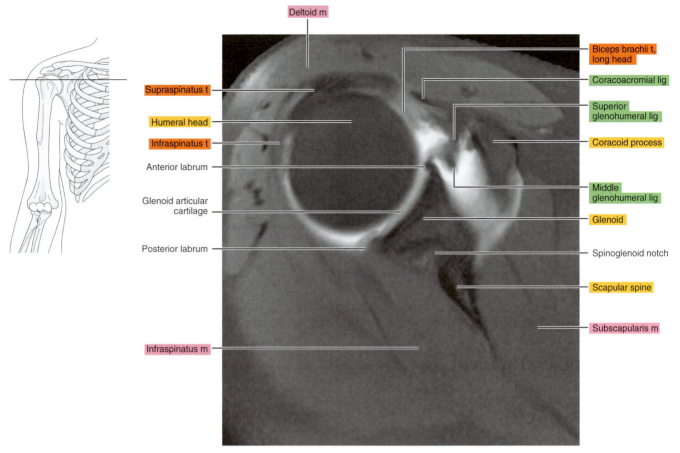

Deltoid m
Biceps brachii t, long head
Coracoacromial lig
Supraspinatus t
Superior glenohumeral lig
Humeral head
Coracoid process
Infraspinatus t
Anterior labrum
Middle glenohumeral lig
Glenoid articular cartilage
Glenoid
Posterior labrum
Spinoglenoid notch
Scapular spine
Subscapularis m
Infraspinatus m

Figure 7.1.4

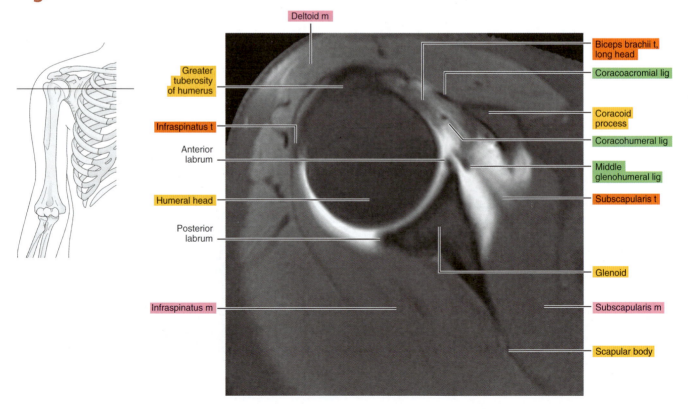

Deltoid m
Biceps brachii t, long head
Coracoacromial lig
Greater tuberosity of humerus
Coracoid process
Infraspinatus t
Coracohumeral lig
Anterior labrum
Middle glenohumeral lig
Humeral head
Subscapularis t
Posterior labrum
Glenoid
Infraspinatus m
Subscapularis m
Scapular body

Figure 7.1.5

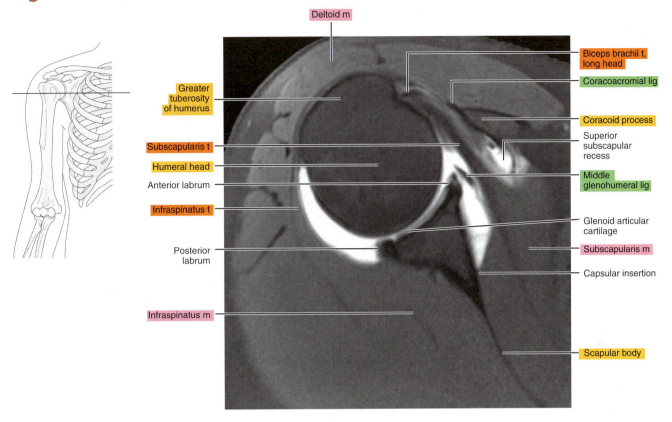

Deltoid m

Biceps brachii t, long head

Coracoacromial lig

Greater tuberosity of humerus

Coracoid process

Superior subscapular recess

Subscapularis t

Humeral head

Middle glenohumeral lig

Anterior labrum

Infraspinatus t

Glenoid articular cartilage

Subscapularis m

Posterior labrum

Capsular insertion

Infraspinatus m

Scapular body

Figure 7.1.6

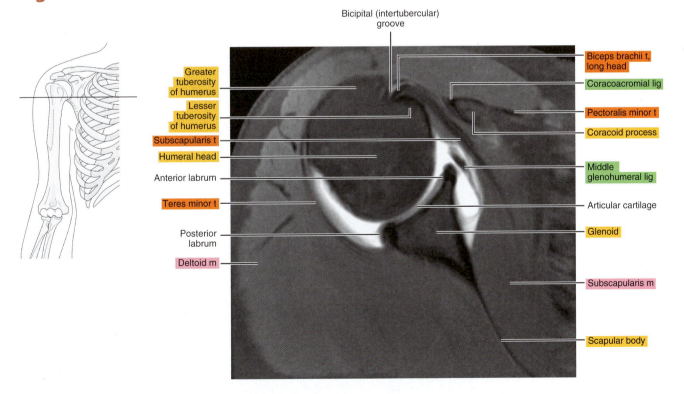

Bicipital (intertubercular) groove

Biceps brachii t, long head

Greater tuberosity of humerus

Coracoacromial lig

Lesser tuberosity of humerus

Pectoralis minor t

Subscapularis t

Coracoid process

Humeral head

Anterior labrum

Middle glenohumeral lig

Teres minor t

Articular cartilage

Posterior labrum

Glenoid

Deltoid m

Subscapularis m

Scapular body

Figure 7.1.7

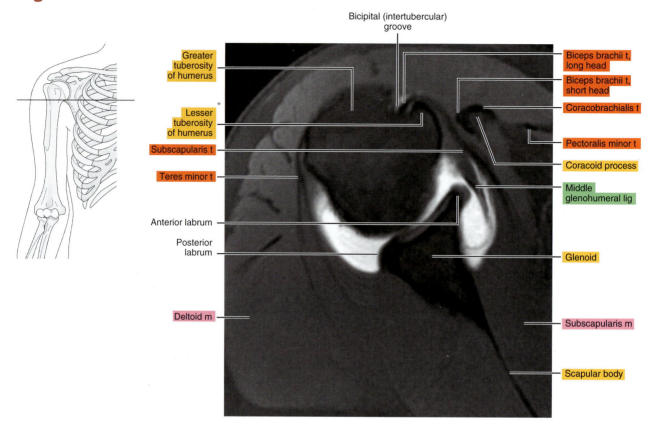

Greater tuberosity of humerus

Lesser tuberosity of humerus

Subscapularis t

Teres minor t

Anterior labrum

Posterior labrum

Deltoid m

Bicipital (intertubercular) groove

Biceps brachii t, long head

Biceps brachii t, short head

Coracobrachialis t

Pectoralis minor t

Coracoid process

Middle glenohumeral lig

Glenoid

Subscapularis m

Scapular body

Figure 7.1.8

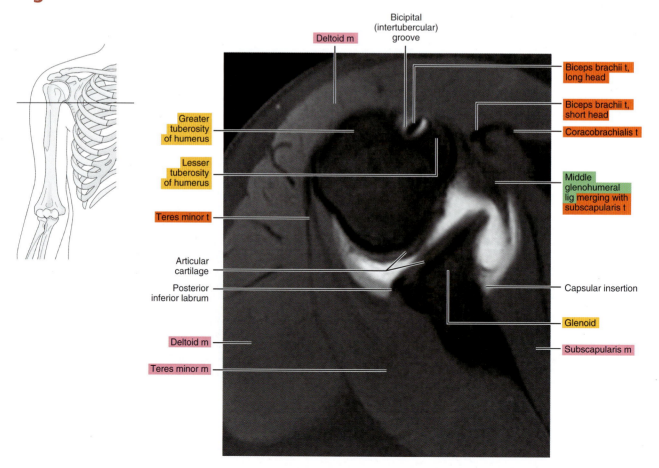

Deltoid m

Bicipital (intertubercular) groove

Greater tuberosity of humerus

Lesser tuberosity of humerus

Teres minor t

Articular cartilage

Posterior inferior labrum

Deltoid m

Teres minor m

Biceps brachii t, long head

Biceps brachii t, short head

Coracobrachialis t

Middle glenohumeral lig merging with subscapularis t

Capsular insertion

Glenoid

Subscapularis m

Figure 7.1.9

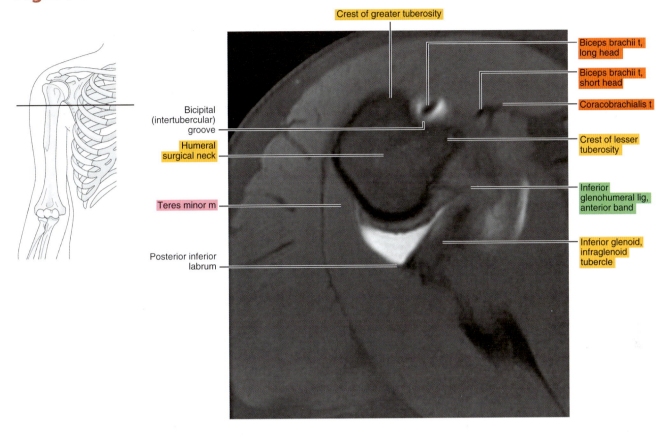

Crest of greater tuberosity

Biceps brachii t, long head

Biceps brachii t, short head

Coracobrachialis t

Bicipital (intertubercular) groove

Crest of lesser tuberosity

Humeral surgical neck

Inferior glenohumeral lig, anterior band

Teres minor m

Inferior glenoid, infraglenoid tubercle

Posterior inferior labrum

Figure 7.1.10

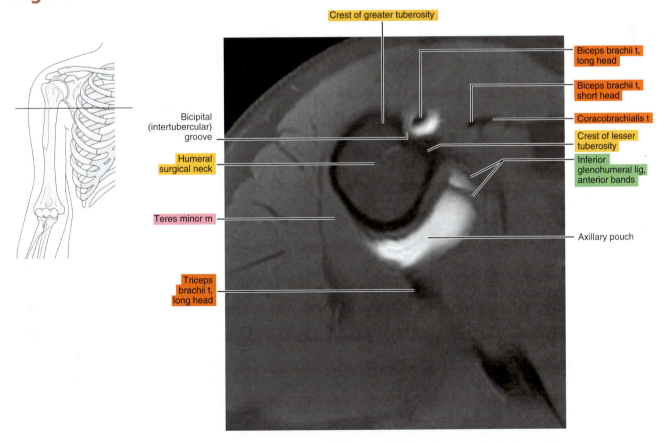

Crest of greater tuberosity

Biceps brachii t, long head

Biceps brachii t, short head

Coracobrachialis t

Bicipital (intertubercular) groove

Crest of lesser tuberosity

Humeral surgical neck

Inferior glenohumeral lig, anterior bands

Teres minor m

Axillary pouch

Triceps brachii t, long head

OBLIQUE SAGITTAL
Figure 7.2.1

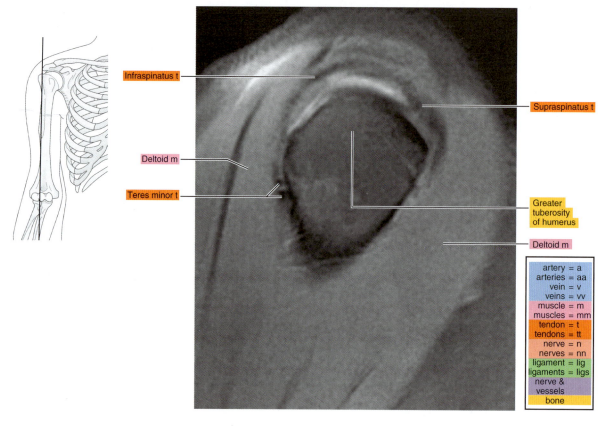

Infraspinatus t

Deltoid m

Teres minor t

Supraspinatus t

Greater tuberosity of humerus

Deltoid m

artery	= a
arteries	= aa
vein	= v
veins	= vv
muscle	= m
muscles	= mm
tendon	= t
tendons	= tt
nerve	= n
nerves	= nn
ligament	= lig
ligaments	= ligs
nerve & vessels	
bone	

Figure 7.2.2

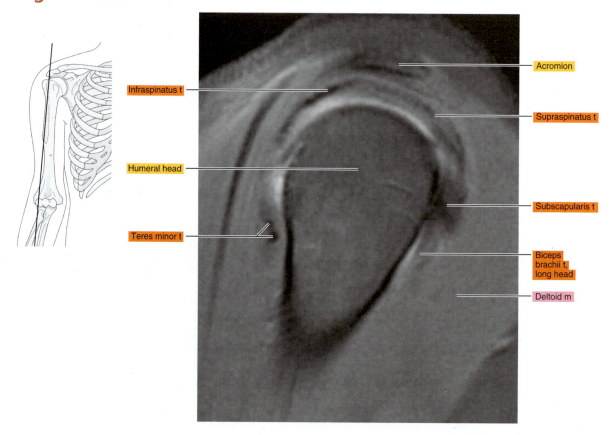

Infraspinatus t

Humeral head

Teres minor t

Acromion

Supraspinatus t

Subscapularis t

Biceps brachii t, long head

Deltoid m

Figure 7.2.3

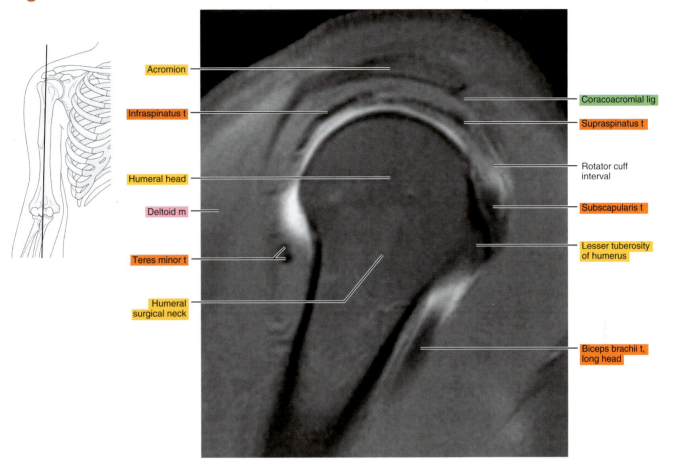

Acromion
Infraspinatus t
Humeral head
Deltoid m
Teres minor t
Humeral surgical neck
Coracoacromial lig
Supraspinatus t
Rotator cuff interval
Subscapularis t
Lesser tuberosity of humerus
Biceps brachii t, long head

Figure 7.2.4

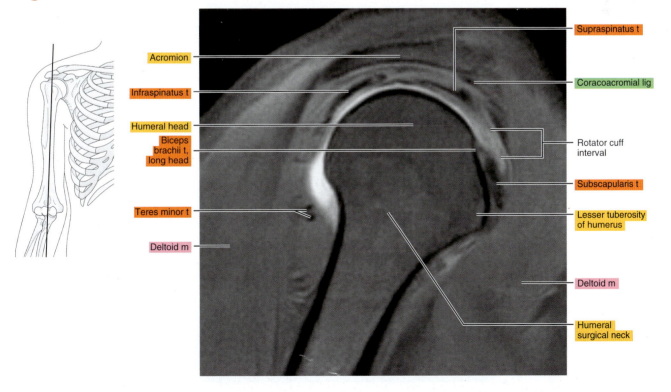

Acromion
Infraspinatus t
Humeral head
Biceps brachii t, long head
Teres minor t
Deltoid m
Supraspinatus t
Coracoacromial lig
Rotator cuff interval
Subscapularis t
Lesser tuberosity of humerus
Deltoid m
Humeral surgical neck

Figure 7.2.5

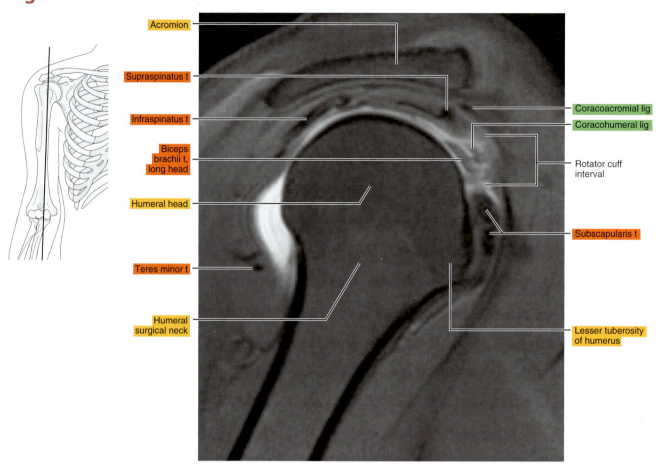

Acromion

Supraspinatus t

Infraspinatus t

Biceps brachii t, long head

Humeral head

Teres minor t

Humeral surgical neck

Coracoacromial lig

Coracohumeral lig

Rotator cuff interval

Subscapularis t

Lesser tuberosity of humerus

Figure 7.2.6

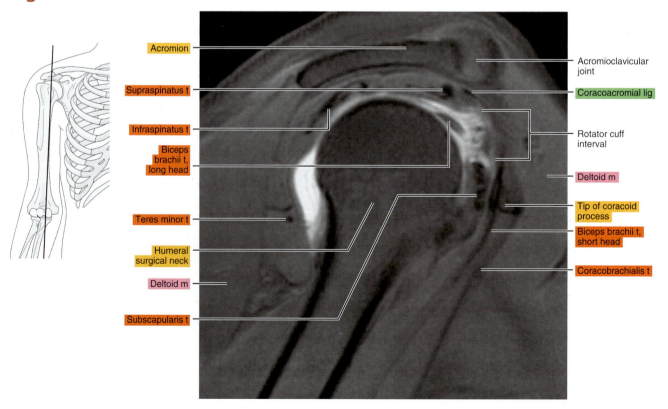

Acromion

Supraspinatus t

Infraspinatus t

Biceps brachii t, long head

Teres minor t

Humeral surgical neck

Deltoid m

Subscapularis t

Acromioclavicular joint

Coracoacromial lig

Rotator cuff interval

Deltoid m

Tip of coracoid process

Biceps brachii t, short head

Coracobrachialis t

Figure 7.2.7

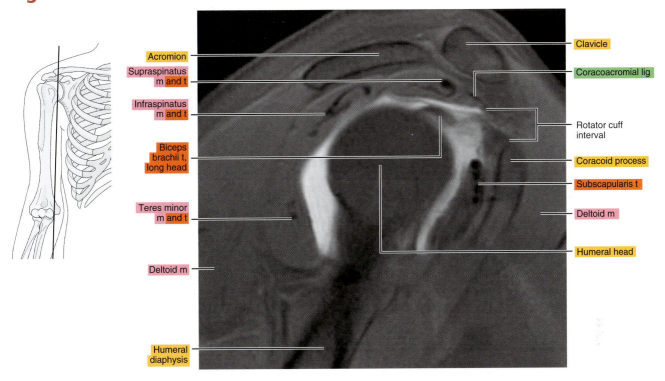

Acromion

Supraspinatus m and t

Infraspinatus m and t

Biceps brachii t, long head

Teres minor m and t

Deltoid m

Humeral diaphysis

Clavicle

Coracoacromial lig

Rotator cuff interval

Coracoid process

Subscapularis t

Deltoid m

Humeral head

Figure 7.2.8

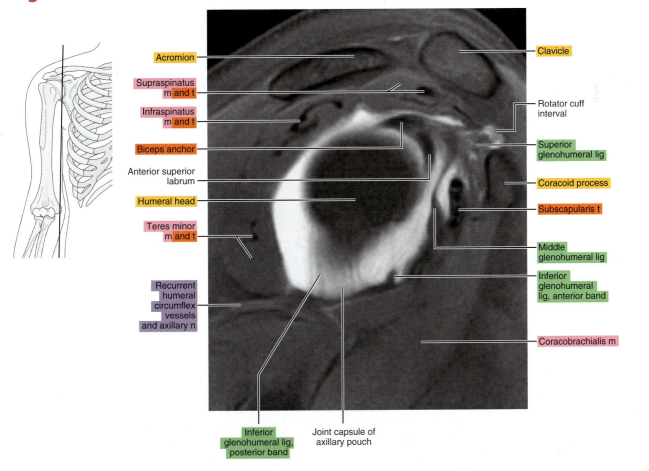

Acromion

Supraspinatus m and t

Infraspinatus m and t

Biceps anchor

Anterior superior labrum

Humeral head

Teres minor m and t

Recurrent humeral circumflex vessels and axillary n

Clavicle

Rotator cuff interval

Superior glenohumeral lig

Coracoid process

Subscapularis t

Middle glenohumeral lig

Inferior glenohumeral lig, anterior band

Coracobrachialis m

Inferior glenohumeral lig, posterior band

Joint capsule of axillary pouch

Figure 7.2.9

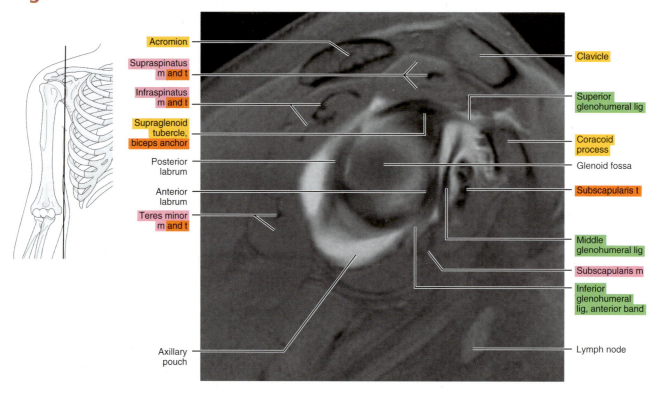

Acromion

Supraspinatus m and t

Infraspinatus m and t

Supraglenoid tubercle, biceps anchor

Posterior labrum

Anterior labrum

Teres minor m and t

Axillary pouch

Clavicle

Superior glenohumeral lig

Coracoid process

Glenoid fossa

Subscapularis t

Middle glenohumeral lig

Subscapularis m

Inferior glenohumeral lig, anterior band

Lymph node

Figure 7.2.10

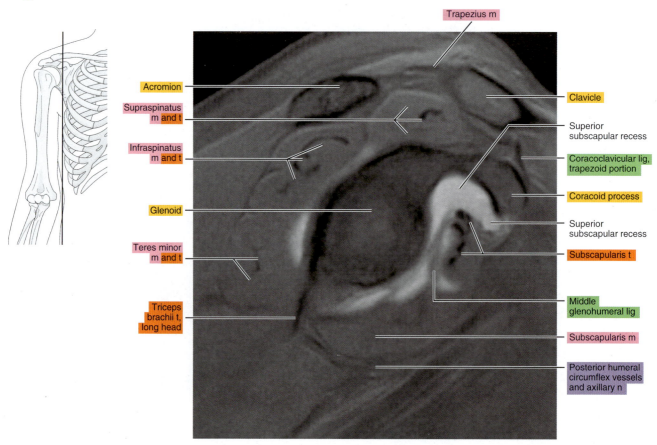

Trapezius m

Acromion

Supraspinatus m and t

Infraspinatus m and t

Glenoid

Teres minor m and t

Triceps brachii t, long head

Clavicle

Superior subscapular recess

Coracoclavicular lig, trapezoid portion

Coracoid process

Superior subscapular recess

Subscapularis t

Middle glenohumeral lig

Subscapularis m

Posterior humeral circumflex vessels and axillary n

Figure 7.2.11

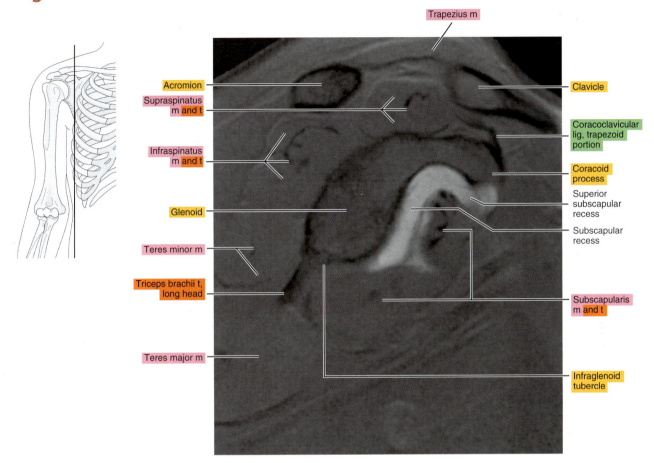

Trapezius m

Acromion

Supraspinatus
m and t

Infraspinatus
m and t

Glenoid

Teres minor m

Triceps brachii t,
long head

Teres major m

Clavicle

Coracoclavicular
lig, trapezoid
portion

Coracoid
process

Superior
subscapular
recess

Subscapular
recess

Subscapularis
m and t

Infraglenoid
tubercle

OBLIQUE CORONAL
Figure 7.3.1

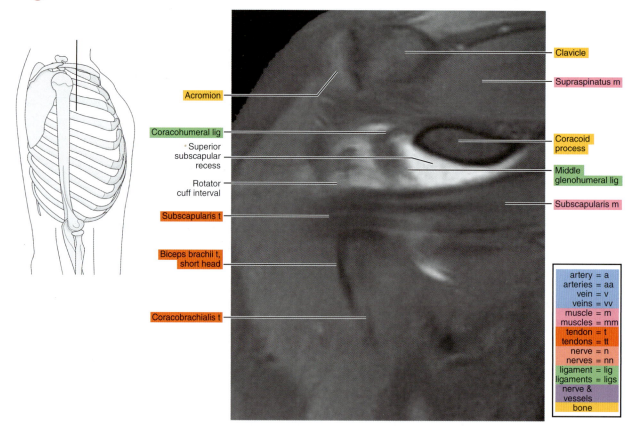

Acromion

Coracohumeral lig

• Superior subscapular recess

Rotator cuff interval

Subscapularis t

Biceps brachii t, short head

Coracobrachialis t

Clavicle

Supraspinatus m

Coracoid process

Middle glenohumeral lig

Subscapularis m

artery = a
arteries = aa
vein = v
veins = vv
muscle = m
muscles = mm
tendon = t
tendons = tt
nerve = n
nerves = nn
ligament = lig
ligaments = ligs
nerve & vessels
bone

Figure 7.3.2

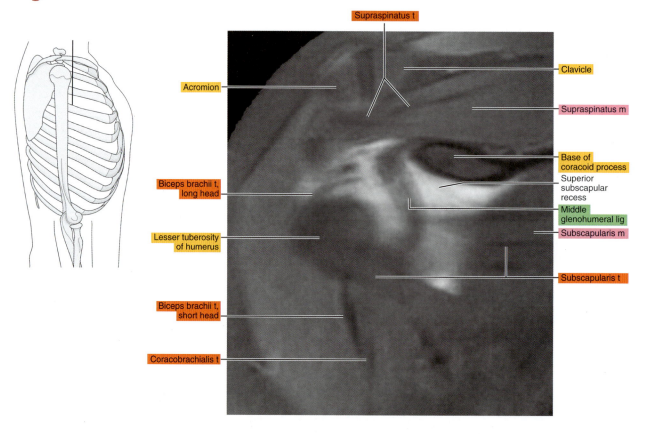

Supraspinatus t

Acromion

Biceps brachii t, long head

Lesser tuberosity of humerus

Biceps brachii t, short head

Coracobrachialis t

Clavicle

Supraspinatus m

Base of coracoid process

Superior subscapular recess

Middle glenohumeral lig

Subscapularis m

Subscapularis t

Figure 7.3.3

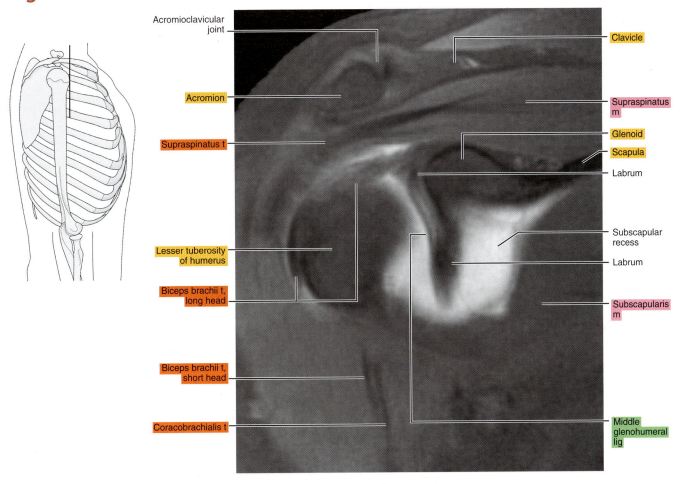

Acromioclavicular joint

Clavicle

Acromion

Supraspinatus m

Supraspinatus t

Glenoid

Scapula

Labrum

Subscapular recess

Labrum

Lesser tuberosity of humerus

Biceps brachii t, long head

Subscapularis m

Biceps brachii t, short head

Coracobrachialis t

Middle glenohumeral lig

Figure 7.3.4

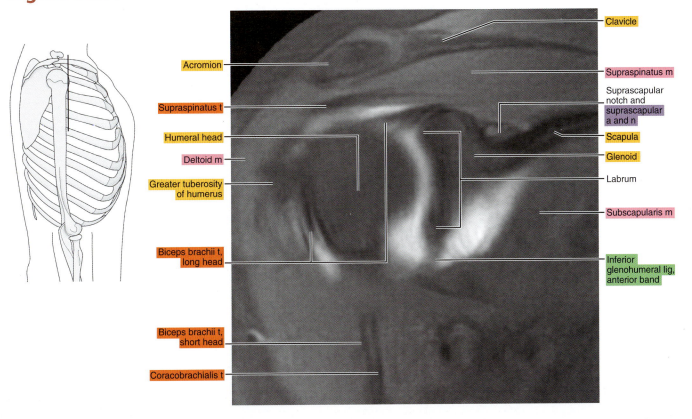

Clavicle

Acromion

Supraspinatus m

Supraspinatus t

Suprascapular notch and suprascapular a and n

Humeral head

Scapula

Deltoid m

Glenoid

Greater tuberosity of humerus

Labrum

Subscapularis m

Biceps brachii t, long head

Inferior glenohumeral lig, anterior band

Biceps brachii t, short head

Coracobrachialis t

Figure 7.3.5

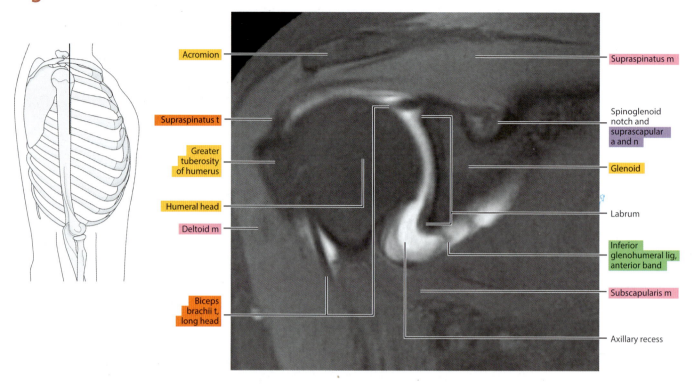

Acromion

Supraspinatus t

Greater tuberosity of humerus

Humeral head

Deltoid m

Biceps brachii t, long head

Supraspinatus m

Spinoglenoid notch and suprascapular a and n

Glenoid

Labrum

Inferior glenohumeral lig, anterior band

Subscapularis m

Axillary recess

Figure 7.3.6

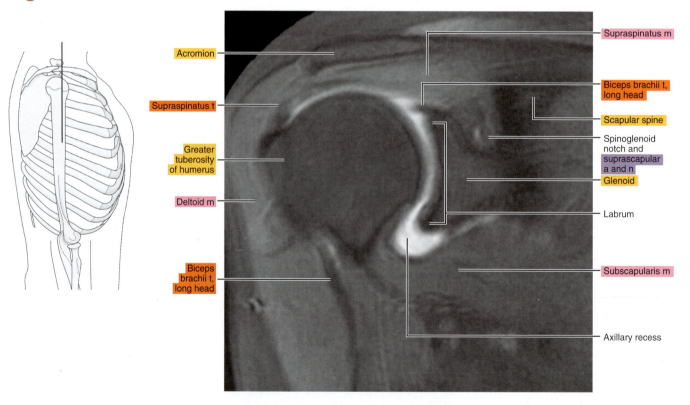

Acromion

Supraspinatus t

Greater tuberosity of humerus

Deltoid m

Biceps brachii t, long head

Supraspinatus m

Biceps brachii t, long head

Scapular spine

Spinoglenoid notch and suprascapular a and n

Glenoid

Labrum

Subscapularis m

Axillary recess

Figure 7.3.7

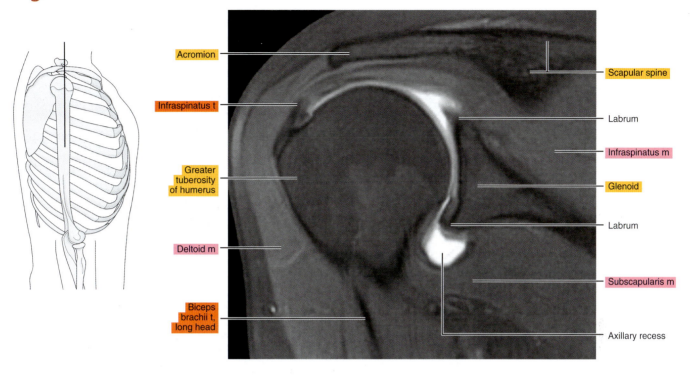

Figure 7.3.8

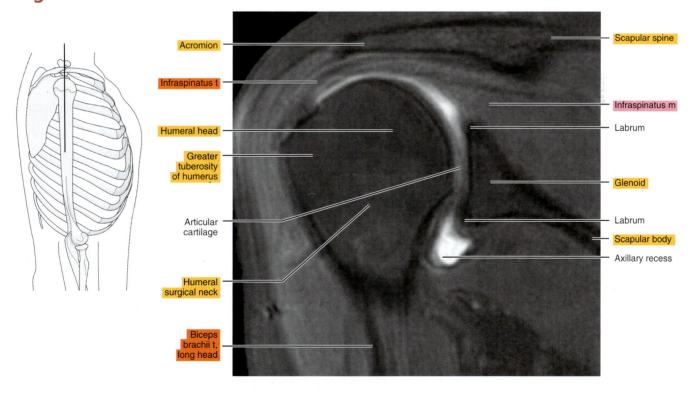

Figure 7.3.9

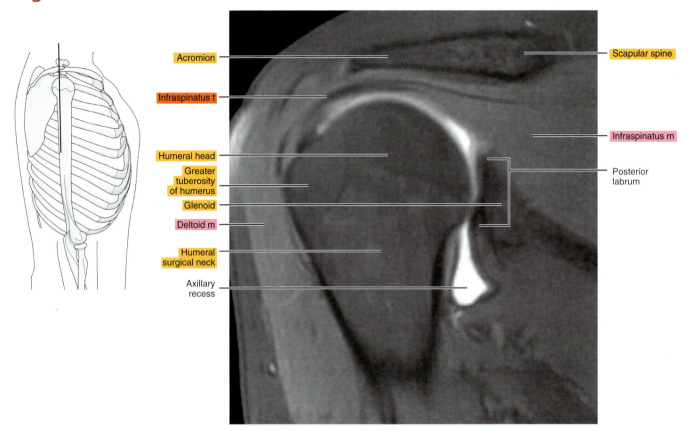

Acromion

Infraspinatus t

Humeral head

Greater tuberosity of humerus

Glenoid

Deltoid m

Humeral surgical neck

Axillary recess

Scapular spine

Infraspinatus m

Posterior labrum

Figure 7.3.10

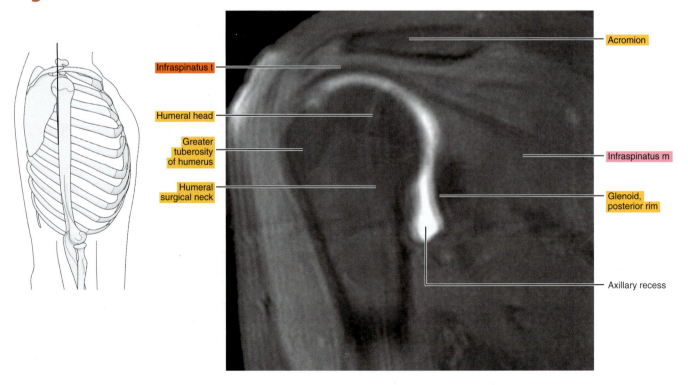

Infraspinatus t

Humeral head

Greater tuberosity of humerus

Humeral surgical neck

Acromion

Infraspinatus m

Glenoid, posterior rim

Axillary recess

Figure 7.3.11

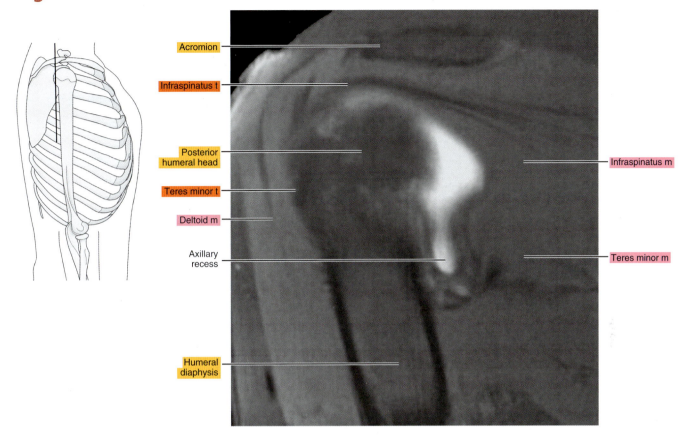

Acromion
Infraspinatus t
Posterior humeral head
Teres minor t
Deltoid m
Axillary recess
Humeral diaphysis
Infraspinatus m
Teres minor m

Figure 7.3.12

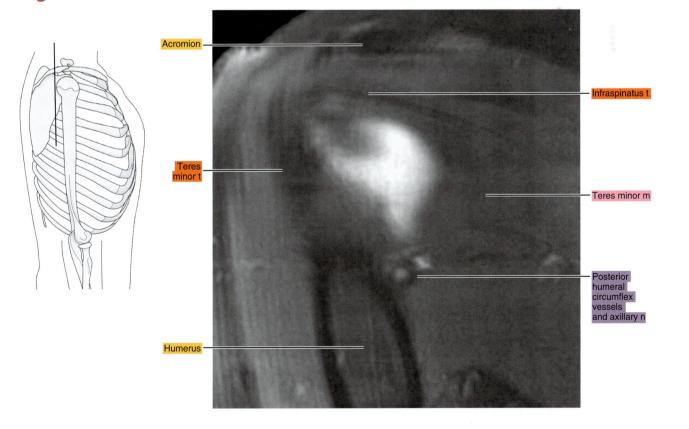

Acromion
Teres minor t
Humerus
Infraspinatus t
Teres minor m
Posterior humeral circumflex vessels and axillary n

ABER (ABDUCTION AND EXTERNAL ROTATION)
Figure 7.4.1

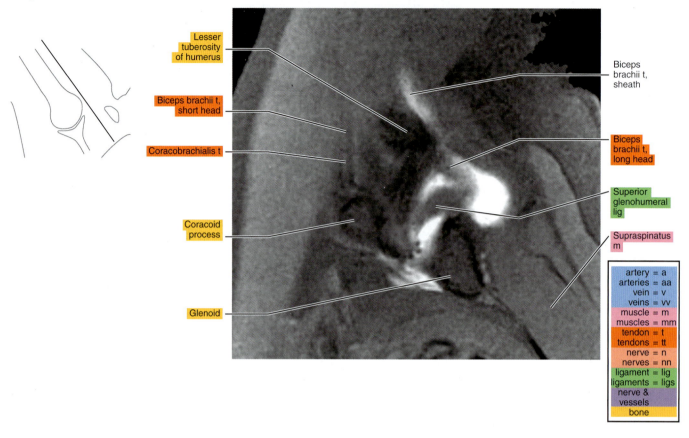

Lesser tuberosity of humerus

Biceps brachii t, short head

Coracobrachialis t

Coracoid process

Glenoid

Biceps brachii t, sheath

Biceps brachii t, long head

Superior glenohumeral lig

Supraspinatus m

artery	= a
arteries	= aa
vein	= v
veins	= vv
muscle	= m
muscles	= mm
tendon	= t
tendons	= tt
nerve	= n
nerves	= nn
ligament	= lig
ligaments	= ligs
nerve & vessels	
bone	

Figure 7.4.2

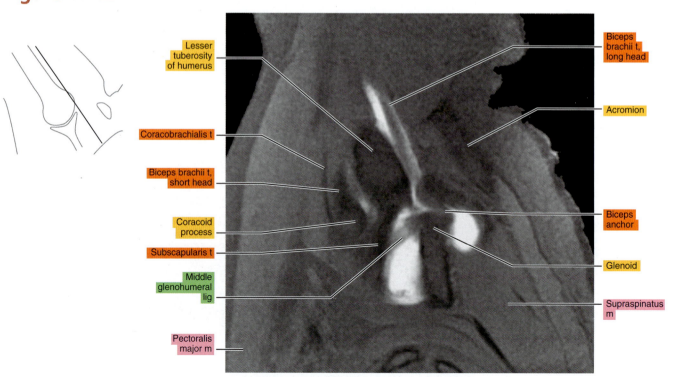

Lesser tuberosity of humerus

Coracobrachialis t

Biceps brachii t, short head

Coracoid process

Subscapularis t

Middle glenohumeral lig

Pectoralis major m

Biceps brachii t, long head

Acromion

Biceps anchor

Glenoid

Supraspinatus m

Figure 7.4.3

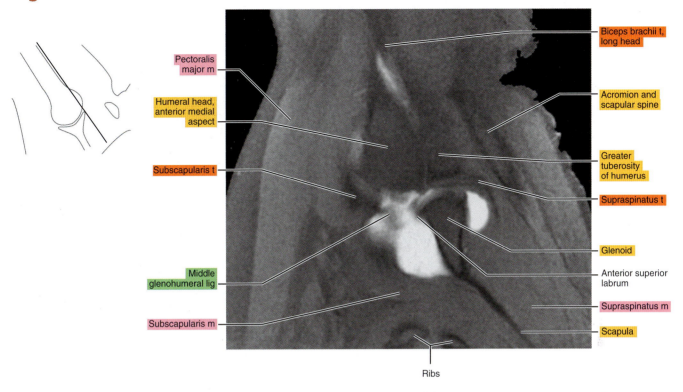

Pectoralis major m

Humeral head, anterior medial aspect

Subscapularis t

Middle glenohumeral lig

Subscapularis m

Biceps brachii t, long head

Acromion and scapular spine

Greater tuberosity of humerus

Supraspinatus t

Glenoid

Anterior superior labrum

Supraspinatus m

Scapula

Ribs

Figure 7.4.4

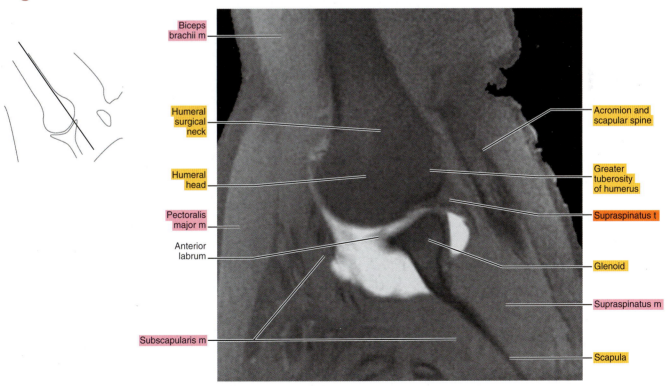

Biceps brachii m

Humeral surgical neck

Humeral head

Pectoralis major m

Anterior labrum

Subscapularis m

Acromion and scapular spine

Greater tuberosity of humerus

Supraspinatus t

Glenoid

Supraspinatus m

Scapula

Figure 7.4.5

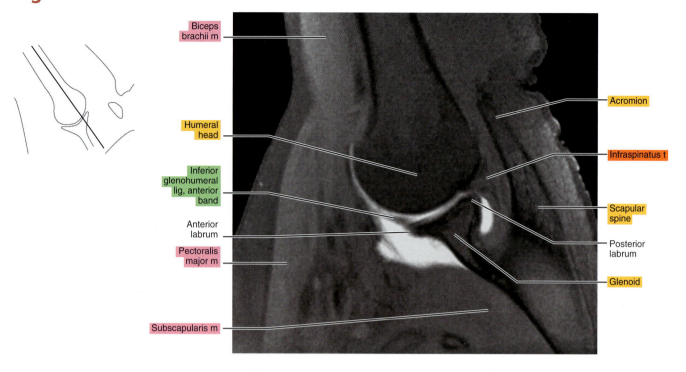

- Biceps brachii m
- Humeral head
- Inferior glenohumeral lig, anterior band
- Anterior labrum
- Pectoralis major m
- Subscapularis m
- Acromion
- Infraspinatus t
- Scapular spine
- Posterior labrum
- Glenoid

Figure 7.4.6

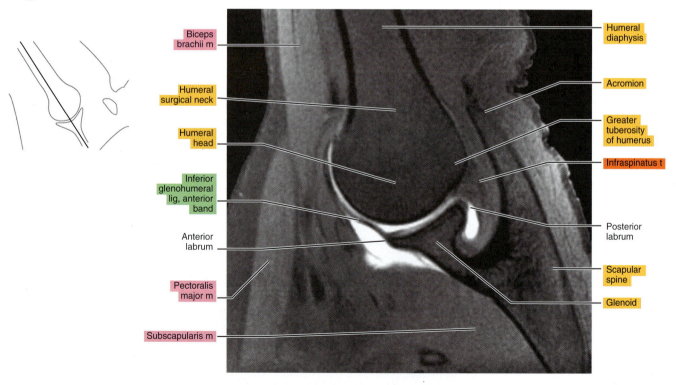

- Biceps brachii m
- Humeral surgical neck
- Humeral head
- Inferior glenohumeral lig, anterior band
- Anterior labrum
- Pectoralis major m
- Subscapularis m
- Humeral diaphysis
- Acromion
- Greater tuberosity of humerus
- Infraspinatus t
- Posterior labrum
- Scapular spine
- Glenoid

Figure 7.4.7

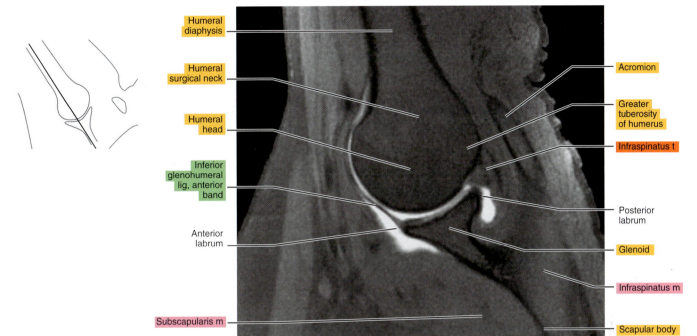

- Humeral diaphysis
- Humeral surgical neck
- Humeral head
- Inferior glenohumeral lig, anterior band
- Anterior labrum
- Subscapularis m
- Acromion
- Greater tuberosity of humerus
- Infraspinatus t
- Posterior labrum
- Glenoid
- Infraspinatus m
- Scapular body

Figure 7.4.8

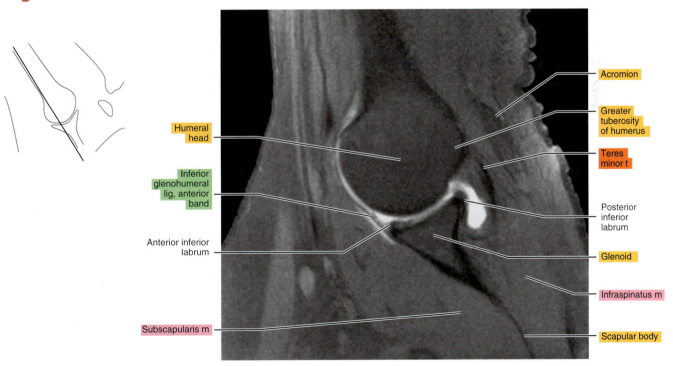

- Humeral head
- Inferior glenohumeral lig, anterior band
- Anterior inferior labrum
- Subscapularis m
- Acromion
- Greater tuberosity of humerus
- Teres minor t
- Posterior inferior labrum
- Glenoid
- Infraspinatus m
- Scapular body

Figure 7.4.9

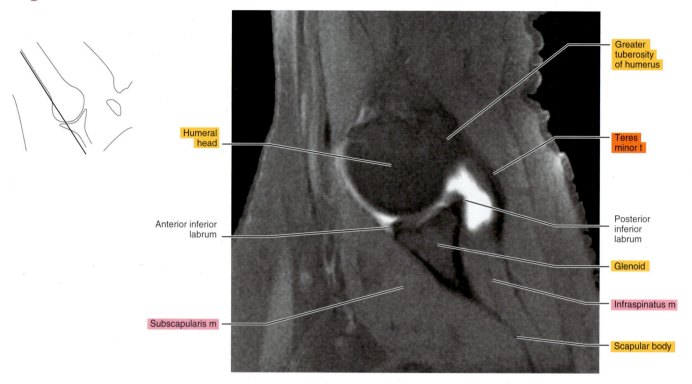

Greater tuberosity of humerus

Humeral head

Teres minor t

Anterior inferior labrum

Posterior inferior labrum

Glenoid

Infraspinatus m

Subscapularis m

Scapular body

Figure 7.4.10

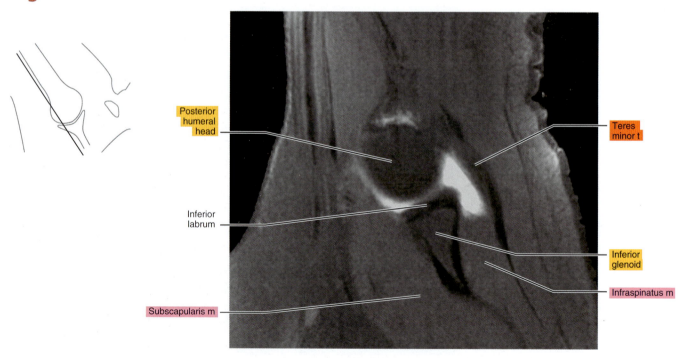

Posterior humeral head

Teres minor t

Inferior labrum

Subscapularis m

Inferior glenoid

Infraspinatus m

Figure 7.4.11

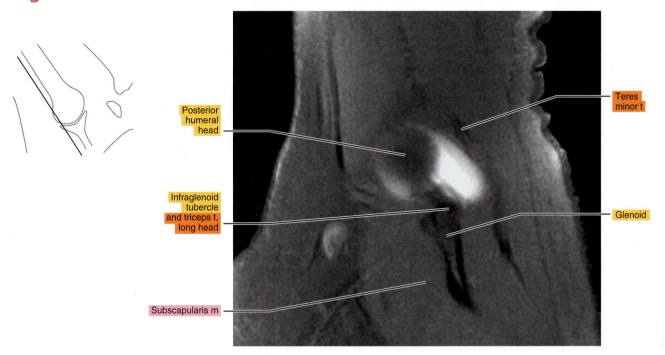

Posterior humeral head

Teres minor t

Infraglenoid tubercle and triceps t, long head

Glenoid

Subscapularis m

Chapter

8

MRI of the Arm

AXIAL
Figure 8.1.1

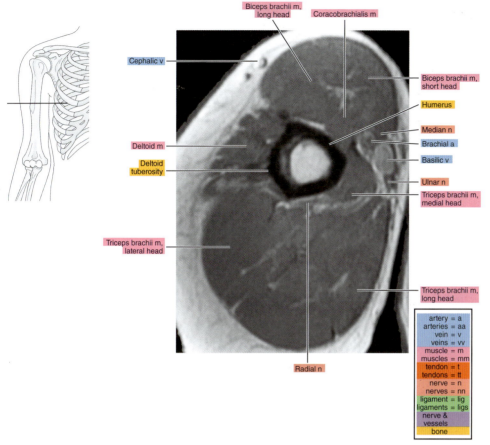

Biceps brachii m, long head
Coracobrachialis m
Cephalic v
Biceps brachii m, short head
Humerus
Median n
Brachial a
Deltoid m
Basilic v
Deltoid tuberosity
Ulnar n
Triceps brachii m, medial head
Triceps brachii m, lateral head
Triceps brachii m, long head
Radial n

artery	= a
arteries	= aa
vein	= v
veins	= vv
muscle	= m
muscles	= mm
tendon	= t
tendons	= tt
nerve	= n
nerves	= nn
ligament	= lig
ligaments	= ligs
nerve & vessels	
bone	

Figure 8.1.2

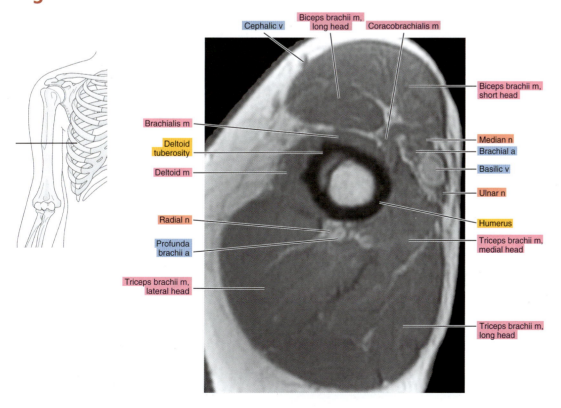

Biceps brachii m, long head
Cephalic v
Coracobrachialis m
Biceps brachii m, short head
Brachialis m
Median n
Deltoid tuberosity
Brachial a
Deltoid m
Basilic v
Ulnar n
Radial n
Humerus
Profunda brachii a
Triceps brachii m, medial head
Triceps brachii m, lateral head
Triceps brachii m, long head

Figure 8.1.3

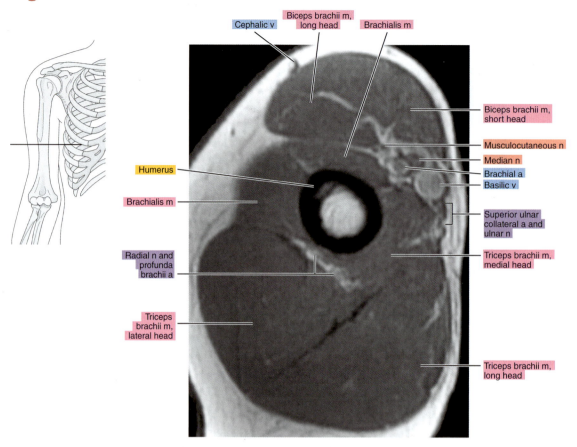

Cephalic v
Biceps brachii m, long head
Brachialis m
Biceps brachii m, short head
Musculocutaneous n
Median n
Brachial a
Basilic v
Humerus
Brachialis m
Superior ulnar collateral a and ulnar n
Radial n and profunda brachii a
Triceps brachii m, medial head
Triceps brachii m, lateral head
Triceps brachii m, long head

Figure 8.1.4

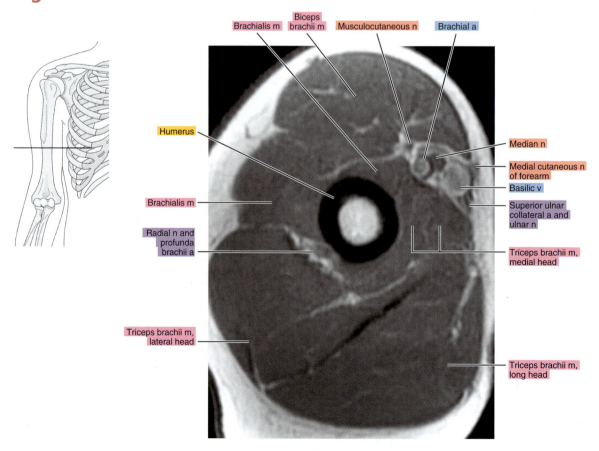

Brachialis m
Biceps brachii m
Musculocutaneous n
Brachial a
Humerus
Median n
Medial cutaneous n of forearm
Basilic v
Brachialis m
Superior ulnar collateral a and ulnar n
Radial n and profunda brachii a
Triceps brachii m, medial head
Triceps brachii m, lateral head
Triceps brachii m, long head

Figure 8.1.5

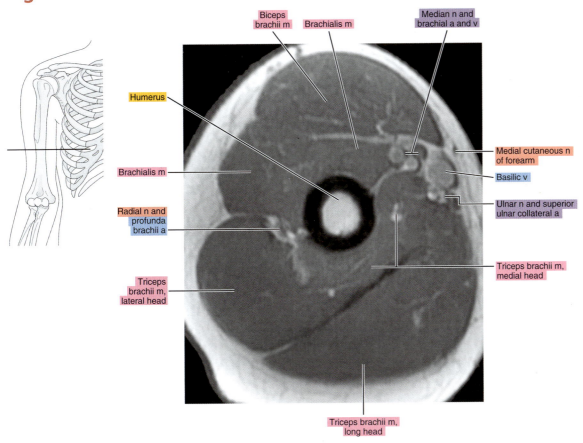

- Biceps brachii m
- Brachialis m
- Median n and brachial a and v
- Humerus
- Brachialis m
- Medial cutaneous n of forearm
- Basilic v
- Radial n and profunda brachii a
- Ulnar n and superior ulnar collateral a
- Triceps brachii m, medial head
- Triceps brachii m, lateral head
- Triceps brachii m, long head

Figure 8.1.6

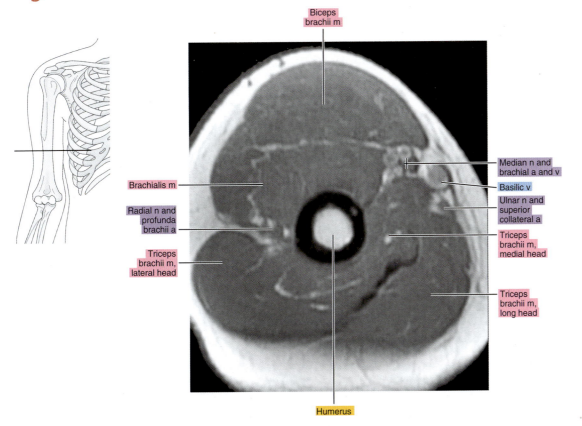

- Biceps brachii m
- Median n and brachial a and v
- Brachialis m
- Basilic v
- Radial n and profunda brachii a
- Ulnar n and superior collateral a
- Triceps brachii m, medial head
- Triceps brachii m, lateral head
- Triceps brachii m, long head
- Humerus

Figure 8.1.7

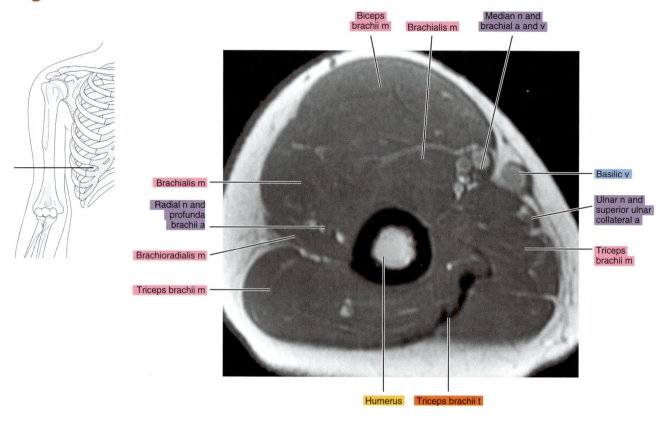

Biceps brachii m

Brachialis m

Median n and brachial a and v

Brachialis m

Radial n and profunda brachii a

Brachioradialis m

Triceps brachii m

Basilic v

Ulnar n and superior ulnar collateral a

Triceps brachii m

Humerus Triceps brachii t

Figure 8.1.8

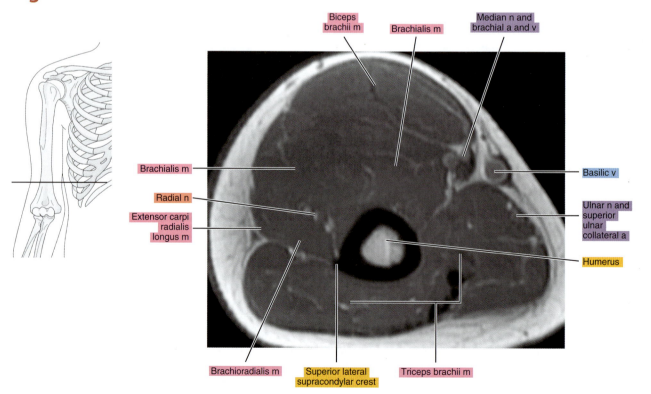

Biceps brachii m

Brachialis m

Median n and brachial a and v

Brachialis m

Radial n

Extensor carpi radialis longus m

Basilic v

Ulnar n and superior ulnar collateral a

Humerus

Brachioradialis m

Superior lateral supracondylar crest

Triceps brachii m

Figure 8.1.9

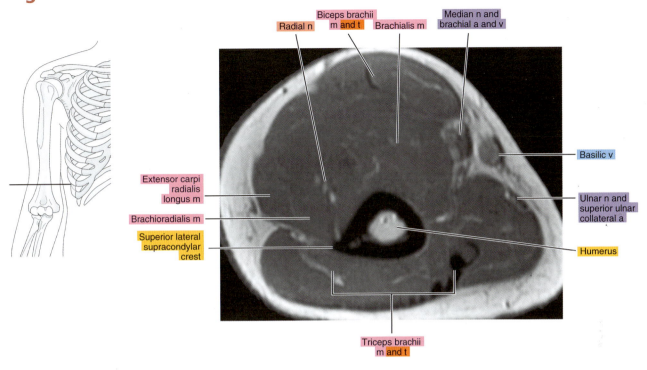

Radial n

Biceps brachii m and t

Brachialis m

Median n and brachial a and v

Extensor carpi radialis longus m

Brachioradialis m

Superior lateral supracondylar crest

Basilic v

Ulnar n and superior ulnar collateral a

Humerus

Triceps brachii m and t

Figure 8.1.10

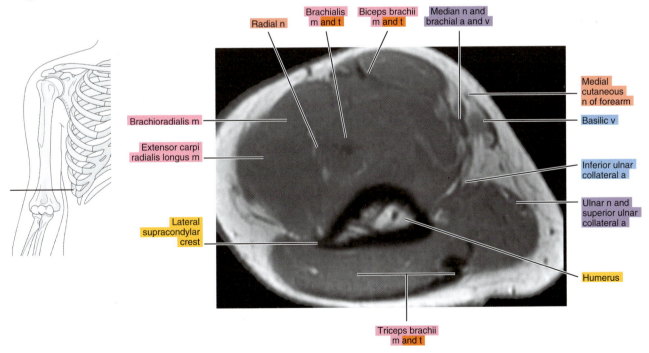

Radial n

Brachialis m and t

Biceps brachii m and t

Median n and brachial a and v

Brachioradialis m

Extensor carpi radialis longus m

Lateral supracondylar crest

Medial cutaneous n of forearm

Basilic v

Inferior ulnar collateral a

Ulnar n and superior ulnar collateral a

Humerus

Triceps brachii m and t

Figure 8.1.11

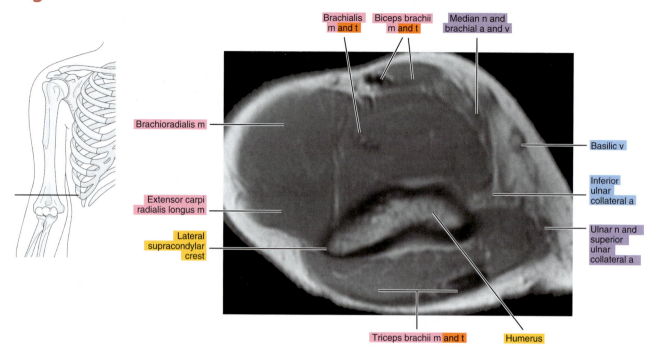

Brachialis m and t

Biceps brachii m and t

Median n and brachial a and v

Brachioradialis m

Extensor carpi radialis longus m

Lateral supracondylar crest

Basilic v

Inferior ulnar collateral a

Ulnar n and superior ulnar collateral a

Triceps brachii m and t

Humerus

SAGITTAL
Figure 8.2.1

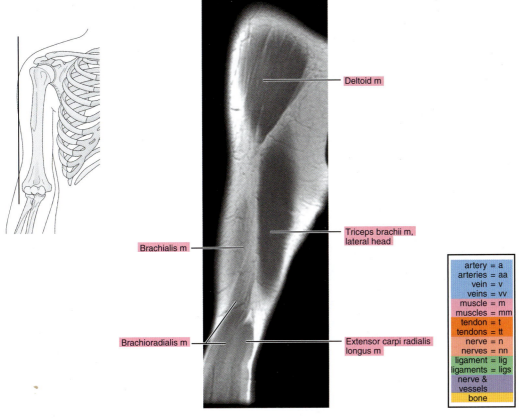

Deltoid m

Triceps brachii m, lateral head

Brachialis m

Brachioradialis m

Extensor carpi radialis longus m

artery = a	
arteries = aa	
vein = v	
veins = vv	
muscle = m	
muscles = mm	
tendon = t	
tendons = tt	
nerve = n	
nerves = nn	
ligament = lig	
ligaments = ligs	
nerve & vessels	
bone	

Figure 8.2.2

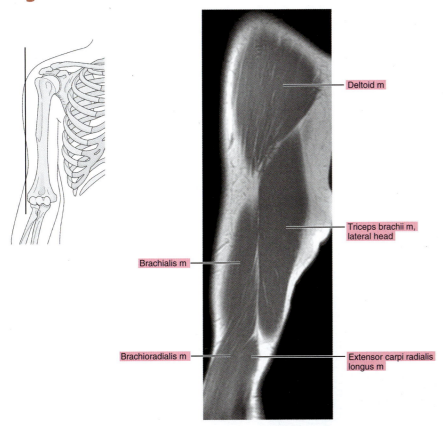

Deltoid m

Triceps brachii m, lateral head

Brachialis m

Brachioradialis m

Extensor carpi radialis longus m

Figure 8.2.3

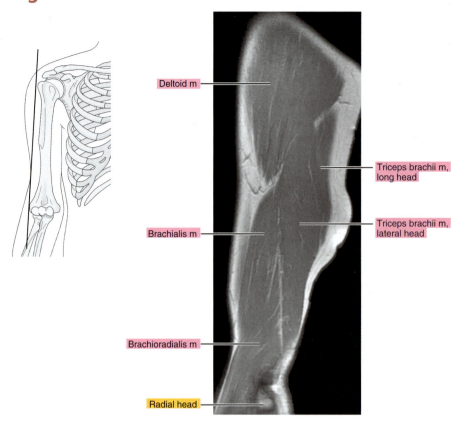

Deltoid m

Triceps brachii m, long head

Triceps brachii m, lateral head

Brachialis m

Brachioradialis m

Radial head

Figure 8.2.4

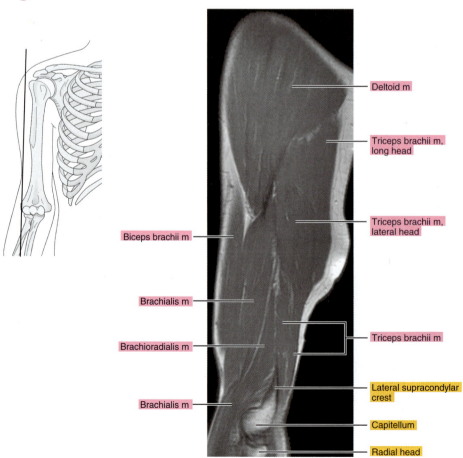

Deltoid m

Triceps brachii m, long head

Triceps brachii m, lateral head

Biceps brachii m

Brachialis m

Triceps brachii m

Brachioradialis m

Lateral supracondylar crest

Brachialis m

Capitellum

Radial head

Figure 8.2.5

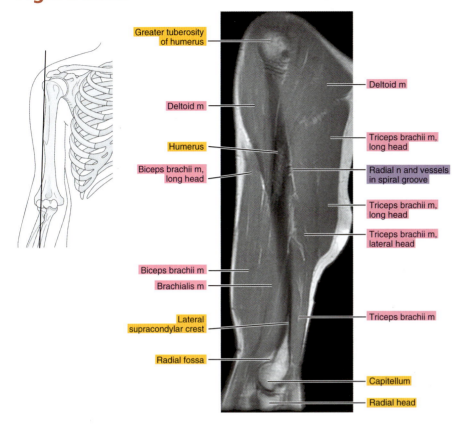

Greater tuberosity of humerus

Deltoid m

Humerus

Biceps brachii m, long head

Biceps brachii m

Brachialis m

Lateral supracondylar crest

Radial fossa

Deltoid m

Triceps brachii m, long head

Radial n and vessels in spiral groove

Triceps brachii m, long head

Triceps brachii m, lateral head

Triceps brachii m

Capitellum

Radial head

Figure 8.2.6

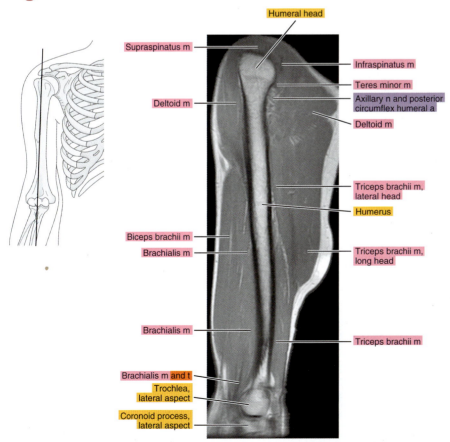

Humeral head

Supraspinatus m

Deltoid m

Biceps brachii m

Brachialis m

Brachialis m

Brachialis m and t

Trochlea, lateral aspect

Coronoid process, lateral aspect

Infraspinatus m

Teres minor m

Axillary n and posterior circumflex humeral a

Deltoid m

Triceps brachii m, lateral head

Humerus

Triceps brachii m, long head

Triceps brachii m

Figure 8.2.7

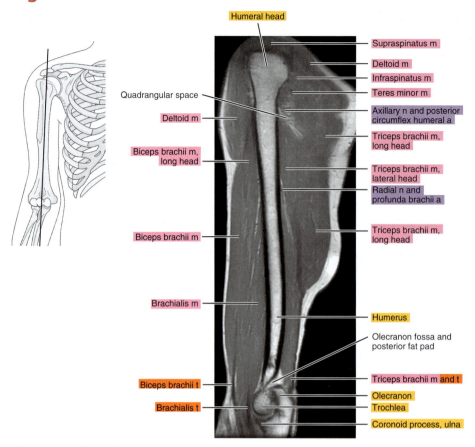

Humeral head

Supraspinatus m

Deltoid m

Infraspinatus m

Teres minor m

Quadrangular space

Deltoid m

Axillary n and posterior circumflex humeral a

Triceps brachii m, long head

Biceps brachii m, long head

Triceps brachii m, lateral head

Radial n and profunda brachii a

Biceps brachii m

Triceps brachii m, long head

Brachialis m

Humerus

Olecranon fossa and posterior fat pad

Biceps brachii t

Triceps brachii m and t

Olecranon

Brachialis t

Trochlea

Coronoid process, ulna

Figure 8.2.8

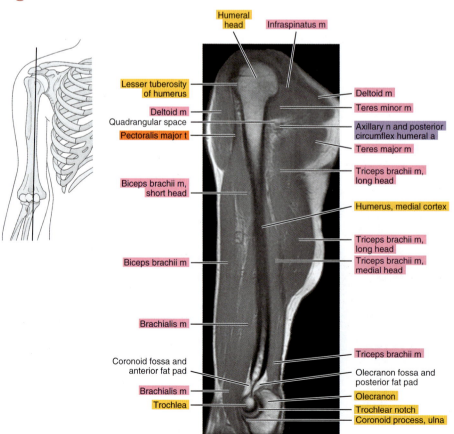

Humeral head

Infraspinatus m

Lesser tuberosity of humerus

Deltoid m

Teres minor m

Deltoid m

Quadrangular space

Axillary n and posterior circumflex humeral a

Pectoralis major t

Teres major m

Biceps brachii m, short head

Triceps brachii m, long head

Humerus, medial cortex

Triceps brachii m, long head

Biceps brachii m

Triceps brachii m, medial head

Brachialis m

Triceps brachii m

Coronoid fossa and anterior fat pad

Olecranon fossa and posterior fat pad

Brachialis m

Olecranon

Trochlea

Trochlear notch

Coronoid process, ulna

Figure 8.2.9

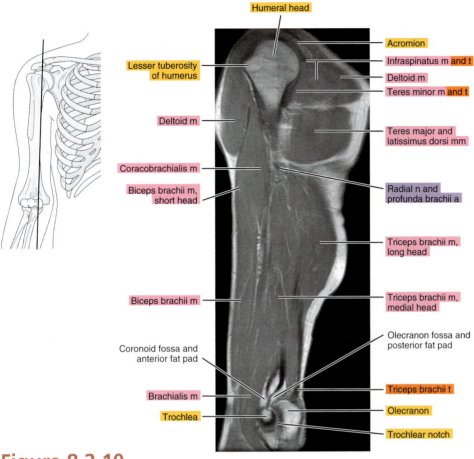

Humeral head

Acromion

Lesser tuberosity of humerus

Infraspinatus m and t

Deltoid m

Teres minor m and t

Deltoid m

Teres major and latissimus dorsi mm

Coracobrachialis m

Biceps brachii m, short head

Radial n and profunda brachii a

Triceps brachii m, long head

Biceps brachii m

Triceps brachii m, medial head

Coronoid fossa and anterior fat pad

Olecranon fossa and posterior fat pad

Brachialis m

Triceps brachii t

Trochlea

Olecranon

Trochlear notch

Figure 8.2.10

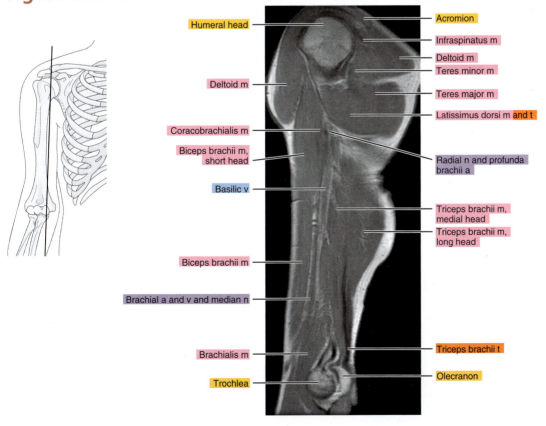

Humeral head

Acromion

Infraspinatus m

Deltoid m

Teres minor m

Deltoid m

Teres major m

Coracobrachialis m

Latissimus dorsi m and t

Biceps brachii m, short head

Radial n and profunda brachii a

Basilic v

Triceps brachii m, medial head

Triceps brachii m, long head

Biceps brachii m

Brachial a and v and median n

Brachialis m

Triceps brachii t

Trochlea

Olecranon

Figure 8.2.11

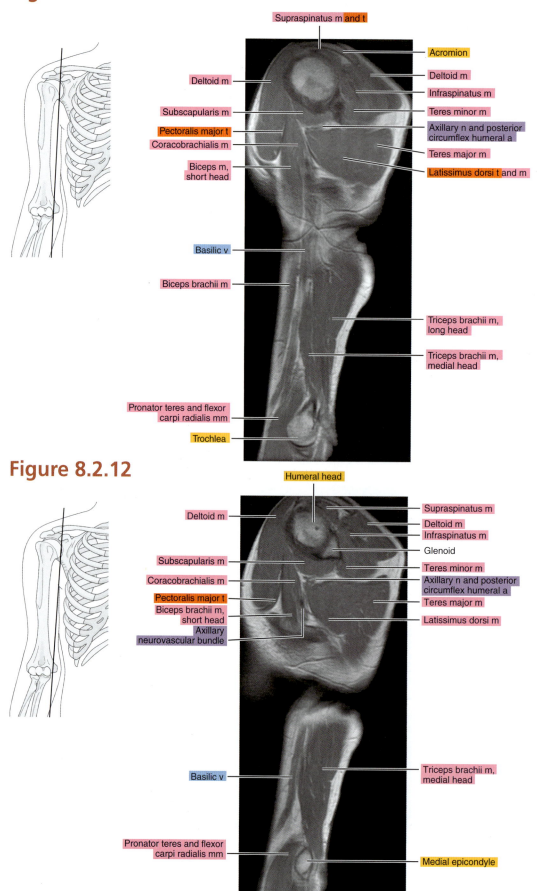

Supraspinatus m and t

Acromion

Deltoid m

Deltoid m

Infraspinatus m

Subscapularis m

Teres minor m

Pectoralis major t

Axillary n and posterior circumflex humeral a

Coracobrachialis m

Teres major m

Biceps m, short head

Latissimus dorsi t and m

Basilic v

Biceps brachii m

Triceps brachii m, long head

Triceps brachii m, medial head

Pronator teres and flexor carpi radialis mm

Trochlea

Figure 8.2.12

Humeral head

Deltoid m

Supraspinatus m

Deltoid m

Infraspinatus m

Subscapularis m

Glenoid

Coracobrachialis m

Teres minor m

Pectoralis major t

Axillary n and posterior circumflex humeral a

Biceps brachii m, short head

Teres major m

Axillary neurovascular bundle

Latissimus dorsi m

Basilic v

Triceps brachii m, medial head

Pronator teres and flexor carpi radialis mm

Medial epicondyle

Figure 8.2.13

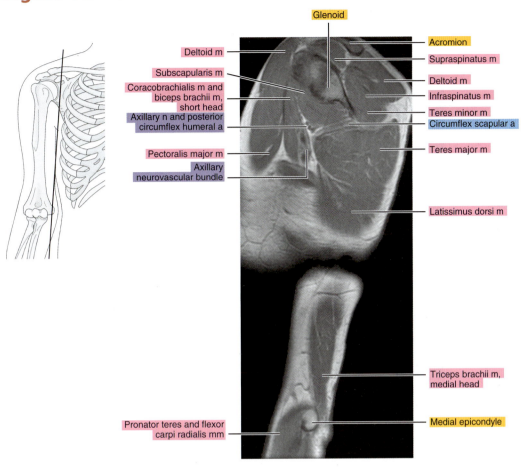

Glenoid

Deltoid m

Subscapularis m

Coracobrachialis m and biceps brachii m, short head

Axillary n and posterior circumflex humeral a

Pectoralis major m

Axillary neurovascular bundle

Acromion

Supraspinatus m

Deltoid m

Infraspinatus m

Teres minor m

Circumflex scapular a

Teres major m

Latissimus dorsi m

Triceps brachii m, medial head

Pronator teres and flexor carpi radialis mm

Medial epicondyle

CORONAL
Figure 8.3.1

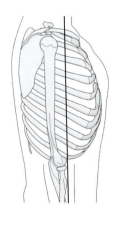

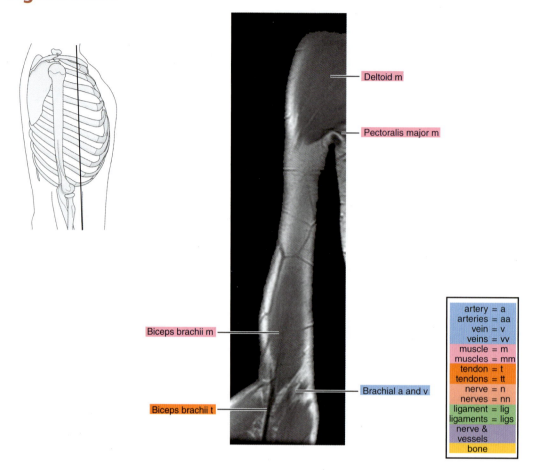

Deltoid m

Pectoralis major m

Biceps brachii m

Brachial a and v

Biceps brachii t

artery	= a
arteries	= aa
vein	= v
veins	= vv
muscle	= m
muscles	= mm
tendon	= t
tendons	= tt
nerve	= n
nerves	= nn
ligament	= lig
ligaments	= ligs
nerve & vessels	
bone	

Figure 8.3.2

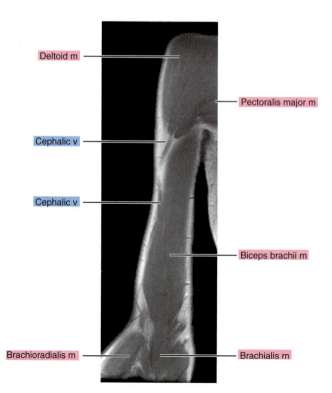

Deltoid m

Pectoralis major m

Cephalic v

Cephalic v

Biceps brachii m

Brachioradialis m

Brachialis m

Figure 8.3.3

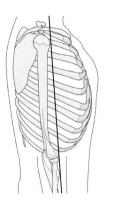
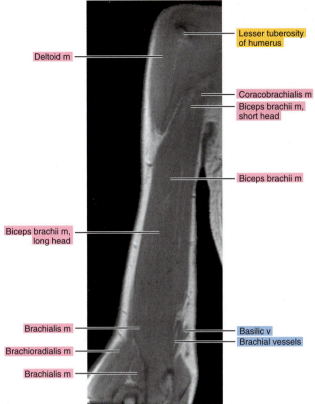

Deltoid m

Lesser tuberosity of humerus

Coracobrachialis m
Biceps brachii m, short head

Biceps brachii m

Biceps brachii m, long head

Brachialis m

Brachioradialis m

Brachialis m

Basilic v
Brachial vessels

Figure 8.3.4

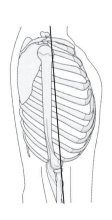
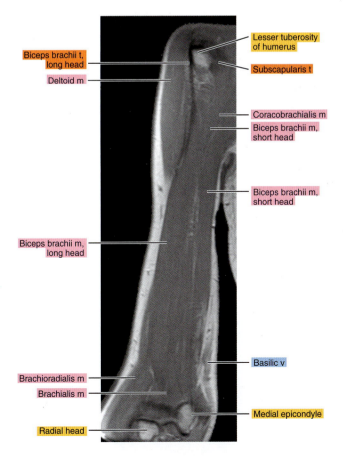

Biceps brachii t, long head

Deltoid m

Biceps brachii m, long head

Brachioradialis m

Brachialis m

Radial head

Lesser tuberosity of humerus

Subscapularis t

Coracobrachialis m
Biceps brachii m, short head

Biceps brachii m, short head

Basilic v

Medial epicondyle

Figure 8.3.5

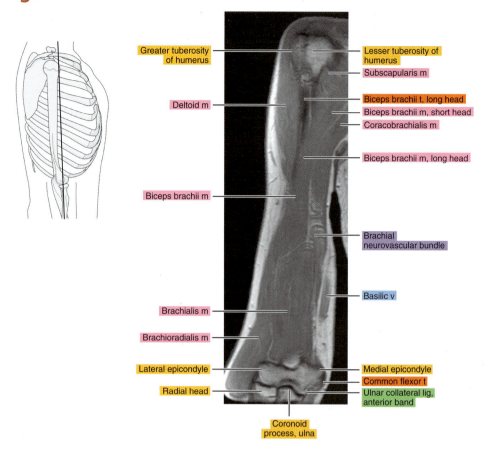

Greater tuberosity of humerus
Lesser tuberosity of humerus
Subscapularis m
Deltoid m
Biceps brachii t, long head
Biceps brachii m, short head
Coracobrachialis m
Biceps brachii m, long head
Biceps brachii m
Brachial neurovascular bundle
Basilic v
Brachialis m
Brachioradialis m
Lateral epicondyle
Medial epicondyle
Common flexor t
Radial head
Ulnar collateral lig, anterior band
Coronoid process, ulna

Figure 8.3.6

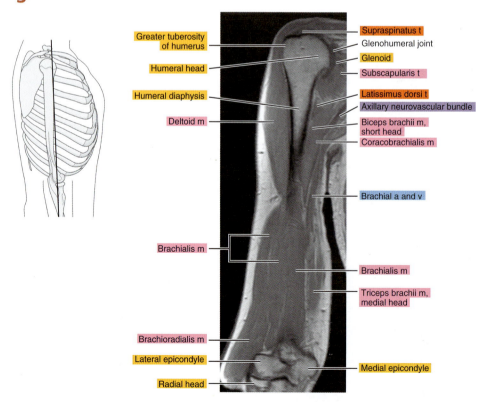

Supraspinatus t
Greater tuberosity of humerus
Glenohumeral joint
Humeral head
Glenoid
Subscapularis t
Humeral diaphysis
Latissimus dorsi t
Axillary neurovascular bundle
Deltoid m
Biceps brachii m, short head
Coracobrachialis m
Brachial a and v
Brachialis m
Brachialis m
Triceps brachii m, medial head
Brachioradialis m
Lateral epicondyle
Medial epicondyle
Radial head

Figure 8.3.7

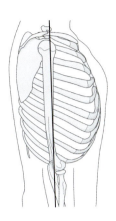

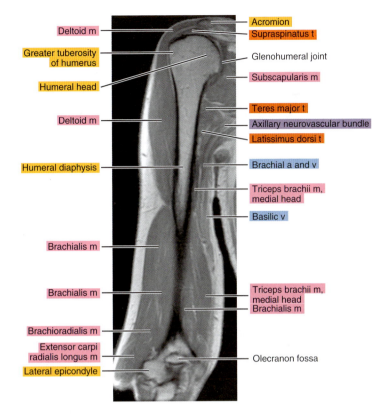

Acromion
Deltoid m
Supraspinatus t
Greater tuberosity of humerus
Glenohumeral joint
Humeral head
Subscapularis m
Deltoid m
Teres major t
Axillary neurovascular bundle
Latissimus dorsi t
Humeral diaphysis
Brachial a and v
Triceps brachii m, medial head
Basilic v
Brachialis m
Brachialis m
Triceps brachii m, medial head
Brachialis m
Brachioradialis m
Extensor carpi radialis longus m
Olecranon fossa
Lateral epicondyle

Figure 8.3.8

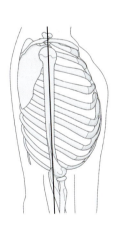

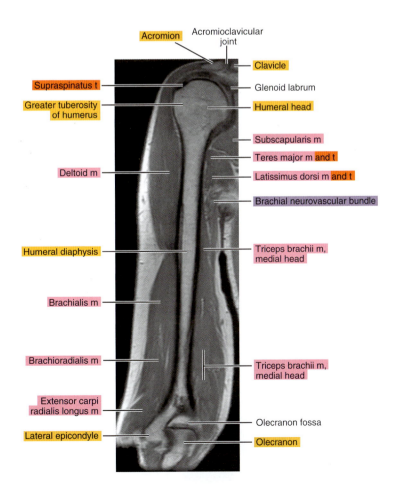

Acromion
Acromioclavicular joint
Clavicle
Supraspinatus t
Glenoid labrum
Greater tuberosity of humerus
Humeral head
Subscapularis m
Deltoid m
Teres major m and t
Latissimus dorsi m and t
Brachial neurovascular bundle
Humeral diaphysis
Triceps brachii m, medial head
Brachialis m
Brachioradialis m
Triceps brachii m, medial head
Extensor carpi radialis longus m
Olecranon fossa
Lateral epicondyle
Olecranon

Figure 8.3.9

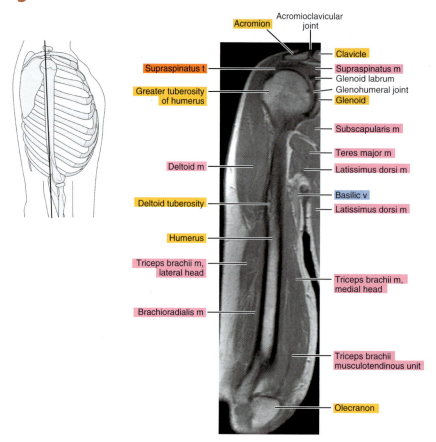

Acromion
Acromioclavicular joint
Clavicle
Supraspinatus t
Supraspinatus m
Glenoid labrum
Glenohumeral joint
Greater tuberosity of humerus
Glenoid
Subscapularis m
Teres major m
Deltoid m
Latissimus dorsi m
Basilic v
Deltoid tuberosity
Latissimus dorsi m
Humerus
Triceps brachii m, lateral head
Triceps brachii m, medial head
Brachioradialis m
Triceps brachii musculotendinous unit
Olecranon

Figure 8.3.10

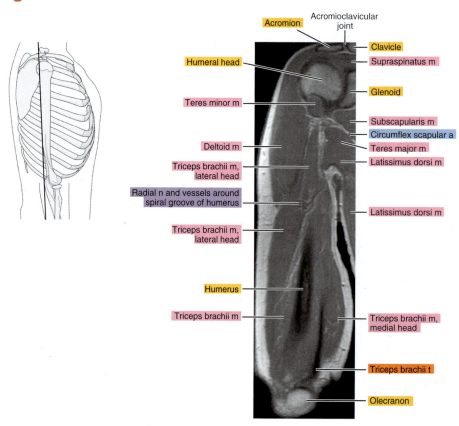

Acromion
Acromioclavicular joint
Clavicle
Humeral head
Supraspinatus m
Teres minor m
Glenoid
Subscapularis m
Circumflex scapular a
Deltoid m
Teres major m
Triceps brachii m, lateral head
Latissimus dorsi m
Radial n and vessels around spiral groove of humerus
Latissimus dorsi m
Triceps brachii m, lateral head
Humerus
Triceps brachii m
Triceps brachii m, medial head
Triceps brachii t
Olecranon

Figure 8.3.11

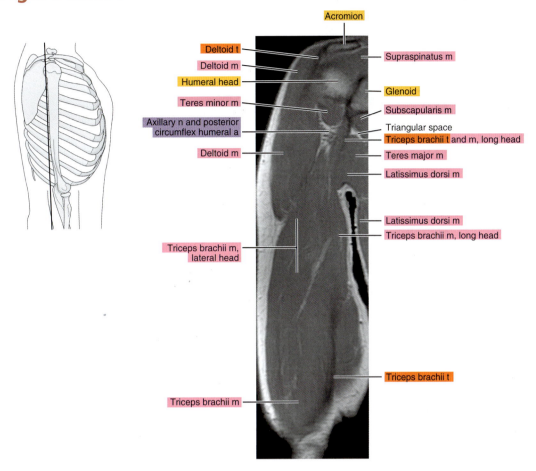

Acromion
Deltoid t
Deltoid m
Humeral head
Teres minor m
Axillary n and posterior circumflex humeral a
Deltoid m
Triceps brachii m, lateral head
Triceps brachii m
Supraspinatus m
Glenoid
Subscapularis m
Triangular space
Triceps brachii t and m, long head
Teres major m
Latissimus dorsi m
Latissimus dorsi m
Triceps brachii m, long head
Triceps brachii t

Figure 8.3.12

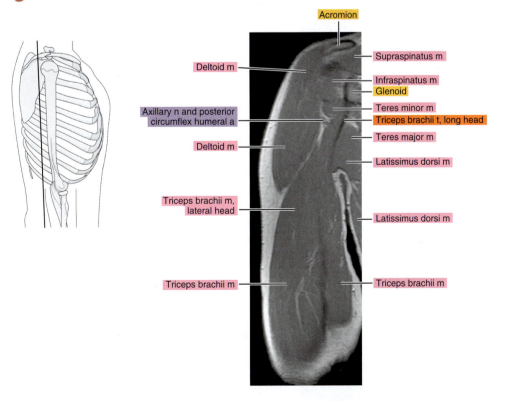

Acromion
Deltoid m
Axillary n and posterior circumflex humeral a
Deltoid m
Triceps brachii m, lateral head
Triceps brachii m
Supraspinatus m
Infraspinatus m
Glenoid
Teres minor m
Triceps brachii t, long head
Teres major m
Latissimus dorsi m
Latissimus dorsi m
Triceps brachii m

Figure 8.3.13

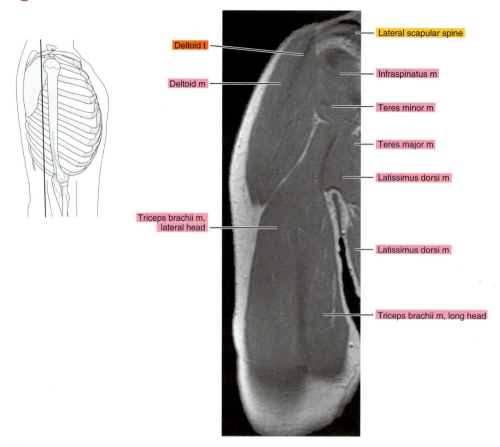

Lateral scapular spine

Deltoid t

Infraspinatus m

Deltoid m

Teres minor m

Teres major m

Latissimus dorsi m

Triceps brachii m, lateral head

Latissimus dorsi m

Triceps brachii m, long head

Figure 8.3.14

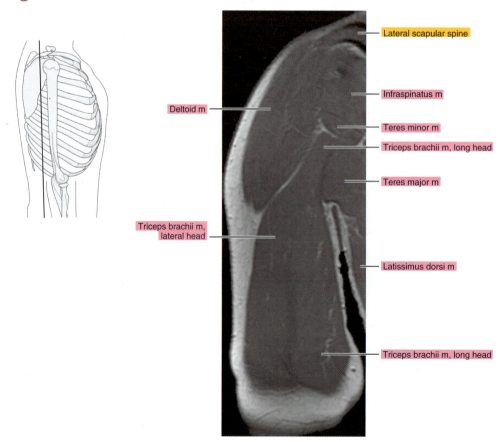

Lateral scapular spine

Infraspinatus m

Deltoid m

Teres minor m

Triceps brachii m, long head

Teres major m

Triceps brachii m, lateral head

Latissimus dorsi m

Triceps brachii m, long head

Figure 8.3.15

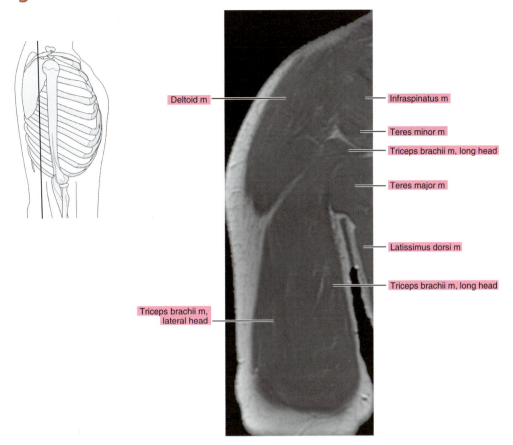

Deltoid m

Infraspinatus m

Teres minor m

Triceps brachii m, long head

Teres major m

Latissimus dorsi m

Triceps brachii m, long head

Triceps brachii m, lateral head

Figure 8.3.16

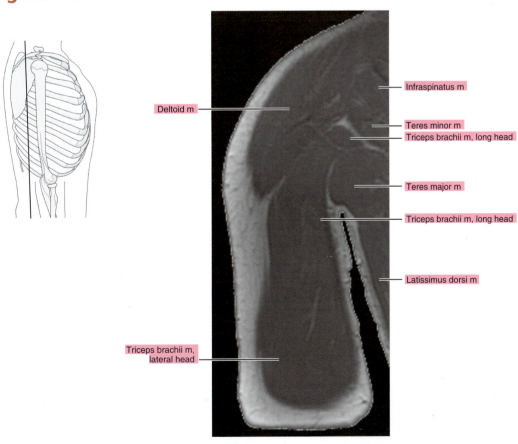

Infraspinatus m

Deltoid m

Teres minor m

Triceps brachii m, long head

Teres major m

Triceps brachii m, long head

Latissimus dorsi m

Triceps brachii m, lateral head

Figure 8.3.17

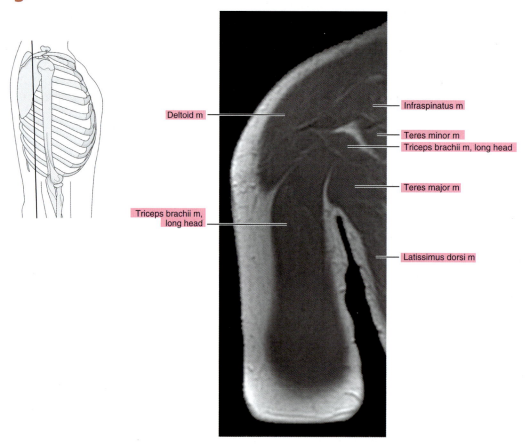

Deltoid m

Infraspinatus m

Teres minor m
Triceps brachii m, long head

Teres major m

Triceps brachii m, long head

Latissimus dorsi m

Figure 8.3.18

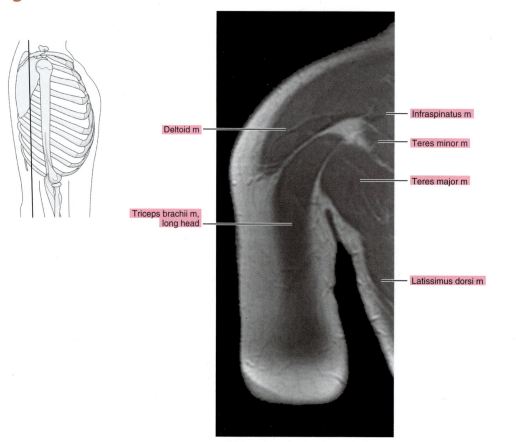

Deltoid m

Infraspinatus m

Teres minor m

Teres major m

Triceps brachii m, long head

Latissimus dorsi m

Table 8-1. **Muscles of the Upper Arm**

MUSCLE	ORIGIN	INSERTION	NERVE SUPPLY
Coracobrachialis	Coracoid process	Shaft of the humerus above the middle of the bone	Musculocutaneous (C5, C6, and C7)
Biceps brachii	Short head, coracoid process; long head, supraglenoid tubercle; and superior part of the glenoid labrum	Tuberosity of the radius and by aponeurotic expansion to the fascia on the ulnar side of the forearm	Musculocutaneous (C5 and C6)
Brachialis	Distal half of the anterior surface of the humerus	Coronoid process and tuberosity of the ulna	Musculocutaneous (C5 and C6)
Triceps	Long head, infraglenoid tuberosity of the scapula; lateral head, from the posterior surface of the humerus; and medial head, from the posterior surface of the humerus below the radial groove and dorsal surfaces of the medial and lateral intermuscular septa	Primary tendon inserts onto the olecranon process of the ulna and laterally, by expansion over the anconeus, into the dorsal fascia of the forearm	Radial (C6, C7, and C8)

Chapter

9

MRI of the Elbow

AXIAL
Figure 9.1.1

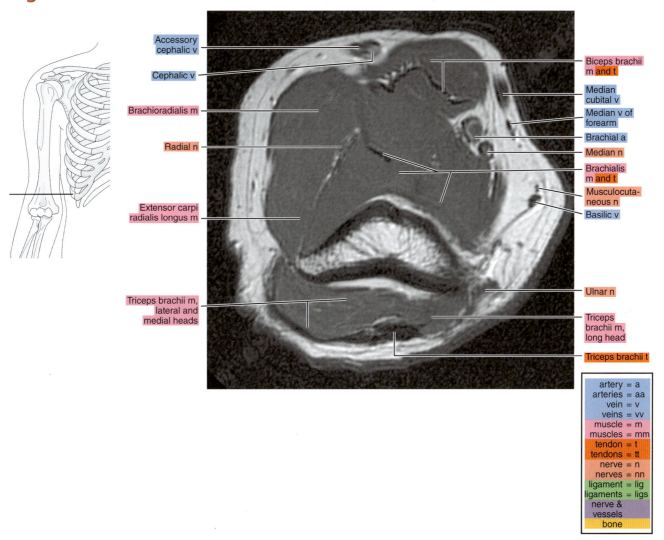

Accessory cephalic v

Cephalic v

Brachioradialis m

Radial n

Extensor carpi radialis longus m

Triceps brachii m, lateral and medial heads

Biceps brachii m and t

Median cubital v

Median v of forearm

Brachial a

Median n

Brachialis m and t

Musculocutaneous n

Basilic v

Ulnar n

Triceps brachii m, long head

Triceps brachii t

artery	= a
arteries	= aa
vein	= v
veins	= vv
muscle	= m
muscles	= mm
tendon	= t
tendons	= tt
nerve	= n
nerves	= nn
ligament	= lig
ligaments	= ligs
nerve & vessels	
bone	

Figure 9.1.2

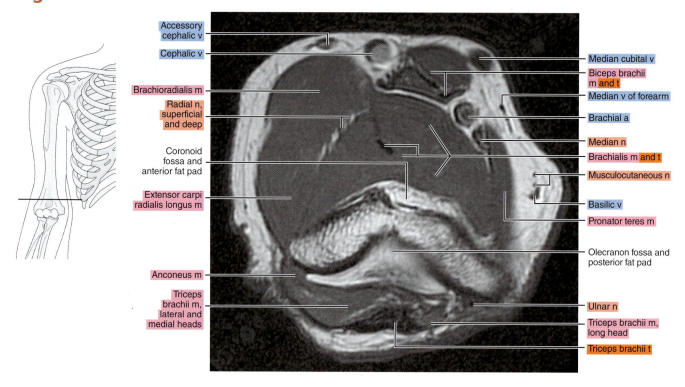

Accessory cephalic v

Cephalic v

Brachioradialis m

Radial n, superficial and deep

Coronoid fossa and anterior fat pad

Extensor carpi radialis longus m

Anconeus m

Triceps brachii m, lateral and medial heads

Median cubital v

Biceps brachii m and t

Median v of forearm

Brachial a

Median n

Brachialis m and t

Musculocutaneous n

Basilic v

Pronator teres m

Olecranon fossa and posterior fat pad

Ulnar n

Triceps brachii m, long head

Triceps brachii t

Figure 9.1.3

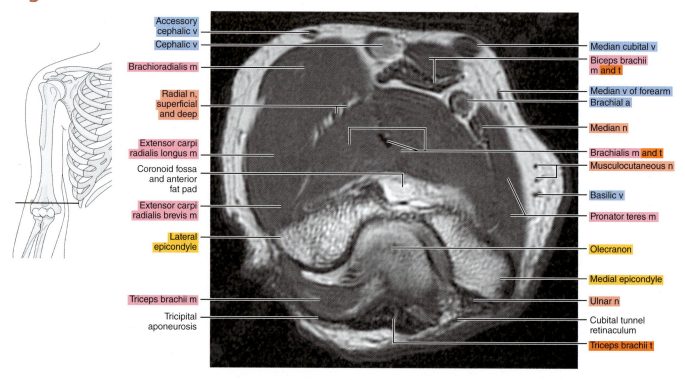

Accessory cephalic v

Cephalic v

Brachioradialis m

Radial n, superficial and deep

Extensor carpi radialis longus m

Coronoid fossa and anterior fat pad

Extensor carpi radialis brevis m

Lateral epicondyle

Triceps brachii m

Tricipital aponeurosis

Median cubital v

Biceps brachii m and t

Median v of forearm

Brachial a

Median n

Brachialis m and t

Musculocutaneous n

Basilic v

Pronator teres m

Olecranon

Medial epicondyle

Ulnar n

Cubital tunnel retinaculum

Triceps brachii t

Figure 9.1.4

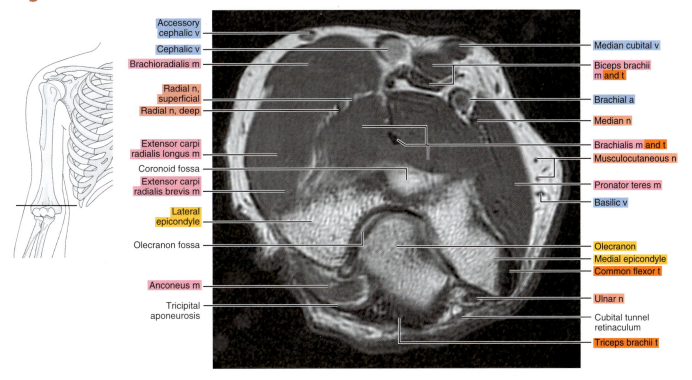

Accessory cephalic v
Cephalic v
Brachioradialis m
Radial n, superficial
Radial n, deep
Extensor carpi radialis longus m
Coronoid fossa
Extensor carpi radialis brevis m
Lateral epicondyle
Olecranon fossa
Anconeus m
Tricipital aponeurosis

Median cubital v
Biceps brachii m and t
Brachial a
Median n
Brachialis m and t
Musculocutaneous n
Pronator teres m
Basilic v
Olecranon
Medial epicondyle
Common flexor t
Ulnar n
Cubital tunnel retinaculum
Triceps brachii t

Figure 9.1.5

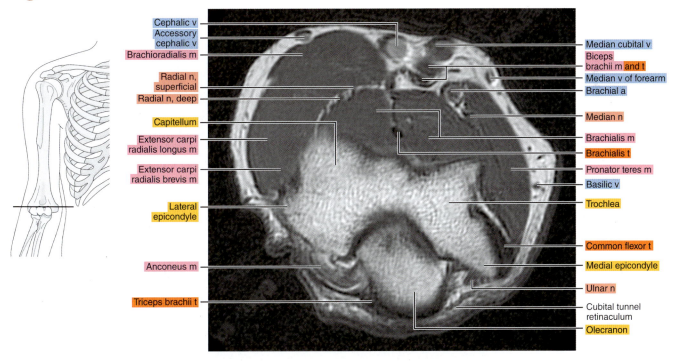

Cephalic v
Accessory cephalic v
Brachioradialis m
Radial n, superficial
Radial n, deep
Capitellum
Extensor carpi radialis longus m
Extensor carpi radialis brevis m
Lateral epicondyle
Anconeus m
Triceps brachii t

Median cubital v
Biceps brachii m and t
Median v of forearm
Brachial a
Median n
Brachialis m
Brachialis t
Pronator teres m
Basilic v
Trochlea
Common flexor t
Medial epicondyle
Ulnar n
Cubital tunnel retinaculum
Olecranon

Figure 9.1.6

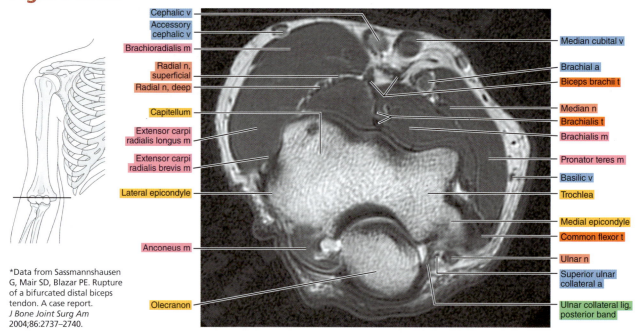

Cephalic v
Accessory cephalic v
Brachioradialis m
Radial n, superficial
Radial n, deep
Capitellum
Extensor carpi radialis longus m
Extensor carpi radialis brevis m
Lateral epicondyle
Anconeus m
Olecranon

Median cubital v
Brachial a
Biceps brachii t
Median n
Brachialis t
Brachialis m
Pronator teres m
Basilic v
Trochlea
Medial epicondyle
Common flexor t
Ulnar n
Superior ulnar collateral a
Ulnar collateral lig, posterior band

*Data from Sassmannshausen G, Mair SD, Blazar PE. Rupture of a bifurcated distal biceps tendon. A case report. *J Bone Joint Surg Am* 2004;86:2737–2740.

Figure 9.1.7

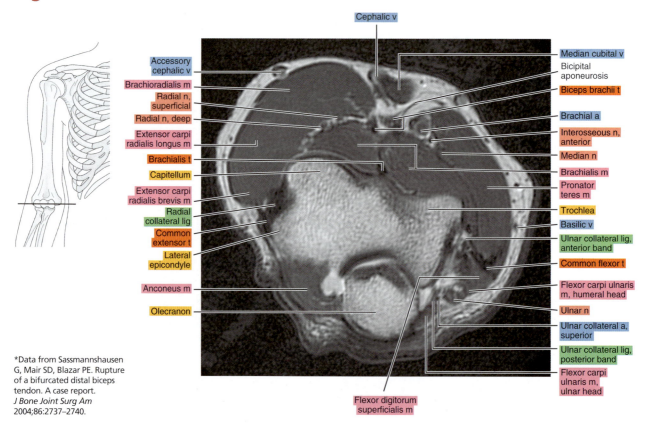

Cephalic v
Accessory cephalic v
Brachioradialis m
Radial n, superficial
Radial n, deep
Extensor carpi radialis longus m
Brachialis t
Capitellum
Extensor carpi radialis brevis m
Radial collateral lig
Common extensor t
Lateral epicondyle
Anconeus m
Olecranon
Flexor digitorum superficialis m

Median cubital v
Bicipital aponeurosis
Biceps brachii t
Brachial a
Interosseous n, anterior
Median n
Brachialis m
Pronator teres m
Trochlea
Basilic v
Ulnar collateral lig, anterior band
Common flexor t
Flexor carpi ulnaris m, humeral head
Ulnar n
Ulnar collateral a, superior
Ulnar collateral lig, posterior band
Flexor carpi ulnaris m, ulnar head

*Data from Sassmannshausen G, Mair SD, Blazar PE. Rupture of a bifurcated distal biceps tendon. A case report. *J Bone Joint Surg Am* 2004;86:2737–2740.

Figure 9.1.8

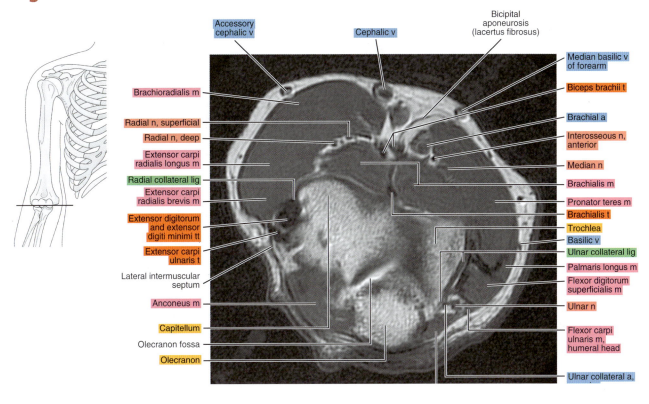

Accessory cephalic v
Cephalic v
Bicipital aponeurosis (lacertus fibrosus)
Brachioradialis m
Radial n, superficial
Radial n, deep
Extensor carpi radialis longus m
Radial collateral lig
Extensor carpi radialis brevis m
Extensor digitorum and extensor digiti minimi tt
Extensor carpi ulnaris t
Lateral intermuscular septum
Anconeus m
Capitellum
Olecranon fossa
Olecranon
Median basilic v of forearm
Biceps brachii t
Brachial a
Interosseous n, anterior
Median n
Brachialis m
Pronator teres m
Brachialis t
Trochlea
Basilic v
Ulnar collateral lig
Palmaris longus m
Flexor digitorum superficialis m
Ulnar n
Flexor carpi ulnaris m, humeral head
Ulnar collateral a,

Figure 9.1.9

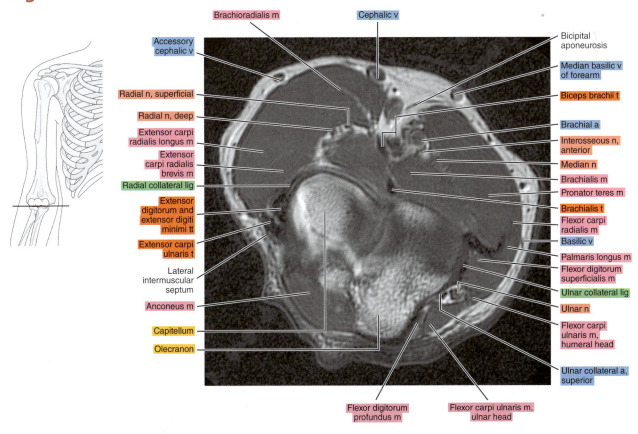

Brachioradialis m
Cephalic v
Accessory cephalic v
Radial n, superficial
Radial n, deep
Extensor carpi radialis longus m
Extensor carpi radialis brevis m
Radial collateral lig
Extensor digitorum and extensor digiti minimi tt
Extensor carpi ulnaris t
Lateral intermuscular septum
Anconeus m
Capitellum
Olecranon
Bicipital aponeurosis
Median basilic v of forearm
Biceps brachii t
Brachial a
Interosseous n, anterior
Median n
Brachialis m
Pronator teres m
Brachialis t
Flexor carpi radialis m
Basilic v
Palmaris longus m
Flexor digitorum superficialis m
Ulnar collateral lig
Ulnar n
Flexor carpi ulnaris m, humeral head
Ulnar collateral a, superior
Flexor digitorum profundus m
Flexor carpi ulnaris m, ulnar head

Figure 9.1.10

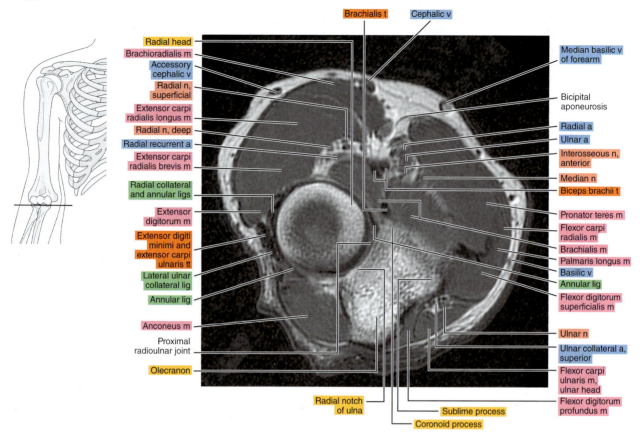

Brachialis t
Cephalic v
Radial head
Brachioradialis m
Accessory cephalic v
Radial n, superficial
Extensor carpi radialis longus m
Radial n, deep
Radial recurrent a
Extensor carpi radialis brevis m
Radial collateral and annular ligs
Extensor digitorum m
Extensor digiti minimi and extensor carpi ulnaris tt
Lateral ulnar collateral lig
Annular lig
Anconeus m
Proximal radioulnar joint
Olecranon
Radial notch of ulna
Coronoid process
Sublime process

Median basilic v of forearm
Bicipital aponeurosis
Radial a
Ulnar a
Interosseous n, anterior
Median n
Biceps brachii t
Pronator teres m
Flexor carpi radialis m
Brachialis m
Palmaris longus m
Basilic v
Annular lig
Flexor digitorum superficialis m
Ulnar n
Ulnar collateral a, superior
Flexor carpi ulnaris m, ulnar head
Flexor digitorum profundus m

Figure 9.1.11

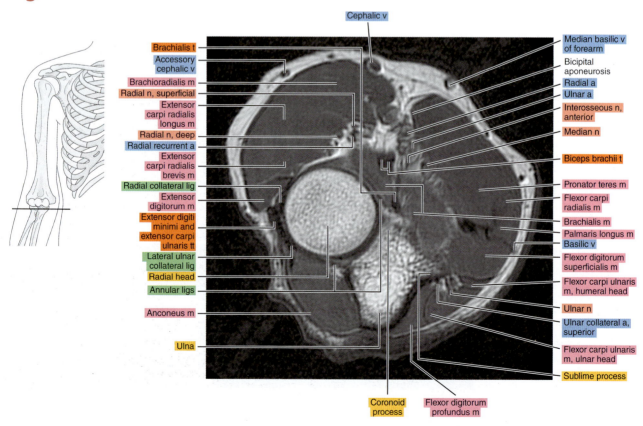

Cephalic v
Brachialis t
Accessory cephalic v
Brachioradialis m
Radial n, superficial
Extensor carpi radialis longus m
Radial n, deep
Radial recurrent a
Extensor carpi radialis brevis m
Radial collateral lig
Extensor digitorum m
Extensor digiti minimi and extensor carpi ulnaris tt
Lateral ulnar collateral lig
Radial head
Annular ligs
Anconeus m
Ulna
Coronoid process
Flexor digitorum profundus m

Median basilic v of forearm
Bicipital aponeurosis
Radial a
Ulnar a
Interosseous n, anterior
Median n
Biceps brachii t
Pronator teres m
Flexor carpi radialis m
Brachialis m
Palmaris longus m
Basilic v
Flexor digitorum superficialis m
Flexor carpi ulnaris m, humeral head
Ulnar n
Ulnar collateral a, superior
Flexor carpi ulnaris m, ulnar head
Sublime process

Figure 9.1.12

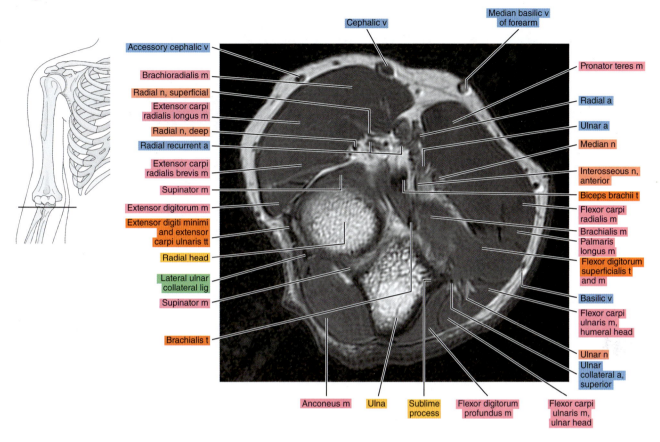

Cephalic v

Median basilic v of forearm

Accessory cephalic v

Pronator teres m

Brachioradialis m

Radial a

Radial n, superficial

Ulnar a

Extensor carpi radialis longus m

Median n

Radial n, deep

Interosseous n, anterior

Radial recurrent a

Biceps brachii t

Extensor carpi radialis brevis m

Flexor carpi radialis m

Supinator m

Brachialis m

Extensor digitorum m

Palmaris longus m

Extensor digiti minimi and extensor carpi ulnaris tt

Flexor digitorum superficialis t and m

Radial head

Lateral ulnar collateral lig

Basilic v

Supinator m

Flexor carpi ulnaris m, humeral head

Brachialis t

Ulnar n

Ulnar collateral a, superior

Anconeus m   Ulna   Sublime process   Flexor digitorum profundus m   Flexor carpi ulnaris m, ulnar head

Figure 9.1.13

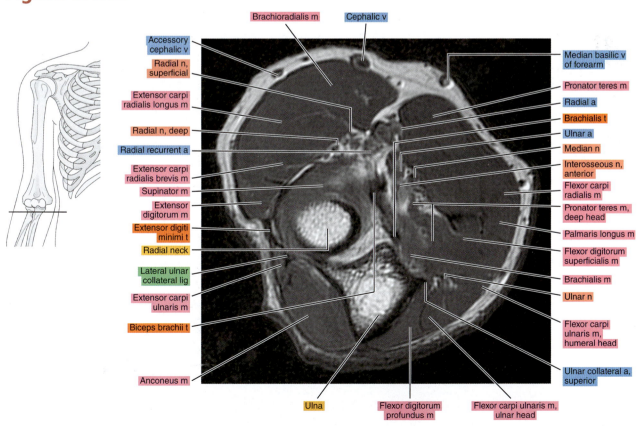

Brachioradialis m   Cephalic v

Accessory cephalic v

Median basilic v of forearm

Radial n, superficial

Pronator teres m

Extensor carpi radialis longus m

Radial a

Brachialis t

Radial n, deep

Ulnar a

Radial recurrent a

Median n

Extensor carpi radialis brevis m

Interosseous n, anterior

Supinator m

Flexor carpi radialis m

Extensor digitorum m

Pronator teres m, deep head

Extensor digiti minimi t

Palmaris longus m

Radial neck

Flexor digitorum superficialis m

Lateral ulnar collateral lig

Brachialis m

Extensor carpi ulnaris m

Ulnar n

Biceps brachii t

Flexor carpi ulnaris m, humeral head

Anconeus m

Ulnar collateral a, superior

Ulna   Flexor digitorum profundus m   Flexor carpi ulnaris m, ulnar head

Figure 9.1.14

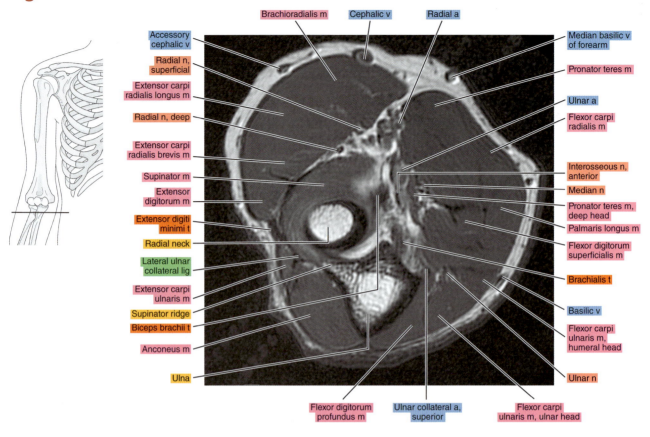

Brachioradialis m — Cephalic v — Radial a

Accessory cephalic v

Radial n, superficial

Extensor carpi radialis longus m

Radial n, deep

Extensor carpi radialis brevis m

Supinator m

Extensor digitorum m

Extensor digiti minimi t

Radial neck

Lateral ulnar collateral lig

Extensor carpi ulnaris m

Supinator ridge

Biceps brachii t

Anconeus m

Ulna

Median basilic v of forearm

Pronator teres m

Ulnar a

Flexor carpi radialis m

Interosseous n, anterior

Median n

Pronator teres m, deep head

Palmaris longus m

Flexor digitorum superficialis m

Brachialis t

Basilic v

Flexor carpi ulnaris m, humeral head

Ulnar n

Flexor digitorum profundus m — Ulnar collateral a, superior — Flexor carpi ulnaris m, ulnar head

Figure 9.1.15

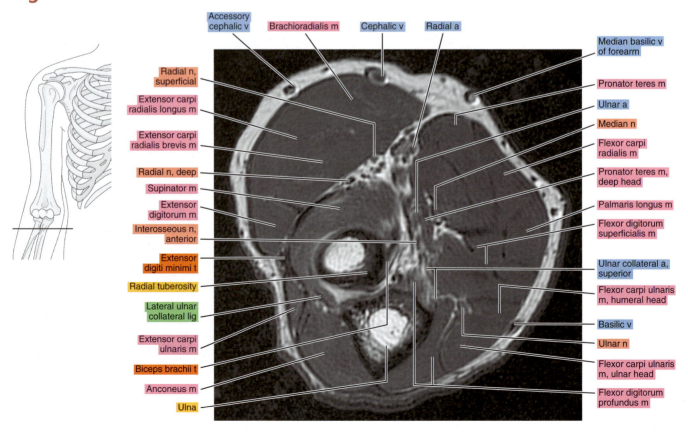

Accessory cephalic v — Brachioradialis m — Cephalic v — Radial a

Radial n, superficial

Extensor carpi radialis longus m

Extensor carpi radialis brevis m

Radial n, deep

Supinator m

Extensor digitorum m

Interosseous n, anterior

Extensor digiti minimi t

Radial tuberosity

Lateral ulnar collateral lig

Extensor carpi ulnaris m

Biceps brachii t

Anconeus m

Ulna

Median basilic v of forearm

Pronator teres m

Ulnar a

Median n

Flexor carpi radialis m

Pronator teres m, deep head

Palmaris longus m

Flexor digitorum superficialis m

Ulnar collateral a, superior

Flexor carpi ulnaris m, humeral head

Basilic v

Ulnar n

Flexor carpi ulnaris m, ulnar head

Flexor digitorum profundus m

Figure 9.1.16

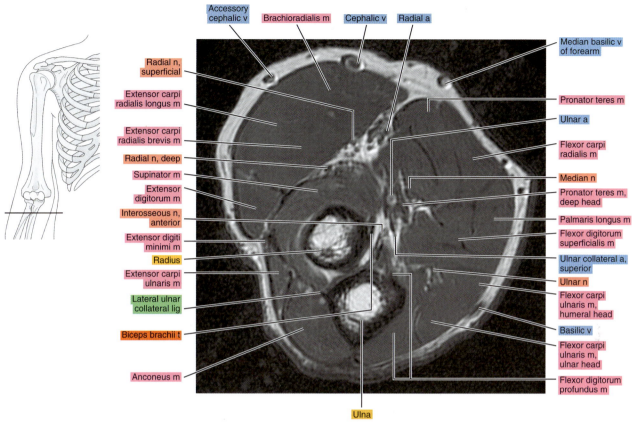

Accessory cephalic v
Brachioradialis m
Cephalic v
Radial a
Median basilic v of forearm
Radial n, superficial
Extensor carpi radialis longus m
Pronator teres m
Extensor carpi radialis brevis m
Ulnar a
Radial n, deep
Flexor carpi radialis m
Supinator m
Extensor digitorum m
Median n
Interosseous n, anterior
Pronator teres m, deep head
Extensor digiti minimi m
Palmaris longus m
Radius
Flexor digitorum superficialis m
Extensor carpi ulnaris m
Ulnar collateral a, superior
Lateral ulnar collateral lig
Ulnar n
Flexor carpi ulnaris m, humeral head
Biceps brachii t
Basilic v
Flexor carpi ulnaris m, ulnar head
Anconeus m
Flexor digitorum profundus m
Ulna

Figure 9.1.17

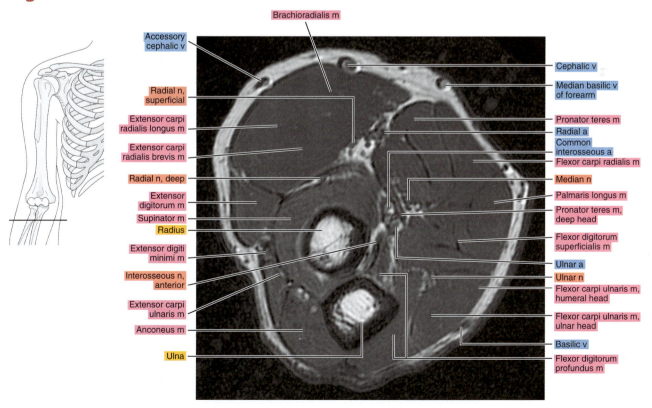

Brachioradialis m
Accessory cephalic v
Cephalic v
Radial n, superficial
Median basilic v of forearm
Extensor carpi radialis longus m
Pronator teres m
Radial a
Extensor carpi radialis brevis m
Common interosseous a
Flexor carpi radialis m
Radial n, deep
Median n
Extensor digitorum m
Palmaris longus m
Supinator m
Pronator teres m, deep head
Radius
Flexor digitorum superficialis m
Extensor digiti minimi m
Interosseous n, anterior
Ulnar a
Ulnar n
Flexor carpi ulnaris m, humeral head
Extensor carpi ulnaris m
Flexor carpi ulnaris m, ulnar head
Anconeus m
Basilic v
Ulna
Flexor digitorum profundus m

Figure 9.1.18

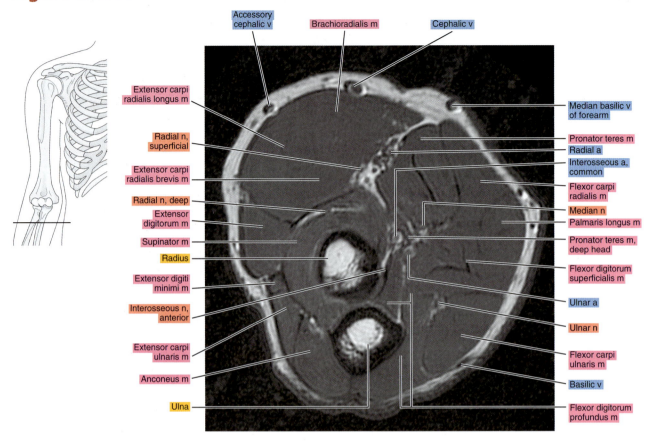

Figure 9.1.19

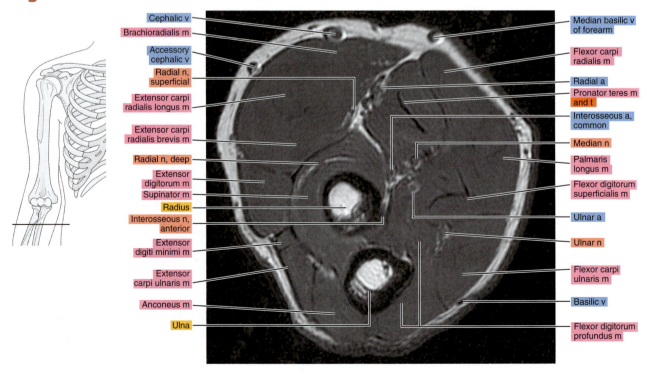

Figure 9.1.20

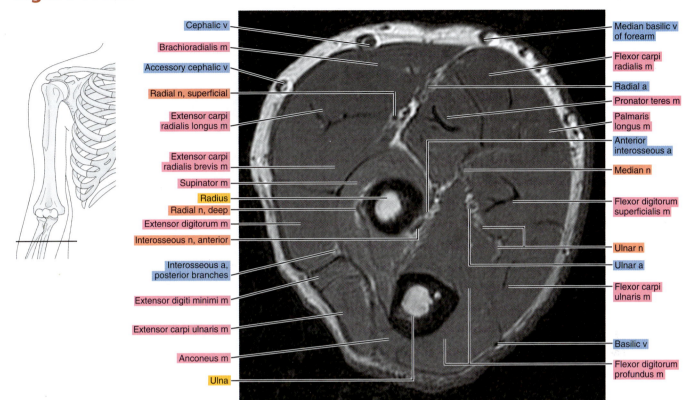

Cephalic v

Brachioradialis m

Accessory cephalic v

Radial n, superficial

Extensor carpi
radialis longus m

Extensor carpi
radialis brevis m

Supinator m

Radius

Radial n, deep

Extensor digitorum m

Interosseous n, anterior

Interosseous a,
posterior branches

Extensor digiti minimi m

Extensor carpi ulnaris m

Anconeus m

Ulna

Median basilic v
of forearm

Flexor carpi
radialis m

Radial a

Pronator teres m

Palmaris
longus m

Anterior
interosseous a

Median n

Flexor digitorum
superficialis m

Ulnar n

Ulnar a

Flexor carpi
ulnaris m

Basilic v

Flexor digitorum
profundus m

OBLIQUE SAGITTAL
Figure 9.2.1

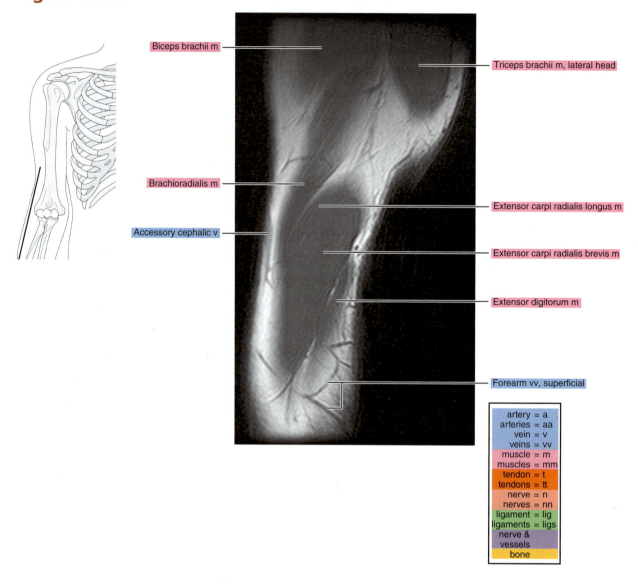

Biceps brachii m

Triceps brachii m, lateral head

Brachioradialis m

Extensor carpi radialis longus m

Accessory cephalic v

Extensor carpi radialis brevis m

Extensor digitorum m

Forearm vv, superficial

artery = a	
arteries = aa	
vein = v	
veins = vv	
muscle = m	
muscles = mm	
tendon = t	
tendons = tt	
nerve = n	
nerves = nn	
ligament = lig	
ligaments = ligs	
nerve & vessels	
bone	

Figure 9.2.2

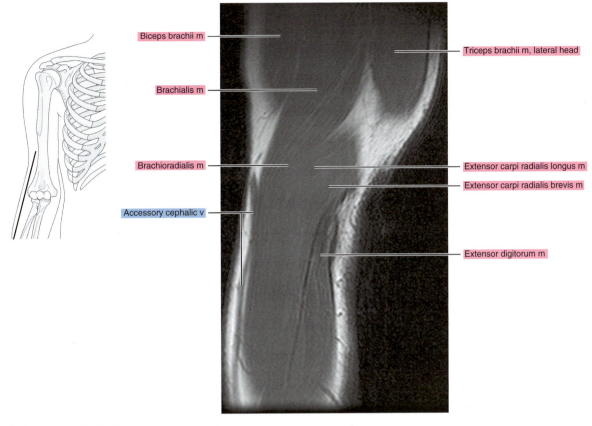

Biceps brachii m

Brachialis m

Brachioradialis m

Accessory cephalic v

Triceps brachii m, lateral head

Extensor carpi radialis longus m

Extensor carpi radialis brevis m

Extensor digitorum m

Figure 9.2.3

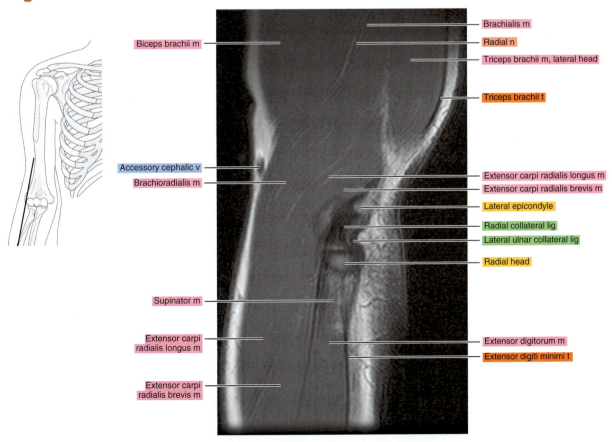

Biceps brachii m

Accessory cephalic v

Brachioradialis m

Supinator m

Extensor carpi
radialis longus m

Extensor carpi
radialis brevis m

Brachialis m

Radial n

Triceps brachii m, lateral head

Triceps brachii t

Extensor carpi radialis longus m

Extensor carpi radialis brevis m

Lateral epicondyle

Radial collateral lig

Lateral ulnar collateral lig

Radial head

Extensor digitorum m

Extensor digiti minimi t

Figure 9.2.4

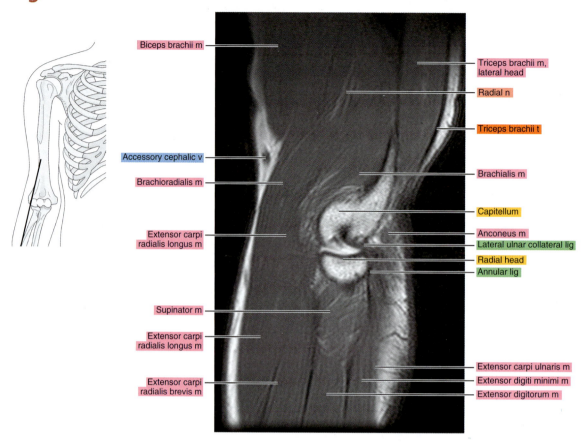

Biceps brachii m

Triceps brachii m, lateral head

Radial n

Triceps brachii t

Accessory cephalic v

Brachialis m

Brachioradialis m

Capitellum

Extensor carpi radialis longus m

Anconeus m

Lateral ulnar collateral lig

Radial head

Annular lig

Supinator m

Extensor carpi radialis longus m

Extensor carpi radialis brevis m

Extensor carpi ulnaris m

Extensor digiti minimi m

Extensor digitorum m

Figure 9.2.5

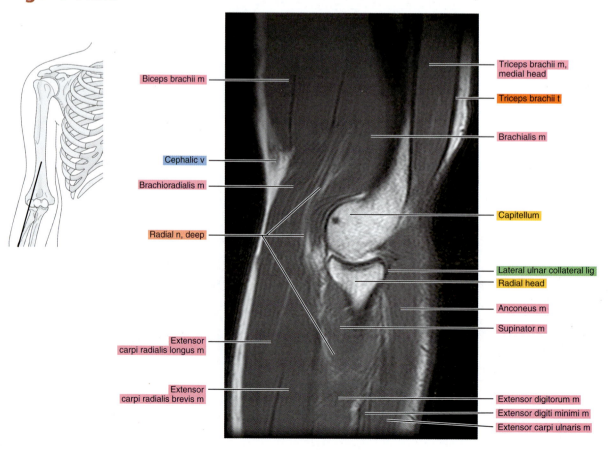

Biceps brachii m

Triceps brachii m, medial head

Triceps brachii t

Brachialis m

Cephalic v

Brachioradialis m

Capitellum

Radial n, deep

Lateral ulnar collateral lig

Radial head

Anconeus m

Supinator m

Extensor carpi radialis longus m

Extensor carpi radialis brevis m

Extensor digitorum m

Extensor digiti minimi m

Extensor carpi ulnaris m

Figure 9.2.6

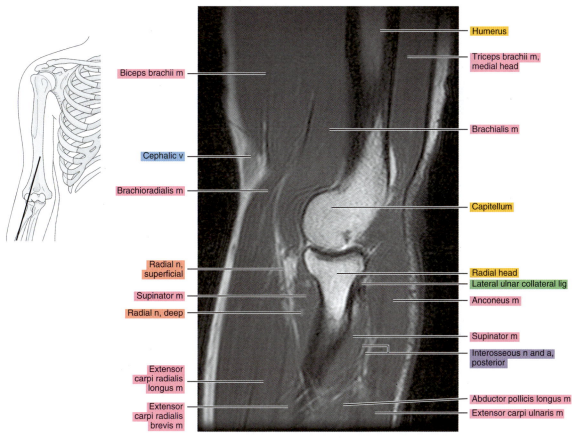

Humerus

Triceps brachii m, medial head

Biceps brachii m

Brachialis m

Cephalic v

Brachioradialis m

Capitellum

Radial n, superficial

Radial head
Lateral ulnar collateral lig

Supinator m

Anconeus m

Radial n, deep

Supinator m

Interosseous n and a, posterior

Extensor carpi radialis longus m

Extensor carpi radialis brevis m

Abductor pollicis longus m

Extensor carpi ulnaris m

Figure 9.2.7

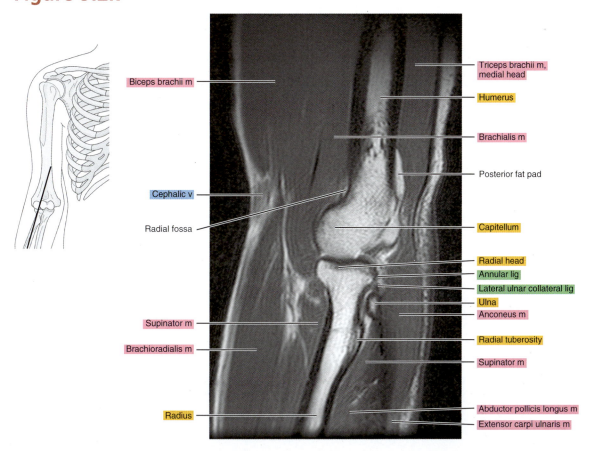

Triceps brachii m, medial head

Biceps brachii m

Humerus

Brachialis m

Posterior fat pad

Cephalic v

Radial fossa

Capitellum

Radial head
Annular lig
Lateral ulnar collateral lig
Ulna
Anconeus m

Supinator m

Radial tuberosity

Brachioradialis m

Supinator m

Radius

Abductor pollicis longus m

Extensor carpi ulnaris m

Figure 9.2.8

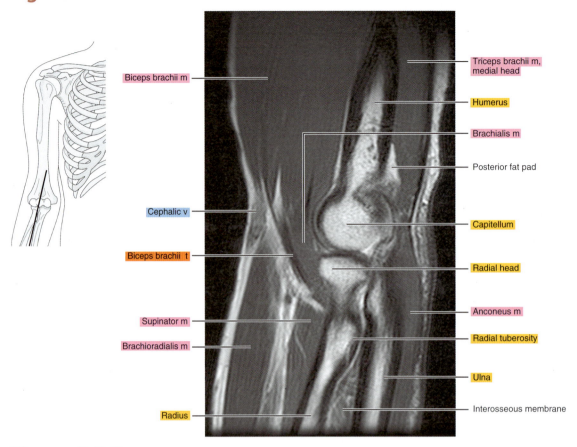

Biceps brachii m

Triceps brachii m, medial head

Humerus

Brachialis m

Posterior fat pad

Cephalic v

Capitellum

Biceps brachii t

Radial head

Supinator m

Anconeus m

Brachioradialis m

Radial tuberosity

Ulna

Radius

Interosseous membrane

Figure 9.2.9

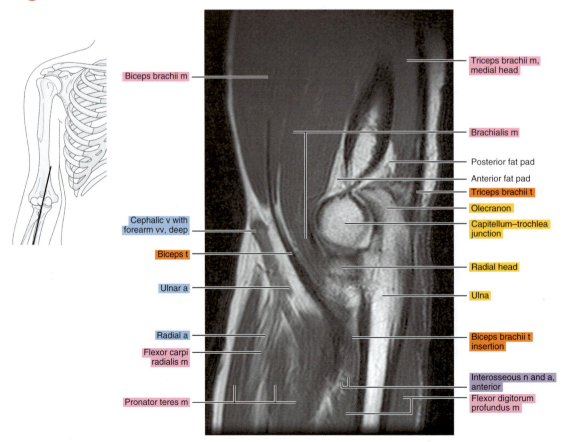

Biceps brachii m

Triceps brachii m, medial head

Brachialis m

Posterior fat pad

Anterior fat pad

Triceps brachii t

Olecranon

Cephalic v with forearm vv, deep

Capitellum–trochlea junction

Biceps t

Radial head

Ulnar a

Ulna

Radial a

Biceps brachii t insertion

Flexor carpi radialis m

Interosseous n and a, anterior

Pronator teres m

Flexor digitorum profundus m

Figure 9.2.10

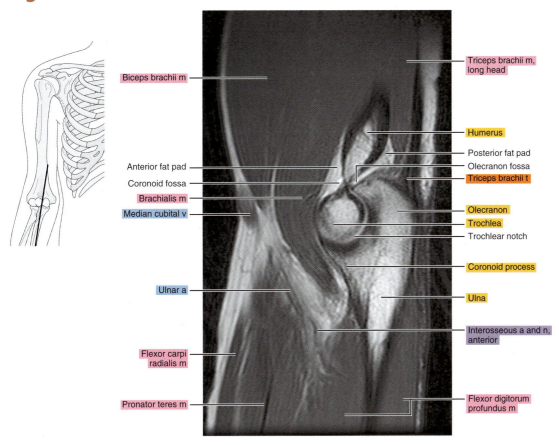

Biceps brachii m

Anterior fat pad
Coronoid fossa
Brachialis m
Median cubital v

Ulnar a

Flexor carpi
radialis m

Pronator teres m

Triceps brachii m,
long head

Humerus
Posterior fat pad
Olecranon fossa
Triceps brachii t

Olecranon
Trochlea
Trochlear notch

Coronoid process

Ulna

Interosseous a and n,
anterior

Flexor digitorum
profundus m

Figure 9.2.11

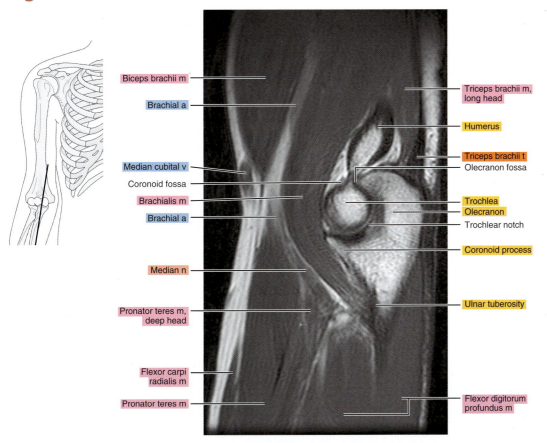

Biceps brachii m

Brachial a

Median cubital v
Coronoid fossa
Brachialis m
Brachial a

Median n

Pronator teres m,
deep head

Flexor carpi
radialis m

Pronator teres m

Triceps brachii m,
long head

Humerus

Triceps brachii t
Olecranon fossa

Trochlea
Olecranon
Trochlear notch

Coronoid process

Ulnar tuberosity

Flexor digitorum
profundus m

Figure 9.2.12

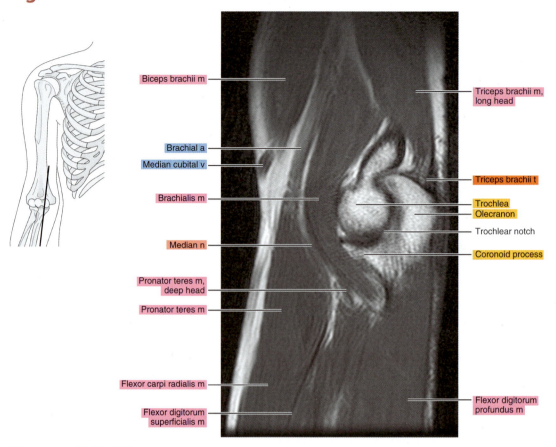

Biceps brachii m

Brachial a
Median cubital v

Brachialis m

Median n

Pronator teres m, deep head

Pronator teres m

Flexor carpi radialis m

Flexor digitorum superficialis m

Triceps brachii m, long head

Triceps brachii t

Trochlea
Olecranon
Trochlear notch
Coronoid process

Flexor digitorum profundus m

Figure 9.2.13

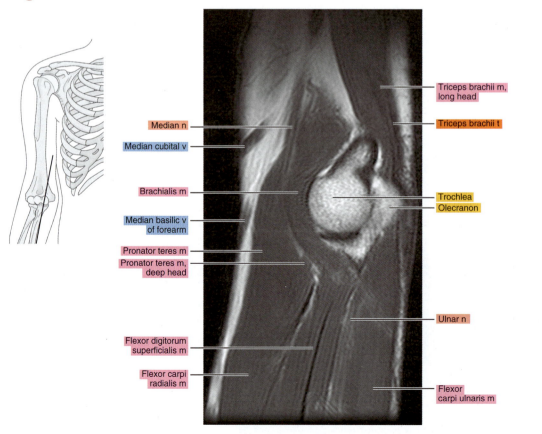

Median n

Median cubital v

Brachialis m

Median basilic v of forearm

Pronator teres m
Pronator teres m, deep head

Flexor digitorum superficialis m

Flexor carpi radialis m

Triceps brachii m, long head

Triceps brachii t

Trochlea
Olecranon

Ulnar n

Flexor carpi ulnaris m

Figure 9.2.14

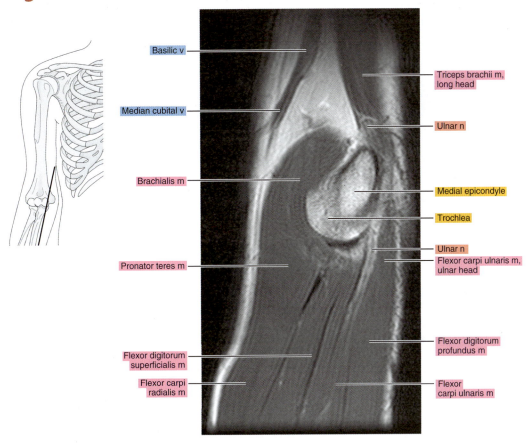

Basilic v

Median cubital v

Brachialis m

Pronator teres m

Flexor digitorum superficialis m

Flexor carpi radialis m

Triceps brachii m, long head

Ulnar n

Medial epicondyle

Trochlea

Ulnar n

Flexor carpi ulnaris m, ulnar head

Flexor digitorum profundus m

Flexor carpi ulnaris m

Figure 9.2.15

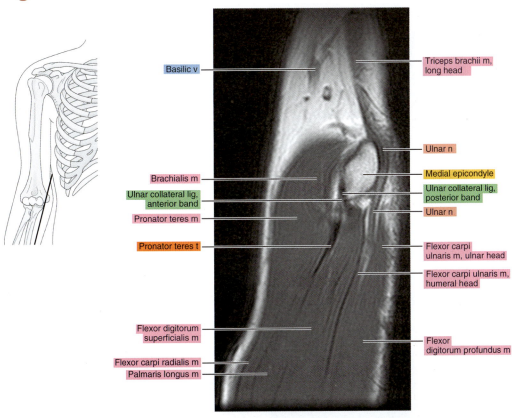

Basilic v

Brachialis m

Ulnar collateral lig, anterior band

Pronator teres m

Pronator teres t

Flexor digitorum superficialis m

Flexor carpi radialis m

Palmaris longus m

Triceps brachii m, long head

Ulnar n

Medial epicondyle

Ulnar collateral lig, posterior band

Ulnar n

Flexor carpi ulnaris m, ulnar head

Flexor carpi ulnaris m, humeral head

Flexor digitorum profundus m

Figure 9.2.16

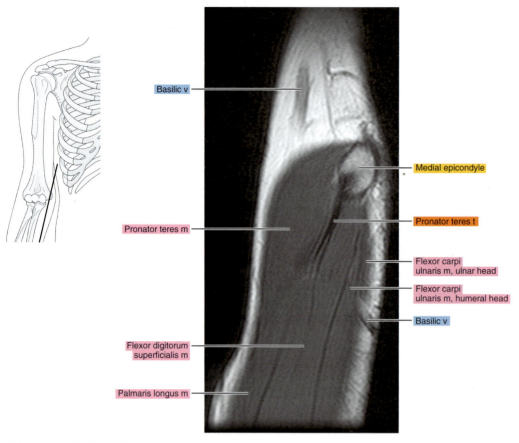

Basilic v

Medial epicondyle

Pronator teres m

Pronator teres t

Flexor carpi
ulnaris m, ulnar head

Flexor carpi
ulnaris m, humeral head

Basilic v

Flexor digitorum
superficialis m

Palmaris longus m

Figure 9.2.17

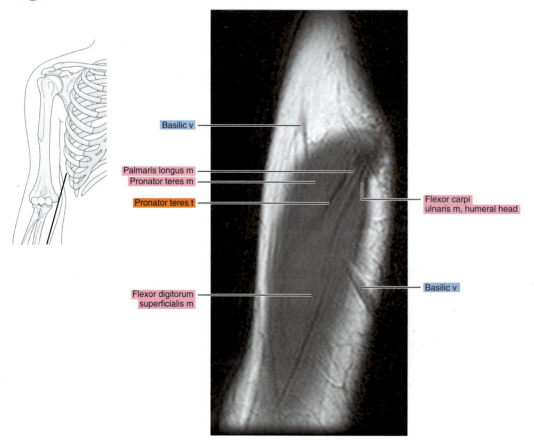

Basilic v

Palmaris longus m

Pronator teres m

Pronator teres t

Flexor carpi
ulnaris m, humeral head

Flexor digitorum
superficialis m

Basilic v

OBLIQUE CORONAL
Figure 9.3.1

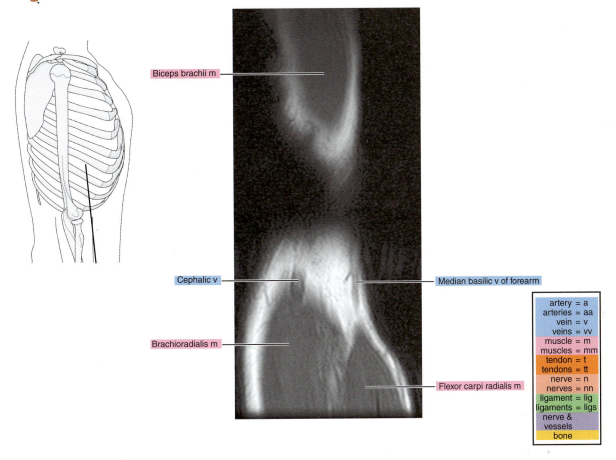

Biceps brachii m

Cephalic v

Median basilic v of forearm

Brachioradialis m

Flexor carpi radialis m

artery	= a
arteries	= aa
vein	= v
veins	= vv
muscle	= m
muscles	= mm
tendon	= t
tendons	= tt
nerve	= n
nerves	= nn
ligament	= lig
ligaments	= ligs
nerve & vessels	
bone	

Figure 9.3.2

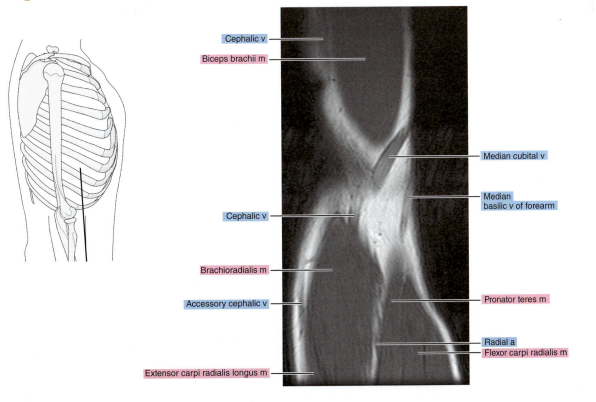

Cephalic v

Biceps brachii m

Median cubital v

Median basilic v of forearm

Cephalic v

Brachioradialis m

Accessory cephalic v

Pronator teres m

Radial a

Flexor carpi radialis m

Extensor carpi radialis longus m

Figure 9.3.3

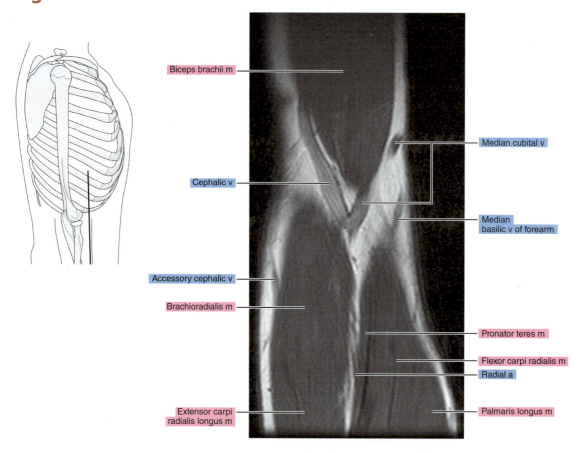

Biceps brachii m

Cephalic v

Accessory cephalic v

Brachioradialis m

Extensor carpi
radialis longus m

Median cubital v

Median
basilic v of forearm

Pronator teres m

Flexor carpi radialis m

Radial a

Palmaris longus m

Figure 9.3.4

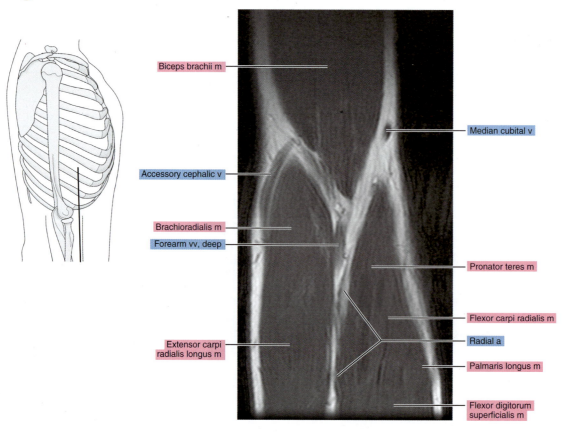

Biceps brachii m

Accessory cephalic v

Brachioradialis m

Forearm vv, deep

Extensor carpi
radialis longus m

Median cubital v

Pronator teres m

Flexor carpi radialis m

Radial a

Palmaris longus m

Flexor digitorum
superficialis m

Figure 9.3.5

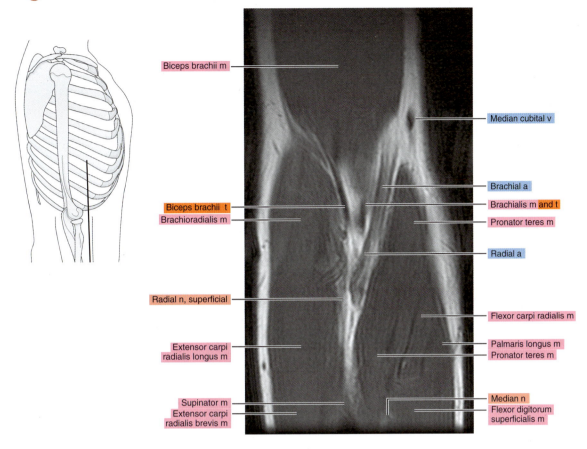

- Biceps brachii m
- Median cubital v
- Brachial a
- Biceps brachii t
- Brachialis m and t
- Brachioradialis m
- Pronator teres m
- Radial a
- Radial n, superficial
- Flexor carpi radialis m
- Extensor carpi radialis longus m
- Palmaris longus m
- Pronator teres m
- Supinator m
- Median n
- Extensor carpi radialis brevis m
- Flexor digitorum superficialis m

Figure 9.3.6

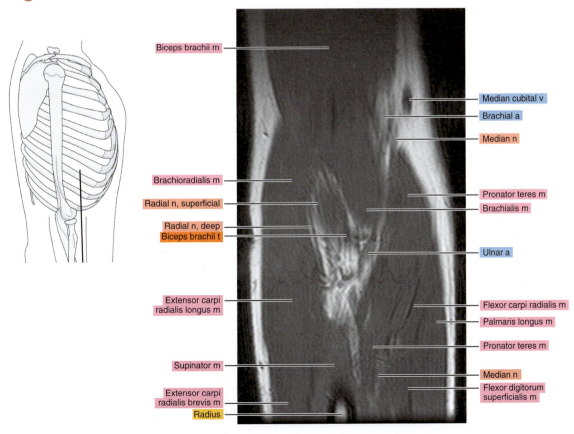

- Biceps brachii m
- Median cubital v
- Brachial a
- Median n
- Brachioradialis m
- Pronator teres m
- Radial n, superficial
- Brachialis m
- Radial n, deep
- Biceps brachii t
- Ulnar a
- Extensor carpi radialis longus m
- Flexor carpi radialis m
- Palmaris longus m
- Pronator teres m
- Supinator m
- Median n
- Extensor carpi radialis brevis m
- Flexor digitorum superficialis m
- Radius

Figure 9.3.7

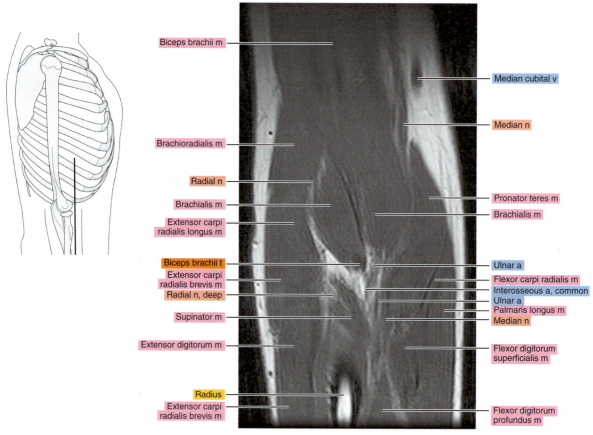

Biceps brachii m
Median cubital v
Median n
Brachioradialis m
Radial n
Pronator teres m
Brachialis m
Brachialis m
Extensor carpi radialis longus m
Biceps brachii t
Ulnar a
Extensor carpi radialis brevis m
Flexor carpi radialis m
Interosseous a, common
Radial n, deep
Ulnar a
Palmaris longus m
Supinator m
Median n
Extensor digitorum m
Flexor digitorum superficialis m
Radius
Extensor carpi radialis brevis m
Flexor digitorum profundus m

Figure 9.3.8

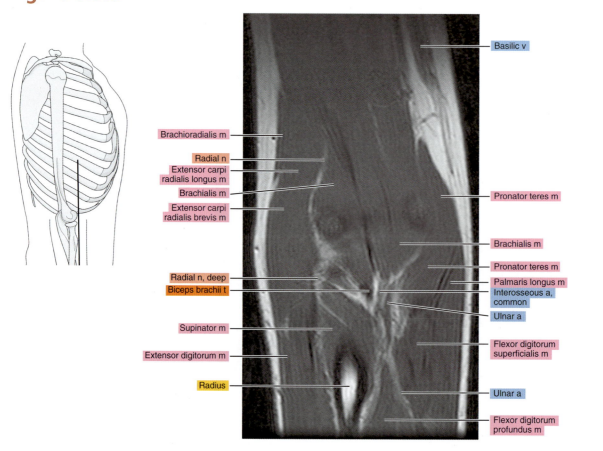

Basilic v
Brachioradialis m
Radial n
Extensor carpi radialis longus m
Brachialis m
Pronator teres m
Extensor carpi radialis brevis m
Brachialis m
Pronator teres m
Radial n, deep
Palmaris longus m
Biceps brachii t
Interosseous a, common
Ulnar a
Supinator m
Flexor digitorum superficialis m
Extensor digitorum m
Radius
Ulnar a
Flexor digitorum profundus m

Figure 9.3.9

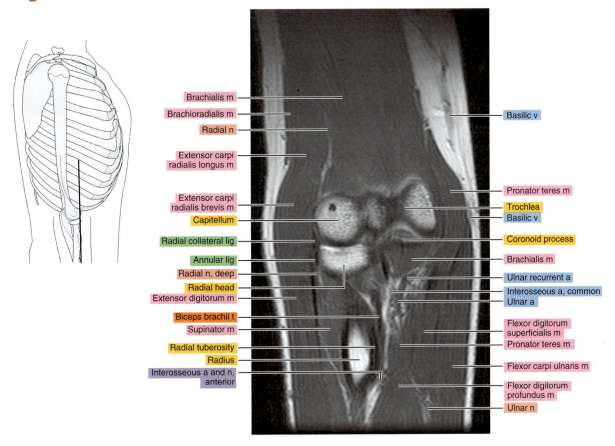

Brachialis m
Brachioradialis m
Radial n
Extensor carpi radialis longus m
Extensor carpi radialis brevis m
Capitellum
Radial collateral lig
Annular lig
Radial n, deep
Radial head
Extensor digitorum m
Biceps brachii t
Supinator m
Radial tuberosity
Radius
Interosseous a and n, anterior

Basilic v
Pronator teres m
Trochlea
Basilic v
Coronoid process
Brachialis m
Ulnar recurrent a
Interosseous a, common
Ulnar a
Flexor digitorum superficialis m
Pronator teres m
Flexor carpi ulnaris m
Flexor digitorum profundus m
Ulnar n

Figure 9.3.10

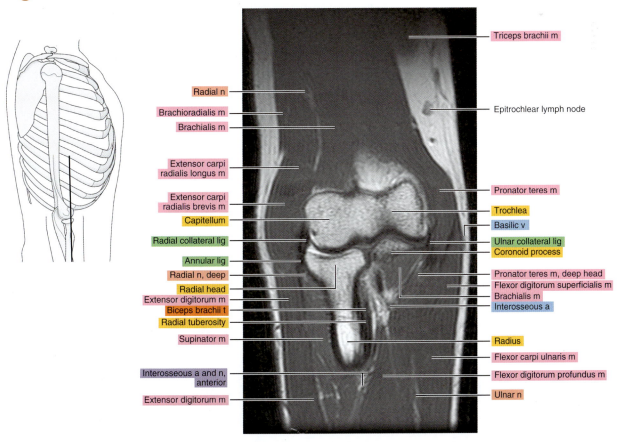

Radial n
Brachioradialis m
Brachialis m
Extensor carpi radialis longus m
Extensor carpi radialis brevis m
Capitellum
Radial collateral lig
Annular lig
Radial n, deep
Radial head
Extensor digitorum m
Biceps brachii t
Radial tuberosity
Supinator m
Interosseous a and n, anterior
Extensor digitorum m

Triceps brachii m
Epitrochlear lymph node
Pronator teres m
Trochlea
Basilic v
Ulnar collateral lig
Coronoid process
Pronator teres m, deep head
Flexor digitorum superficialis m
Brachialis m
Interosseous a
Radius
Flexor carpi ulnaris m
Flexor digitorum profundus m
Ulnar n

Figure 9.3.11

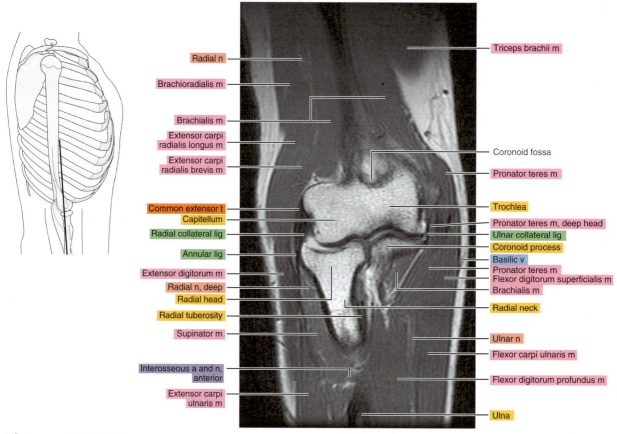

Radial n
Brachioradialis m
Brachialis m
Extensor carpi radialis longus m
Extensor carpi radialis brevis m
Common extensor t
Capitellum
Radial collateral lig
Annular lig
Extensor digitorum m
Radial n, deep
Radial head
Radial tuberosity
Supinator m
Interosseous a and n, anterior
Extensor carpi ulnaris m

Triceps brachii m
Coronoid fossa
Pronator teres m
Trochlea
Pronator teres m, deep head
Ulnar collateral lig
Coronoid process
Basilic v
Pronator teres m
Flexor digitorum superficialis m
Brachialis m
Radial neck
Ulnar n
Flexor carpi ulnaris m
Flexor digitorum profundus m
Ulna

Figure 9.3.12

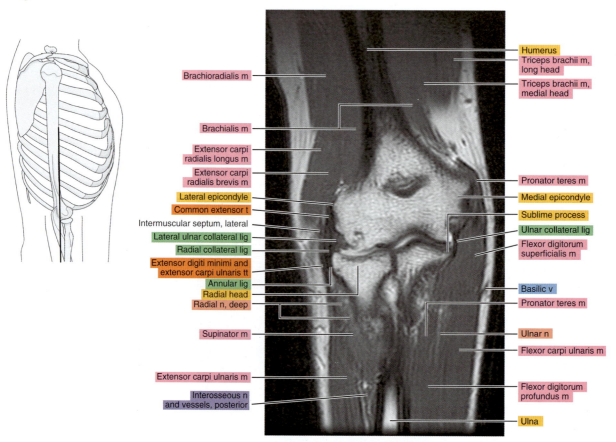

Brachioradialis m
Brachialis m
Extensor carpi radialis longus m
Extensor carpi radialis brevis m
Lateral epicondyle
Common extensor t
Intermuscular septum, lateral
Lateral ulnar collateral lig
Radial collateral lig
Extensor digiti minimi and extensor carpi ulnaris tt
Annular lig
Radial head
Radial n, deep
Supinator m
Extensor carpi ulnaris m
Interosseous n and vessels, posterior

Humerus
Triceps brachii m, long head
Triceps brachii m, medial head
Pronator teres m
Medial epicondyle
Sublime process
Ulnar collateral lig
Flexor digitorum superficialis m
Basilic v
Pronator teres m
Ulnar n
Flexor carpi ulnaris m
Flexor digitorum profundus m
Ulna

Figure 9.3.13

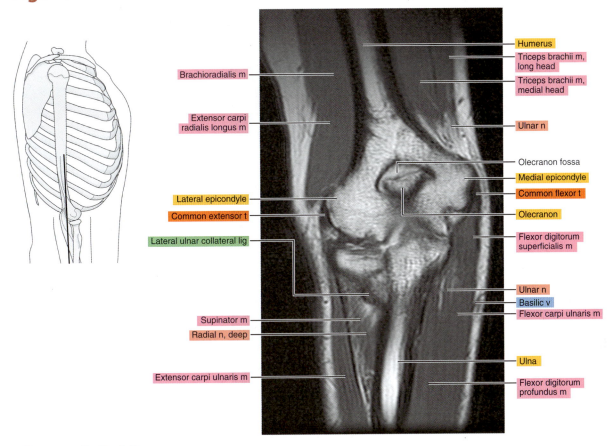

Brachioradialis m

Extensor carpi
radialis longus m

Lateral epicondyle

Common extensor t

Lateral ulnar collateral lig

Supinator m

Radial n, deep

Extensor carpi ulnaris m

Humerus

Triceps brachii m,
long head

Triceps brachii m,
medial head

Ulnar n

Olecranon fossa

Medial epicondyle

Common flexor t

Olecranon

Flexor digitorum
superficialis m

Ulnar n

Basilic v

Flexor carpi ulnaris m

Ulna

Flexor digitorum
profundus m

Figure 9.3.14

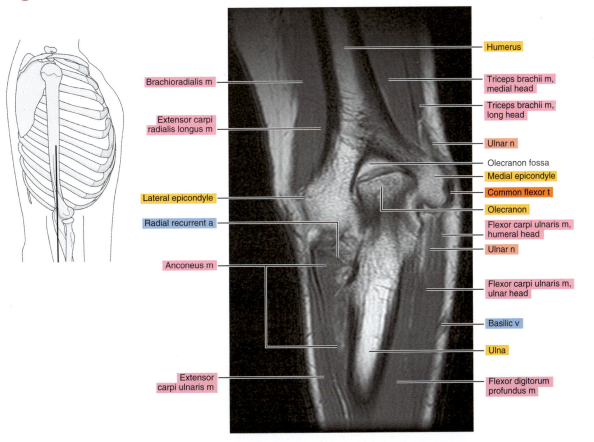

Brachioradialis m

Extensor carpi
radialis longus m

Lateral epicondyle

Radial recurrent a

Anconeus m

Extensor
carpi ulnaris m

Humerus

Triceps brachii m,
medial head

Triceps brachii m,
long head

Ulnar n

Olecranon fossa

Medial epicondyle

Common flexor t

Olecranon

Flexor carpi ulnaris m,
humeral head

Ulnar n

Flexor carpi ulnaris m,
ulnar head

Basilic v

Ulna

Flexor digitorum
profundus m

Figure 9.3.15

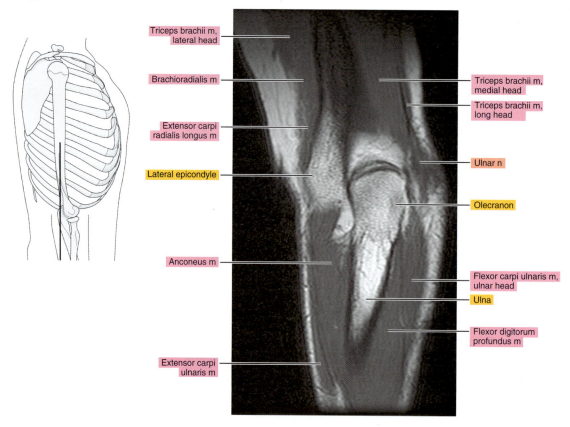

Triceps brachii m, lateral head

Brachioradialis m

Extensor carpi radialis longus m

Lateral epicondyle

Anconeus m

Extensor carpi ulnaris m

Triceps brachii m, medial head

Triceps brachii m, long head

Ulnar n

Olecranon

Flexor carpi ulnaris m, ulnar head

Ulna

Flexor digitorum profundus m

Figure 9.3.16

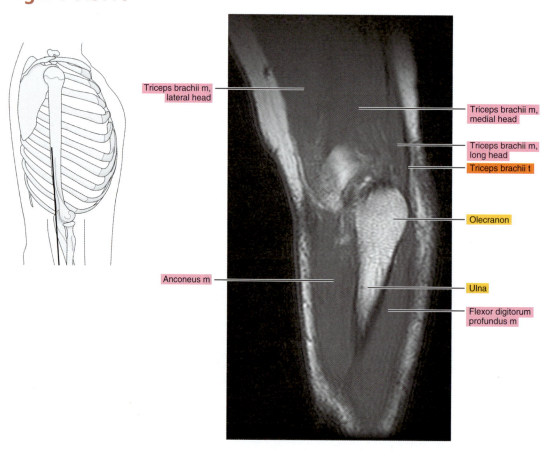

Triceps brachii m, lateral head

Anconeus m

Triceps brachii m, medial head

Triceps brachii m, long head

Triceps brachii t

Olecranon

Ulna

Flexor digitorum profundus m

Figure 9.3.17

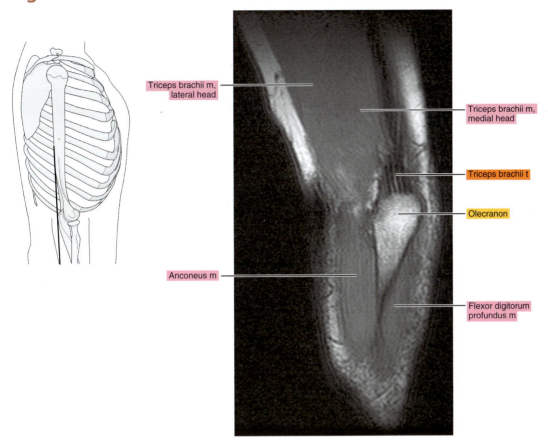

Triceps brachii m, lateral head

Triceps brachii m, medial head

Triceps brachii t

Olecranon

Anconeus m

Flexor digitorum profundus m

Chapter 10

MRI of the Forearm

AXIAL
Figure 10.1.1

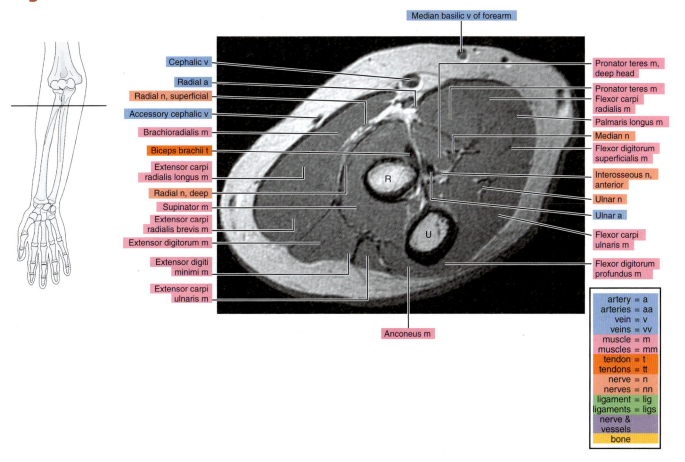

Median basilic v of forearm

Cephalic v
Radial a
Radial n, superficial
Accessory cephalic v
Brachioradialis m
Biceps brachii t
Extensor carpi radialis longus m
Radial n, deep
Supinator m
Extensor carpi radialis brevis m
Extensor digitorum m
Extensor digiti minimi m
Extensor carpi ulnaris m

Pronator teres m, deep head
Pronator teres m
Flexor carpi radialis m
Palmaris longus m
Median n
Flexor digitorum superficialis m
Interosseous n, anterior
Ulnar n
Ulnar a
Flexor carpi ulnaris m
Flexor digitorum profundus m

R
U

Anconeus m

artery	= a
arteries	= aa
vein	= v
veins	= vv
muscle	= m
muscles	= mm
tendon	= t
tendons	= tt
nerve	= n
nerves	= nn
ligament	= lig
ligaments	= ligs
nerve & vessels	
bone	

Figure 10.1.2

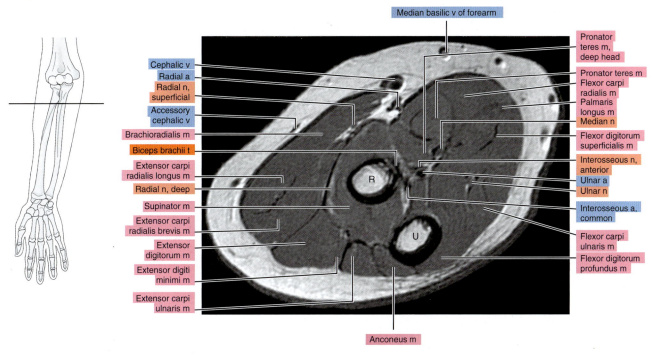

Median basilic v of forearm

Cephalic v
Radial a
Radial n, superficial
Accessory cephalic v
Brachioradialis m
Biceps brachii t
Extensor carpi radialis longus m
Radial n, deep
Supinator m
Extensor carpi radialis brevis m
Extensor digitorum m
Extensor digiti minimi m
Extensor carpi ulnaris m

Pronator teres m, deep head
Pronator teres m
Flexor carpi radialis m
Palmaris longus m
Median n
Flexor digitorum superficialis m
Interosseous n, anterior
Ulnar a
Ulnar n
Interosseous a, common
Flexor carpi ulnaris m
Flexor digitorum profundus m

R
U

Anconeus m

Figure 10.1.3

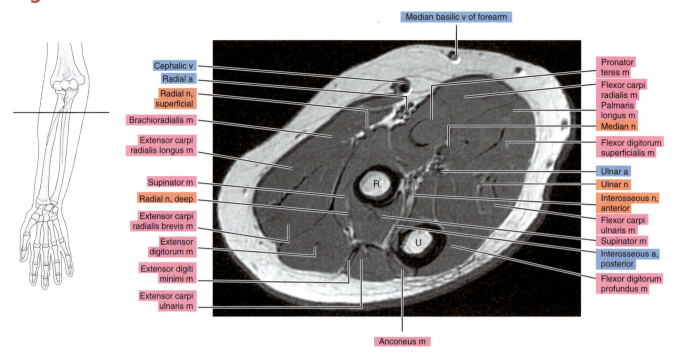

Labels for Figure 10.1.3:
- Median basilic v of forearm
- Cephalic v
- Radial a
- Radial n, superficial
- Brachioradialis m
- Extensor carpi radialis longus m
- Supinator m
- Radial n, deep
- Extensor carpi radialis brevis m
- Extensor digitorum m
- Extensor digiti minimi m
- Extensor carpi ulnaris m
- Pronator teres m
- Flexor carpi radialis m
- Palmaris longus m
- Median n
- Flexor digitorum superficialis m
- Ulnar a
- Ulnar n
- Interosseous n, anterior
- Flexor carpi ulnaris m
- Supinator m
- Interosseous a, posterior
- Flexor digitorum profundus m
- Anconeus m

Figure 10.1.4

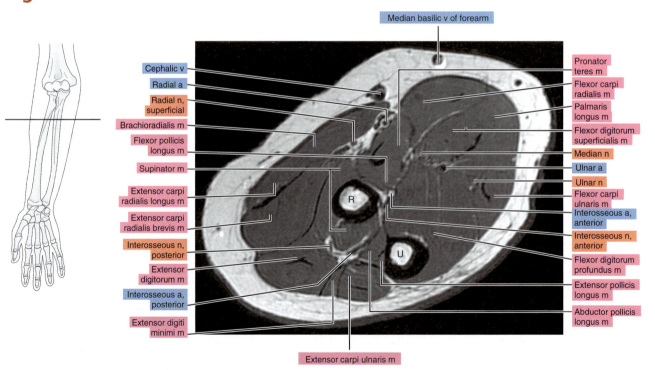

Labels for Figure 10.1.4:
- Median basilic v of forearm
- Cephalic v
- Radial a
- Radial n, superficial
- Brachioradialis m
- Flexor pollicis longus m
- Supinator m
- Extensor carpi radialis longus m
- Extensor carpi radialis brevis m
- Interosseous n, posterior
- Extensor digitorum m
- Interosseous a, posterior
- Extensor digiti minimi m
- Pronator teres m
- Flexor carpi radialis m
- Palmaris longus m
- Flexor digitorum superficialis m
- Median n
- Ulnar a
- Ulnar n
- Flexor carpi ulnaris m
- Interosseous a, anterior
- Interosseous n, anterior
- Flexor digitorum profundus m
- Extensor pollicis longus m
- Abductor pollicis longus m
- Extensor carpi ulnaris m

Figure 10.1.5

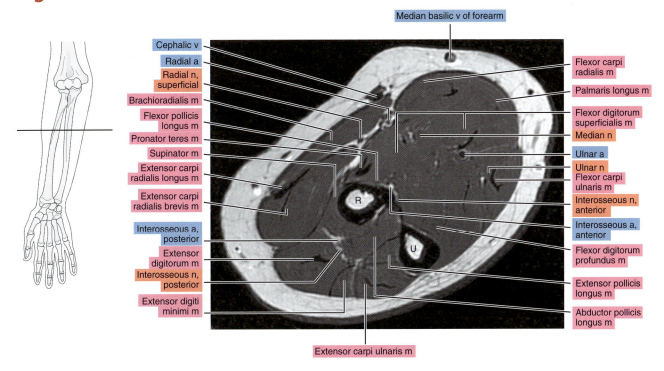

Median basilic v of forearm

Cephalic v

Radial a

Radial n, superficial

Brachioradialis m

Flexor pollicis longus m

Pronator teres m

Supinator m

Extensor carpi radialis longus m

Extensor carpi radialis brevis m

Interosseous a, posterior

Extensor digitorum m

Interosseous n, posterior

Extensor digiti minimi m

Flexor carpi radialis m

Palmaris longus m

Flexor digitorum superficialis m

Median n

Ulnar a

Ulnar n

Flexor carpi ulnaris m

Interosseous n, anterior

Interosseous a, anterior

Flexor digitorum profundus m

Extensor pollicis longus m

Abductor pollicis longus m

Extensor carpi ulnaris m

Figure 10.1.6

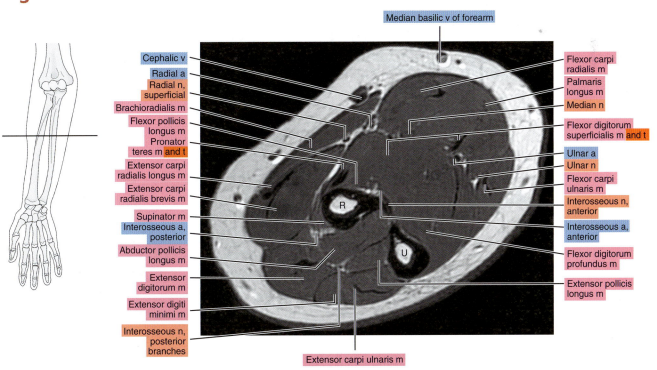

Median basilic v of forearm

Cephalic v

Radial a

Radial n, superficial

Brachioradialis m

Flexor pollicis longus m

Pronator teres m and t

Extensor carpi radialis longus m

Extensor carpi radialis brevis m

Supinator m

Interosseous a, posterior

Abductor pollicis longus m

Extensor digitorum m

Extensor digiti minimi m

Interosseous n, posterior branches

Flexor carpi radialis m

Palmaris longus m

Median n

Flexor digitorum superficialis m and t

Ulnar a

Ulnar n

Flexor carpi ulnaris m

Interosseous n, anterior

Interosseous a, anterior

Flexor digitorum profundus m

Extensor pollicis longus m

Extensor carpi ulnaris m

Figure 10.1.7

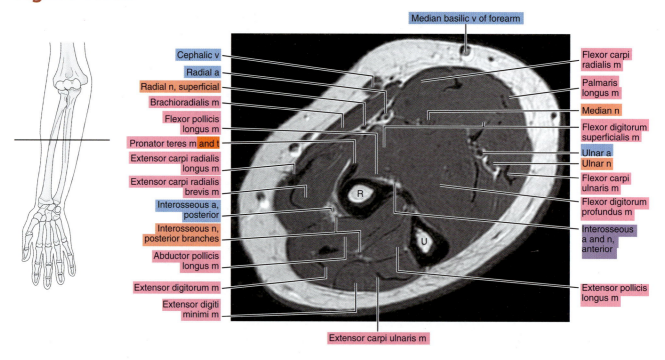

Median basilic v of forearm

Cephalic v

Radial a

Radial n, superficial

Brachioradialis m

Flexor pollicis longus m

Pronator teres m and t

Extensor carpi radialis longus m

Extensor carpi radialis brevis m

Interosseous a, posterior

Interosseous n, posterior branches

Abductor pollicis longus m

Extensor digitorum m

Extensor digiti minimi m

Extensor carpi ulnaris m

Flexor carpi radialis m

Palmaris longus m

Median n

Flexor digitorum superficialis m

Ulnar a

Ulnar n

Flexor carpi ulnaris m

Flexor digitorum profundus m

Interosseous a and n, anterior

Extensor pollicis longus m

R

U

Figure 10.1.8

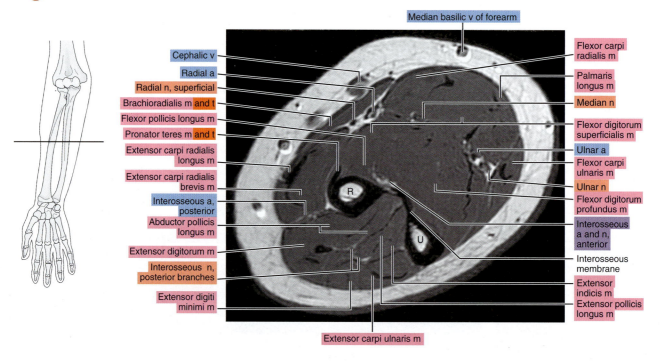

Median basilic v of forearm

Cephalic v

Radial a

Radial n, superficial

Brachioradialis m and t

Flexor pollicis longus m

Pronator teres m and t

Extensor carpi radialis longus m

Extensor carpi radialis brevis m

Interosseous a, posterior

Abductor pollicis longus m

Extensor digitorum m

Interosseous n, posterior branches

Extensor digiti minimi m

Extensor carpi ulnaris m

Flexor carpi radialis m

Palmaris longus m

Median n

Flexor digitorum superficialis m

Ulnar a

Flexor carpi ulnaris m

Ulnar n

Flexor digitorum profundus m

Interosseous a and n, anterior

Interosseous membrane

Extensor indicis m

Extensor pollicis longus m

R

U

Figure 10.1.9

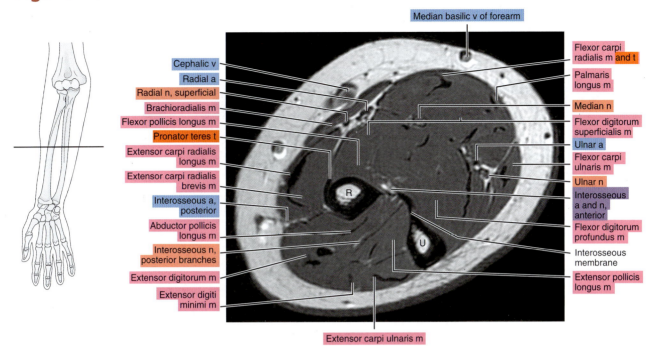

Median basilic v of forearm

Cephalic v
Radial a
Radial n, superficial
Brachioradialis m
Flexor pollicis longus m
Pronator teres t
Extensor carpi radialis longus m
Extensor carpi radialis brevis m
Interosseous a, posterior
Abductor pollicis longus m
Interosseous n, posterior branches
Extensor digitorum m
Extensor digiti minimi m

Flexor carpi radialis m and t
Palmaris longus m
Median n
Flexor digitorum superficialis m
Ulnar a
Flexor carpi ulnaris m
Ulnar n
Interosseous a and n, anterior
Flexor digitorum profundus m
Interosseous membrane
Extensor pollicis longus m

Extensor carpi ulnaris m

Figure 10.1.10

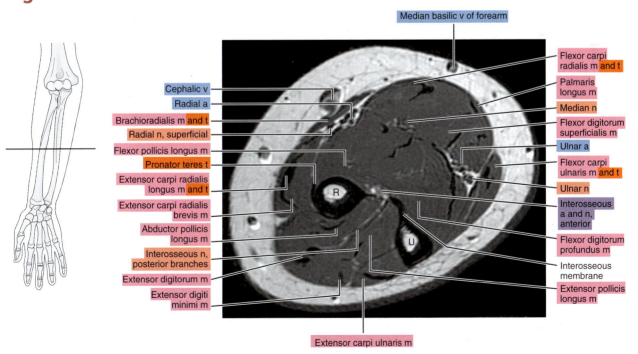

Median basilic v of forearm

Cephalic v
Radial a
Brachioradialis m and t
Radial n, superficial
Flexor pollicis longus m
Pronator teres t
Extensor carpi radialis longus m and t
Extensor carpi radialis brevis m
Abductor pollicis longus m
Interosseous n, posterior branches
Extensor digitorum m
Extensor digiti minimi m

Flexor carpi radialis m and t
Palmaris longus m
Median n
Flexor digitorum superficialis m
Ulnar a
Flexor carpi ulnaris m and t
Ulnar n
Interosseous a and n, anterior
Flexor digitorum profundus m
Interosseous membrane
Extensor pollicis longus m

Extensor carpi ulnaris m

Figure 10.1.11

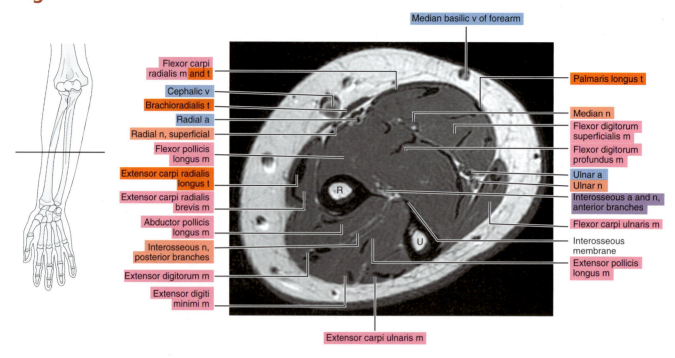

Median basilic v of forearm

Flexor carpi radialis m and t

Cephalic v

Brachioradialis t

Radial a

Radial n, superficial

Flexor pollicis longus m

Extensor carpi radialis longus t

Extensor carpi radialis brevis m

Abductor pollicis longus m

Interosseous n, posterior branches

Extensor digitorum m

Extensor digiti minimi m

Palmaris longus t

Median n

Flexor digitorum superficialis m

Flexor digitorum profundus m

Ulnar a

Ulnar n

Interosseous a and n, anterior branches

Flexor carpi ulnaris m

Interosseous membrane

Extensor pollicis longus m

Extensor carpi ulnaris m

Figure 10.1.12

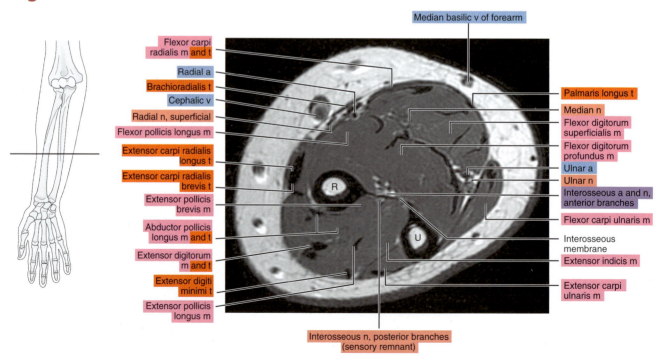

Median basilic v of forearm

Flexor carpi radialis m and t

Radial a

Brachioradialis t

Cephalic v

Radial n, superficial

Flexor pollicis longus m

Extensor carpi radialis longus t

Extensor carpi radialis brevis t

Extensor pollicis brevis m

Abductor pollicis longus m and t

Extensor digitorum m and t

Extensor digiti minimi t

Extensor pollicis longus m

Palmaris longus t

Median n

Flexor digitorum superficialis m

Flexor digitorum profundus m

Ulnar a

Ulnar n

Interosseous a and n, anterior branches

Flexor carpi ulnaris m

Interosseous membrane

Extensor indicis m

Extensor carpi ulnaris m

Interosseous n, posterior branches (sensory remnant)

Figure 10.1.13

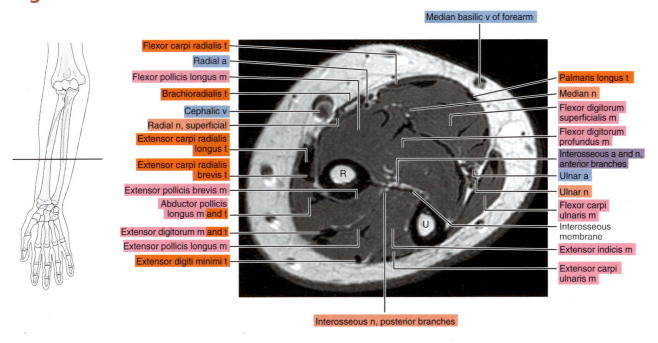

Flexor carpi radialis t
Radial a
Flexor pollicis longus m
Brachioradialis t
Cephalic v
Radial n, superficial
Extensor carpi radialis longus t
Extensor carpi radialis brevis t
Extensor pollicis brevis m
Abductor pollicis longus m and t
Extensor digitorum m and t
Extensor pollicis longus m
Extensor digiti minimi t

Median basilic v of forearm

Palmaris longus t
Median n
Flexor digitorum superficialis m
Flexor digitorum profundus m
Interosseous a and n, anterior branches
Ulnar a
Ulnar n
Flexor carpi ulnaris m
Interosseous membrane
Extensor indicis m
Extensor carpi ulnaris m

Interosseous n, posterior branches

Figure 10.1.14

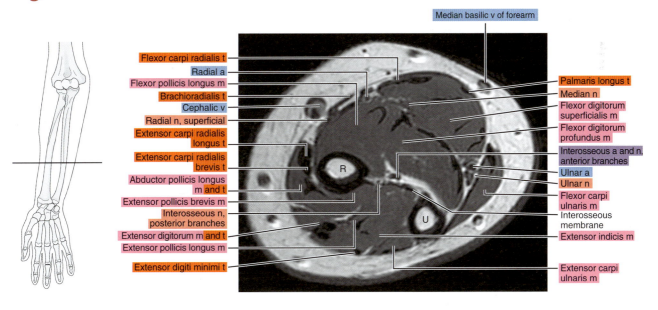

Flexor carpi radialis t
Radial a
Flexor pollicis longus m
Brachioradialis t
Cephalic v
Radial n, superficial
Extensor carpi radialis longus t
Extensor carpi radialis brevis t
Abductor pollicis longus m and t
Extensor pollicis brevis m
Interosseous n, posterior branches
Extensor digitorum m and t
Extensor pollicis longus m
Extensor digiti minimi t

Median basilic v of forearm

Palmaris longus t
Median n
Flexor digitorum superficialis m
Flexor digitorum profundus m
Interosseous a and n, anterior branches
Ulnar a
Ulnar n
Flexor carpi ulnaris m
Interosseous membrane
Extensor indicis m
Extensor carpi ulnaris m

Figure 10.1.15

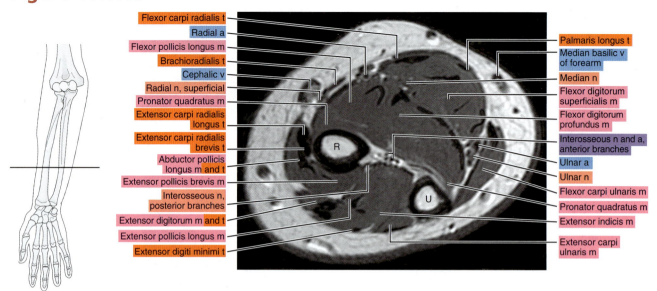

Flexor carpi radialis t
Radial a
Flexor pollicis longus m
Brachioradialis t
Cephalic v
Radial n, superficial
Pronator quadratus m
Extensor carpi radialis longus t
Extensor carpi radialis brevis t
Abductor pollicis longus m and t
Extensor pollicis brevis m
Interosseous n, posterior branches
Extensor digitorum m and t
Extensor pollicis longus m
Extensor digiti minimi t

Palmaris longus t
Median basilic v of forearm
Median n
Flexor digitorum superficialis m
Flexor digitorum profundus m
Interosseous n and a, anterior branches
Ulnar a
Ulnar n
Flexor carpi ulnaris m
Pronator quadratus m
Extensor indicis m
Extensor carpi ulnaris m

Figure 10.1.16

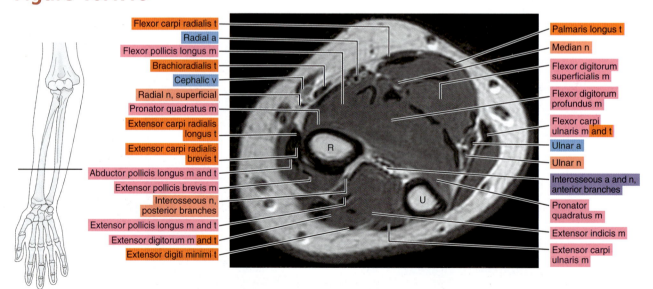

Flexor carpi radialis t
Radial a
Flexor pollicis longus m
Brachioradialis t
Cephalic v
Radial n, superficial
Pronator quadratus m
Extensor carpi radialis longus t
Extensor carpi radialis brevis t
Abductor pollicis longus m and t
Extensor pollicis brevis m
Interosseous n, posterior branches
Extensor pollicis longus m and t
Extensor digitorum m and t
Extensor digiti minimi t

Palmaris longus t
Median n
Flexor digitorum superficialis m
Flexor digitorum profundus m
Flexor carpi ulnaris m and t
Ulnar a
Ulnar n
Interosseous a and n, anterior branches
Pronator quadratus m
Extensor indicis m
Extensor carpi ulnaris m

Figure 10.1.17

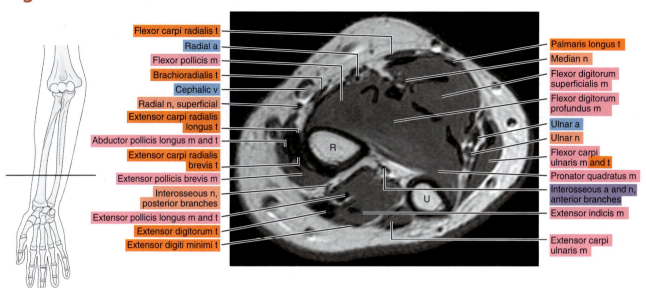

Flexor carpi radialis t
Radial a
Flexor pollicis m
Brachioradialis t
Cephalic v
Radial n, superficial
Extensor carpi radialis longus t
Abductor pollicis longus m and t
Extensor carpi radialis brevis t
Extensor pollicis brevis m
Interosseous n, posterior branches
Extensor pollicis longus m and t
Extensor digitorum t
Extensor digiti minimi t

Palmaris longus t
Median n
Flexor digitorum superficialis m
Flexor digitorum profundus m
Ulnar a
Ulnar n
Flexor carpi ulnaris m and t
Pronator quadratus m
Interosseous a and n, anterior branches
Extensor indicis m
Extensor carpi ulnaris m

R
U

Figure 10.1.18

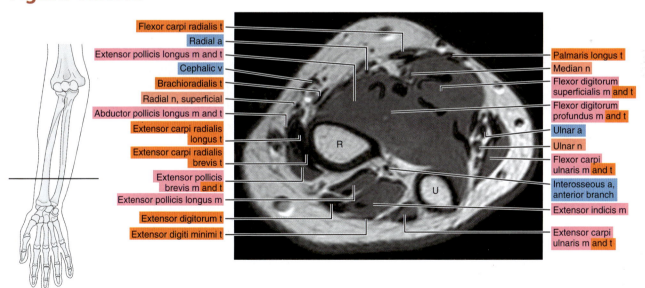

Flexor carpi radialis t
Radial a
Extensor pollicis longus m and t
Cephalic v
Brachioradialis t
Radial n, superficial
Abductor pollicis longus m and t
Extensor carpi radialis longus t
Extensor carpi radialis brevis t
Extensor pollicis brevis m and t
Extensor pollicis longus m
Extensor digitorum t
Extensor digiti minimi t

Palmaris longus t
Median n
Flexor digitorum superficialis m and t
Flexor digitorum profundus m and t
Ulnar a
Ulnar n
Flexor carpi ulnaris m and t
Interosseous a, anterior branch
Extensor indicis m
Extensor carpi ulnaris m and t

R
U

Figure 10.1.19

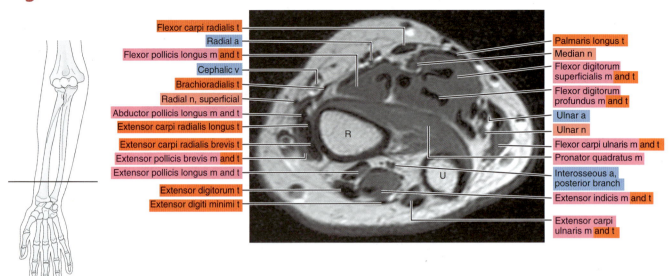

Flexor carpi radialis t
Radial a
Flexor pollicis longus m and t
Cephalic v
Brachioradialis t
Radial n, superficial
Abductor pollicis longus m and t
Extensor carpi radialis longus t
Extensor carpi radialis brevis t
Extensor pollicis brevis m and t
Extensor pollicis longus m and t
Extensor digitorum t
Extensor digiti minimi t

Palmaris longus t
Median n
Flexor digitorum superficialis m and t
Flexor digitorum profundus m and t
Ulnar a
Ulnar n
Flexor carpi ulnaris m and t
Pronator quadratus m
Interosseous a, posterior branch
Extensor indicis m and t
Extensor carpi ulnaris m and t

R
U

Figure 10.1.20

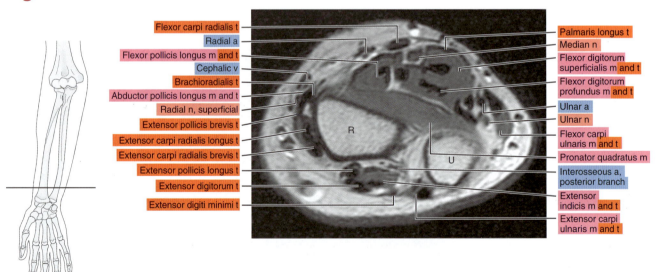

Flexor carpi radialis t
Radial a
Flexor pollicis longus m and t
Cephalic v
Brachioradialis t
Abductor pollicis longus m and t
Radial n, superficial
Extensor pollicis brevis t
Extensor carpi radialis longus t
Extensor carpi radialis brevis t
Extensor pollicis longus t
Extensor digitorum t
Extensor digiti minimi t

Palmaris longus t
Median n
Flexor digitorum superficialis m and t
Flexor digitorum profundus m and t
Ulnar a
Ulnar n
Flexor carpi ulnaris m and t
Pronator quadratus m
Interosseous a, posterior branch
Extensor indicis m and t
Extensor carpi ulnaris m and t

R
U

SAGITTAL
Figure 10.2.1

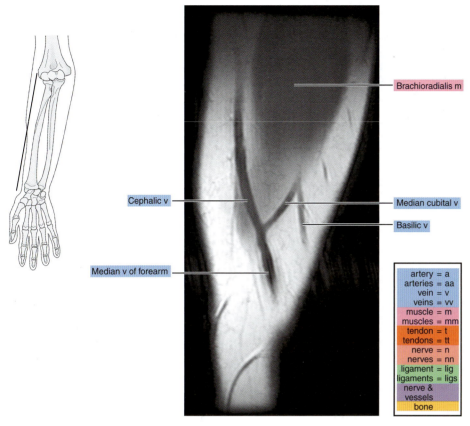

Brachioradialis m

Cephalic v

Median cubital v

Basilic v

Median v of forearm

artery = a	
arteries = aa	
vein = v	
veins = vv	
muscle = m	
muscles = mm	
tendon = t	
tendons = tt	
nerve = n	
nerves = nn	
ligament = lig	
ligaments = ligs	
nerve & vessels	
bone	

Figure 10.2.2

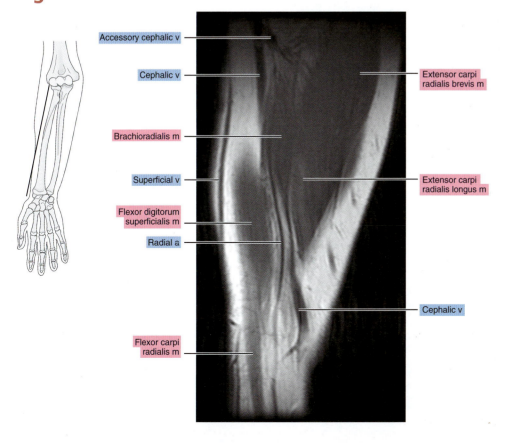

Accessory cephalic v

Cephalic v

Extensor carpi radialis brevis m

Brachioradialis m

Superficial v

Extensor carpi radialis longus m

Flexor digitorum superficialis m

Radial a

Cephalic v

Flexor carpi radialis m

Figure 10.2.3

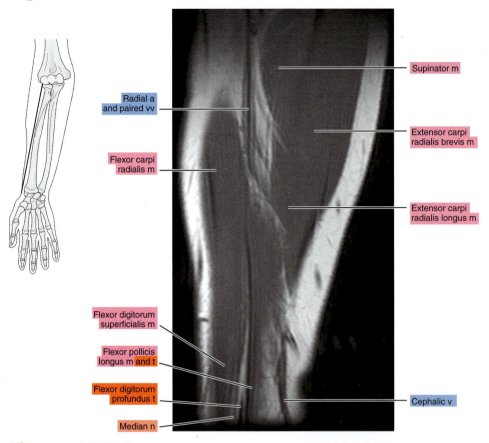

Supinator m

Radial a and paired vv

Extensor carpi radialis brevis m

Flexor carpi radialis m

Extensor carpi radialis longus m

Flexor digitorum superficialis m

Flexor pollicis longus m and t

Flexor digitorum profundus t

Cephalic v

Median n

Figure 10.2.4

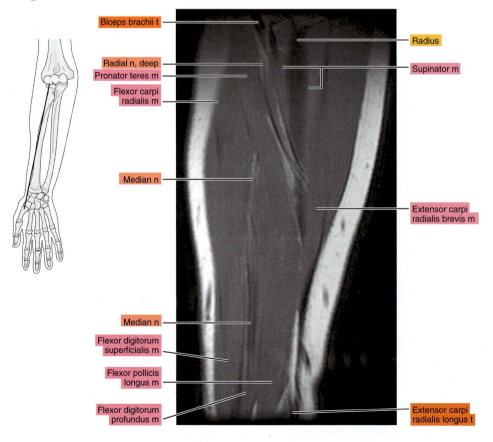

Biceps brachii t

Radius

Radial n, deep

Supinator m

Pronator teres m

Flexor carpi radialis m

Median n

Extensor carpi radialis brevis m

Median n

Flexor digitorum superficialis m

Flexor pollicis longus m

Flexor digitorum profundus m

Extensor carpi radialis longus t

Figure 10.2.5

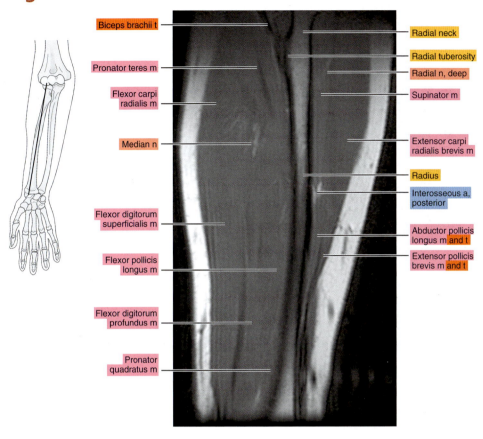

Biceps brachii t
Pronator teres m
Flexor carpi radialis m
Median n
Flexor digitorum superficialis m
Flexor pollicis longus m
Flexor digitorum profundus m
Pronator quadratus m

Radial neck
Radial tuberosity
Radial n, deep
Supinator m
Extensor carpi radialis brevis m
Radius
Interosseous a, posterior
Abductor pollicis longus m and t
Extensor pollicis brevis m and t

Figure 10.2.6

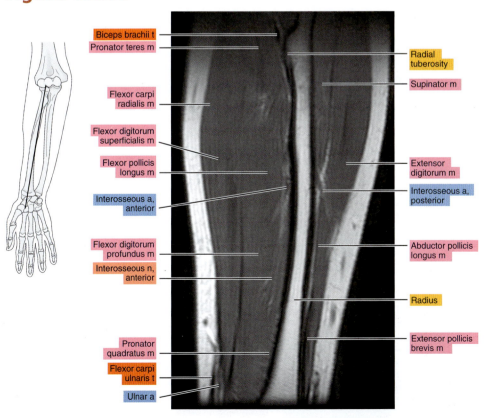

Biceps brachii t
Pronator teres m
Flexor carpi radialis m
Flexor digitorum superficialis m
Flexor pollicis longus m
Interosseous a, anterior
Flexor digitorum profundus m
Interosseous n, anterior
Pronator quadratus m
Flexor carpi ulnaris t
Ulnar a

Radial tuberosity
Supinator m
Extensor digitorum m
Interosseous a, posterior
Abductor pollicis longus m
Radius
Extensor pollicis brevis m

Figure 10.2.7

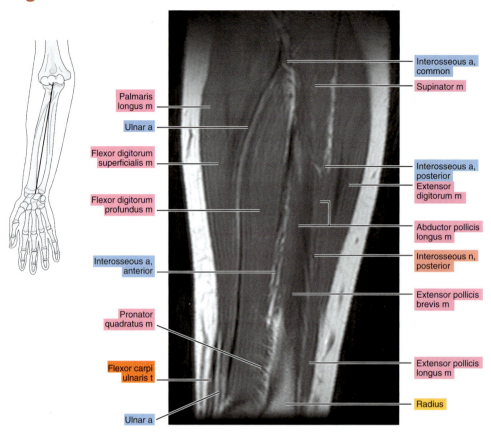

Palmaris longus m

Ulnar a

Flexor digitorum superficialis m

Flexor digitorum profundus m

Interosseous a, anterior

Pronator quadratus m

Flexor carpi ulnaris t

Ulnar a

Interosseous a, common

Supinator m

Interosseous a, posterior

Extensor digitorum m

Abductor pollicis longus m

Interosseous n, posterior

Extensor pollicis brevis m

Extensor pollicis longus m

Radius

Figure 10.2.8

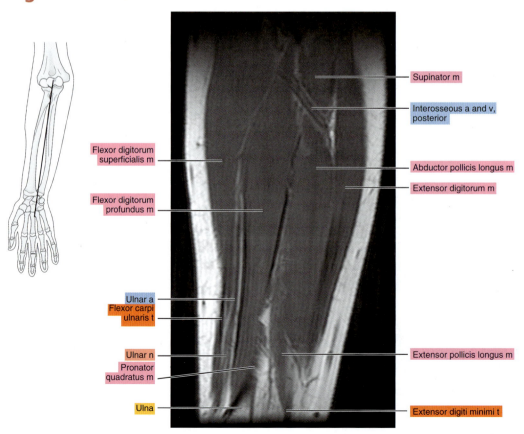

Flexor digitorum superficialis m

Flexor digitorum profundus m

Ulnar a

Flexor carpi ulnaris t

Ulnar n

Pronator quadratus m

Ulna

Supinator m

Interosseous a and v, posterior

Abductor pollicis longus m

Extensor digitorum m

Extensor pollicis longus m

Extensor digiti minimi t

Figure 10.2.9

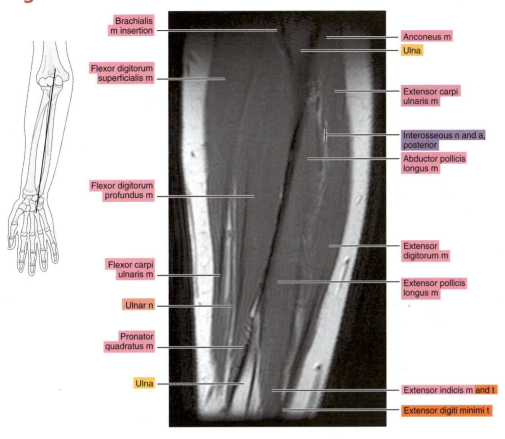

Brachialis m insertion

Flexor digitorum superficialis m

Flexor digitorum profundus m

Flexor carpi ulnaris m

Ulnar n

Pronator quadratus m

Ulna

Anconeus m

Ulna

Extensor carpi ulnaris m

Interosseous n and a, posterior

Abductor pollicis longus m

Extensor digitorum m

Extensor pollicis longus m

Extensor indicis m and t

Extensor digiti minimi t

Figure 10.2.10

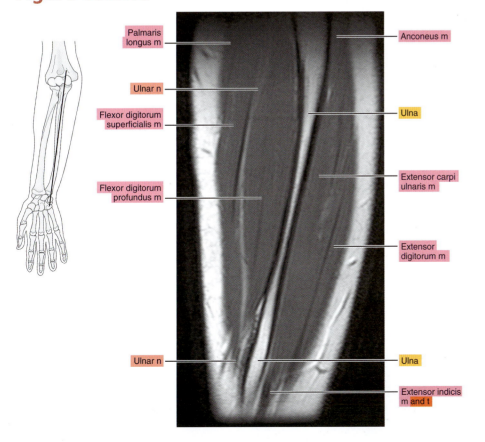

Palmaris longus m

Ulnar n

Flexor digitorum superficialis m

Flexor digitorum profundus m

Ulnar n

Anconeus m

Ulna

Extensor carpi ulnaris m

Extensor digitorum m

Ulna

Extensor indicis m and t

Figure 10.2.11

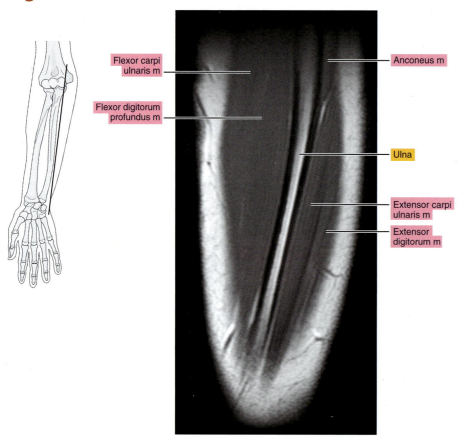

Flexor carpi ulnaris m

Flexor digitorum profundus m

Anconeus m

Ulna

Extensor carpi ulnaris m

Extensor digitorum m

Figure 10.2.12

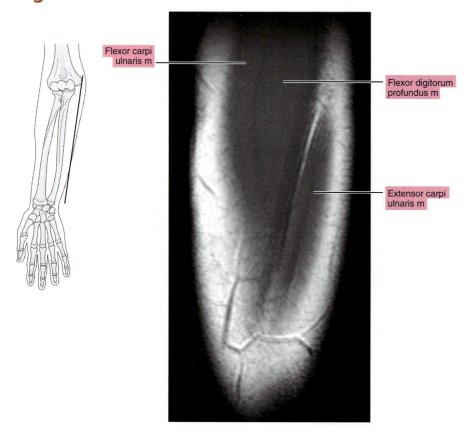

Flexor carpi ulnaris m

Flexor digitorum profundus m

Extensor carpi ulnaris m

CORONAL
Figure 10.3.1

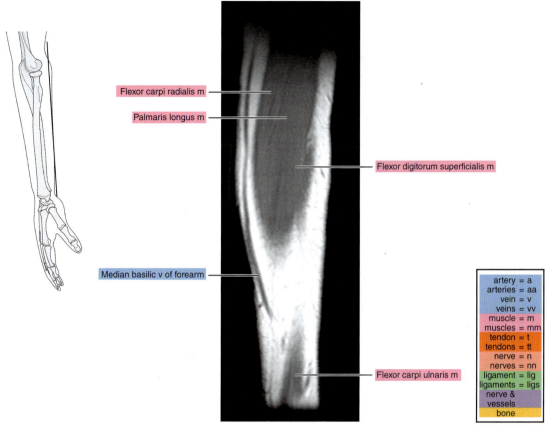

Flexor carpi radialis m

Palmaris longus m

Flexor digitorum superficialis m

Median basilic v of forearm

Flexor carpi ulnaris m

artery = a	
arteries = aa	
vein = v	
veins = vv	
muscle = m	
muscles = mm	
tendon = t	
tendons = tt	
nerve = n	
nerves = nn	
ligament = lig	
ligaments = ligs	
nerve & vessels	
bone	

Figure 10.3.2

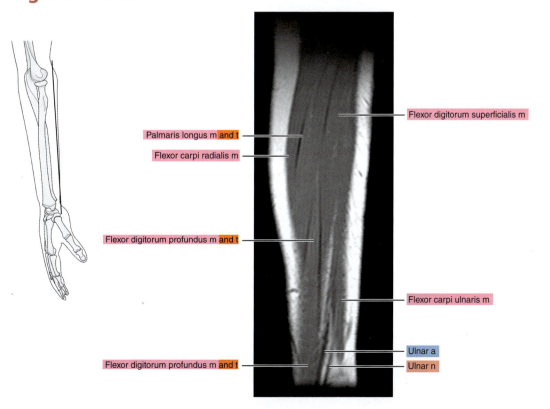

Flexor digitorum superficialis m

Palmaris longus m and t

Flexor carpi radialis m

Flexor digitorum profundus m and t

Flexor carpi ulnaris m

Ulnar a

Ulnar n

Flexor digitorum profundus m and t

Figure 10.3.3

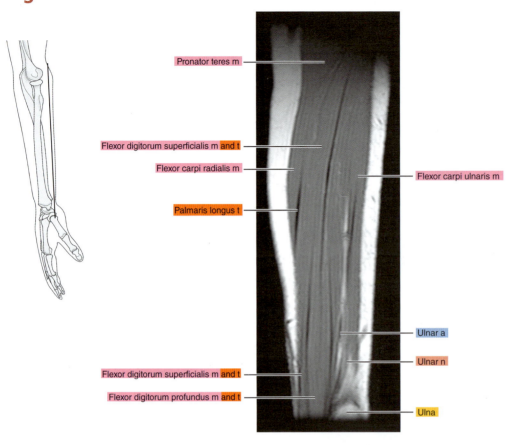

Pronator teres m

Flexor digitorum superficialis m and t

Flexor carpi radialis m

Palmaris longus t

Flexor carpi ulnaris m

Ulnar a

Ulnar n

Flexor digitorum superficialis m and t

Flexor digitorum profundus m and t

Ulna

Figure 10.3.4

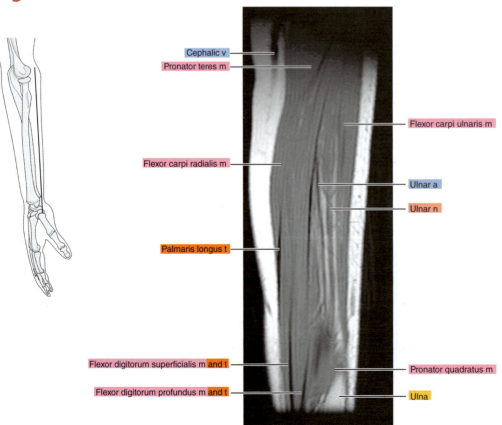

Cephalic v

Pronator teres m

Flexor carpi ulnaris m

Flexor carpi radialis m

Ulnar a

Ulnar n

Palmaris longus t

Flexor digitorum superficialis m and t

Pronator quadratus m

Flexor digitorum profundus m and t

Ulna

Figure 10.3.5

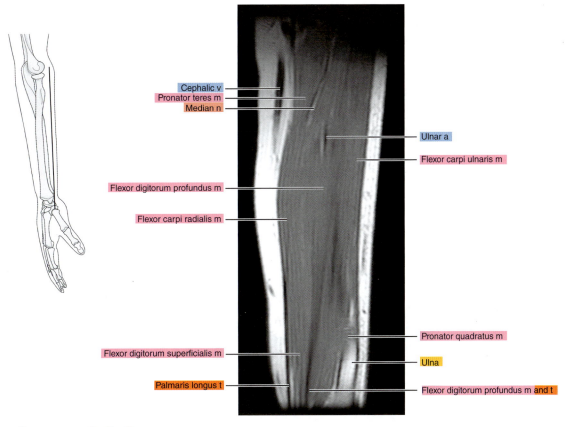

- Cephalic v
- Pronator teres m
- Median n
- Ulnar a
- Flexor carpi ulnaris m
- Flexor digitorum profundus m
- Flexor carpi radialis m
- Pronator quadratus m
- Flexor digitorum superficialis m
- Ulna
- Palmaris longus t
- Flexor digitorum profundus m and t

Figure 10.3.6

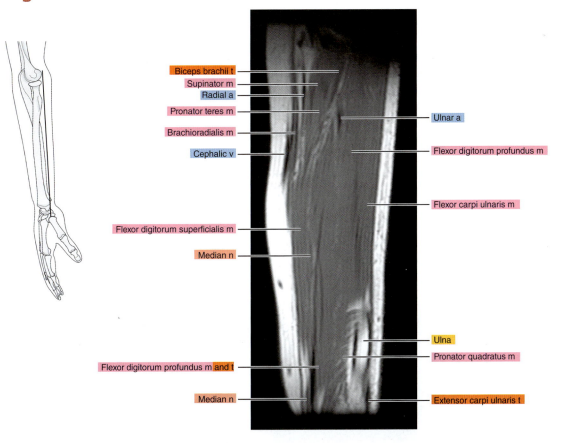

- Biceps brachii t
- Supinator m
- Radial a
- Pronator teres m
- Brachioradialis m
- Cephalic v
- Ulnar a
- Flexor digitorum profundus m
- Flexor carpi ulnaris m
- Flexor digitorum superficialis m
- Median n
- Flexor digitorum profundus m and t
- Ulna
- Pronator quadratus m
- Median n
- Extensor carpi ulnaris t

Figure 10.3.7

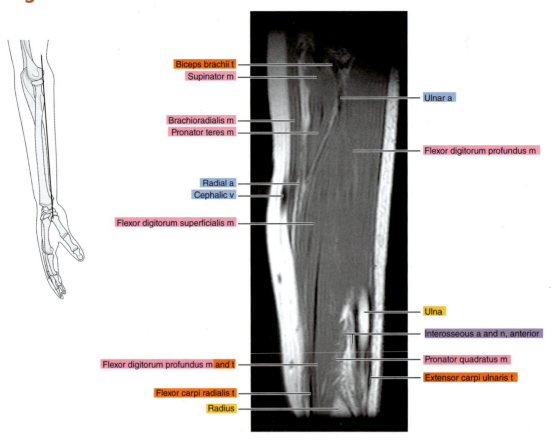

Biceps brachii t
Supinator m
Ulnar a
Brachioradialis m
Pronator teres m
Flexor digitorum profundus m
Radial a
Cephalic v
Flexor digitorum superficialis m
Ulna
Interosseous a and n, anterior
Flexor digitorum profundus m and t
Pronator quadratus m
Flexor carpi radialis t
Extensor carpi ulnaris t
Radius

Figure 10.3.8

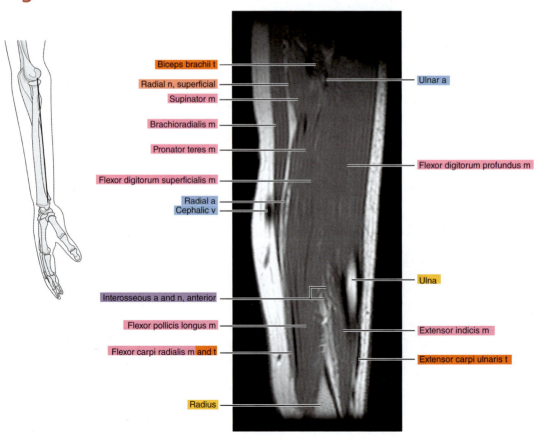

Biceps brachii t
Radial n, superficial
Supinator m
Ulnar a
Brachioradialis m
Pronator teres m
Flexor digitorum profundus m
Flexor digitorum superficialis m
Radial a
Cephalic v
Ulna
Interosseous a and n, anterior
Flexor pollicis longus m
Extensor indicis m
Flexor carpi radialis m and t
Extensor carpi ulnaris t
Radius

Figure 10.3.9

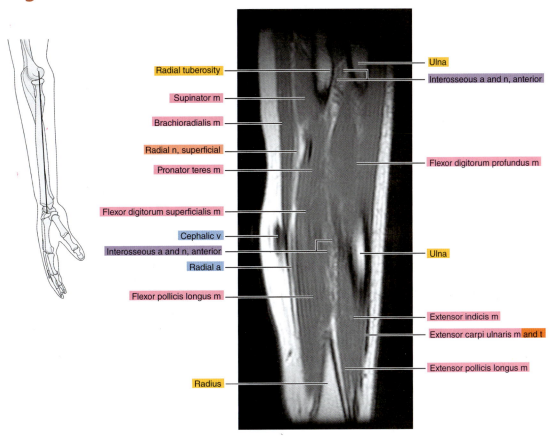

Radial tuberosity

Supinator m

Brachioradialis m

Radial n, superficial

Pronator teres m

Flexor digitorum superficialis m

Cephalic v

Interosseous a and n, anterior

Radial a

Flexor pollicis longus m

Radius

Ulna

Interosseous a and n, anterior

Flexor digitorum profundus m

Ulna

Extensor indicis m

Extensor carpi ulnaris m and t

Extensor pollicis longus m

Figure 10.3.10

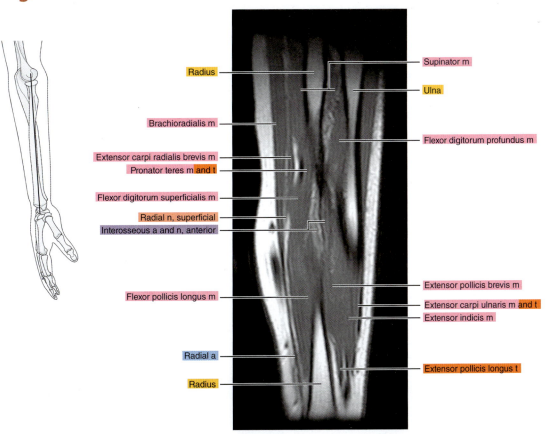

Radius

Brachioradialis m

Extensor carpi radialis brevis m

Pronator teres m and t

Flexor digitorum superficialis m

Radial n, superficial

Interosseous a and n, anterior

Flexor pollicis longus m

Radial a

Radius

Supinator m

Ulna

Flexor digitorum profundus m

Extensor pollicis brevis m

Extensor carpi ulnaris m and t

Extensor indicis m

Extensor pollicis longus t

Figure 10.3.11

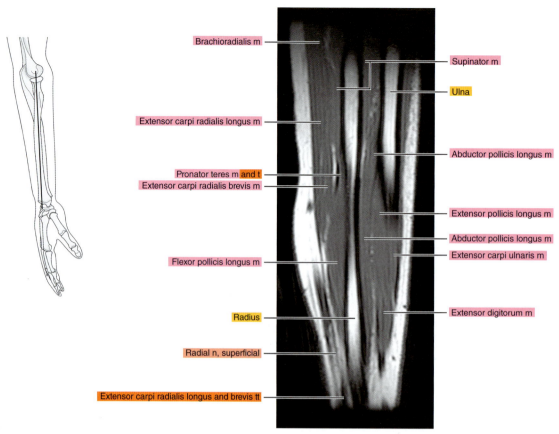

Brachioradialis m

Supinator m

Ulna

Extensor carpi radialis longus m

Abductor pollicis longus m

Pronator teres m and t
Extensor carpi radialis brevis m

Extensor pollicis longus m

Abductor pollicis longus m
Extensor carpi ulnaris m

Flexor pollicis longus m

Extensor digitorum m

Radius

Radial n, superficial

Extensor carpi radialis longus and brevis tt

Figure 10.3.12

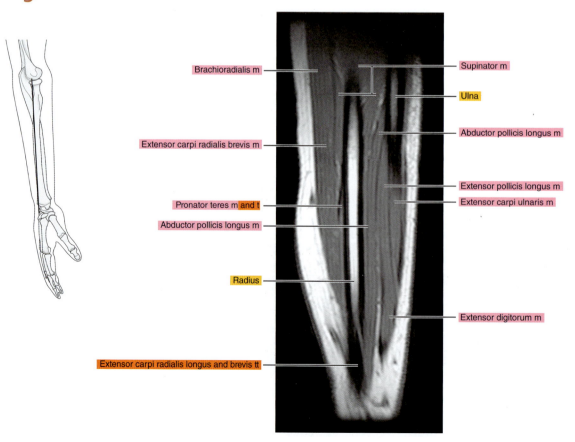

Brachioradialis m

Supinator m

Ulna

Abductor pollicis longus m

Extensor carpi radialis brevis m

Extensor pollicis longus m

Pronator teres m and t

Extensor carpi ulnaris m

Abductor pollicis longus m

Radius

Extensor digitorum m

Extensor carpi radialis longus and brevis tt

Figure 10.3.13

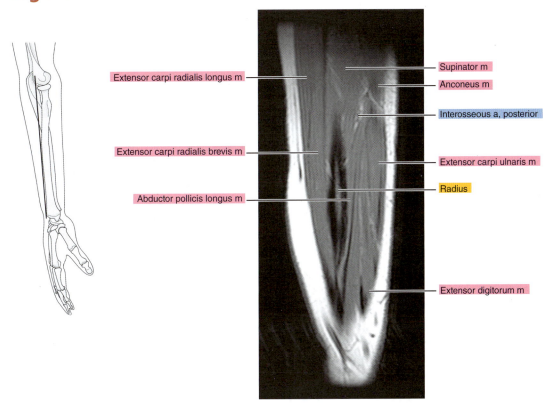

Extensor carpi radialis longus m

Extensor carpi radialis brevis m

Abductor pollicis longus m

Supinator m

Anconeus m

Interosseous a, posterior

Extensor carpi ulnaris m

Radius

Extensor digitorum m

Figure 10.3.14

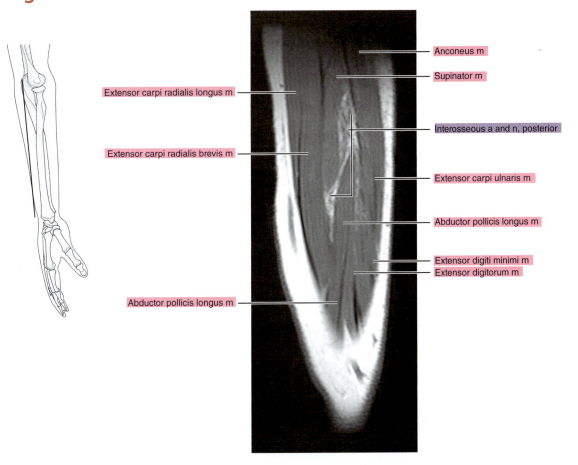

Extensor carpi radialis longus m

Extensor carpi radialis brevis m

Abductor pollicis longus m

Anconeus m

Supinator m

Interosseous a and n, posterior

Extensor carpi ulnaris m

Abductor pollicis longus m

Extensor digiti minimi m

Extensor digitorum m

Figure 10.3.15

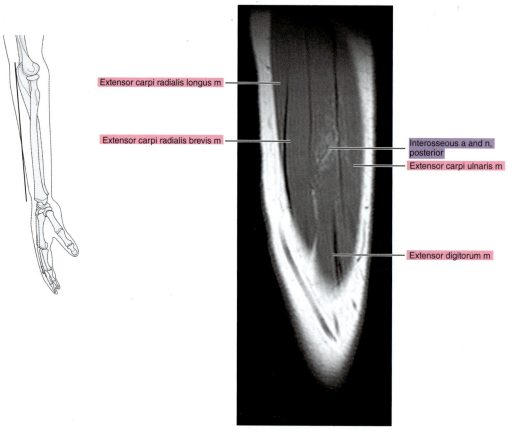

Extensor carpi radialis longus m

Extensor carpi radialis brevis m

Interosseous a and n, posterior

Extensor carpi ulnaris m

Extensor digitorum m

Figure 10.3.16

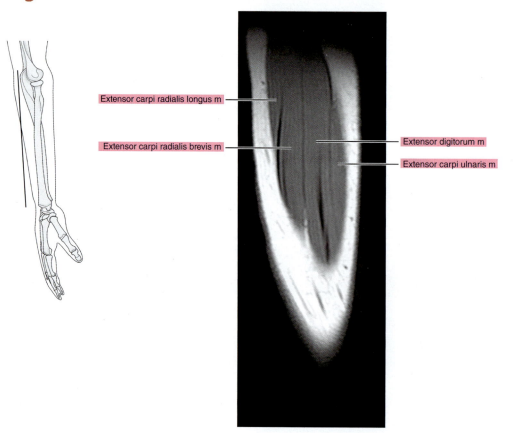

Extensor carpi radialis longus m

Extensor carpi radialis brevis m

Extensor digitorum m

Extensor carpi ulnaris m

Table 10-1. Muscles of the Forearm

MUSCLE	ORIGIN	INSERTION	NERVE SUPPLY
Anconeus	Posterior surface of the lateral epicondyle and adjacent capsular ligament of the elbow	Onto the radial side of the olecranon and adjacent shaft of the ulna	Nerve to anconeus (C7, C8, and T1)
Brachioradialis	Upper two-thirds of the lateral epicondylar ridge of the humerus and the anterior surface of the lateral intermuscular septum	Lateral side of the base of the styloid process of the radius	Radial (C5, C6, and C7)
Extensor carpi radialis longus	Lower third of the lateral epicondylar ridge, lateral intermuscular septum, and extensor tendons from the lateral epicondyle	Lateral aspect of the base of the second metacarpal	Radial (C5, C6, and C7)
Extensor carpi radialis brevis	Common extensor tendon from the lateral epicondyle, intermuscular septa, and radial collateral ligament of the elbow joint	Dorsal aspect of the base of the third metacarpal	Radial or deep radial (posterior interosseus) (C7 and C8)
Extensor digitorum	Common extensor tendon	Dorsal digital fibrous expansion covering the dorsum of the proximal phalanx and sides of its base, base of the middle, and distal phalanges	Deep radial (posterior interosseus) (C7 and C8)
Extensor digiti minimi	Intermuscular septa, overlying fascia, and common extensor tendon	Base of the proximal phalanx of the little finger	Deep radial (posterior interosseus) (C7 and C8)
Extensor carpi ulnaris	Two heads: (1) distal dorsal aspect of the lateral epicondyle and (2) proximal three-fourths of the dorsal border of the ulna	Onto a tubercle at the base of the fifth metacarpal	Deep radial (posterior interosseus) (C7 and C8)
Supinator	Dorsal aspect of the lateral epicondyle, ulnar depression distal to the radial notch, and supinator crest	Lateral surface of the radius between the anterior and posterior oblique lines	Deep radial (posterior interosseous) (C5 and C6)
Abductor pollicis longus	Lateral edge of the proximal part of the middle third of the ulna, adjacent interosseous membrane, dorsal surface of the radius, and, occasionally, the intermuscular septa	Radial side of the ventral aspect of the base of the first metacarpal	Deep radial (posterior interosseus) (C7 and C8)
Extensor pollicis brevis	Distal end of the middle third of the radius in its dorsal surface, interosseous membrane, and, occasionally, the ulna	Base of the proximal phalanx of the thumb or into the capsule of the metacarpophalangeal joint	Deep radial (posterior interosseus) (C7 and C8)
Extensor pollicis longus	Middle third of the dorsal surface of the ulna adjacent to the interosseous membrane	Base of the distal phalanx of the thumb	Deep radial (posterior interosseus) (C7 and C8)
Extensor indicis	Proximal part of the distal third of the posterior surface of the ulna interosseous membrane	Dorsal aponeurosis on the ulnar side of the index finger, adjacent to the base of the proximal phalanx	Deep radial (posterior interosseus) (C7 and C8)

continued

Table 10-1. Muscles of the Forearm–cont'd

MUSCLE	ORIGIN	INSERTION	NERVE SUPPLY
Pronator teres	Two heads: (1) humeral head (superior half of the ventral surface of the medial epicondyle) and (2) ulnar head (medial border of the coronoid process)	Onto the middle third of the lateral surface of the radius	Median (C6 and C7)
Flexor carpi radialis	Medial epicondyle of the humerus	Base of the second metacarpal and, usually, base of the third metacarpal	Median (C6 and C7)
Palmaris longus	Medial epicondyle	Flexor retinaculum and palmar aponeurosis	Median (C7 and C8)
Flexor carpi ulnaris	Two heads: (1) medial epicondyle and (2) medial side of the olecranon, upper two-thirds of the dorsal border of the ulna	Primarily onto the pisiform	Ulnar (C7 and C8)
Flexor digitorum superficialis	Two heads: (1) ulnar (ventral surface of the medial epicondyle, ulnar collateral ligament, ulnar tuberosity, medial border of coronoid process) and (2) radial (anterior oblique line and ventral border below the radial oblique line)	Ventral surface of the shaft of the middle phalanx of each finger	Median (C7, C8, and T1)
Flexor digitorum profundus	Proximal three-fourths of the medial and anterior surface of the ulna and interosseous membrane	Bases of the distal phalanges of the second to fifth digits	Median, anterior interosseous branch (C8 and T1)
Flexor pollicis longus	Ventral surface of the radius, oblique line, and adjacent interosseus membrane	Base of the distal phalanx of the thumb	Median, anterior interosseous branch (C8 and T1)
Pronator quadratus	Medial side and ventral surface of the distal fourth of the ulna	Distal quarter of the ventral surface of the radius	Median, anterior interosseous branch (C8 and T1)

Chapter 11

MRI of the Wrist

AXIAL
Figure 11.1.1

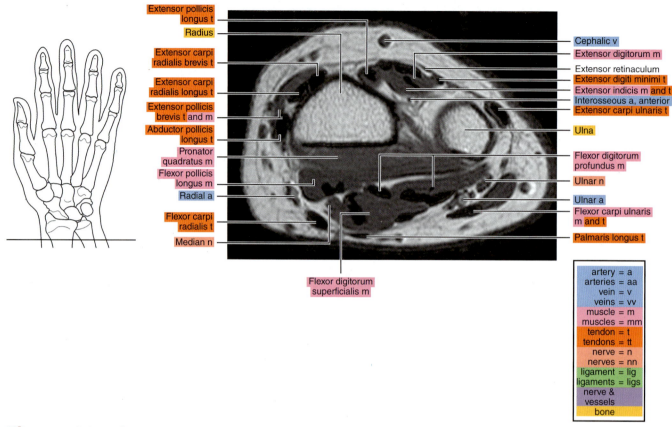

Extensor pollicis longus t
Radius
Extensor carpi radialis brevis t
Extensor carpi radialis longus t
Extensor pollicis brevis t and m
Abductor pollicis longus t
Pronator quadratus m
Flexor pollicis longus m
Radial a
Flexor carpi radialis t
Median n
Flexor digitorum superficialis m

Cephalic v
Extensor digitorum m
Extensor retinaculum
Extensor digiti minimi t
Extensor indicis m and t
Interosseous a, anterior
Extensor carpi ulnaris t
Ulna
Flexor digitorum profundus m
Ulnar n
Ulnar a
Flexor carpi ulnaris m and t
Palmaris longus t

artery = a
arteries = aa
vein = v
veins = vv
muscle = m
muscles = mm
tendon = t
tendons = tt
nerve = n
nerves = nn
ligament = lig
ligaments = ligs
nerve & vessels
bone

Figure 11.1.2

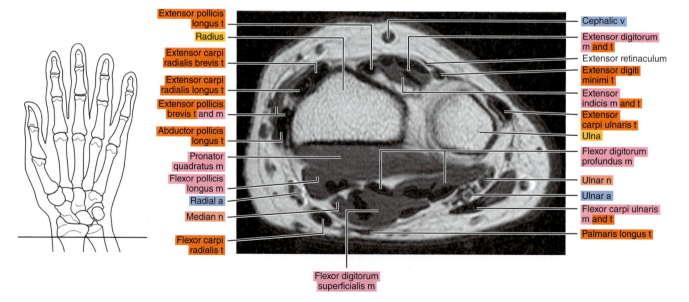

Extensor pollicis longus t
Radius
Extensor carpi radialis brevis t
Extensor carpi radialis longus t
Extensor pollicis brevis t and m
Abductor pollicis longus t
Pronator quadratus m
Flexor pollicis longus m
Radial a
Median n
Flexor carpi radialis t
Flexor digitorum superficialis m

Cephalic v
Extensor digitorum m and t
Extensor retinaculum
Extensor digiti minimi t
Extensor indicis m and t
Extensor carpi ulnaris t
Ulna
Flexor digitorum profundus m
Ulnar n
Ulnar a
Flexor carpi ulnaris m and t
Palmaris longus t

Figure 11.1.3

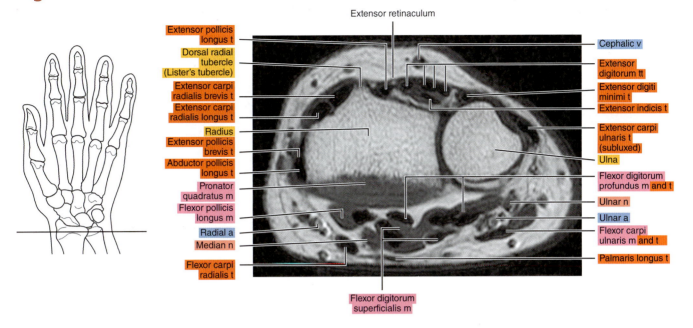

Extensor pollicis longus t
Dorsal radial tubercle (Lister's tubercle)
Extensor carpi radialis brevis t
Extensor carpi radialis longus t
Radius
Extensor pollicis brevis t
Abductor pollicis longus t
Pronator quadratus m
Flexor pollicis longus m
Radial a
Median n
Flexor carpi radialis t

Extensor retinaculum

Cephalic v
Extensor digitorum tt
Extensor digiti minimi t
Extensor indicis t
Extensor carpi ulnaris t (subluxed)
Ulna
Flexor digitorum profundus m and t
Ulnar n
Ulnar a
Flexor carpi ulnaris m and t
Palmaris longus t

Flexor digitorum superficialis m

Figure 11.1.4

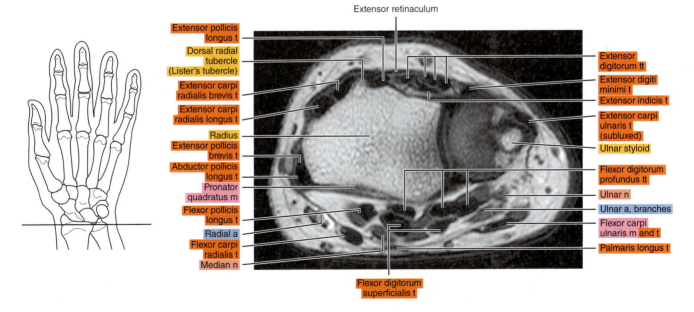

Extensor pollicis longus t
Dorsal radial tubercle (Lister's tubercle)
Extensor carpi radialis brevis t
Extensor carpi radialis longus t
Radius
Extensor pollicis brevis t
Abductor pollicis longus t
Pronator quadratus m
Flexor pollicis longus t
Radial a
Flexor carpi radialis t
Median n

Extensor retinaculum

Extensor digitorum tt
Extensor digiti minimi t
Extensor indicis t
Extensor carpi ulnaris t (subluxed)
Ulnar styloid
Flexor digitorum profundus tt
Ulnar n
Ulnar a, branches
Flexor carpi ulnaris m and t
Palmaris longus t

Flexor digitorum superficialis t

Figure 11.1.5

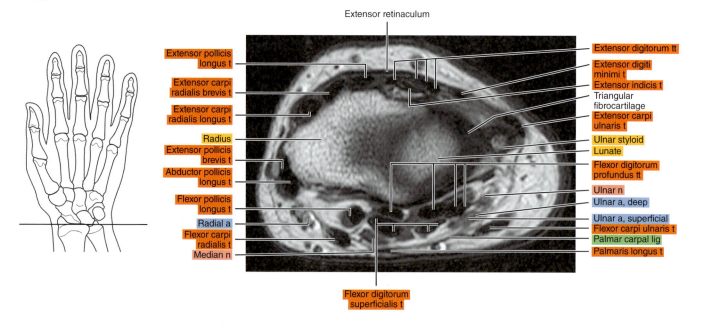

Extensor retinaculum

Extensor pollicis longus t
Extensor carpi radialis brevis t
Extensor carpi radialis longus t
Radius
Extensor pollicis brevis t
Abductor pollicis longus t
Flexor pollicis longus t
Radial a
Flexor carpi radialis t
Median n

Extensor digitorum tt
Extensor digiti minimi t
Extensor indicis t
Triangular fibrocartilage
Extensor carpi ulnaris t
Ulnar styloid
Lunate
Flexor digitorum profundus tt
Ulnar n
Ulnar a, deep
Ulnar a, superficial
Flexor carpi ulnaris t
Palmar carpal lig
Palmaris longus t

Flexor digitorum superficialis t

Figure 11.1.6

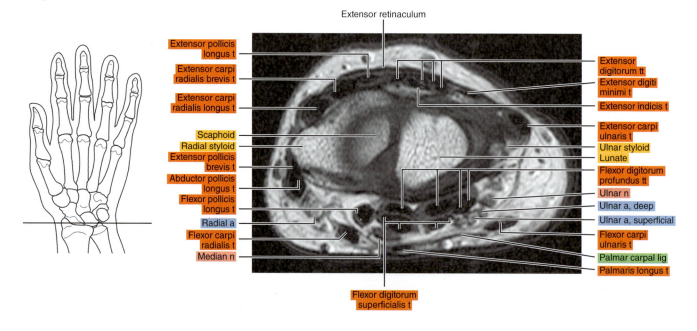

Extensor retinaculum

Extensor pollicis longus t
Extensor carpi radialis brevis t
Extensor carpi radialis longus t
Scaphoid
Radial styloid
Extensor pollicis brevis t
Abductor pollicis longus t
Flexor pollicis longus t
Radial a
Flexor carpi radialis t
Median n

Extensor digitorum tt
Extensor digiti minimi t
Extensor indicis t
Extensor carpi ulnaris t
Ulnar styloid
Lunate
Flexor digitorum profundus tt
Ulnar n
Ulnar a, deep
Ulnar a, superficial
Flexor carpi ulnaris t
Palmar carpal lig
Palmaris longus t

Flexor digitorum superficialis t

Figure 11.1.7

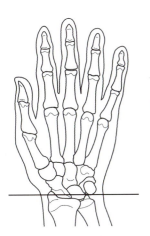

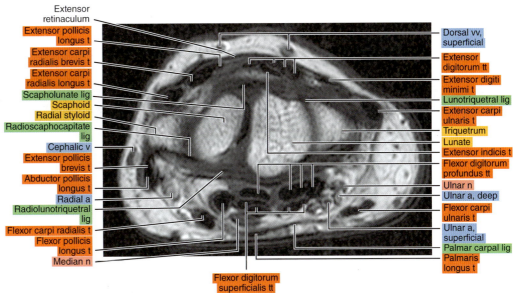

Extensor retinaculum
Extensor pollicis longus t
Extensor carpi radialis brevis t
Extensor carpi radialis longus t
Scapholunate lig
Scaphoid
Radial styloid
Radioscaphocapitate lig
Cephalic v
Extensor pollicis brevis t
Abductor pollicis longus t
Radial a
Radiolunotriquetral lig
Flexor carpi radialis t
Flexor pollicis longus t
Median n

Dorsal vv, superficial
Extensor digitorum tt
Extensor digiti minimi t
Lunotriquetral lig
Extensor carpi ulnaris t
Triquetrum
Lunate
Extensor indicis t
Flexor digitorum profundus tt
Ulnar n
Ulnar a, deep
Flexor carpi ulnaris t
Ulnar a, superficial
Palmar carpal lig
Palmaris longus t

Flexor digitorum superficialis tt

Figure 11.1.8

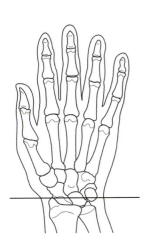

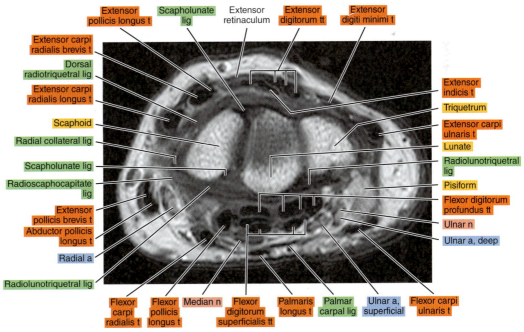

Extensor pollicis longus t
Scapholunate lig
Extensor retinaculum
Extensor digitorum tt
Extensor digiti minimi t

Extensor carpi radialis brevis t
Dorsal radiotriquetral lig
Extensor carpi radialis longus t
Scaphoid
Radial collateral lig
Scapholunate lig
Radioscaphocapitate lig
Extensor pollicis brevis t
Abductor pollicis longus t
Radial a
Radiolunotriquetral lig

Extensor indicis t
Triquetrum
Extensor carpi ulnaris t
Lunate
Radiolunotriquetral lig
Pisiform
Flexor digitorum profundus tt
Ulnar n
Ulnar a, deep

Flexor carpi radialis t
Flexor pollicis longus t
Median n
Flexor digitorum superficialis tt
Palmaris longus t
Palmar carpal lig
Ulnar a, superficial
Flexor carpi ulnaris t

Figure 11.1.9

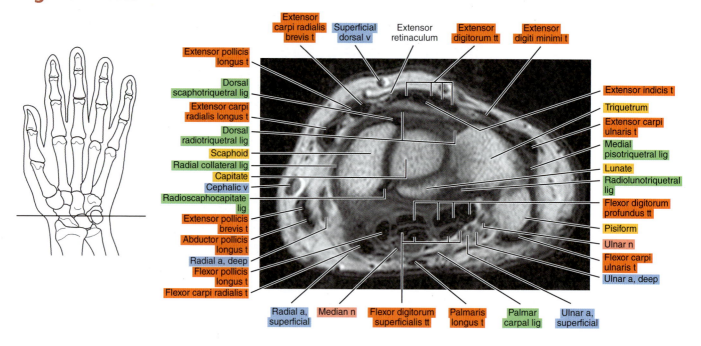

Figure 11.1.10

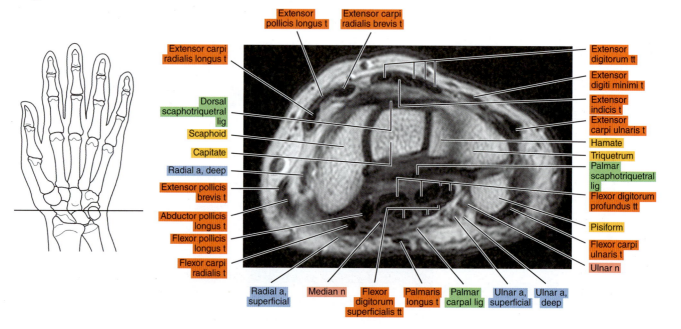

Figure 11.1.11

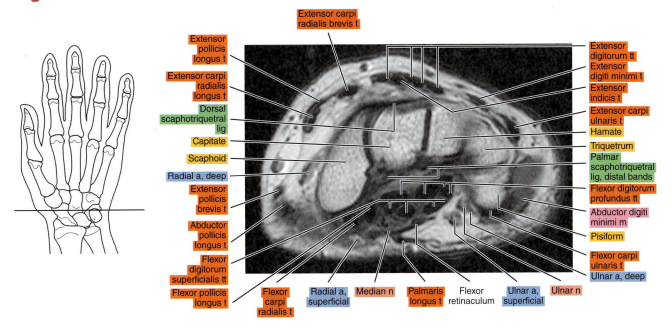

Extensor carpi radialis brevis t

Extensor pollicis longus t

Extensor carpi radialis longus t

Dorsal scaphotriquetral lig

Capitate

Scaphoid

Radial a, deep

Extensor pollicis brevis t

Abductor pollicis longus t

Flexor digitorum superficialis tt

Flexor pollicis longus t

Extensor digitorum tt

Extensor digiti minimi t

Extensor indicis t

Extensor carpi ulnaris t

Hamate

Triquetrum

Palmar scaphotriquetral lig, distal bands

Flexor digitorum profundus tt

Abductor digiti minimi m

Pisiform

Flexor carpi ulnaris t

Ulnar a, deep

Flexor carpi radialis t

Radial a, superficial

Median n

Palmaris longus t

Flexor retinaculum

Ulnar a, superficial

Ulnar n

Figure 11.1.12

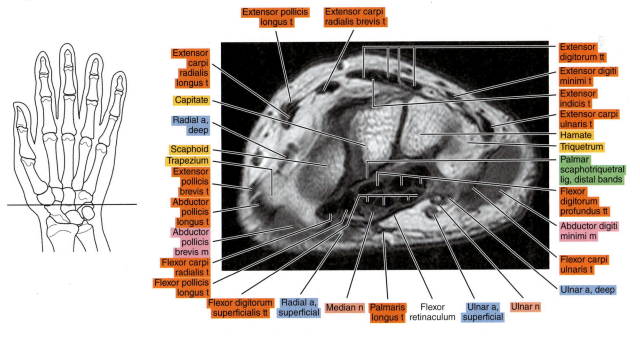

Extensor pollicis longus t

Extensor carpi radialis brevis t

Extensor carpi radialis longus t

Capitate

Radial a, deep

Scaphoid

Trapezium

Extensor pollicis brevis t

Abductor pollicis longus t

Abductor pollicis brevis m

Flexor carpi radialis t

Flexor pollicis longus t

Extensor digitorum tt

Extensor digiti minimi t

Extensor indicis t

Extensor carpi ulnaris t

Hamate

Triquetrum

Palmar scaphotriquetral lig, distal bands

Flexor digitorum profundus tt

Abductor digiti minimi m

Flexor carpi ulnaris t

Ulnar a, deep

Flexor digitorum superficialis tt

Radial a, superficial

Median n

Palmaris longus t

Flexor retinaculum

Ulnar a, superficial

Ulnar n

Figure 11.1.13

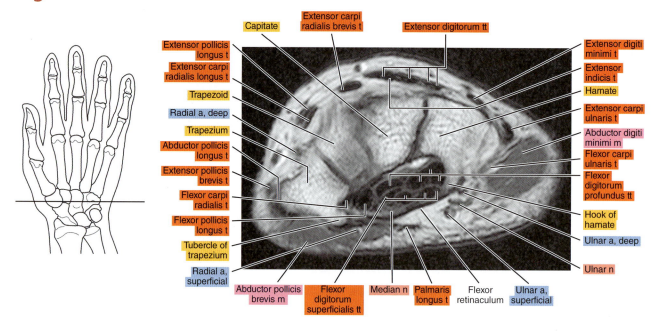

Figure 11.1.14

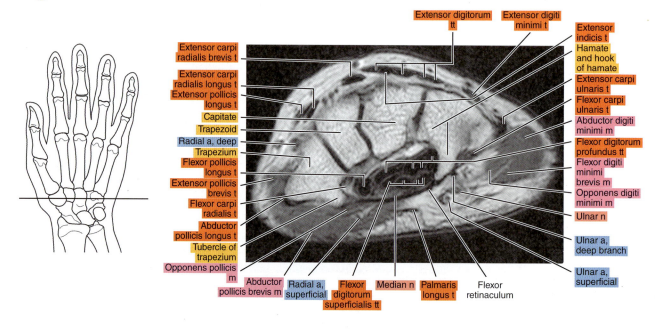

Figure 11.1.15

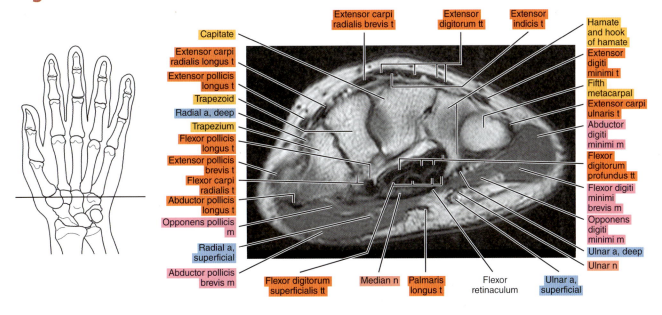

Capitate
Extensor carpi radialis longus t
Extensor pollicis longus t
Trapezoid
Radial a, deep
Trapezium
Flexor pollicis longus t
Extensor pollicis brevis t
Flexor carpi radialis t
Abductor pollicis longus t
Opponens pollicis m
Radial a, superficial
Abductor pollicis brevis m

Extensor carpi radialis brevis t
Extensor digitorum tt
Extensor indicis t

Hamate and hook of hamate
Extensor digiti minimi t
Fifth metacarpal
Extensor carpi ulnaris t
Abductor digiti minimi m
Flexor digitorum profundus tt
Flexor digiti minimi brevis m
Opponens digiti minimi m
Ulnar a, deep
Ulnar n

Flexor digitorum superficialis tt
Median n
Palmaris longus t
Flexor retinaculum
Ulnar a, superficial

Figure 11.1.16

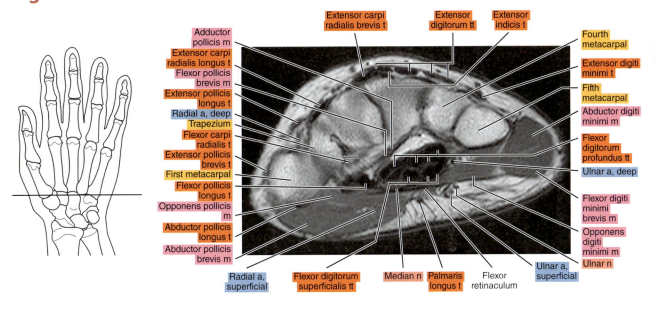

Adductor pollicis m
Extensor carpi radialis longus t
Flexor pollicis brevis m
Extensor pollicis longus t
Radial a, deep
Trapezium
Flexor carpi radialis t
Extensor pollicis brevis t
First metacarpal
Flexor pollicis longus t
Opponens pollicis m
Abductor pollicis longus t
Abductor pollicis brevis m

Extensor carpi radialis brevis t
Extensor digitorum tt
Extensor indicis t

Fourth metacarpal
Extensor digiti minimi t
Fifth metacarpal
Abductor digiti minimi m
Flexor digitorum profundus tt
Ulnar a, deep
Flexor digiti minimi brevis m
Opponens digiti minimi m
Ulnar n

Radial a, superficial
Flexor digitorum superficialis tt
Median n
Palmaris longus t
Flexor retinaculum
Ulnar a, superficial

Figure 11.1.17

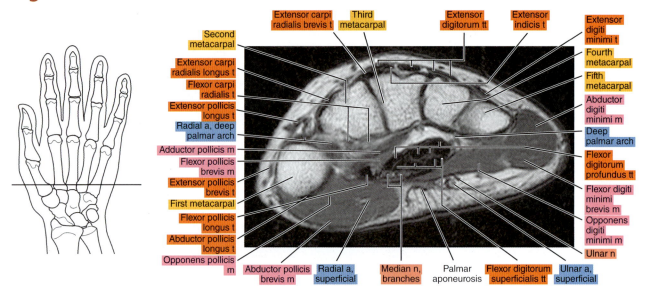

Figure 11.1.18

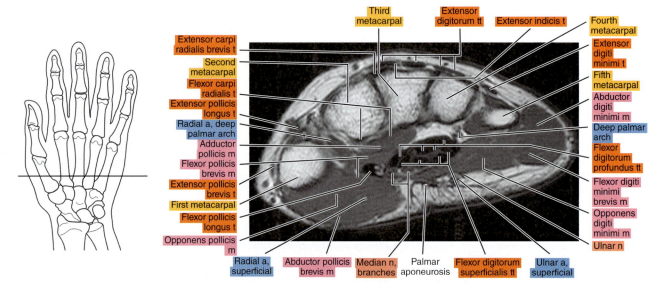

SAGITTAL
Figure 11.2.1

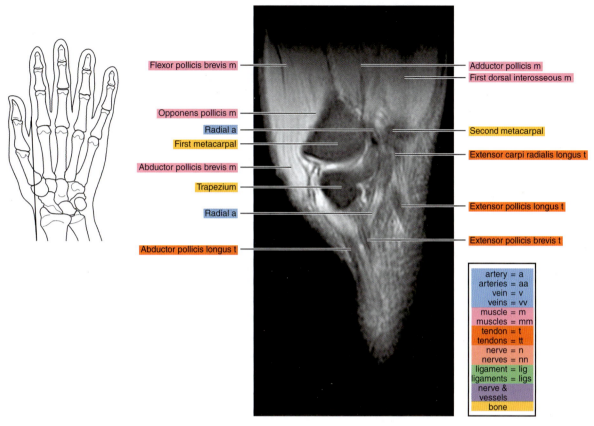

Flexor pollicis brevis m

Opponens pollicis m

Radial a

First metacarpal

Abductor pollicis brevis m

Trapezium

Radial a

Abductor pollicis longus t

Adductor pollicis m

First dorsal interosseous m

Second metacarpal

Extensor carpi radialis longus t

Extensor pollicis longus t

Extensor pollicis brevis t

artery = a	
arteries = aa	
vein = v	
veins = vv	
muscle = m	
muscles = mm	
tendon = t	
tendons = tt	
nerve = n	
nerves = nn	
ligament = lig	
ligaments = ligs	
nerve & vessels	
bone	

Figure 11.2.2

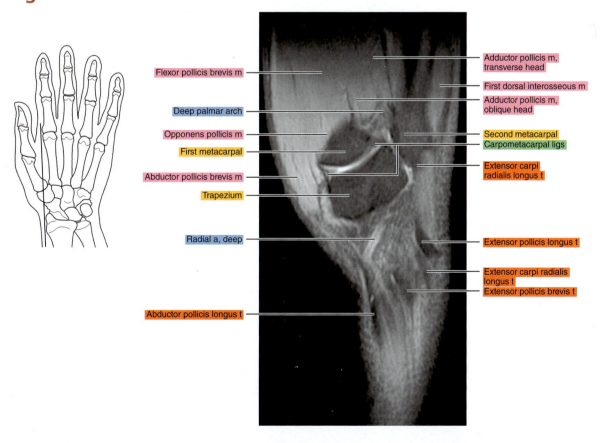

Flexor pollicis brevis m

Deep palmar arch

Opponens pollicis m

First metacarpal

Abductor pollicis brevis m

Trapezium

Radial a, deep

Abductor pollicis longus t

Adductor pollicis m, transverse head

First dorsal interosseous m

Adductor pollicis m, oblique head

Second metacarpal

Carpometacarpal ligs

Extensor carpi radialis longus t

Extensor pollicis longus t

Extensor carpi radialis longus t

Extensor pollicis brevis t

Figure 11.2.3

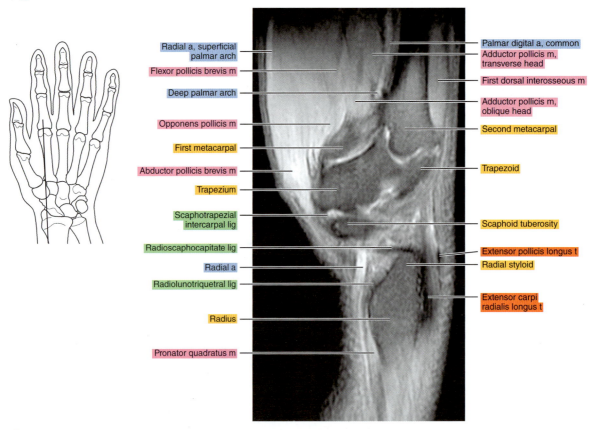

Radial a, superficial palmar arch
Flexor pollicis brevis m
Deep palmar arch
Opponens pollicis m
First metacarpal
Abductor pollicis brevis m
Trapezium
Scaphotrapezial intercarpal lig
Radioscaphocapitate lig
Radial a
Radiolunotriquetral lig
Radius
Pronator quadratus m

Palmar digital a, common
Adductor pollicis m, transverse head
First dorsal interosseous m
Adductor pollicis m, oblique head
Second metacarpal
Trapezoid
Scaphoid tuberosity
Extensor pollicis longus t
Radial styloid
Extensor carpi radialis longus t

Figure 11.2.4

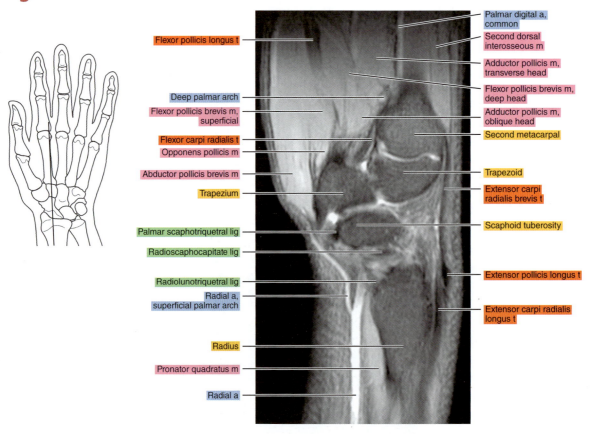

Flexor pollicis longus t
Deep palmar arch
Flexor pollicis brevis m, superficial
Flexor carpi radialis t
Opponens pollicis m
Abductor pollicis brevis m
Trapezium
Palmar scaphotriquetral lig
Radioscaphocapitate lig
Radiolunotriquetral lig
Radial a, superficial palmar arch
Radius
Pronator quadratus m
Radial a

Palmar digital a, common
Second dorsal interosseous m
Adductor pollicis m, transverse head
Flexor pollicis brevis m, deep head
Adductor pollicis m, oblique head
Second metacarpal
Trapezoid
Extensor carpi radialis brevis t
Scaphoid tuberosity
Extensor pollicis longus t
Extensor carpi radialis longus t

Figure 11.2.5

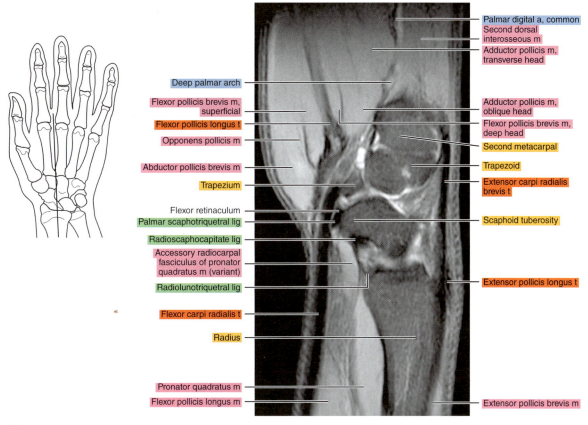

Palmar digital a, common
Second dorsal interosseous m
Adductor pollicis m, transverse head
Deep palmar arch
Flexor pollicis brevis m, superficial
Flexor pollicis longus t
Opponens pollicis m
Adductor pollicis m, oblique head
Flexor pollicis brevis m, deep head
Second metacarpal
Abductor pollicis brevis m
Trapezium
Trapezoid
Extensor carpi radialis brevis t
Flexor retinaculum
Palmar scaphotriquetral lig
Radioscaphocapitate lig
Accessory radiocarpal fasciculus of pronator quadratus m (variant)
Scaphoid tuberosity
Radiolunotriquetral lig
Flexor carpi radialis t
Radius
Extensor pollicis longus t
Pronator quadratus m
Flexor pollicis longus m
Extensor pollicis brevis m

Figure 11.2.6

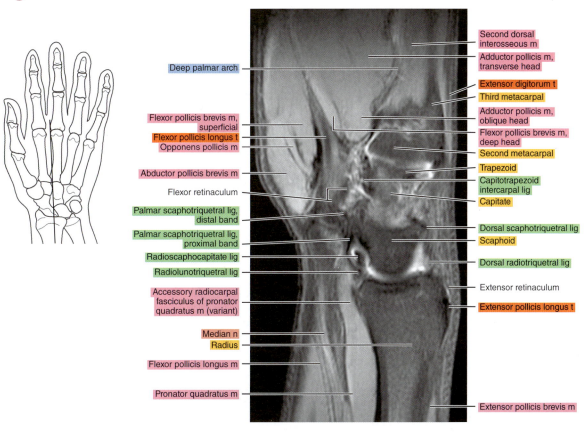

Second dorsal interosseous m
Adductor pollicis m, transverse head
Deep palmar arch
Extensor digitorum t
Third metacarpal
Adductor pollicis m, oblique head
Flexor pollicis brevis m, superficial
Flexor pollicis longus t
Opponens pollicis m
Flexor pollicis brevis m, deep head
Second metacarpal
Abductor pollicis brevis m
Trapezoid
Flexor retinaculum
Capitotrapezoid intercarpal lig
Palmar scaphotriquetral lig, distal band
Capitate
Palmar scaphotriquetral lig, proximal band
Dorsal scaphotriquetral lig
Scaphoid
Radioscaphocapitate lig
Radiolunotriquetral lig
Dorsal radiotriquetral lig
Accessory radiocarpal fasciculus of pronator quadratus m (variant)
Extensor retinaculum
Extensor pollicis longus t
Median n
Radius
Flexor pollicis longus m
Pronator quadratus m
Extensor pollicis brevis m

Figure 11.2.7

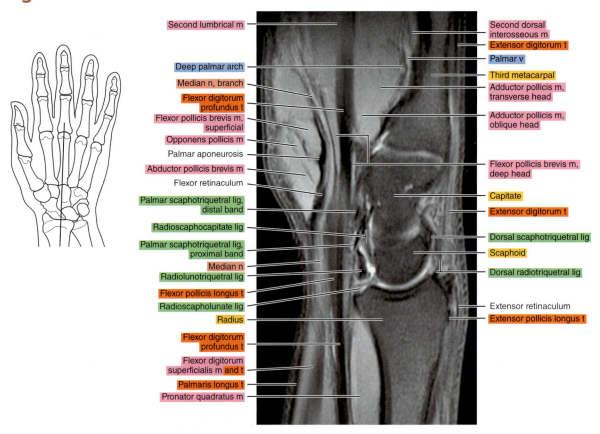

Second lumbrical m

Deep palmar arch

Median n, branch

Flexor digitorum profundus t

Flexor pollicis brevis m, superficial

Opponens pollicis m

Palmar aponeurosis

Abductor pollicis brevis m

Flexor retinaculum

Palmar scaphotriquetral lig, distal band

Radioscaphocapitate lig

Palmar scaphotriquetral lig, proximal band

Median n

Radiolunotriquetral lig

Flexor pollicis longus t

Radioscapholunate lig

Radius

Flexor digitorum profundus t

Flexor digitorum superficialis m and t

Palmaris longus t

Pronator quadratus m

Second dorsal interosseous m

Extensor digitorum t

Palmar v

Third metacarpal

Adductor pollicis m, transverse head

Adductor pollicis m, oblique head

Flexor pollicis brevis m, deep head

Capitate

Extensor digitorum t

Dorsal scaphotriquetral lig

Scaphoid

Dorsal radiotriquetral lig

Extensor retinaculum

Extensor pollicis longus t

Figure 11.2.8

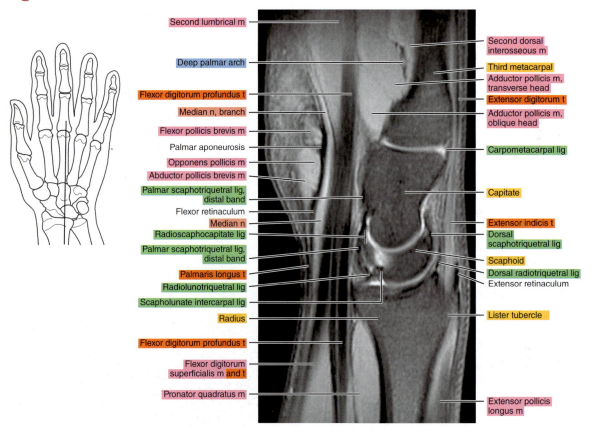

Second lumbrical m

Deep palmar arch

Flexor digitorum profundus t

Median n, branch

Flexor pollicis brevis m

Palmar aponeurosis

Opponens pollicis m

Abductor pollicis brevis m

Palmar scaphotriquetral lig, distal band

Flexor retinaculum

Median n

Radioscaphocapitate lig

Palmar scaphotriquetral lig, distal band

Palmaris longus t

Radiolunotriquetral lig

Scapholunate intercarpal lig

Radius

Flexor digitorum profundus t

Flexor digitorum superficialis m and t

Pronator quadratus m

Second dorsal interosseous m

Third metacarpal

Adductor pollicis m, transverse head

Extensor digitorum t

Adductor pollicis m, oblique head

Carpometacarpal lig

Capitate

Extensor indicis t

Dorsal scaphotriquetral lig

Scaphoid

Dorsal radiotriquetral lig

Extensor retinaculum

Lister tubercle

Extensor pollicis longus m

Figure 11.2.9

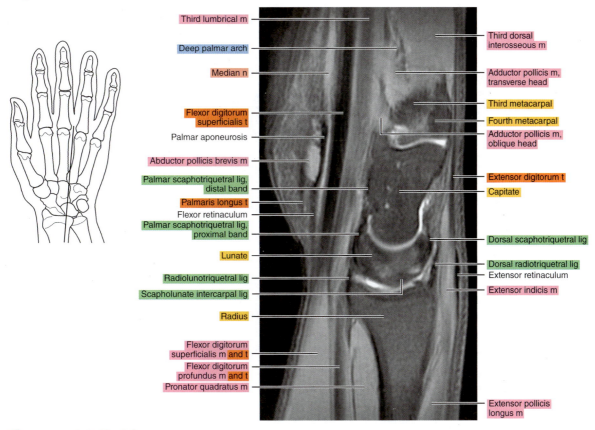

Third lumbrical m
Deep palmar arch
Median n
Flexor digitorum superficialis t
Palmar aponeurosis
Abductor pollicis brevis m
Palmar scaphotriquetral lig, distal band
Palmaris longus t
Flexor retinaculum
Palmar scaphotriquetral lig, proximal band
Lunate
Radiolunotriquetral lig
Scapholunate intercarpal lig
Radius
Flexor digitorum superficialis m and t
Flexor digitorum profundus m and t
Pronator quadratus m

Third dorsal interosseous m
Adductor pollicis m, transverse head
Third metacarpal
Fourth metacarpal
Adductor pollicis m, oblique head
Extensor digitorum t
Capitate
Dorsal scaphotriquetral lig
Dorsal radiotriquetral lig
Extensor retinaculum
Extensor indicis m
Extensor pollicis longus m

Figure 11.2.10

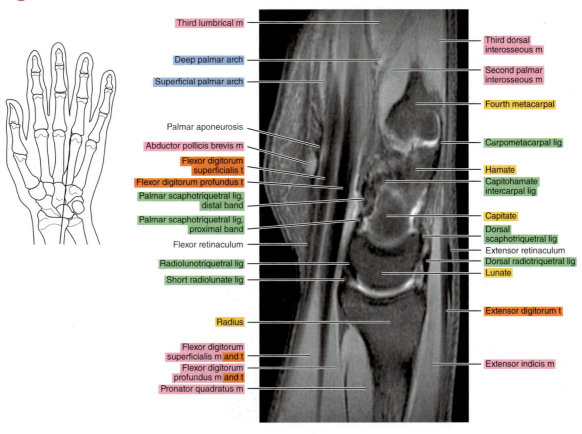

Third lumbrical m
Deep palmar arch
Superficial palmar arch
Palmar aponeurosis
Abductor pollicis brevis m
Flexor digitorum superficialis t
Flexor digitorum profundus t
Palmar scaphotriquetral lig, distal band
Palmar scaphotriquetral lig, proximal band
Flexor retinaculum
Radiolunotriquetral lig
Short radiolunate lig
Radius
Flexor digitorum superficialis m and t
Flexor digitorum profundus m and t
Pronator quadratus m

Third dorsal interosseous m
Second palmar interosseous m
Fourth metacarpal
Carpometacarpal lig
Hamate
Capitohamate intercarpal lig
Capitate
Dorsal scaphotriquetral lig
Extensor retinaculum
Dorsal radiotriquetral lig
Lunate
Extensor digitorum t
Extensor indicis m

Figure 11.2.11

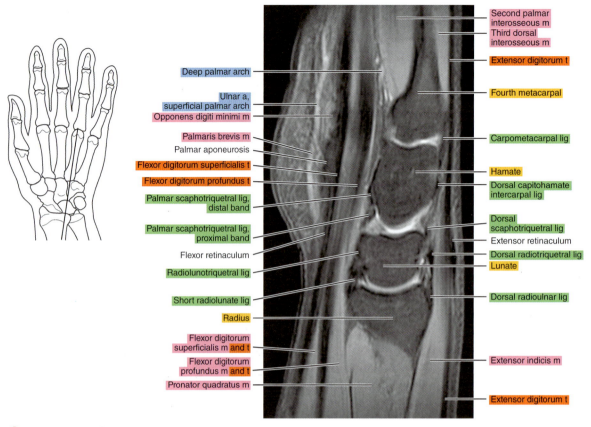

Deep palmar arch
Ulnar a, superficial palmar arch
Opponens digiti minimi m
Palmaris brevis m
Palmar aponeurosis
Flexor digitorum superficialis t
Flexor digitorum profundus t
Palmar scaphotriquetral lig, distal band
Palmar scaphotriquetral lig, proximal band
Flexor retinaculum
Radiolunotriquetral lig
Short radiolunate lig
Radius
Flexor digitorum superficialis m and t
Flexor digitorum profundus m and t
Pronator quadratus m

Second palmar interosseous m
Third dorsal interosseous m
Extensor digitorum t
Fourth metacarpal
Carpometacarpal lig
Hamate
Dorsal capitohamate intercarpal lig
Dorsal scaphotriquetral lig
Extensor retinaculum
Dorsal radiotriquetral lig
Lunate
Dorsal radioulnar lig
Extensor indicis m
Extensor digitorum t

Figure 11.2.12

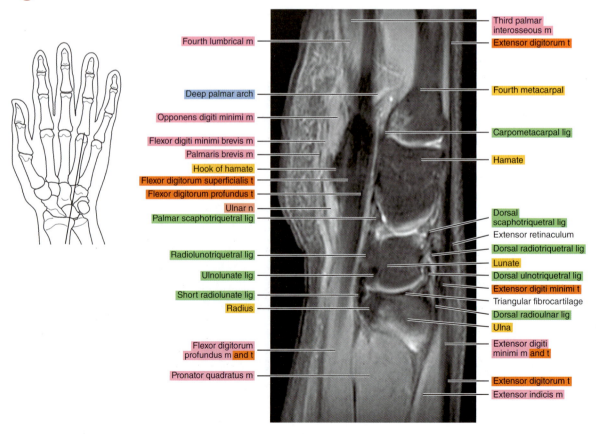

Fourth lumbrical m
Deep palmar arch
Opponens digiti minimi m
Flexor digiti minimi brevis m
Palmaris brevis m
Hook of hamate
Flexor digitorum superficialis t
Flexor digitorum profundus t
Ulnar n
Palmar scaphotriquetral lig
Radiolunotriquetral lig
Ulnolunate lig
Short radiolunate lig
Radius
Flexor digitorum profundus m and t
Pronator quadratus m

Third palmar interosseous m
Extensor digitorum t
Fourth metacarpal
Carpometacarpal lig
Hamate
Dorsal scaphotriquetral lig
Extensor retinaculum
Dorsal radiotriquetral lig
Lunate
Dorsal ulnotriquetral lig
Extensor digiti minimi t
Triangular fibrocartilage
Dorsal radioulnar lig
Ulna
Extensor digiti minimi m and t
Extensor digitorum t
Extensor indicis m

Figure 11.2.13

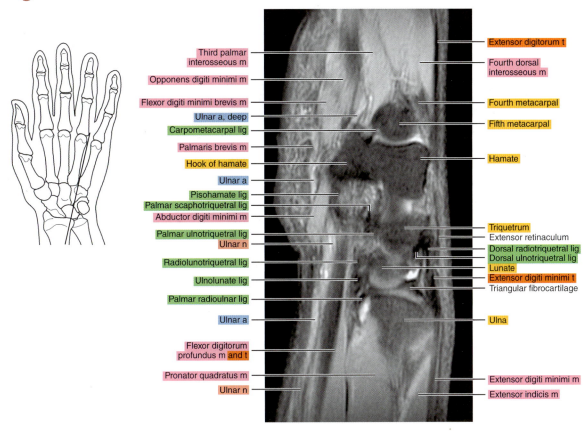

Third palmar interosseous m
Opponens digiti minimi m
Flexor digiti minimi brevis m
Ulnar a, deep
Carpometacarpal lig
Palmaris brevis m
Hook of hamate
Ulnar a
Pisohamate lig
Palmar scaphotriquetral lig
Abductor digiti minimi m
Palmar ulnotriquetral lig
Ulnar n
Radiolunotriquetral lig
Ulnolunate lig
Palmar radioulnar lig
Ulnar a
Flexor digitorum profundus m and t
Pronator quadratus m
Ulnar n

Extensor digitorum t
Fourth dorsal interosseous m
Fourth metacarpal
Fifth metacarpal
Hamate
Triquetrum
Extensor retinaculum
Dorsal radiotriquetral lig
Dorsal ulnotriquetral lig
Lunate
Extensor digiti minimi t
Triangular fibrocartilage
Ulna
Extensor digiti minimi m
Extensor indicis m

Figure 11.2.14

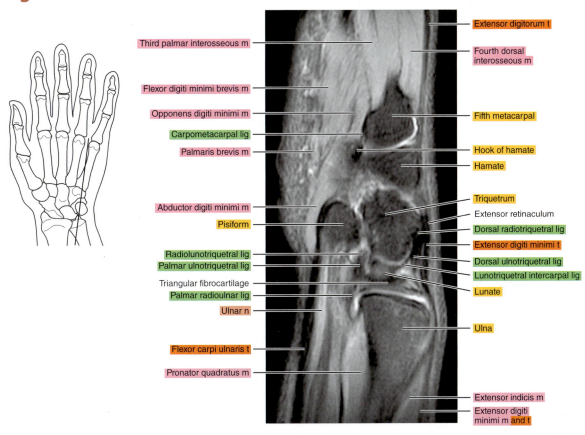

Third palmar interosseous m
Flexor digiti minimi brevis m
Opponens digiti minimi m
Carpometacarpal lig
Palmaris brevis m
Abductor digiti minimi m
Pisiform
Radiolunotriquetral lig
Palmar ulnotriquetral lig
Triangular fibrocartilage
Palmar radioulnar lig
Ulnar n
Flexor carpi ulnaris t
Pronator quadratus m

Extensor digitorum t
Fourth dorsal interosseous m
Fifth metacarpal
Hook of hamate
Hamate
Triquetrum
Extensor retinaculum
Dorsal radiotriquetral lig
Extensor digiti minimi t
Dorsal ulnotriquetral lig
Lunotriquetral intercarpal lig
Lunate
Ulna
Extensor indicis m
Extensor digiti minimi m and t

Figure 11.2.15

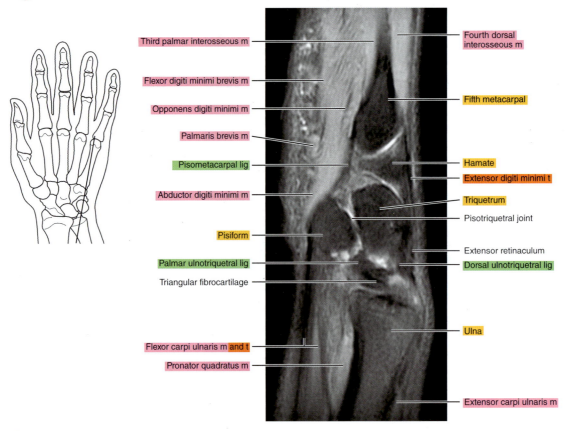

Third palmar interosseous m

Flexor digiti minimi brevis m

Opponens digiti minimi m

Palmaris brevis m

Pisometacarpal lig

Abductor digiti minimi m

Pisiform

Palmar ulnotriquetral lig

Triangular fibrocartilage

Flexor carpi ulnaris m and t

Pronator quadratus m

Fourth dorsal interosseous m

Fifth metacarpal

Hamate

Extensor digiti minimi t

Triquetrum

Pisotriquetral joint

Extensor retinaculum

Dorsal ulnotriquetral lig

Ulna

Extensor carpi ulnaris m

Figure 11.2.16

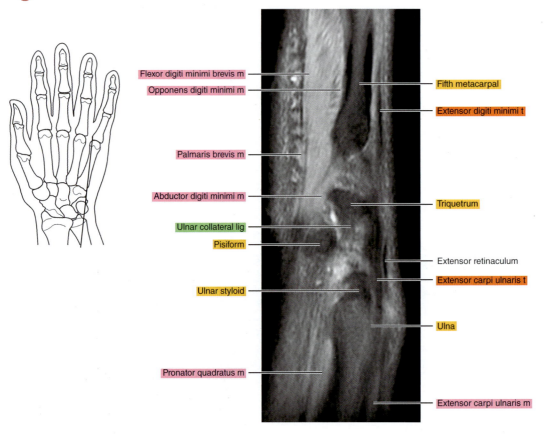

Flexor digiti minimi brevis m

Opponens digiti minimi m

Palmaris brevis m

Abductor digiti minimi m

Ulnar collateral lig

Pisiform

Ulnar styloid

Pronator quadratus m

Fifth metacarpal

Extensor digiti minimi t

Triquetrum

Extensor retinaculum

Extensor carpi ulnaris t

Ulna

Extensor carpi ulnaris m

Figure 11.2.17

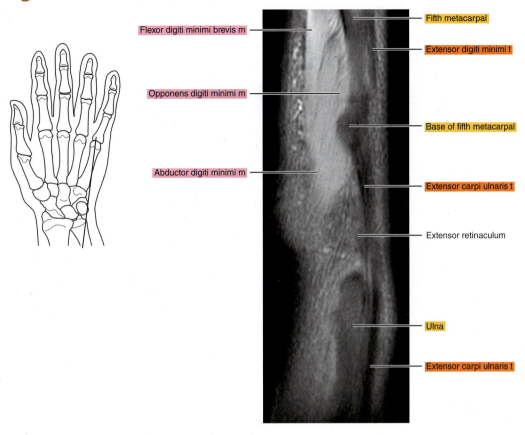

Flexor digiti minimi brevis m

Opponens digiti minimi m

Abductor digiti minimi m

Fifth metacarpal

Extensor digiti minimi t

Base of fifth metacarpal

Extensor carpi ulnaris t

Extensor retinaculum

Ulna

Extensor carpi ulnaris t

CORONAL
Figure 11.3.1

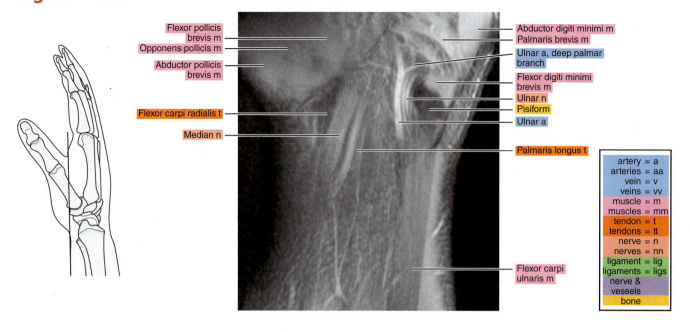

Flexor pollicis brevis m
Opponens pollicis m
Abductor pollicis brevis m
Flexor carpi radialis t
Median n

Abductor digiti minimi m
Palmaris brevis m
Ulnar a, deep palmar branch
Flexor digiti minimi brevis m
Ulnar n
Pisiform
Ulnar a
Palmaris longus t
Flexor carpi ulnaris m

artery = a
arteries = aa
vein = v
veins = vv
muscle = m
muscles = mm
tendon = t
tendons = tt
nerve = n
nerves = nn
ligament = lig
ligaments = ligs
nerve & vessels
bone

Figure 11.3.2

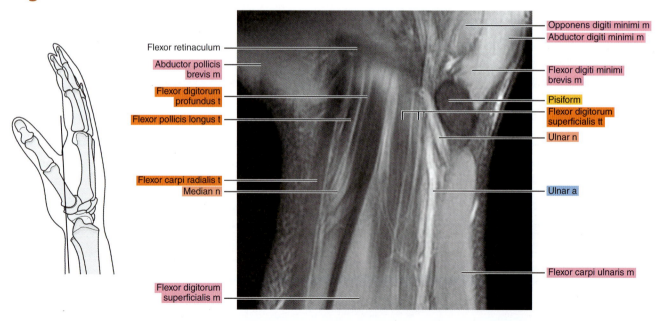

Flexor retinaculum
Abductor pollicis brevis m
Flexor digitorum profundus t
Flexor pollicis longus t
Flexor carpi radialis t
Median n
Flexor digitorum superficialis m

Opponens digiti minimi m
Abductor digiti minimi m
Flexor digiti minimi brevis m
Pisiform
Flexor digitorum superficialis tt
Ulnar n
Ulnar a
Flexor carpi ulnaris m

Figure 11.3.3

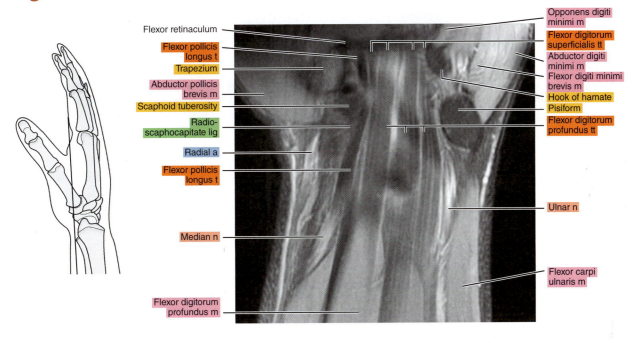

Flexor retinaculum

Flexor pollicis longus t

Trapezium

Abductor pollicis brevis m

Scaphoid tuberosity

Radio-scaphocapitate lig

Radial a

Flexor pollicis longus t

Median n

Flexor digitorum profundus m

Opponens digiti minimi m

Flexor digitorum superficialis tt

Abductor digiti minimi m

Flexor digiti minimi brevis m

Hook of hamate

Pisiform

Flexor digitorum profundus tt

Ulnar n

Flexor carpi ulnaris m

Figure 11.3.4

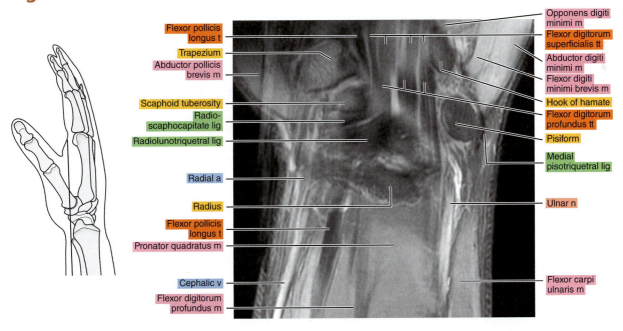

Flexor pollicis longus t

Trapezium

Abductor pollicis brevis m

Scaphoid tuberosity

Radio-scaphocapitate lig

Radiolunotriquetral lig

Radial a

Radius

Flexor pollicis longus t

Pronator quadratus m

Cephalic v

Flexor digitorum profundus m

Opponens digiti minimi m

Flexor digitorum superficialis tt

Abductor digiti minimi m

Flexor digiti minimi brevis m

Hook of hamate

Flexor digitorum profundus tt

Pisiform

Medial pisotriquetral lig

Ulnar n

Flexor carpi ulnaris m

Figure 11.3.5

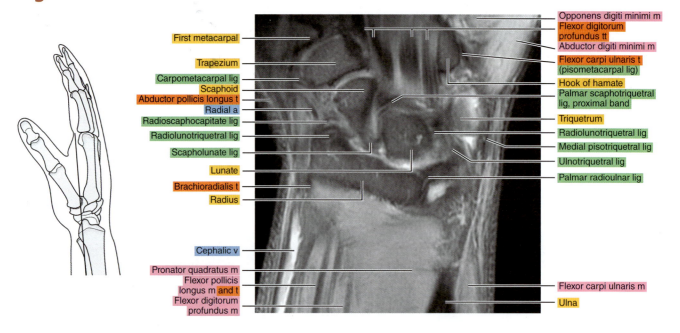

First metacarpal
Trapezium
Carpometacarpal lig
Scaphoid
Abductor pollicis longus t
Radial a
Radioscaphocapitate lig
Radiolunotriquetral lig
Scapholunate lig
Lunate
Brachioradialis t
Radius

Cephalic v

Pronator quadratus m
Flexor pollicis longus m and t
Flexor digitorum profundus m

Opponens digiti minimi m
Flexor digitorum profundus tt
Abductor digiti minimi m
Flexor carpi ulnaris t (pisometacarpal lig)
Hook of hamate
Palmar scaphotriquetral lig, proximal band
Triquetrum
Radiolunotriquetral lig
Medial pisotriquetral lig
Ulnotriquetral lig
Palmar radioulnar lig

Flexor carpi ulnaris m
Ulna

Figure 11.3.6

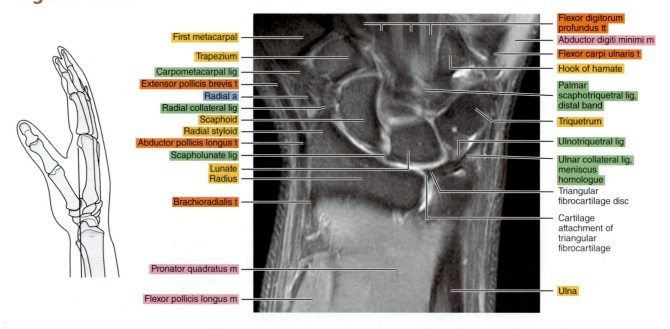

First metacarpal
Trapezium
Carpometacarpal lig
Extensor pollicis brevis t
Radial a
Radial collateral lig
Scaphoid
Radial styloid
Abductor pollicis longus t
Scapholunate lig
Lunate
Radius
Brachioradialis t

Pronator quadratus m

Flexor pollicis longus m

Flexor digitorum profundus tt
Abductor digiti minimi m
Flexor carpi ulnaris t
Hook of hamate
Palmar scaphotriquetral lig, distal band
Triquetrum
Ulnotriquetral lig
Ulnar collateral lig, meniscus homologue
Triangular fibrocartilage disc
Cartilage attachment of triangular fibrocartilage

Ulna

Figure 11.3.7

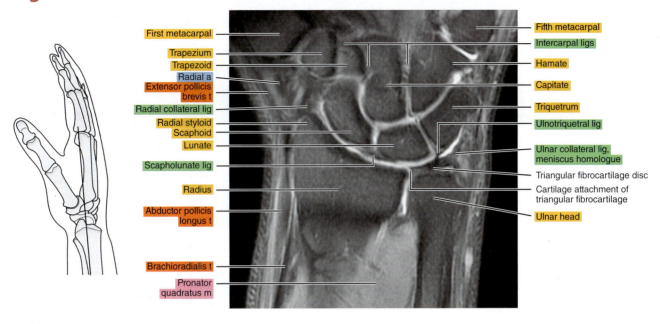

First metacarpal
Trapezium
Trapezoid
Radial a
Extensor pollicis brevis t
Radial collateral lig
Radial styloid
Scaphoid
Lunate
Scapholunate lig
Radius
Abductor pollicis longus t
Brachioradialis t
Pronator quadratus m

Fifth metacarpal
Intercarpal ligs
Hamate
Capitate
Triquetrum
Ulnotriquetral lig
Ulnar collateral lig, meniscus homologue
Triangular fibrocartilage disc
Cartilage attachment of triangular fibrocartilage
Ulnar head

Figure 11.3.8

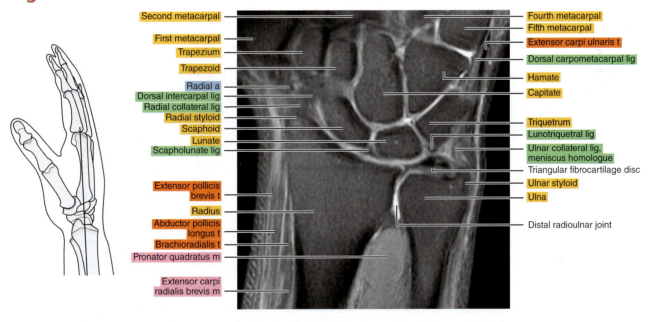

Second metacarpal
First metacarpal
Trapezium
Trapezoid
Radial a
Dorsal intercarpal lig
Radial collateral lig
Radial styloid
Scaphoid
Lunate
Scapholunate lig
Extensor pollicis brevis t
Radius
Abductor pollicis longus t
Brachioradialis t
Pronator quadratus m
Extensor carpi radialis brevis m

Fourth metacarpal
Fifth metacarpal
Extensor carpi ulnaris t
Dorsal carpometacarpal lig
Hamate
Capitate
Triquetrum
Lunotriquetral lig
Ulnar collateral lig, meniscus homologue
Triangular fibrocartilage disc
Ulnar styloid
Ulna
Distal radioulnar joint

Figure 11.3.9

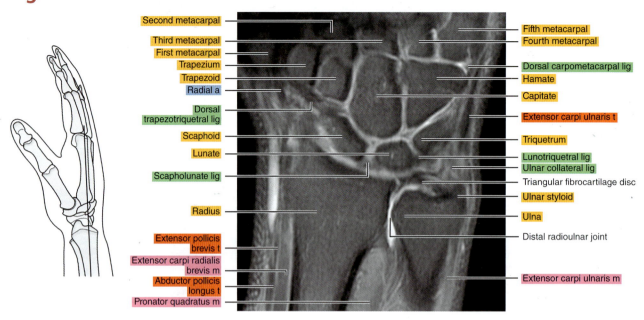

Second metacarpal — Fifth metacarpal
Third metacarpal — Fourth metacarpal
First metacarpal — Dorsal carpometacarpal lig
Trapezium — Hamate
Trapezoid — Capitate
Radial a
Dorsal trapezotriquetral lig — Extensor carpi ulnaris t
Scaphoid — Triquetrum
Lunate — Lunotriquetral lig
Scapholunate lig — Ulnar collateral lig
— Triangular fibrocartilage disc
Radius — Ulnar styloid
— Ulna
Extensor pollicis brevis t — Distal radioulnar joint
Extensor carpi radialis brevis m
Abductor pollicis longus t — Extensor carpi ulnaris m
Pronator quadratus m

Figure 11.3.10

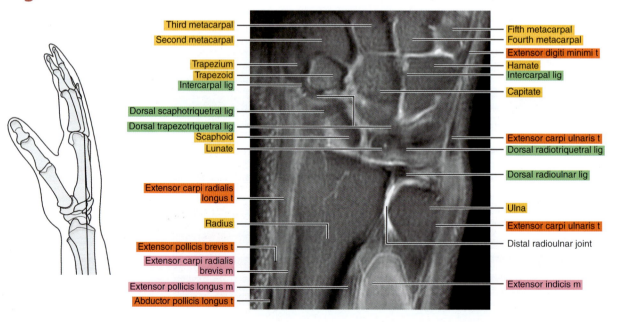

Third metacarpal — Fifth metacarpal
Second metacarpal — Fourth metacarpal
— Extensor digiti minimi t
Trapezium — Hamate
Trapezoid — Intercarpal lig
Intercarpal lig — Capitate
Dorsal scaphotriquetral lig
Dorsal trapezotriquetral lig
Scaphoid — Extensor carpi ulnaris t
Lunate — Dorsal radiotriquetral lig
— Dorsal radioulnar lig
Extensor carpi radialis longus t
Radius — Ulna
Extensor pollicis brevis t — Extensor carpi ulnaris t
Extensor carpi radialis brevis m — Distal radioulnar joint
Extensor pollicis longus m — Extensor indicis m
Abductor pollicis longus t

Figure 11.3.11

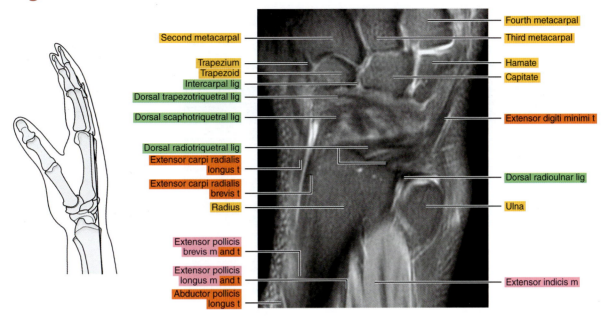

Second metacarpal
Trapezium
Trapezoid
Intercarpal lig
Dorsal trapezotriquetral lig
Dorsal scaphotriquetral lig
Dorsal radiotriquetral lig
Extensor carpi radialis longus t
Extensor carpi radialis brevis t
Radius
Extensor pollicis brevis m and t
Extensor pollicis longus m and t
Abductor pollicis longus t

Fourth metacarpal
Third metacarpal
Hamate
Capitate
Extensor digiti minimi t
Dorsal radioulnar lig
Ulna
Extensor indicis m

Figure 11.3.12

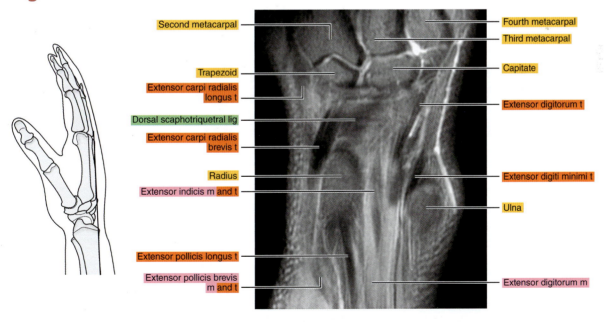

Second metacarpal
Trapezoid
Extensor carpi radialis longus t
Dorsal scaphotriquetral lig
Extensor carpi radialis brevis t
Radius
Extensor indicis m and t
Extensor pollicis longus t
Extensor pollicis brevis m and t

Fourth metacarpal
Third metacarpal
Capitate
Extensor digitorum t
Extensor digiti minimi t
Ulna
Extensor digitorum m

Figure 11.3.13

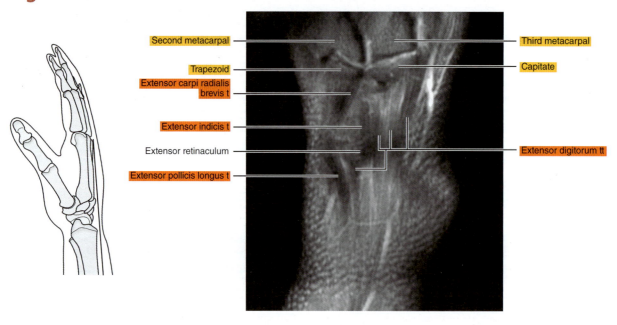

Second metacarpal

Trapezoid

Extensor carpi radialis brevis t

Extensor indicis t

Extensor retinaculum

Extensor pollicis longus t

Third metacarpal

Capitate

Extensor digitorum tt

Chapter 12

MRI of the Hand

AXIAL
Figure 12.1.1

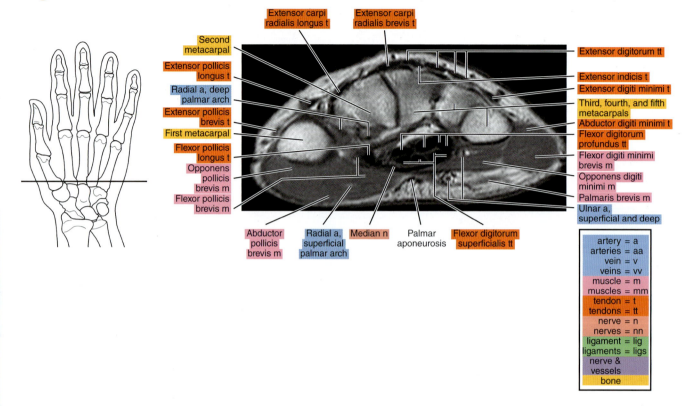

Extensor carpi radialis longus t
Extensor carpi radialis brevis t
Second metacarpal
Extensor pollicis longus t
Radial a, deep palmar arch
Extensor pollicis brevis t
First metacarpal
Flexor pollicis longus t
Opponens pollicis brevis m
Flexor pollicis brevis m
Abductor pollicis brevis m
Radial a, superficial palmar arch
Median n
Palmar aponeurosis
Flexor digitorum superficialis tt
Extensor digitorum tt
Extensor indicis t
Extensor digiti minimi t
Third, fourth, and fifth metacarpals
Abductor digiti minimi t
Flexor digitorum profundus tt
Flexor digiti minimi brevis m
Opponens digiti minimi m
Palmaris brevis m
Ulnar a, superficial and deep

artery = a	
arteries = aa	
vein = v	
veins = vv	
muscle = m	
muscles = mm	
tendon = t	
tendons = tt	
nerve = n	
nerves = nn	
ligament = lig	
ligaments = ligs	
nerve & vessels	
bone	

Figure 12.1.2

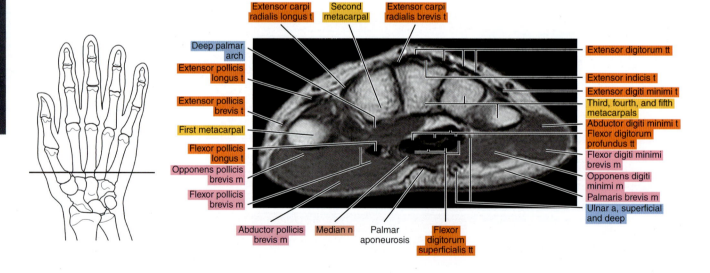

Extensor carpi radialis longus t
Second metacarpal
Extensor carpi radialis brevis t
Deep palmar arch
Extensor pollicis longus t
Extensor pollicis brevis t
First metacarpal
Flexor pollicis longus t
Opponens pollicis brevis m
Flexor pollicis brevis m
Abductor pollicis brevis m
Median n
Palmar aponeurosis
Flexor digitorum superficialis tt
Extensor digitorum tt
Extensor indicis t
Extensor digiti minimi t
Third, fourth, and fifth metacarpals
Abductor digiti minimi t
Flexor digitorum profundus tt
Flexor digiti minimi brevis m
Opponens digiti minimi m
Palmaris brevis m
Ulnar a, superficial and deep

Figure 12.1.3

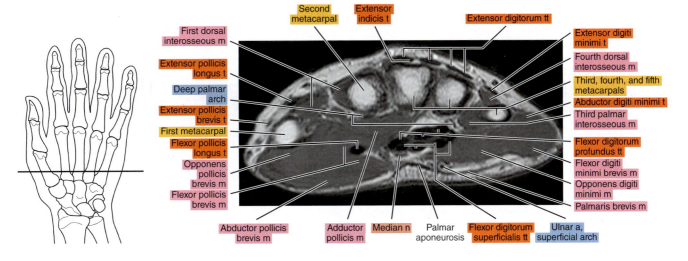

Figure 12.1.4

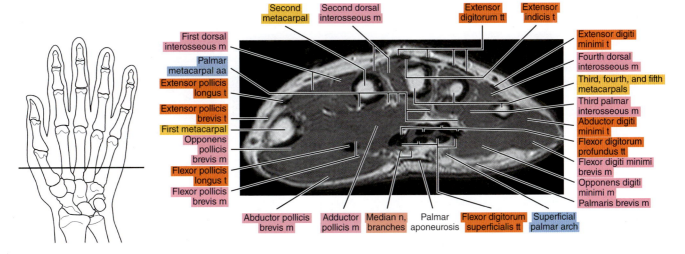

Figure 12.1.5

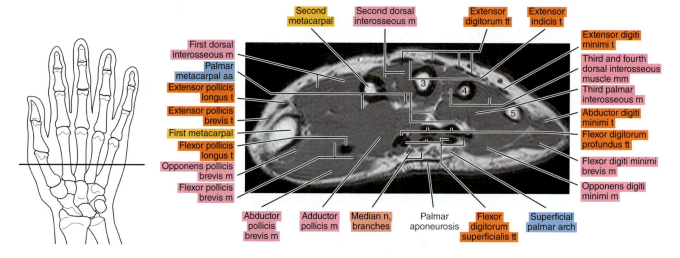

Figure 12.1.6

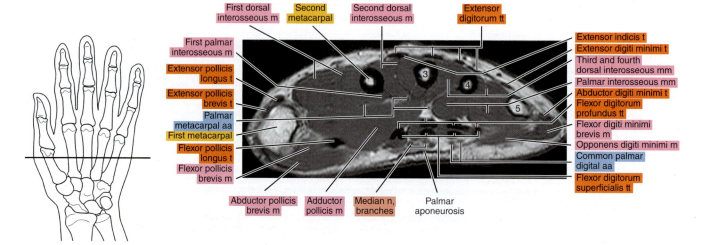

Figure 12.1.7

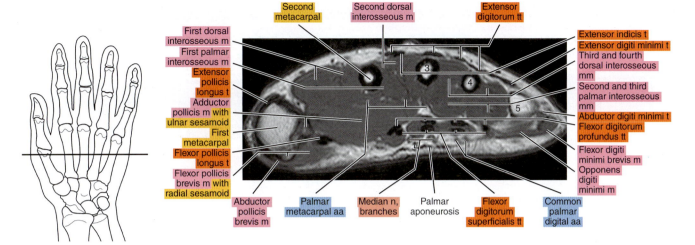

- Second metacarpal
- Second dorsal interosseous m
- Extensor digitorum tt
- Extensor indicis t
- Extensor digiti minimi t
- Third and fourth dorsal interosseous mm
- Second and third palmar interosseous mm
- Abductor digiti minimi t
- Flexor digitorum profundus tt
- Flexor digiti minimi brevis m
- Opponens digiti minimi m
- First dorsal interosseous m
- First palmar interosseous m
- Extensor pollicis longus t
- Adductor pollicis m with ulnar sesamoid
- First metacarpal
- Flexor pollicis longus t
- Flexor pollicis brevis m with radial sesamoid
- Abductor pollicis brevis m
- Palmar metacarpal aa
- Median n, branches
- Palmar aponeurosis
- Flexor digitorum superficialis tt
- Common palmar digital aa

Figure 12.1.8

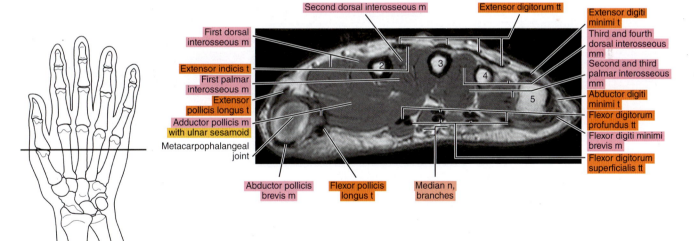

- Second dorsal interosseous m
- Extensor digitorum tt
- Extensor digiti minimi t
- Third and fourth dorsal interosseous mm
- Second and third palmar interosseous mm
- Abductor digiti minimi t
- Flexor digitorum profundus tt
- Flexor digiti minimi brevis m
- Flexor digitorum superficialis tt
- First dorsal interosseous m
- Extensor indicis t
- First palmar interosseous m
- Extensor pollicis longus t
- Adductor pollicis m with ulnar sesamoid
- Metacarpophalangeal joint
- Abductor pollicis brevis m
- Flexor pollicis longus t
- Median n, branches

Figure 12.1.9

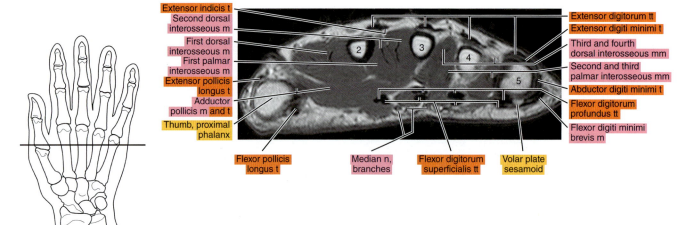

Extensor indicis t
Second dorsal interosseous m
First dorsal interosseous m
First palmar interosseous m
Extensor pollicis longus t
Adductor pollicis m and t
Thumb, proximal phalanx

Extensor digitorum tt
Extensor digiti minimi t
Third and fourth dorsal interosseous mm
Second and third palmar interosseous mm
Abductor digiti minimi t
Flexor digitorum profundus tt
Flexor digiti minimi brevis m

Flexor pollicis longus t
Median n, branches
Flexor digitorum superficialis tt
Volar plate sesamoid

Figure 12.1.10

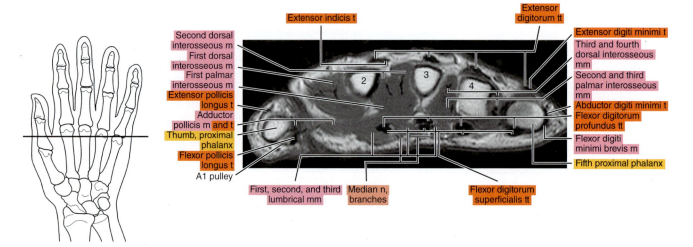

Extensor indicis t
Extensor digitorum tt

Second dorsal interosseous m
First dorsal interosseous m
First palmar interosseous m
Extensor pollicis longus t
Adductor pollicis m and t
Thumb, proximal phalanx
Flexor pollicis longus t
A1 pulley

Extensor digiti minimi t
Third and fourth dorsal interosseous mm
Second and third palmar interosseous mm
Abductor digiti minimi t
Flexor digitorum profundus tt
Flexor digiti minimi brevis m
Fifth proximal phalanx

First, second, and third lumbrical mm
Median n, branches
Flexor digitorum superficialis tt

Figure 12.1.11

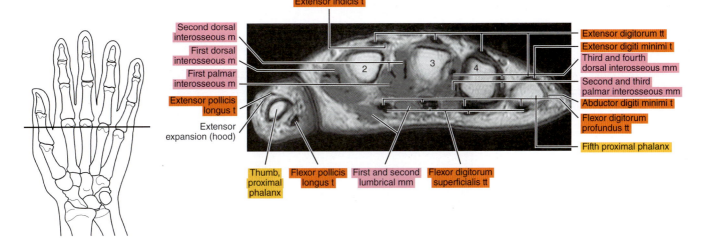

Figure 12.1.12

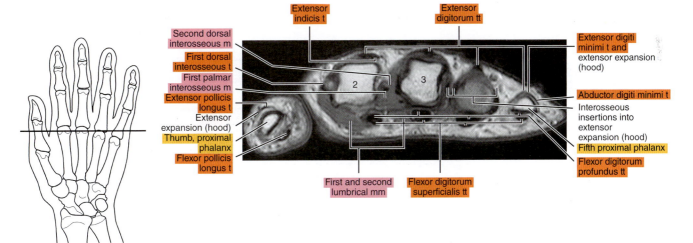

Figure 12.1.13

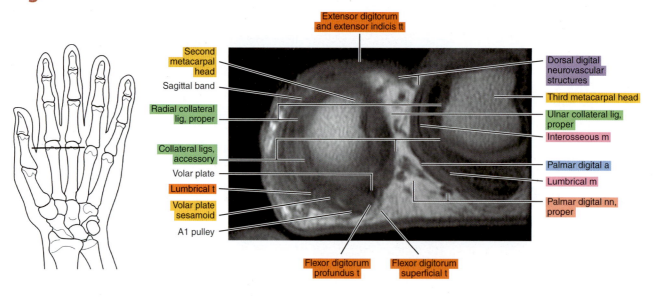

Extensor digitorum and extensor indicis tt

Second metacarpal head

Sagittal band

Radial collateral lig, proper

Collateral ligs, accessory

Volar plate

Lumbrical t

Volar plate sesamoid

A1 pulley

Dorsal digital neurovascular structures

Third metacarpal head

Ulnar collateral lig, proper

Interosseous m

Palmar digital a

Lumbrical m

Palmar digital nn, proper

Flexor digitorum profundus t

Flexor digitorum superficial t

Figure 12.1.14

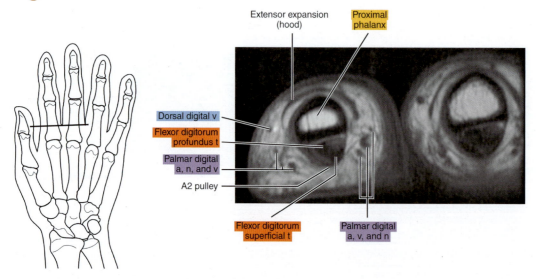

Extensor expansion (hood)

Proximal phalanx

Dorsal digital v

Flexor digitorum profundus t

Palmar digital a, n, and v

A2 pulley

Flexor digitorum superficial t

Palmar digital a, v, and n

SAGITTAL
Figure 12.2.1

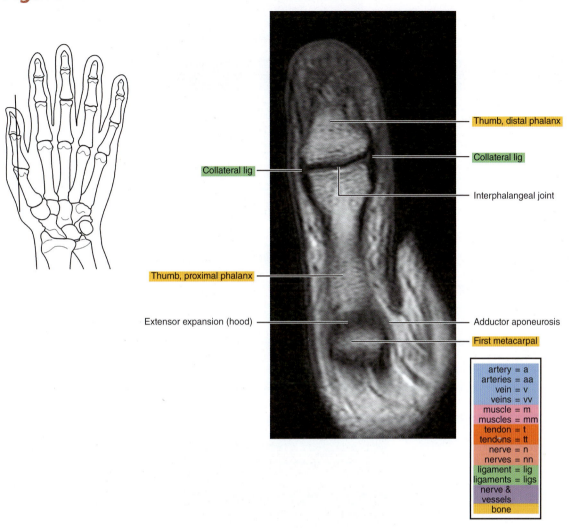

Thumb, distal phalanx

Collateral lig

Interphalangeal joint

Collateral lig

Thumb, proximal phalanx

Extensor expansion (hood)

Adductor aponeurosis

First metacarpal

artery = a	
arteries = aa	
vein = v	
veins = vv	
muscle = m	
muscles = mm	
tendon = t	
tendons = tt	
nerve = n	
nerves = nn	
ligament = lig	
ligaments = ligs	
nerve & vessels	
bone	

Figure 12.2.2

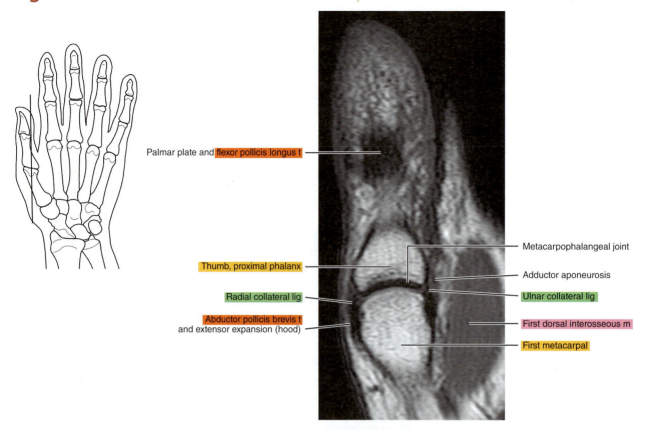

Palmar plate and `flexor pollicis longus t`

Thumb, proximal phalanx

Radial collateral lig

Abductor pollicis brevis t
and extensor expansion (hood)

Metacarpophalangeal joint

Adductor aponeurosis

Ulnar collateral lig

First dorsal interosseous m

First metacarpal

Figure 12.2.3

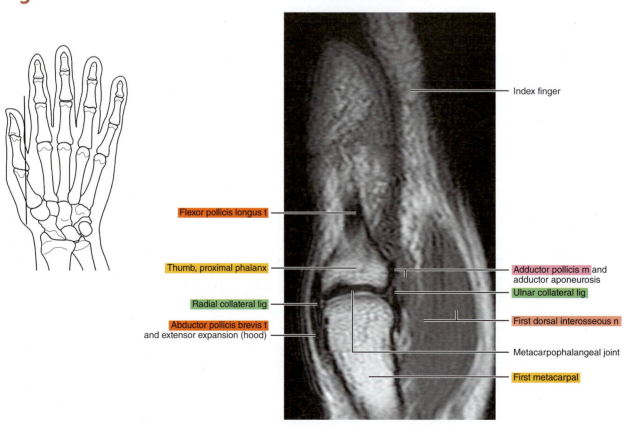

Flexor pollicis longus t

Thumb, proximal phalanx

Radial collateral lig

Abductor pollicis brevis t
and extensor expansion (hood)

Index finger

Adductor pollicis m and
adductor aponeurosis

Ulnar collateral lig

First dorsal interosseous n

Metacarpophalangeal joint

First metacarpal

Figure 12.2.4

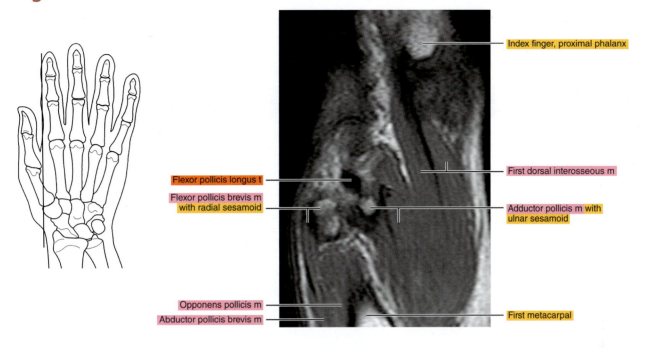

Index finger, proximal phalanx

First dorsal interosseous m

Flexor pollicis longus t

Flexor pollicis brevis m with radial sesamoid

Adductor pollicis m with ulnar sesamoid

Opponens pollicis m

Abductor pollicis brevis m

First metacarpal

Figure 12.2.5

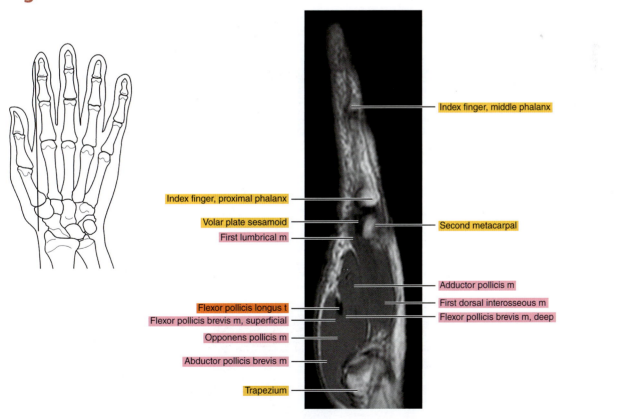

Index finger, middle phalanx

Index finger, proximal phalanx

Volar plate sesamoid

Second metacarpal

First lumbrical m

Adductor pollicis m

First dorsal interosseous m

Flexor pollicis longus t

Flexor pollicis brevis m, superficial

Flexor pollicis brevis m, deep

Opponens pollicis m

Abductor pollicis brevis m

Trapezium

Figure 12.2.6

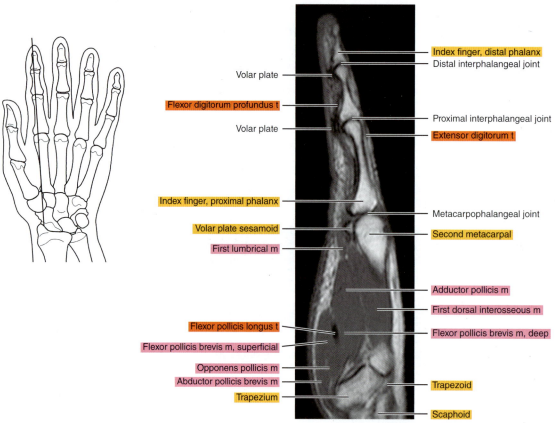

Volar plate

Flexor digitorum profundus t

Volar plate

Index finger, proximal phalanx

Volar plate sesamoid

First lumbrical m

Flexor pollicis longus t

Flexor pollicis brevis m, superficial

Opponens pollicis m

Abductor pollicis brevis m

Trapezium

Index finger, distal phalanx
Distal interphalangeal joint

Proximal interphalangeal joint

Extensor digitorum t

Metacarpophalangeal joint

Second metacarpal

Adductor pollicis m

First dorsal interosseous m

Flexor pollicis brevis m, deep

Trapezoid

Scaphoid

Figure 12.2.7

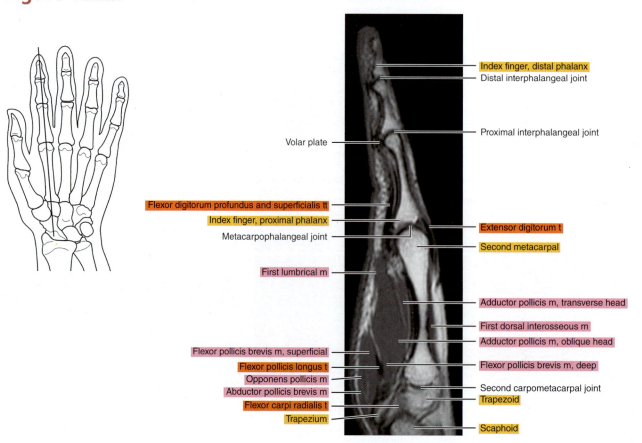

Volar plate

Flexor digitorum profundus and superficialis tt

Index finger, proximal phalanx

Metacarpophalangeal joint

First lumbrical m

Flexor pollicis brevis m, superficial

Flexor pollicis longus t

Opponens pollicis m

Abductor pollicis brevis m

Flexor carpi radialis t

Trapezium

Index finger, distal phalanx
Distal interphalangeal joint

Proximal interphalangeal joint

Extensor digitorum t

Second metacarpal

Adductor pollicis m, transverse head

First dorsal interosseous m

Adductor pollicis m, oblique head

Flexor pollicis brevis m, deep

Second carpometacarpal joint

Trapezoid

Scaphoid

Figure 12.2.8

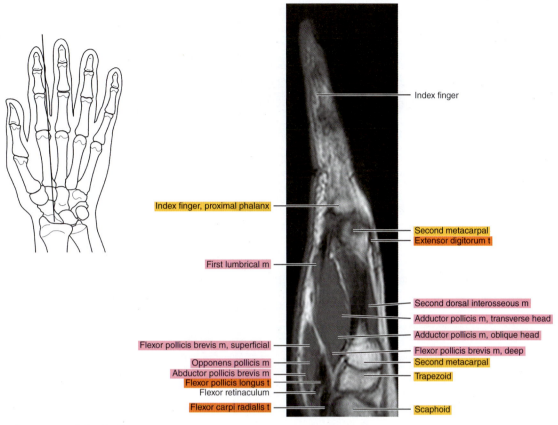

Index finger

Index finger, proximal phalanx

Second metacarpal
Extensor digitorum t

First lumbrical m

Second dorsal interosseous m
Adductor pollicis m, transverse head
Adductor pollicis m, oblique head
Flexor pollicis brevis m, superficial
Flexor pollicis brevis m, deep
Opponens pollicis m
Second metacarpal
Abductor pollicis brevis m
Trapezoid
Flexor pollicis longus t
Flexor retinaculum
Flexor carpi radialis t
Scaphoid

Figure 12.2.9

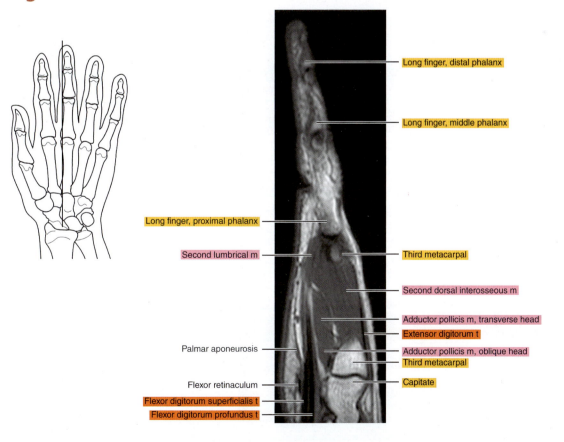

Long finger, distal phalanx

Long finger, middle phalanx

Long finger, proximal phalanx

Second lumbrical m
Third metacarpal

Second dorsal interosseous m

Adductor pollicis m, transverse head
Extensor digitorum t
Palmar aponeurosis
Adductor pollicis m, oblique head
Third metacarpal

Flexor retinaculum
Capitate

Flexor digitorum superficialis t
Flexor digitorum profundus t

Figure 12.2.10

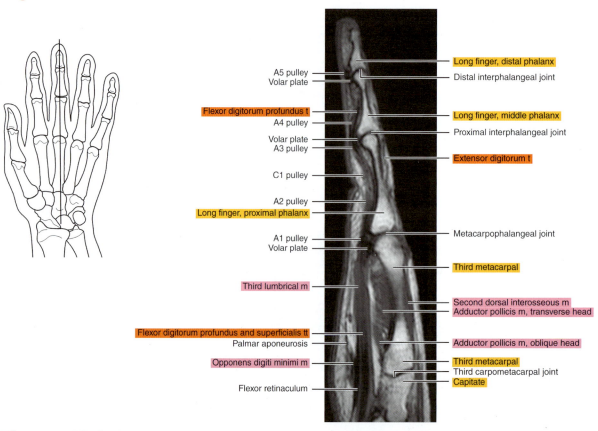

A5 pulley
Volar plate

Long finger, distal phalanx
Distal interphalangeal joint

Flexor digitorum profundus t
A4 pulley

Long finger, middle phalanx
Proximal interphalangeal joint

Volar plate
A3 pulley

Extensor digitorum t

C1 pulley

A2 pulley
Long finger, proximal phalanx

A1 pulley
Volar plate

Metacarpophalangeal joint

Third metacarpal

Third lumbrical m

Second dorsal interosseous m
Adductor pollicis m, transverse head

Flexor digitorum profundus and superficialis tt
Palmar aponeurosis

Adductor pollicis m, oblique head

Opponens digiti minimi m

Third metacarpal
Third carpometacarpal joint
Capitate

Flexor retinaculum

Figure 12.2.11

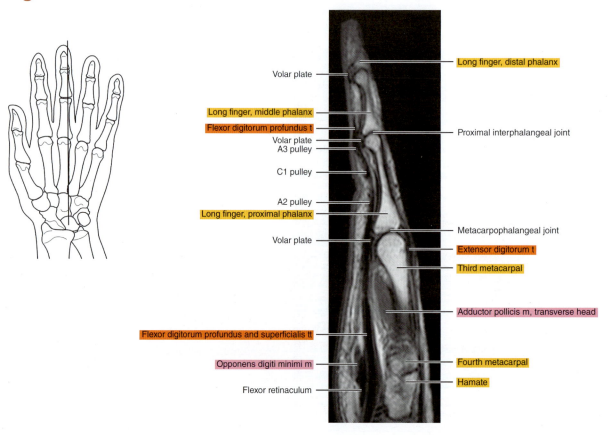

Volar plate

Long finger, distal phalanx

Long finger, middle phalanx
Flexor digitorum profundus t
Volar plate
A3 pulley

Proximal interphalangeal joint

C1 pulley

A2 pulley
Long finger, proximal phalanx

Volar plate

Metacarpophalangeal joint
Extensor digitorum t
Third metacarpal

Adductor pollicis m, transverse head

Flexor digitorum profundus and superficialis tt

Opponens digiti minimi m

Fourth metacarpal

Flexor retinaculum

Hamate

Figure 12.2.12

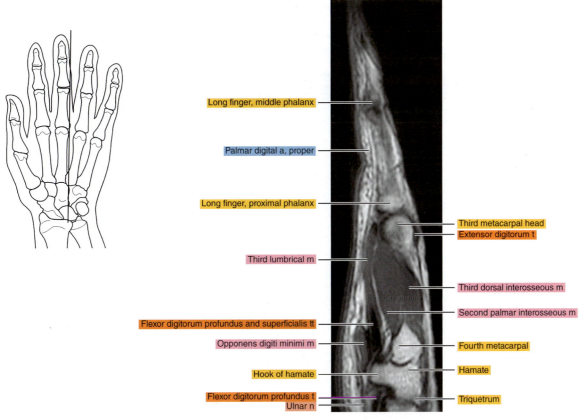

Long finger, middle phalanx

Palmar digital a, proper

Long finger, proximal phalanx

Third metacarpal head
Extensor digitorum t

Third lumbrical m

Third dorsal interosseous m

Second palmar interosseous m

Flexor digitorum profundus and superficialis tt

Opponens digiti minimi m

Fourth metacarpal

Hook of hamate

Hamate

Flexor digitorum profundus t

Triquetrum

Ulnar n

Figure 12.2.13

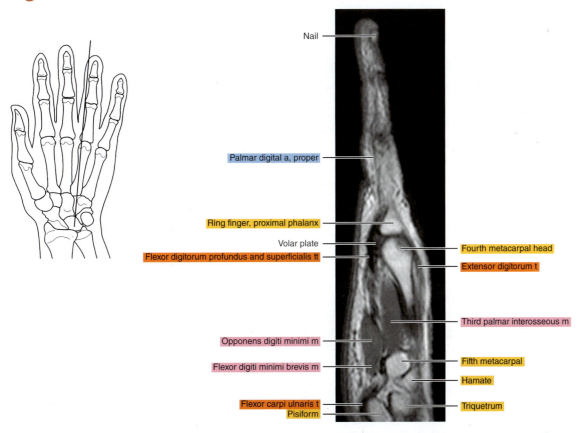

Nail

Palmar digital a, proper

Ring finger, proximal phalanx

Volar plate

Fourth metacarpal head

Flexor digitorum profundus and superficialis tt

Extensor digitorum t

Third palmar interosseous m

Opponens digiti minimi m

Flexor digiti minimi brevis m

Fifth metacarpal

Hamate

Flexor carpi ulnaris t

Triquetrum

Pisiform

Figure 12.2.14

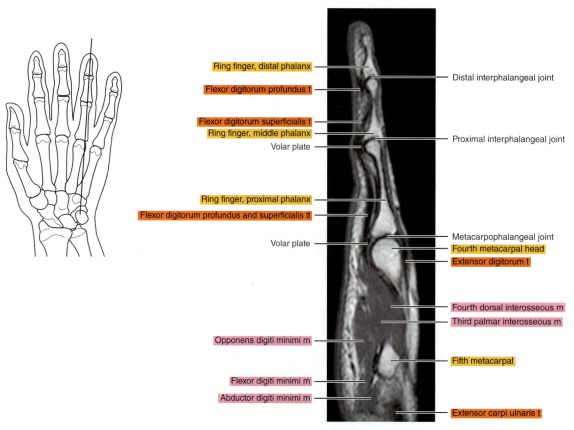

Ring finger, distal phalanx

Flexor digitorum profundus t

Flexor digitorum superficialis t

Ring finger, middle phalanx

Volar plate

Ring finger, proximal phalanx

Flexor digitorum profundus and superficialis tt

Volar plate

Opponens digiti minimi m

Flexor digiti minimi m

Abductor digiti minimi m

Distal interphalangeal joint

Proximal interphalangeal joint

Metacarpophalangeal joint

Fourth metacarpal head

Extensor digitorum t

Fourth dorsal interosseous m

Third palmar interosseous m

Fifth metacarpal

Extensor carpi ulnaris t

Figure 12.2.15

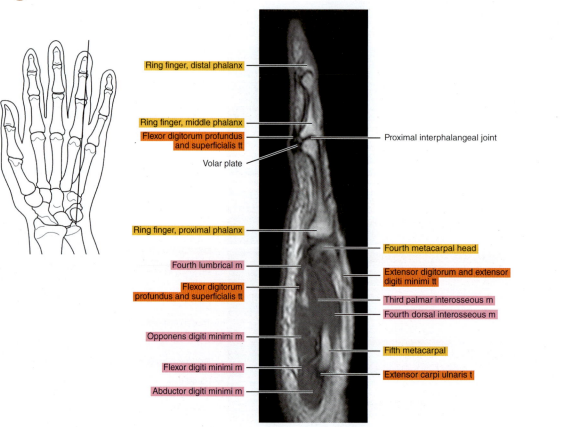

Ring finger, distal phalanx

Ring finger, middle phalanx

Flexor digitorum profundus and superficialis tt

Volar plate

Ring finger, proximal phalanx

Fourth lumbrical m

Flexor digitorum profundus and superficialis tt

Opponens digiti minimi m

Flexor digiti minimi m

Abductor digiti minimi m

Proximal interphalangeal joint

Fourth metacarpal head

Extensor digitorum and extensor digiti minimi tt

Third palmar interosseous m

Fourth dorsal interosseous m

Fifth metacarpal

Extensor carpi ulnaris t

Figure 12.2.16

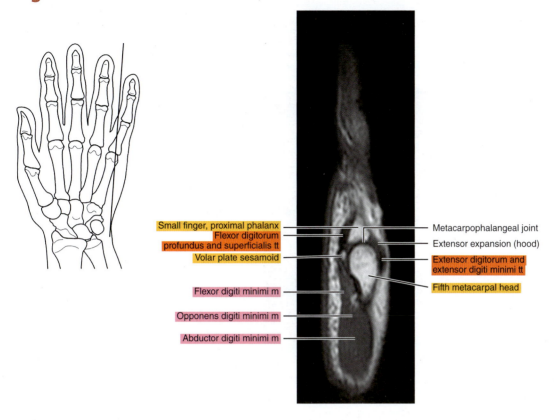

Small finger, proximal phalanx
Flexor digitorum profundus and superficialis tt
Volar plate sesamoid
Flexor digiti minimi m
Opponens digiti minimi m
Abductor digiti minimi m
Metacarpophalangeal joint
Extensor expansion (hood)
Extensor digitorum and extensor digiti minimi tt
Fifth metacarpal head

Figure 12.2.17

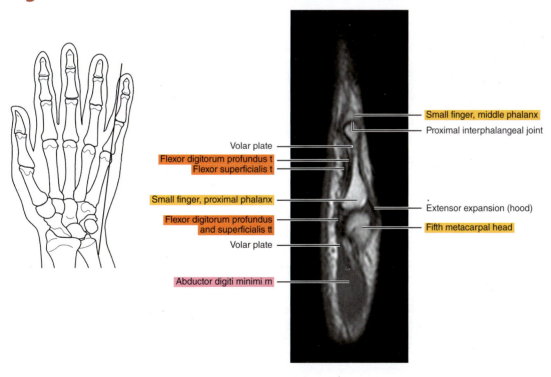

Volar plate
Flexor digitorum profundus t
Flexor superficialis t
Small finger, proximal phalanx
Flexor digitorum profundus and superficialis tt
Volar plate
Abductor digiti minimi m
Small finger, middle phalanx
Proximal interphalangeal joint
Extensor expansion (hood)
Fifth metacarpal head

Figure 12.2.18

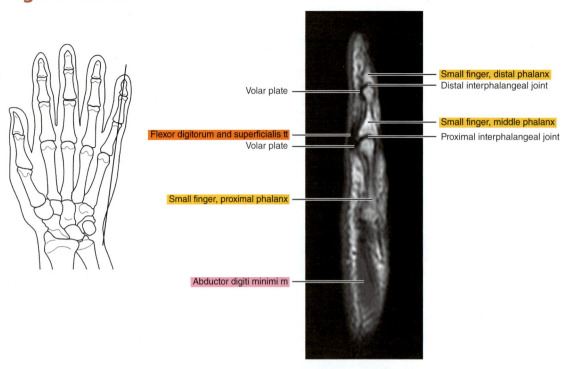

Volar plate

Small finger, distal phalanx
Distal interphalangeal joint

Flexor digitorum and superficialis tt
Volar plate

Small finger, middle phalanx
Proximal interphalangeal joint

Small finger, proximal phalanx

Abductor digiti minimi m

CORONAL
Figure 12.3.1

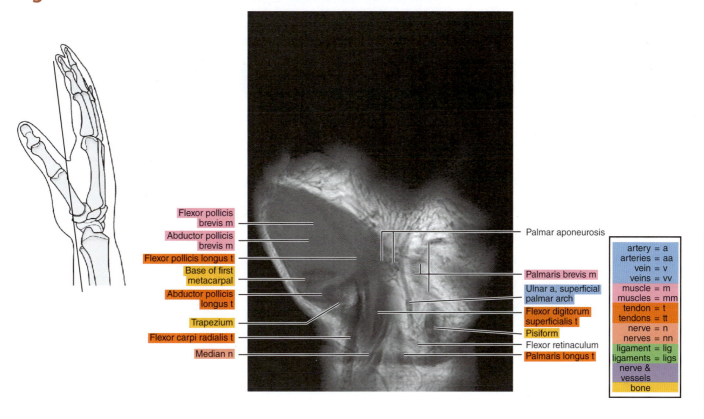

Flexor pollicis brevis m
Abductor pollicis brevis m
Flexor pollicis longus t
Base of first metacarpal
Abductor pollicis longus t
Trapezium
Flexor carpi radialis t
Median n

Palmar aponeurosis
Palmaris brevis m
Ulnar a, superficial palmar arch
Flexor digitorum superficialis t
Pisiform
Flexor retinaculum
Palmaris longus t

artery = a	
arteries = aa	
vein = v	
veins = vv	
muscle = m	
muscles = mm	
tendon = t	
tendons = tt	
nerve = n	
nerves = nn	
ligament = lig	
ligaments = ligs	
nerve & vessels	
bone	

Figure 12.3.2

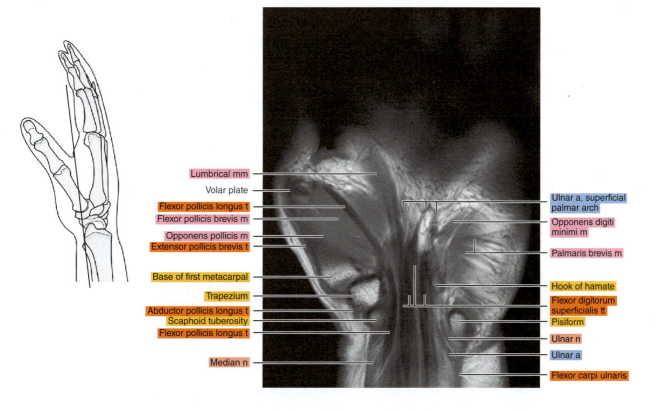

Lumbrical mm
Volar plate
Flexor pollicis longus t
Flexor pollicis brevis m
Opponens pollicis m
Extensor pollicis brevis t
Base of first metacarpal
Trapezium
Abductor pollicis longus t
Scaphoid tuberosity
Flexor pollicis longus t
Median n

Ulnar a, superficial palmar arch
Opponens digiti minimi m
Palmaris brevis m
Hook of hamate
Flexor digitorum superficialis tt
Pisiform
Ulnar n
Ulnar a
Flexor carpi ulnaris

Figure 12.3.3

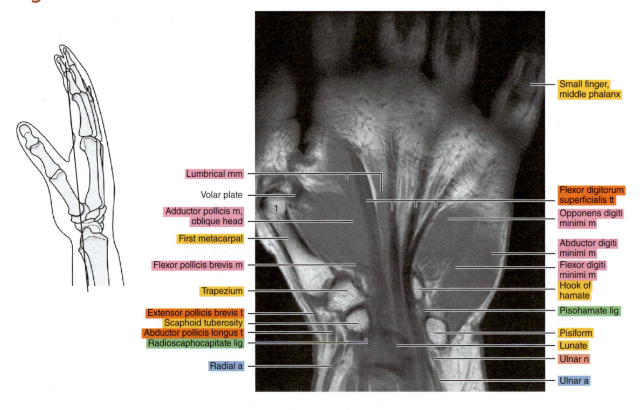

Lumbrical mm
Volar plate
Adductor pollicis m, oblique head
First metacarpal
Flexor pollicis brevis m
Trapezium
Extensor pollicis brevis t
Scaphoid tuberosity
Abductor pollicis longus t
Radioscaphocapitate lig
Radial a

Small finger, middle phalanx
Flexor digitorum superficialis tt
Opponens digiti minimi m
Abductor digiti minimi m
Flexor digiti minimi m
Hook of hamate
Pisohamate lig
Pisiform
Lunate
Ulnar n
Ulnar a

Figure 12.3.4

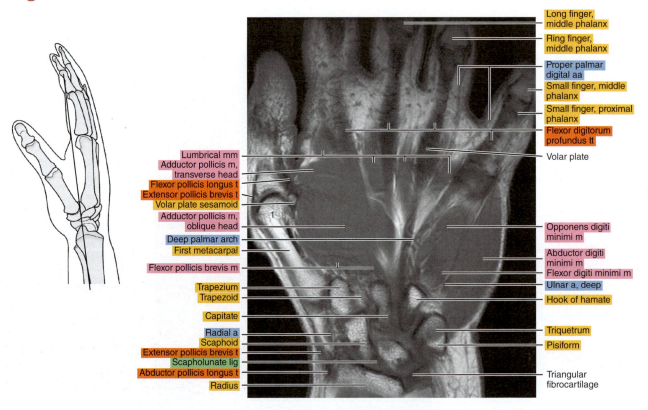

Lumbrical mm
Adductor pollicis m, transverse head
Flexor pollicis longus t
Extensor pollicis brevis t
Volar plate sesamoid
Adductor pollicis m, oblique head
Deep palmar arch
First metacarpal
Flexor pollicis brevis m
Trapezium
Trapezoid
Capitate
Radial a
Scaphoid
Extensor pollicis brevis t
Scapholunate lig
Abductor pollicis longus t
Radius

Long finger, middle phalanx
Ring finger, middle phalanx
Proper palmar digital aa
Small finger, middle phalanx
Small finger, proximal phalanx
Flexor digitorum profundus tt
Volar plate
Opponens digiti minimi m
Abductor digiti minimi m
Flexor digiti minimi m
Ulnar a, deep
Hook of hamate
Triquetrum
Pisiform
Triangular fibrocartilage

Figure 12.3.5

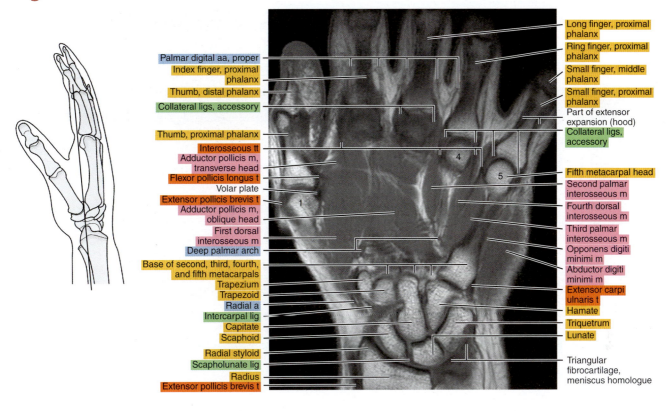

Palmar digital aa, proper
Index finger, proximal phalanx
Thumb, distal phalanx
Collateral ligs, accessory

Thumb, proximal phalanx
Interosseous tt
Adductor pollicis m, transverse head
Flexor pollicis longus t
Volar plate
Extensor pollicis brevis t
Adductor pollicis m, oblique head
First dorsal interosseous m
Deep palmar arch
Base of second, third, fourth, and fifth metacarpals
Trapezium
Trapezoid
Radial a
Intercarpal lig
Capitate
Scaphoid
Radial styloid
Scapholunate lig
Radius
Extensor pollicis brevis t

Long finger, proximal phalanx
Ring finger, proximal phalanx
Small finger, middle phalanx
Small finger, proximal phalanx
Part of extensor expansion (hood)
Collateral ligs, accessory

Fifth metacarpal head
Second palmar interosseous m
Fourth dorsal interosseous m
Third palmar interosseous m
Opponens digiti minimi m
Abductor digiti minimi m
Extensor carpi ulnaris t
Hamate
Triquetrum
Lunate

Triangular fibrocartilage, meniscus homologue

Figure 12.3.6

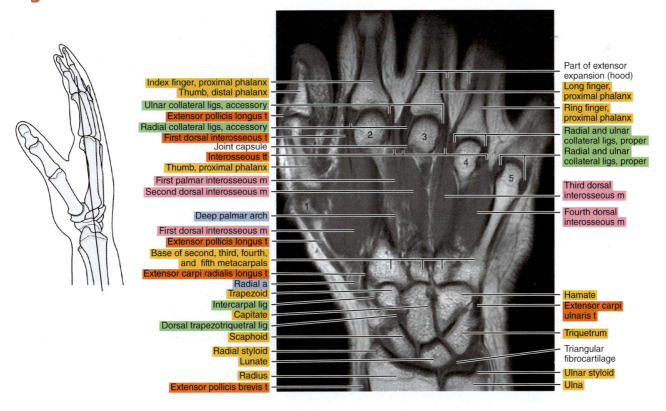

Index finger, proximal phalanx
Thumb, distal phalanx
Ulnar collateral ligs, accessory
Extensor pollicis longus t
Radial collateral ligs, accessory
First dorsal interosseous t
Joint capsule
Interosseous tt
Thumb, proximal phalanx
First palmar interosseous m
Second dorsal interosseous m

Deep palmar arch
First dorsal interosseous m
Extensor pollicis longus t
Base of second, third, fourth, and fifth metacarpals
Extensor carpi radialis longus t
Radial a
Trapezoid
Intercarpal lig
Capitate
Dorsal trapezotriquetral lig
Scaphoid
Radial styloid
Lunate
Radius
Extensor pollicis brevis t

Part of extensor expansion (hood)
Long finger, proximal phalanx
Ring finger, proximal phalanx
Radial and ulnar collateral ligs, proper
Radial and ulnar collateral ligs, proper

Third dorsal interosseous m
Fourth dorsal interosseous m

Hamate
Extensor carpi ulnaris t
Triquetrum
Triangular fibrocartilage
Ulnar styloid
Ulna

Figure 12.3.7

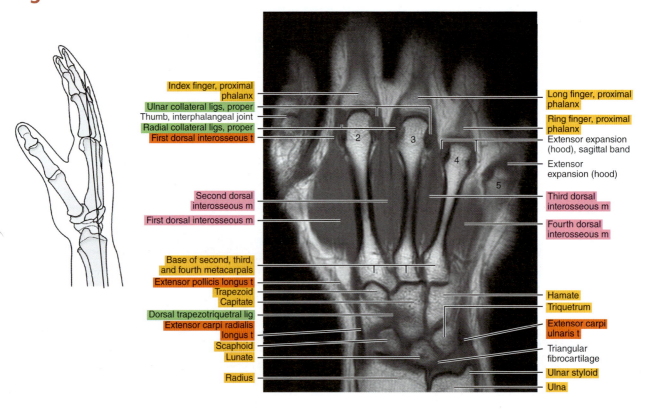

Index finger, proximal phalanx
Ulnar collateral ligs, proper
Thumb, interphalangeal joint
Radial collateral ligs, proper
First dorsal interosseous t

Second dorsal interosseous m
First dorsal interosseous m

Base of second, third, and fourth metacarpals
Extensor pollicis longus t
Trapezoid
Capitate
Dorsal trapezotriquetral lig
Extensor carpi radialis longus t
Scaphoid
Lunate
Radius

Long finger, proximal phalanx
Ring finger, proximal phalanx
Extensor expansion (hood), sagittal band
Extensor expansion (hood)
Third dorsal interosseous m
Fourth dorsal interosseous m

Hamate
Triquetrum
Extensor carpi ulnaris t
Triangular fibrocartilage
Ulnar styloid
Ulna

Figure 12.3.8

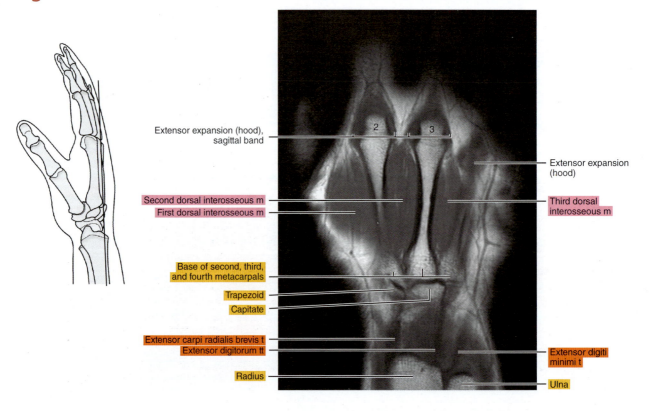

Extensor expansion (hood), sagittal band

Second dorsal interosseous m
First dorsal interosseous m

Base of second, third, and fourth metacarpals
Trapezoid
Capitate

Extensor carpi radialis brevis t
Extensor digitorum tt
Radius

Extensor expansion (hood)
Third dorsal interosseous m

Extensor digiti minimi t
Ulna

Figure 12.3.9

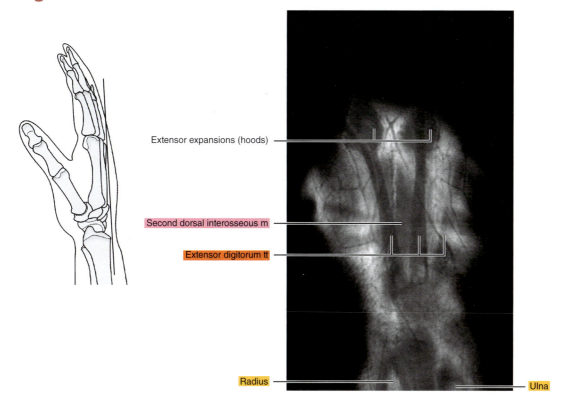

Extensor expansions (hoods)

Second dorsal interosseous m

Extensor digitorum tt

Radius

Ulna

Table 12-1. Muscles of the Hand

MUSCLE	ORIGIN	INSERTION	NERVE SUPPLY
Palmaris brevis	Ulnar border of the palmar aponeurosis.	Deep surface of the skin along the ulnar border of the palm.	Superficial branch of ulnar (C8 and T1)
Abductor pollicis brevis	Palmar surface of the flexor retinaculum, trapezium, and, occasionally, scaphoid.	Radial side of the base of the proximal phalanx of the thumb.	Recurrent branch of median (C8 and T1)
Opponens pollicis	Palmar surface of the flexor retinaculum and tubercle of the trapezium.	Lateral part of the palmar surface of the shaft of the first metacarpal.	Recurrent branch of median (C8 and T1)
Flexor pollicis brevis	Superficial head: trapezium, adjacent part of the flexor retinaculum, and tendon sheath of the flexor carpi radialis; deep head: trapezoid and capitate.	Superficial head: lateral side of the palmar aspect of the base of the proximal phalanx; deep head: into a tendon of the superficial head.	Recurrent branch of median and deep branch of ulnar (C8 and T1)
Adductor pollicis brevis	Carpal head: flexor retinaculum, capitate, bases of the second and third metacarpals; metacarpal head: palmar ridges of the third metacarpal and capsules of the second, third, and fourth metacarpophalangeal articulations.	Ulnar side of the palmar aspect of the base of the proximal phalanx of the thumb.	Recurrent branch of median (C8 and T1)
Abductor digiti minimi	Distal half of the pisiform, pisohamate ligament, tendon of the flexor carpi ulnaris, and, frequently, the flexor retinaculum.	Two tendons: (1) the ulnar side of the base of the proximal phalanx of the little finger and (2) the aponeurosis of the extensor tendon of the little finger.	Deep palmar division of ulnar (C8 and T1)
Flexor digiti minimi brevis	Hook of the hamate and adjacent parts of the flexor retinaculum.	Ulnar side of the base of the proximal phalanx of the little finger.	Superficial or deep palmar branch of ulnar (C8 and T1)
Opponens digiti minimi	Distal border of the hook of the hamate and adjacent flexor retinaculum.	Medial surface of the body and particularly onto the head of the fifth metacarpal.	Deep palmar branch of ulnar (C8 and T1)
Lumbrical	Two lateral lumbricals: radial and palmar sides of the first and second tendons of the flexor digitorum profundus; two medial lumbricals: adjacent side of the second and third tendons, and the third and fourth tendons of the flexor digitorum profundus.	Into the radial border of the tendon of the extensor digitorum on the dorsal aspect of the proximal phalanx.	Median, lateral two or three lumbricals; ulnar, deep palmar branch, medial one or two lumbricals (C8 and T1)
Interosseous	Palmar interosseous: anterior border of the shaft of the first, second, fourth, and fifth metacarpals. The first arises near the base and the others arise from three-fourths of the shaft of the bone. Dorsal interosseous: adjacent sides of the metacarpal bones in each metacarpal interspace.	Into the expansion on the axial side of the corresponding digit. The first palmar interosseous is described frequently as a division of the flexor brevis or adductor pollicis. The first dorsal interosseous usually inserts onto the proximal phalanx. The other three insert into the extensor expansion and proximal phalanx.	Deep palmar branch of ulnar (C8 and T1)

Section IV

Spine and Back

Chapter

13

MRI of the Cervical Spine

AXIAL
Figure 13.1.1

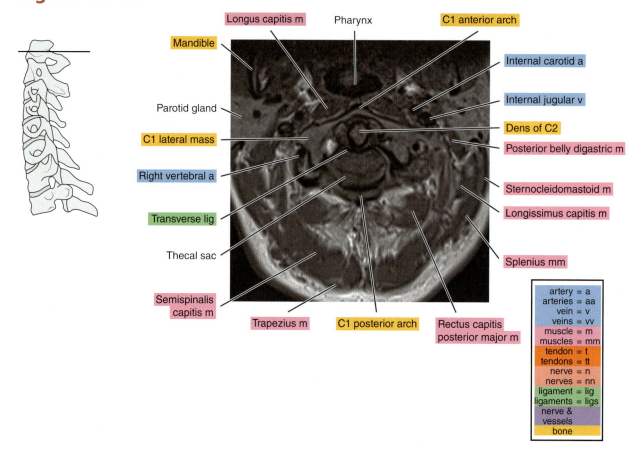

Longus capitis m | Pharynx | C1 anterior arch
Mandible
Internal carotid a
Parotid gland
Internal jugular v
C1 lateral mass
Dens of C2
Posterior belly digastric m
Right vertebral a
Sternocleidomastoid m
Transverse lig
Longissimus capitis m
Thecal sac
Splenius mm
Semispinalis capitis m
Trapezius m | C1 posterior arch | Rectus capitis posterior major m

artery = a
arteries = aa
vein = v
veins = vv
muscle = m
muscles = mm
tendon = t
tendons = tt
nerve = n
nerves = nn
ligament = lig
ligaments = ligs
nerve & vessels
bone

Figure 13.1.2

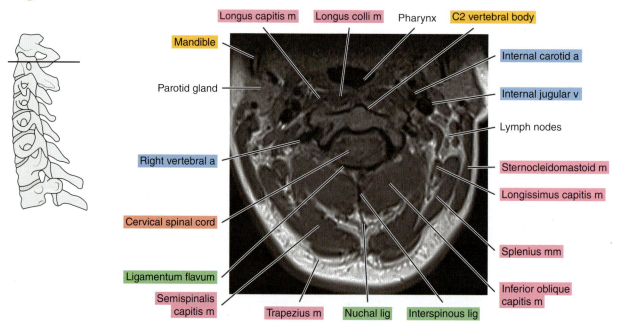

Longus capitis m | Longus colli m | Pharynx | C2 vertebral body
Mandible
Internal carotid a
Parotid gland
Internal jugular v
Lymph nodes
Right vertebral a
Sternocleidomastoid m
Longissimus capitis m
Cervical spinal cord
Splenius mm
Ligamentum flavum
Inferior oblique capitis m
Semispinalis capitis m | Trapezius m | Nuchal lig | Interspinous lig

Figure 13.1.3

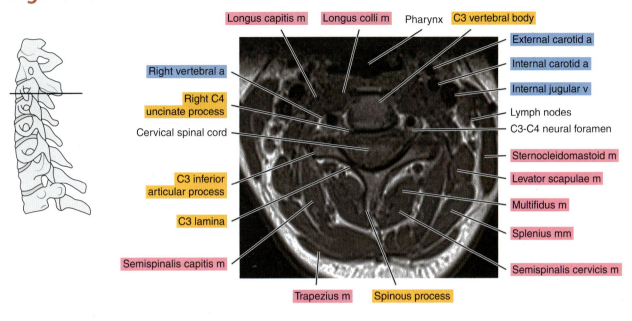

Longus capitis m · Longus colli m · Pharynx · C3 vertebral body · External carotid a · Internal carotid a · Internal jugular v · Right vertebral a · Right C4 uncinate process · Cervical spinal cord · Lymph nodes · C3-C4 neural foramen · Sternocleidomastoid m · Levator scapulae m · C3 inferior articular process · C3 lamina · Multifidus m · Splenius mm · Semispinalis capitis m · Semispinalis cervicis m · Trapezius m · Spinous process

Figure 13.1.4

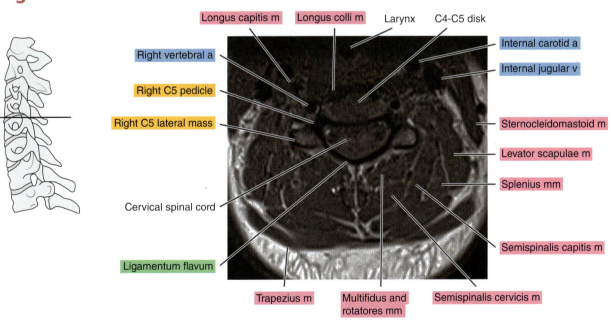

Longus capitis m · Longus colli m · Larynx · C4-C5 disk · Right vertebral a · Internal carotid a · Internal jugular v · Right C5 pedicle · Right C5 lateral mass · Sternocleidomastoid m · Levator scapulae m · Cervical spinal cord · Splenius mm · Ligamentum flavum · Semispinalis capitis m · Semispinalis cervicis m · Trapezius m · Multifidus and rotatores mm

Figure 13.1.5

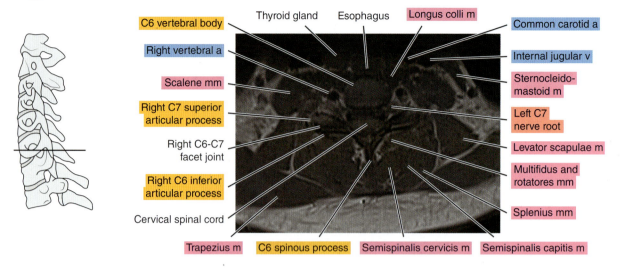

Thyroid gland — Esophagus — Longus colli m — Common carotid a — Internal jugular v — Sternocleido-mastoid m — Left C7 nerve root — Levator scapulae m — Multifidus and rotatores mm — Splenius mm

C6 vertebral body — Right vertebral a — Scalene mm — Right C7 superior articular process — Right C6-C7 facet joint — Right C6 inferior articular process — Cervical spinal cord

Trapezius m — C6 spinous process — Semispinalis cervicis m — Semispinalis capitis m

Figure 13.1.6

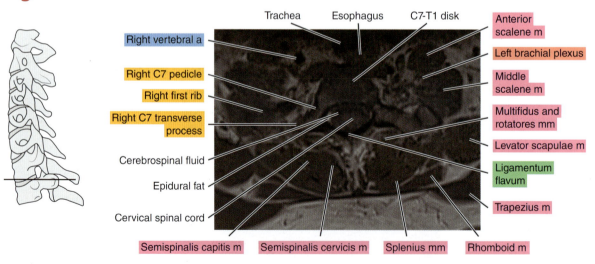

Trachea — Esophagus — C7-T1 disk — Anterior scalene m — Left brachial plexus — Middle scalene m — Multifidus and rotatores mm — Levator scapulae m — Ligamentum flavum — Trapezius m

Right vertebral a — Right C7 pedicle — Right first rib — Right C7 transverse process — Cerebrospinal fluid — Epidural fat — Cervical spinal cord

Semispinalis capitis m — Semispinalis cervicis m — Splenius mm — Rhomboid m

SAGITTAL
Figure 13.2.1

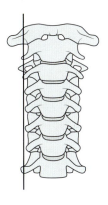

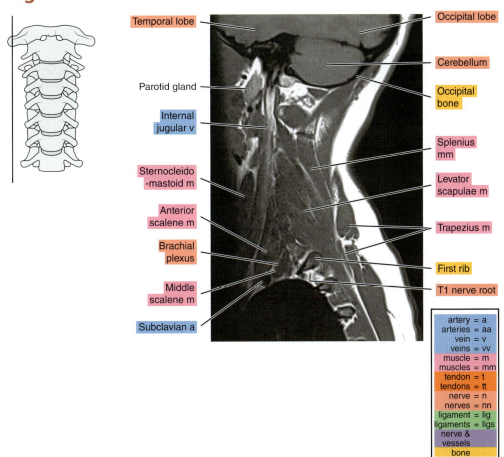

Temporal lobe

Parotid gland

Internal jugular v

Sternocleido -mastoid m

Anterior scalene m

Brachial plexus

Middle scalene m

Subclavian a

Occipital lobe

Cerebellum

Occipital bone

Splenius mm

Levator scapulae m

Trapezius m

First rib

T1 nerve root

| artery = a |
| arteries = aa |
| vein = v |
| veins = vv |
| muscle = m |
| muscles = mm |
| tendon = t |
| tendons = tt |
| nerve = n |
| nerves = nn |
| ligament = lig |
| ligaments = ligs |
| nerve & vessels |
| bone |

Figure 13.2.2

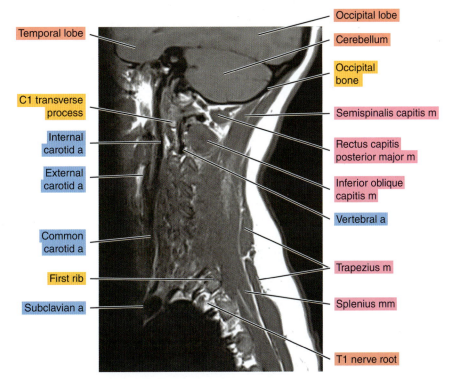

Temporal lobe

C1 transverse process

Internal carotid a

External carotid a

Common carotid a

First rib

Subclavian a

Occipital lobe

Cerebellum

Occipital bone

Semispinalis capitis m

Rectus capitis posterior major m

Inferior oblique capitis m

Vertebral a

Trapezius m

Splenius mm

T1 nerve root

Figure 13.2.3

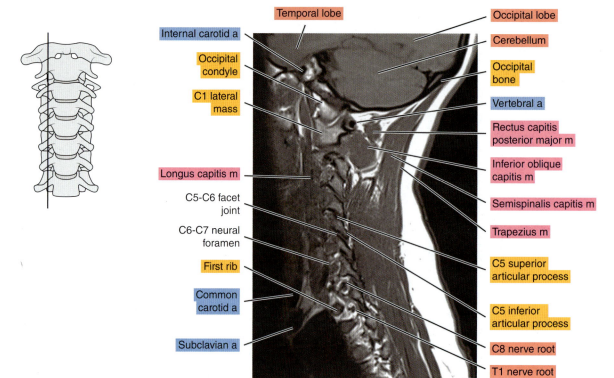

Temporal lobe
Internal carotid a
Occipital condyle
C1 lateral mass
Longus capitis m
C5-C6 facet joint
C6-C7 neural foramen
First rib
Common carotid a
Subclavian a

Occipital lobe
Cerebellum
Occipital bone
Vertebral a
Rectus capitis posterior major m
Inferior oblique capitis m
Semispinalis capitis m
Trapezius m
C5 superior articular process
C5 inferior articular process
C8 nerve root
T1 nerve root

Figure 13.2.4

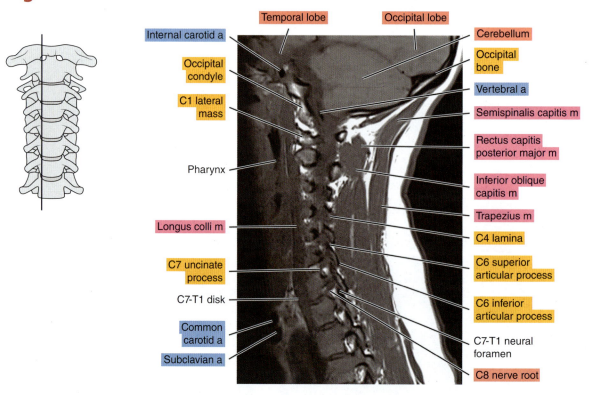

Temporal lobe
Occipital lobe
Internal carotid a
Occipital condyle
C1 lateral mass
Pharynx
Longus colli m
C7 uncinate process
C7-T1 disk
Common carotid a
Subclavian a

Cerebellum
Occipital bone
Vertebral a
Semispinalis capitis m
Rectus capitis posterior major m
Inferior oblique capitis m
Trapezius m
C4 lamina
C6 superior articular process
C6 inferior articular process
C7-T1 neural foramen
C8 nerve root

Figure 13.2.5

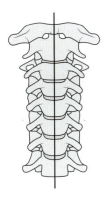

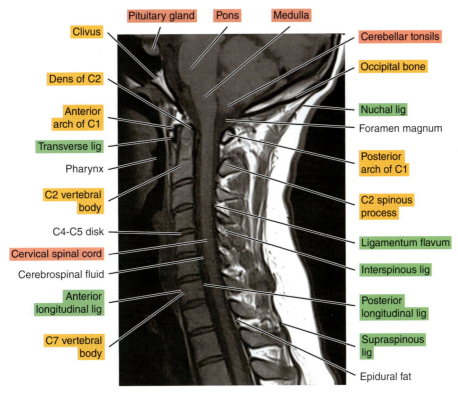

Pituitary gland

Pons

Medulla

Clivus

Cerebellar tonsils

Occipital bone

Dens of C2

Anterior arch of C1

Nuchal lig

Foramen magnum

Transverse lig

Posterior arch of C1

Pharynx

C2 vertebral body

C2 spinous process

C4-C5 disk

Ligamentum flavum

Cervical spinal cord

Interspinous lig

Cerebrospinal fluid

Anterior longitudinal lig

Posterior longitudinal lig

C7 vertebral body

Supraspinous lig

Epidural fat

CORONAL
Figure 13.3.1

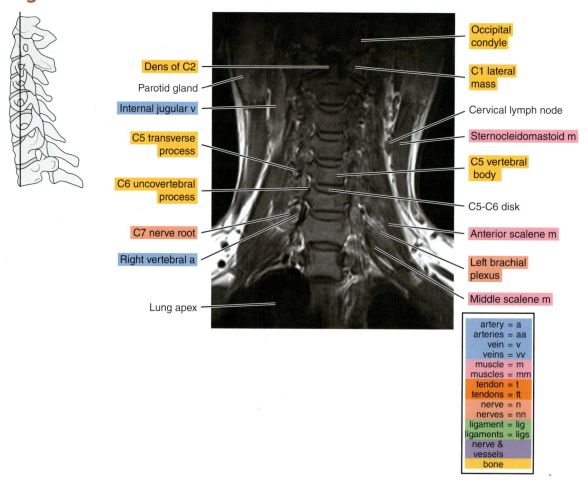

Dens of C2

Parotid gland

Internal jugular v

C5 transverse process

C6 uncovertebral process

C7 nerve root

Right vertebral a

Lung apex

Occipital condyle

C1 lateral mass

Cervical lymph node

Sternocleidomastoid m

C5 vertebral body

C5-C6 disk

Anterior scalene m

Left brachial plexus

Middle scalene m

artery	= a
arteries	= aa
vein	= v
veins	= vv
muscle	= m
muscles	= mm
tendon	= t
tendons	= tt
nerve	= n
nerves	= nn
ligament	= lig
ligaments	= ligs
nerve & vessels	
bone	

Figure 13.3.2

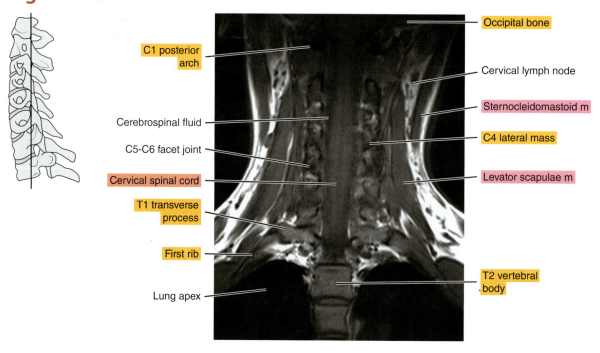

C1 posterior arch

Cerebrospinal fluid

C5-C6 facet joint

Cervical spinal cord

T1 transverse process

First rib

Lung apex

Occipital bone

Cervical lymph node

Sternocleidomastoid m

C4 lateral mass

Levator scapulae m

T2 vertebral body

Figure 13.3.3

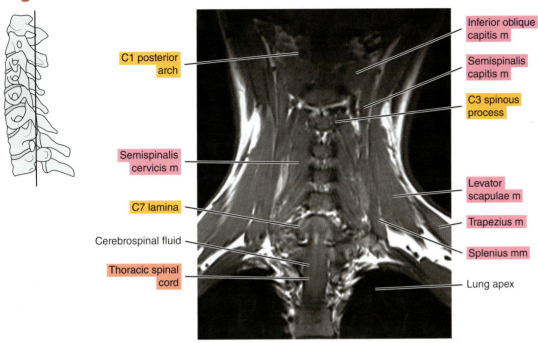

C1 posterior arch

Semispinalis cervicis m

C7 lamina

Cerebrospinal fluid

Thoracic spinal cord

Inferior oblique capitis m

Semispinalis capitis m

C3 spinous process

Levator scapulae m

Trapezius m

Splenius mm

Lung apex

Figure 13.3.4

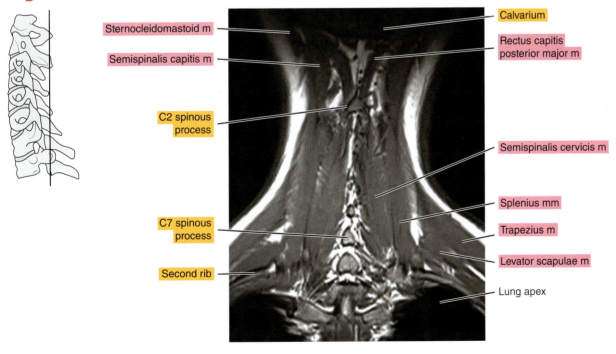

Sternocleidomastoid m

Semispinalis capitis m

C2 spinous process

C7 spinous process

Second rib

Calvarium

Rectus capitis posterior major m

Semispinalis cervicis m

Splenius mm

Trapezius m

Levator scapulae m

Lung apex

Chapter

14

MRI of the Thoracic Spine

AXIAL
Figure 14.1.1

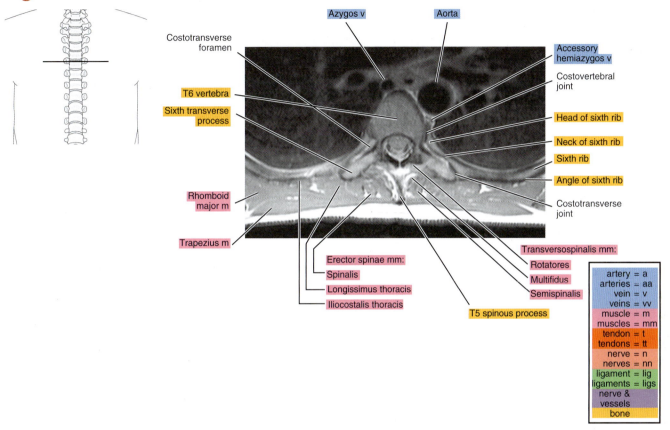

Azygos v
Aorta

Costotransverse foramen

Accessory hemiazygos v

Costovertebral joint

T6 vertebra

Sixth transverse process

Head of sixth rib

Neck of sixth rib

Sixth rib

Angle of sixth rib

Costotransverse joint

Rhomboid major m

Trapezius m

Transversospinalis mm:

Erector spinae mm:

Rotatores

Spinalis

Multifidus

Longissimus thoracis

Semispinalis

Iliocostalis thoracis

T5 spinous process

artery =	a
arteries =	aa
vein =	v
veins =	vv
muscle =	m
muscles =	mm
tendon =	t
tendons =	tt
nerve =	n
nerves =	nn
ligament =	lig
ligaments =	ligs
nerve & vessels	
bone	

Figure 14.1.2

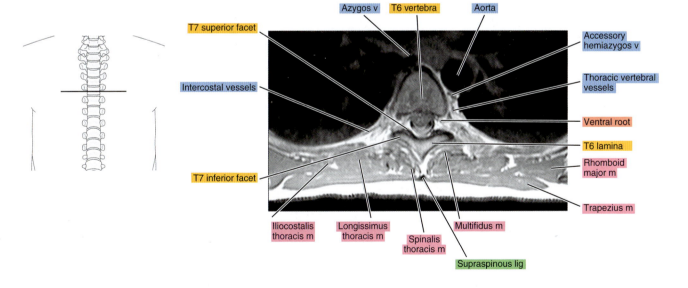

Azygos v   T6 vertebra   Aorta

T7 superior facet

Accessory hemiazygos v

Intercostal vessels

Thoracic vertebral vessels

Ventral root

T6 lamina

Rhomboid major m

T7 inferior facet

Trapezius m

Iliocostalis thoracis m

Longissimus thoracis m

Multifidus m

Spinalis thoracis m

Supraspinous lig

Figure 14.1.3

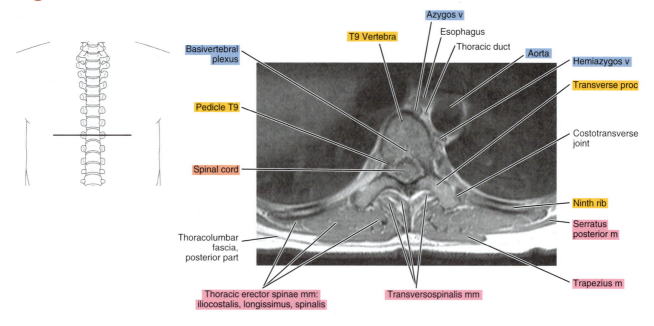

Figure 14.1.4

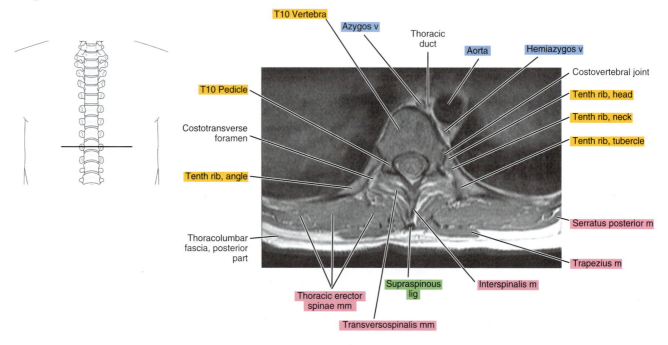

SAGITTAL
Figure 14.2.1

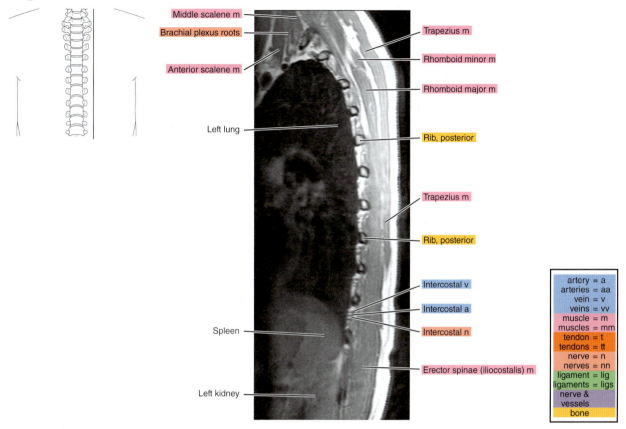

Middle scalene m

Brachial plexus roots

Anterior scalene m

Left lung

Spleen

Left kidney

Trapezius m

Rhomboid minor m

Rhomboid major m

Rib, posterior

Trapezius m

Rib, posterior

Intercostal v

Intercostal a

Intercostal n

Erector spinae (iliocostalis) m

artery	= a
arteries	= aa
vein	= v
veins	= vv
muscle	= m
muscles	= mm
tendon	= t
tendons	= tt
nerve	= n
nerves	= nn
ligament	= lig
ligaments	= ligs
nerve & vessels	
bone	

Figure 14.2.2

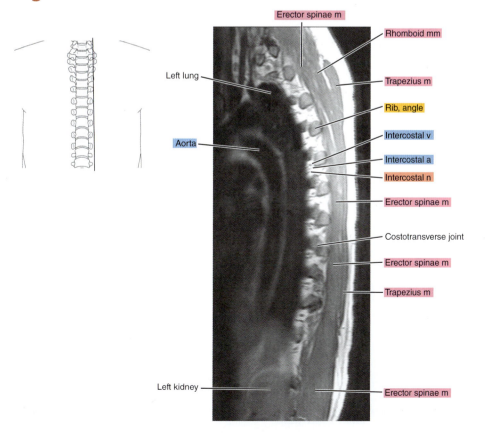

Erector spinae m

Left lung

Aorta

Left kidney

Rhomboid mm

Trapezius m

Rib, angle

Intercostal v

Intercostal a

Intercostal n

Erector spinae m

Costotransverse joint

Erector spinae m

Trapezius m

Erector spinae m

Figure 14.2.3

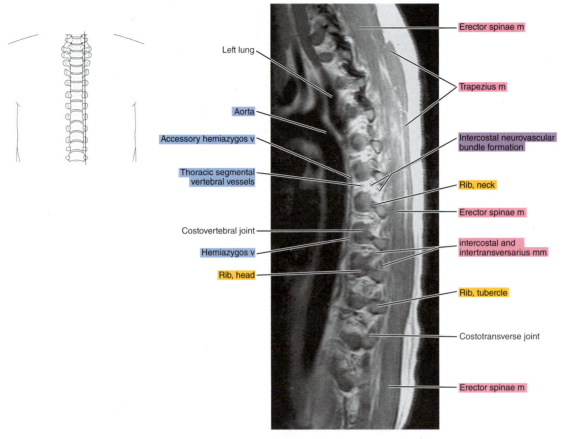

Left lung

Aorta

Accessory hemiazygos v

Thoracic segmental vertebral vessels

Costovertebral joint

Hemiazygos v

Rib, head

Erector spinae m

Trapezius m

Intercostal neurovascular bundle formation

Rib, neck

Erector spinae m

intercostal and intertransversarius mm

Rib, tubercle

Costotransverse joint

Erector spinae m

Figure 14.2.4

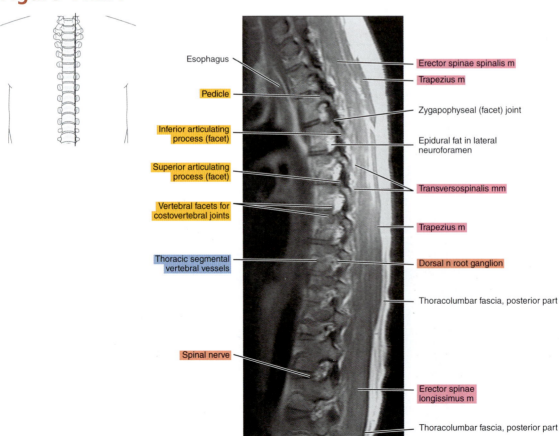

Esophagus

Pedicle

Inferior articulating process (facet)

Superior articulating process (facet)

Vertebral facets for costovertebral joints

Thoracic segmental vertebral vessels

Spinal nerve

Erector spinae spinalis m

Trapezius m

Zygapophyseal (facet) joint

Epidural fat in lateral neuroforamen

Transversospinalis mm

Trapezius m

Dorsal n root ganglion

Thoracolumbar fascia, posterior part

Erector spinae longissimus m

Thoracolumbar fascia, posterior part

Figure 14.2.5

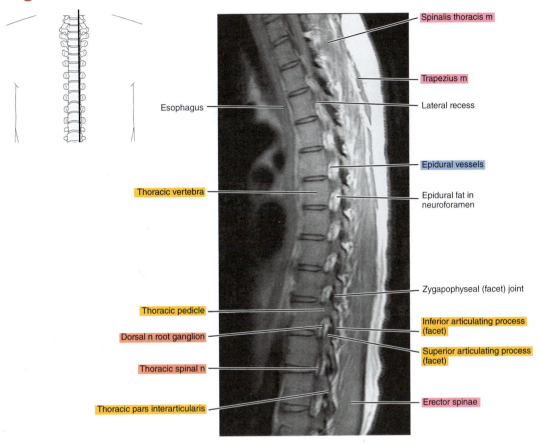

Spinalis thoracis m

Trapezius m

Esophagus

Lateral recess

Epidural vessels

Thoracic vertebra

Epidural fat in neuroforamen

Zygapophyseal (facet) joint

Thoracic pedicle

Inferior articulating process (facet)

Dorsal n root ganglion

Superior articulating process (facet)

Thoracic spinal n

Thoracic pars interarticularis

Erector spinae

Figure 14.2.6

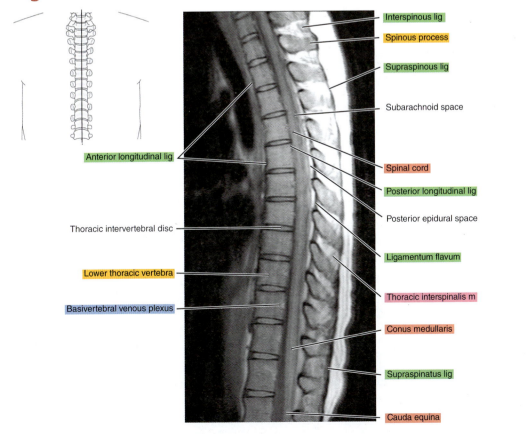

Interspinous lig

Spinous process

Supraspinous lig

Subarachnoid space

Anterior longitudinal lig

Spinal cord

Posterior longitudinal lig

Posterior epidural space

Thoracic intervertebral disc

Ligamentum flavum

Lower thoracic vertebra

Thoracic interspinalis m

Basivertebral venous plexus

Conus medullaris

Supraspinatus lig

Cauda equina

CORONAL
Figure 14.3.1

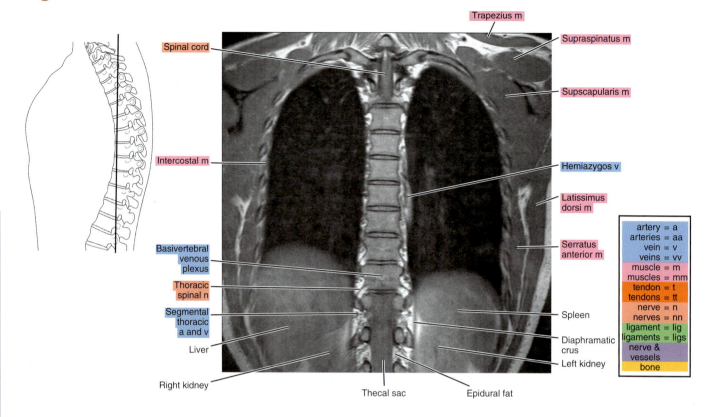

Spinal cord

Trapezius m

Supraspinatus m

Supscapularis m

Intercostal m

Hemiazygos v

Latissimus dorsi m

Serratus anterior m

Basivertebral venous plexus

Thoracic spinal n

Segmental thoracic a and v

Liver

Spleen

Diaphramatic crus

Left kidney

Right kidney

Thecal sac

Epidural fat

artery = a
arteries = aa
vein = v
veins = vv
muscle = m
muscles = mm
tendon = t
tendons = tt
nerve = n
nerves = nn
ligament = lig
ligaments = ligs
nerve & vessels
bone

Figure 14.3.2

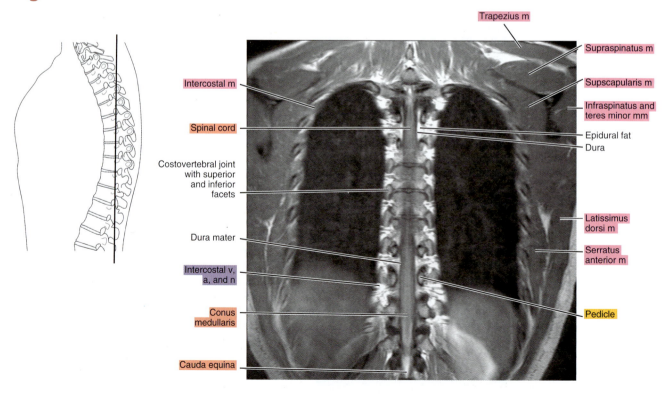

Trapezius m

Supraspinatus m

Supscapularis m

Intercostal m

Infraspinatus and teres minor mm

Spinal cord

Epidural fat
Dura

Costovertebral joint with superior and inferior facets

Dura mater

Latissimus dorsi m

Serratus anterior m

Intercostal v, a, and n

Conus medullaris

Pedicle

Cauda equina

Figure 14.3.3

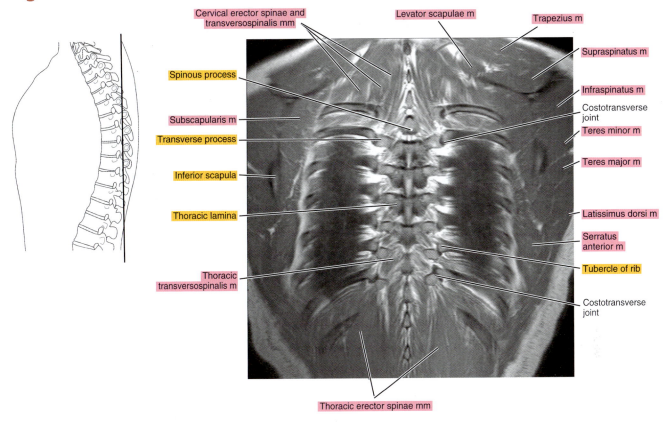

Cervical erector spinae and transversospinalis mm

Levator scapulae m

Trapezius m

Spinous process

Supraspinatus m

Subscapularis m

Infraspinatus m

Costotransverse joint

Transverse process

Teres minor m

Inferior scapula

Teres major m

Thoracic lamina

Latissimus dorsi m

Serratus anterior m

Thoracic transversospinalis m

Tubercle of rib

Costotransverse joint

Thoracic erector spinae mm

Figure 14.3.4

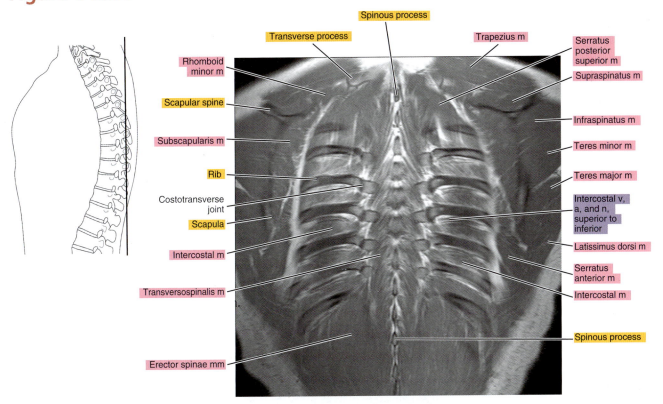

Spinous process

Transverse process

Trapezius m

Serratus posterior superior m

Rhomboid minor m

Supraspinatus m

Scapular spine

Infraspinatus m

Subscapularis m

Teres minor m

Rib

Teres major m

Costotransverse joint

Intercostal v, a, and n, superior to inferior

Scapula

Latissimus dorsi m

Intercostal m

Serratus anterior m

Transversospinalis m

Intercostal m

Spinous process

Erector spinae mm

Figure 14.3.5

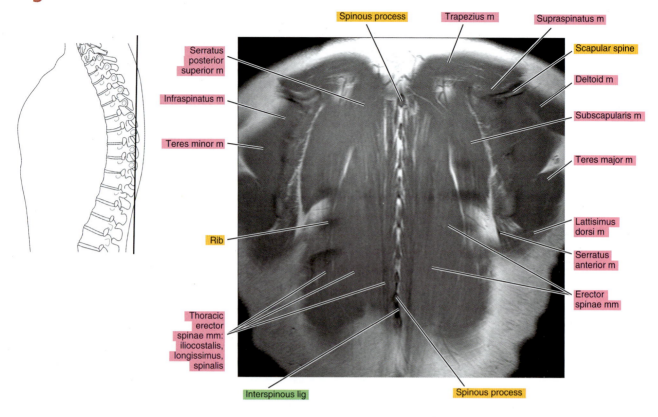

Spinous process — Trapezius m — Supraspinatus m

Serratus posterior superior m

Infraspinatus m

Teres minor m

Rib

Thoracic erector spinae mm: iliocostalis, longissimus, spinalis

Interspinous lig

Scapular spine

Deltoid m

Subscapularis m

Teres major m

Lattisimus dorsi m

Serratus anterior m

Erector spinae mm

Spinous process

Figure 14.3.6

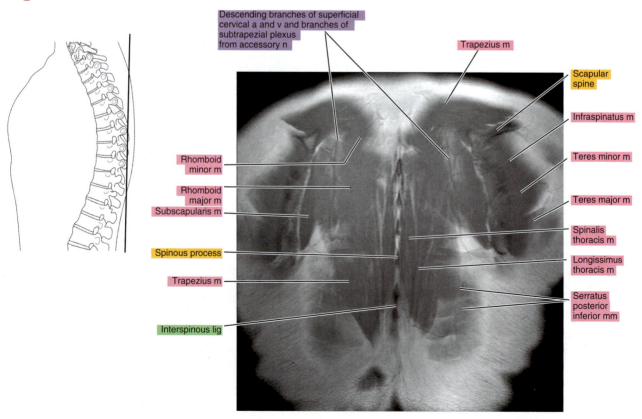

Descending branches of superficial cervical a and v and branches of subtrapezial plexus from accessory n

Trapezius m

Scapular spine

Infraspinatus m

Teres minor m

Teres major m

Rhomboid minor m

Rhomboid major m

Subscapularis m

Spinous process

Trapezius m

Interspinous lig

Spinalis thoracis m

Longissimus thoracis m

Serratus posterior inferior mm

Figure 14.3.7

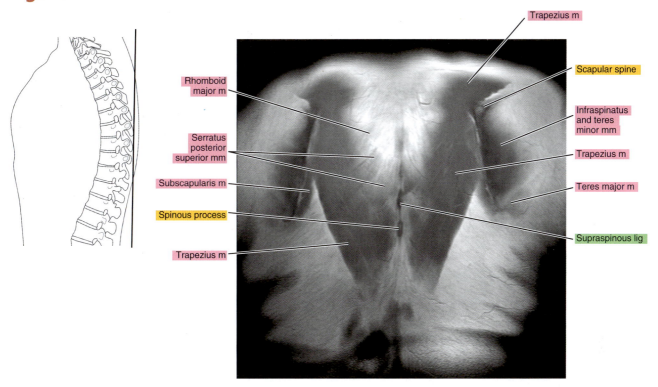

Trapezius m

Scapular spine

Rhomboid major m

Infraspinatus and teres minor mm

Serratus posterior superior mm

Trapezius m

Subscapularis m

Teres major m

Spinous process

Trapezius m

Supraspinous lig

Table 14-1. Muscles of the Back

MUSCLE	ORIGIN	INSERTION	NERVE SUPPLY
Trapezius	Medial third of the superior nuchal line, external occipital protuberance, ligamentum nuchae, spinous processes of the seventh cervical and thoracic vertebrae, and corresponding supraspinous ligaments	Lateral third of the posterior surface of the clavicle, medial side of the acromion, and upper border of the spine of the scapula	Accessory and cervical plexus
Rhomboideus major	Spinous processes and corresponding supraspinous ligaments of the first four thoracic vertebrae	Medial border of the scapula below the scapular spine	Dorsal scapular
Rhomboideus minor	Spinous processes of the sixth and seventh cervical vertebrae	Medial margin of the scapula above the scapular spine	Dorsal scapular
Levator scapulae	Posterior tubercles of the transverse processes of the four upper cervical vertebrae	Superior angle of the scapula	Dorsal scapular
Serratus posterior superior	From spinous processes of the two lower cervical and two upper thoracic vertebrae	Onto the lateral side of the angles of the second to fifth ribs	First to fourth intercostal
Serratus posterior inferior	With latissimus dorsi, from the spinous processes of the two lower thoracic and two upper lumbar vertebrae	Onto the lower borders of the last four ribs	Ninth to 12th intercostal
Serratus anterior	From the center of the lateral aspect of the first eight or nine ribs	Superior and inferior angles and intervening medial margin of the scapula	Long thoracic from brachial plexus
Deltoid	Lateral third of the clavicle, lateral border of the acromion process, and lower border of the scapular spine	Lateral margin of the proximal half of the humeral shaft	Axillary from fifth and sixth cervical nerves through brachial plexus
Latissimus dorsi	Spinous processes of the lower five or six thoracic and lumbar vertebrae, median ridge of the sacrum, and outer lip of the iliac crest	With teres major, onto the medial border of the bicipital groove of the humerus	Thoracodorsal
Infraspinatus	Infraspinous fossa of the scapula	Middle facet of the greater tuberosity of the humerus	Suprascapular from fifth to sixth cervical
Supraspinatus	Supraspinous fossa of the scapula	Greater tuberosity of the humerus	Suprascapular from fifth to sixth cervical
Teres major	Inferior angle and lower third of the border of the scapula	Medial border of the bicipital groove of the humerus	Lower subscapular from fifth and sixth cervical
Teres minor	Upper two-thirds of the lateral border of the scapula	Lower facet of the greater tuberosity of the humerus	Axillary from fifth and sixth cervical
Spinalis capitis	Rarely a separate muscle; it arises with the semispinalis capitis from the upper thoracic spinous process	Inserts with the semispinalis capitis on the occiput	Branches of the dorsal primary divisions of the spinal nerves

Table 14-1. Muscles of the Back

MUSCLE	ORIGIN	INSERTION	NERVE SUPPLY
Spinalis cervicis	Spinous processes of the sixth and seventh cervical vertebrae	Spinous processes of the axis and the third cervical vertebra	Dorsal branches of cervical
Spinalis thoracis	Spinous processes of the upper lumbar and two lower thoracic vertebrae	Spinous processes of the middle and upper thoracic vertebrae	Dorsal branches of thoracic and upper lumbar
Iliocostalis cervicis	Angles of the upper six ribs	Transverse processes of the middle cervical vertebrae	Dorsal branches of upper thoracic
Iliocostalis thoracis	Medial side of the angles of the lower six ribs	Angles of the upper six ribs	Dorsal branches of thoracic
Iliocostalis lumborum	With erector spinae, from the sacrum, ilium, and spines of the lumbar vertebrae	Angles of the lower six ribs	Dorsal branches of thoracic and lumbar nerves
Longissimus capitis	From the transverse processes of the upper thoracic and transverse and articular processes of the lower and middle cervical vertebrae	Onto the mastoid process	Dorsal branches of cervical
Longissimus cervicis	Transverse processes of the upper thoracic vertebrae	Transverse processes of the middle and upper cervical vertebrae	Dorsal branches of lower cervical and upper thoracic
Longissimus thoracis	With the iliocostalis and from the transverse processes of the lower thoracic vertebrae	By lateral slips onto most or all of the ribs between the angles and the tubercles and onto the tips of the transverse processes of the upper lumbar vertebrae, and by medial slips into the accessory processes of the upper lumbar and transverse processes of the thoracic vertebrae	Dorsal branches of thoracic and lumbar
Splenius capitis	From the ligamentum nuchae of the last four cervical vertebrae and the supraspinous ligament of first and second thoracic vertebrae	Lateral half of the superior nuchal line and mastoid process	Dorsal branches of second to sixth cervical
Splenius cervicis	From the supraspinous ligament and the spinous processes of the third to fifth thoracic vertebrae	Posterior tubercles of the transverse processes of the first and second (sometimes third) cervical vertebrae	Dorsal branches of fourth to eighth cervical
Semispinalis capitis	Transverse processes of the five or six upper thoracic and articular processes of the four lower cervical vertebrae	Occipital bone between the superior and inferior nuchal lines	Dorsal branches of cervical
Semispinalis cervicis	Transverse processes of the second to fifth thoracic vertebrae	Spinous processes of the axis and the third to fifth cervical vertebrae	Dorsal branches of cervical and thoracic
Semispinalis thoracis	Transverse processes of the fifth to 11th thoracic vertebrae	Spinous processes of the first four thoracic and fifth and seventh cervical vertebrae	Dorsal branches of cervical and thoracic

continued

Table 14-1. Muscles of the Back–cont'd

MUSCLE	ORIGIN	INSERTION	NERVE SUPPLY
Multifidus	From the sacrum, the sacroiliac ligament, mammillary processes of the lumbar vertebrae, transverse processes of the thoracic vertebrae, and articular processes of the last four cervical vertebrae	Onto the spinous processes of all the vertebrae, up to and including the axis	Dorsal branches of spinal
Rotatores	Primarily developed in the thoracic region from the transverse processes of the vertebrae	Into the root of the spinous processes of the next two or three vertebrae above	Dorsal branches of spinal
Interspinales cervicis	Tubercle of the spinous process of the cervical vertebrae	Tubercle of the spinous process of the next superior vertebra	Dorsal branches of cervical
Interspinales thoracis	Often poorly developed or absent between the spinous processes of the thoracic vertebrae	Spinous processes of thoracic vertebrae	Dorsal branches of thoracic
Interspinales lumborum	Superior margin of the lumbar spinous processes	Inferior margin of the next superior spinous process	Dorsal branches of lumbar
Intertransversarii anteriores cervicis	Anterior tubercle of the cervical transverse process	Anterior tubercle of the next superior transverse process	Ventral branch of cervical
Intertransversarii laterales lumbar	Transverse processes of the lumbar vertebrae	Next superior transverse process	Ventral branches of lumbar
Intertransversarii thoracis	Transverse processes of the thoracic vertebrae	Next superior transverse process	Dorsal branches of thoracic

Chapter 15

MRI of the Lumbar Spine

AXIAL
Figure 15.1.1

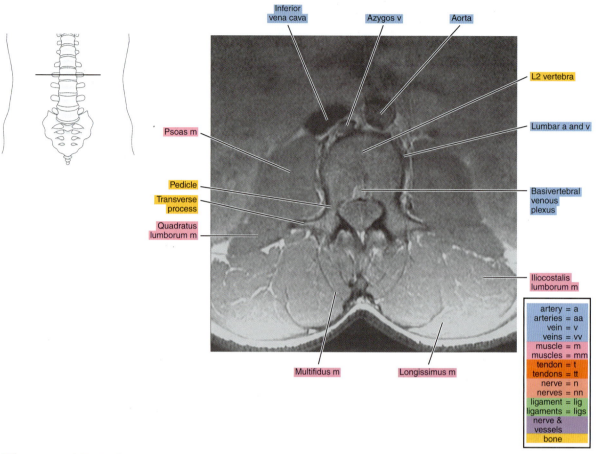

Inferior vena cava

Azygos v

Aorta

L2 vertebra

Psoas m

Lumbar a and v

Pedicle

Transverse process

Quadratus lumborum m

Basivertebral venous plexus

Iliocostalis lumborum m

artery = a	
arteries = aa	
vein = v	
veins = vv	
muscle = m	
muscles = mm	
tendon = t	
tendons = tt	
nerve = n	
nerves = nn	
ligament = lig	
ligaments = ligs	
nerve & vessels	
bone	

Multifidus m

Longissimus m

Figure 15.1.2

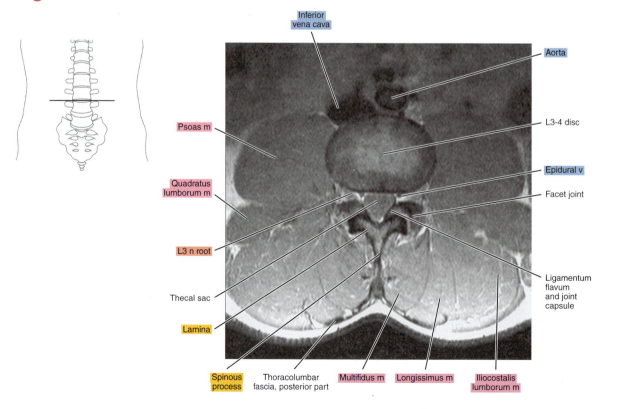

Inferior vena cava

Aorta

Psoas m

L3-4 disc

Quadratus lumborum m

Epidural v

Facet joint

L3 n root

Thecal sac

Ligamentum flavum and joint capsule

Lamina

Spinous process

Thoracolumbar fascia, posterior part

Multifidus m

Longissimus m

Iliocostalis lumborum m

Figure 15.1.3

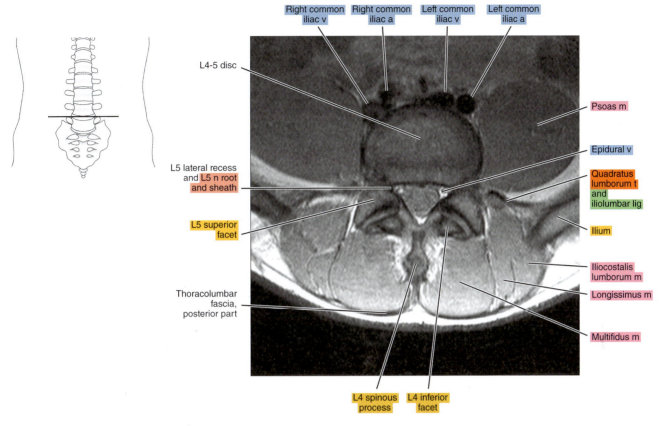

Right common iliac v · Right common iliac a · Left common iliac v · Left common iliac a

L4-5 disc

Psoas m

Epidural v

Quadratus lumborum t and iliolumbar lig

L5 lateral recess and L5 n root and sheath

Ilium

L5 superior facet

Iliocostalis lumborum m

Longissimus m

Thoracolumbar fascia, posterior part

Multifidus m

L4 spinous process · L4 inferior facet

Figure 15.1.4

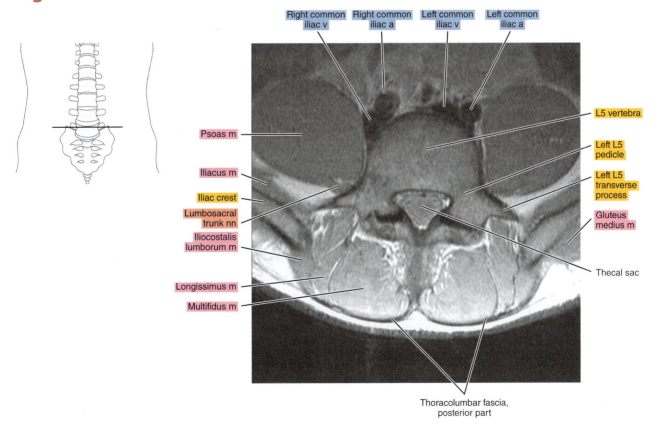

Right common iliac v · Right common iliac a · Left common iliac v · Left common iliac a

Psoas m

L5 vertebra

Iliacus m

Left L5 pedicle

Iliac crest

Left L5 transverse process

Lumbosacral trunk nn

Gluteus medius m

Iliocostalis lumborum m

Longissimus m

Thecal sac

Multifidus m

Thoracolumbar fascia, posterior part

Figure 15.1.5

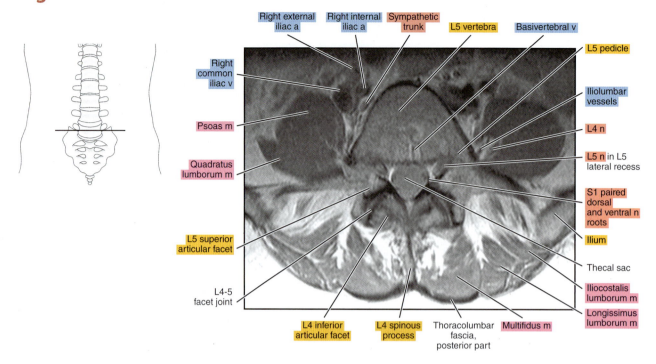

Figure 15.1.6

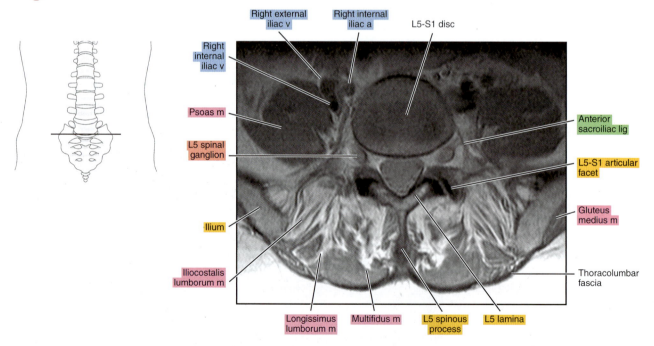

Figure 15.1.7

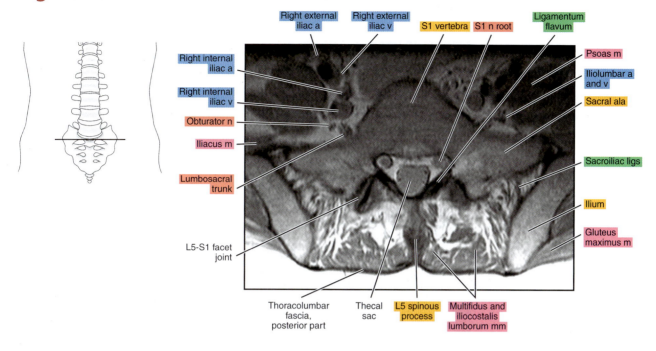

Right external iliac a

Right external iliac v

S1 vertebra

S1 n root

Ligamentum flavum

Right internal iliac a

Right internal iliac v

Obturator n

Iliacus m

Lumbosacral trunk

L5-S1 facet joint

Psoas m

Iliolumbar a and v

Sacral ala

Sacroiliac ligs

Ilium

Gluteus maximus m

Thoracolumbar fascia, posterior part

Thecal sac

L5 spinous process

Multifidus and iliocostalis lumborum mm

Figure 15.1.8

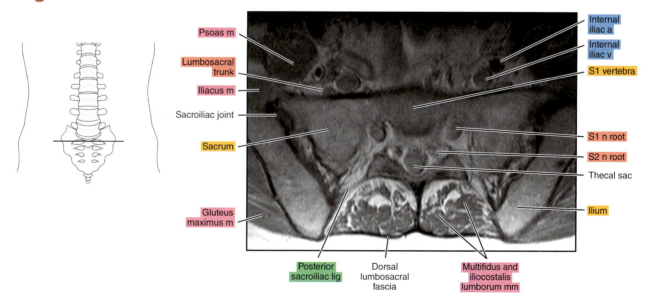

Psoas m

Lumbosacral trunk

Iliacus m

Sacroiliac joint

Sacrum

Gluteus maximus m

Internal iliac a

Internal iliac v

S1 vertebra

S1 n root

S2 n root

Thecal sac

Ilium

Posterior sacroiliac lig

Dorsal lumbosacral fascia

Multifidus and iliocostalis lumborum mm

SAGITTAL
Figure 15.2.1

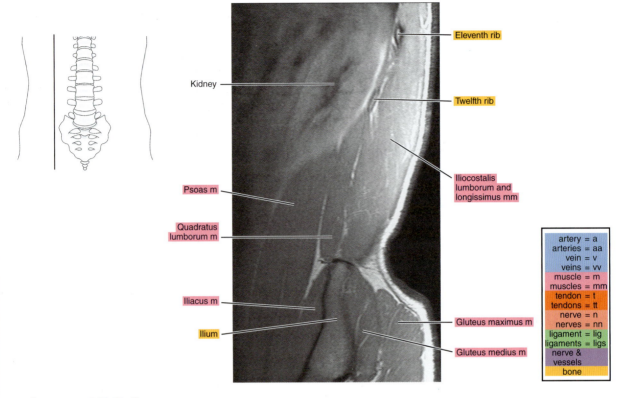

Kidney

Psoas m

Quadratus lumborum m

Iliacus m

Ilium

Eleventh rib

Twelfth rib

Iliocostalis lumborum and longissimus mm

Gluteus maximus m

Gluteus medius m

artery	= a
arteries	= aa
vein	= v
veins	= vv
muscle	= m
muscles	= mm
tendon	= t
tendons	= tt
nerve	= n
nerves	= nn
ligament	= lig
ligaments	= ligs
nerve & vessels	
bone	

Figure 15.2.2

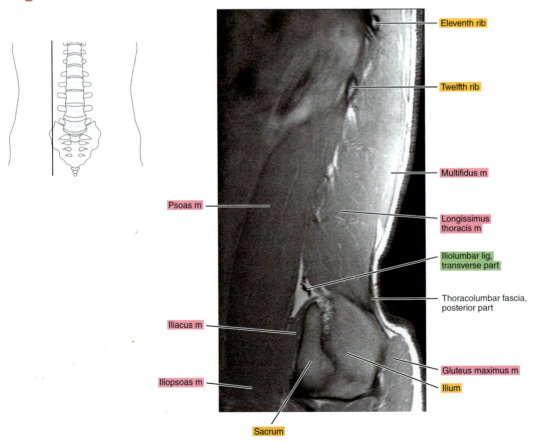

Psoas m

Iliacus m

Iliopsoas m

Sacrum

Eleventh rib

Twelfth rib

Multifidus m

Longissimus thoracis m

Iliolumbar lig, transverse part

Thoracolumbar fascia, posterior part

Gluteus maximus m

Ilium

Figure 15.2.3

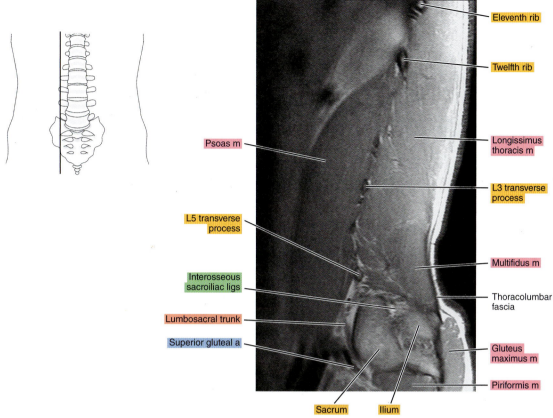

Eleventh rib

Twelfth rib

Longissimus thoracis m

L3 transverse process

Psoas m

Multifidus m

L5 transverse process

Thoracolumbar fascia

Interosseous sacroiliac ligs

Lumbosacral trunk

Superior gluteal a

Gluteus maximus m

Piriformis m

Sacrum   Ilium

Figure 15.2.4

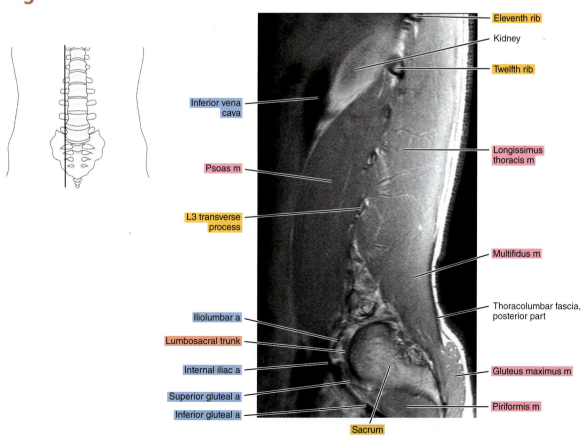

Eleventh rib

Kidney

Twelfth rib

Inferior vena cava

Longissimus thoracis m

Psoas m

L3 transverse process

Multifidus m

Thoracolumbar fascia, posterior part

Iliolumbar a

Lumbosacral trunk

Internal iliac a

Gluteus maximus m

Superior gluteal a

Inferior gluteal a

Piriformis m

Sacrum

Figure 15.2.5

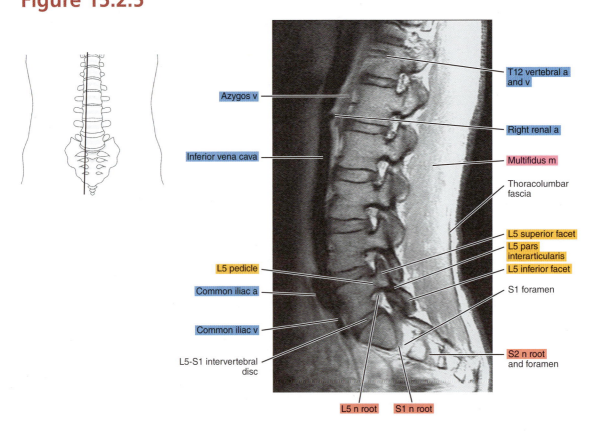

Azygos v

Inferior vena cava

L5 pedicle

Common iliac a

Common iliac v

L5-S1 intervertebral disc

L5 n root   S1 n root

T12 vertebral a and v

Right renal a

Multifidus m

Thoracolumbar fascia

L5 superior facet

L5 pars interarticularis

L5 inferior facet

S1 foramen

S2 n root and foramen

Figure 15.2.6

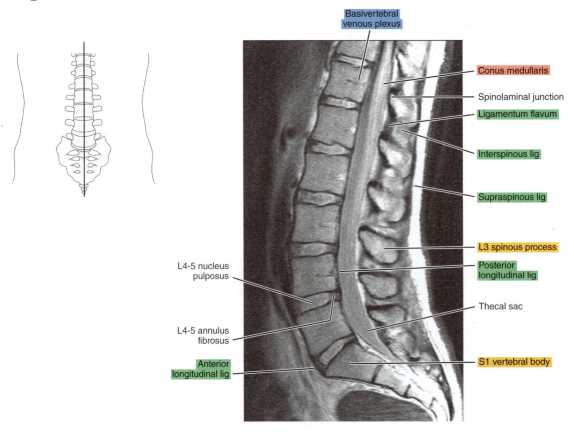

Basivertebral venous plexus

Conus medullaris

Spinolaminal junction

Ligamentum flavum

Interspinous lig

Supraspinous lig

L3 spinous process

Posterior longitudinal lig

Thecal sac

S1 vertebral body

L4-5 nucleus pulposus

L4-5 annulus fibrosus

Anterior longitudinal lig

CORONAL
Figure 15.3.1

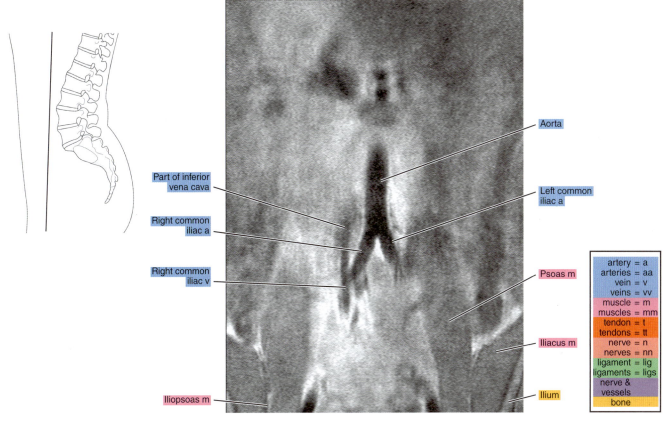

Part of inferior vena cava

Right common iliac a

Right common iliac v

Iliopsoas m

Aorta

Left common iliac a

Psoas m

Iliacus m

Ilium

artery = a	
arteries = aa	
vein = v	
veins = vv	
muscle = m	
muscles = mm	
tendon = t	
tendons = tt	
nerve = n	
nerves = nn	
ligament = lig	
ligaments = ligs	
nerve & vessels	
bone	

Figure 15.3.2

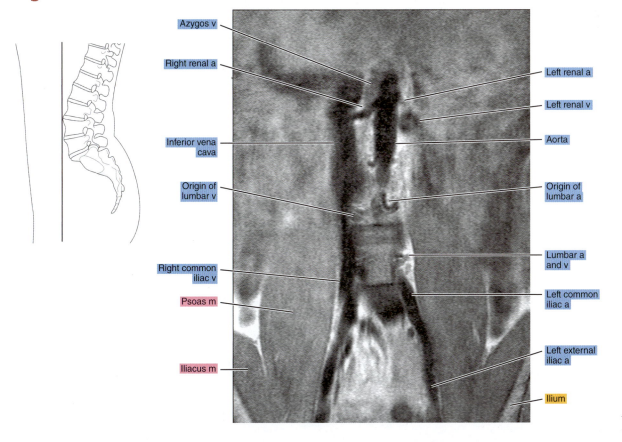

Azygos v

Right renal a

Inferior vena cava

Origin of lumbar v

Right common iliac v

Psoas m

Iliacus m

Left renal a

Left renal v

Aorta

Origin of lumbar a

Lumbar a and v

Left common iliac a

Left external iliac a

Ilium

Figure 15.3.3

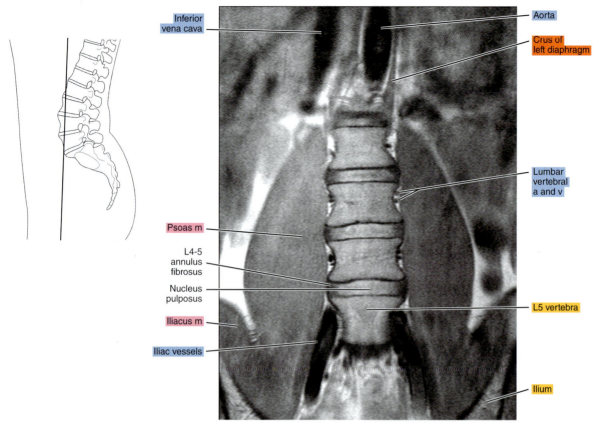

Inferior vena cava

Aorta

Crus of left diaphragm

Lumbar vertebral a and v

Psoas m

L4-5 annulus fibrosus

Nucleus pulposus

L5 vertebra

Iliacus m

Iliac vessels

Ilium

Figure 15.3.4

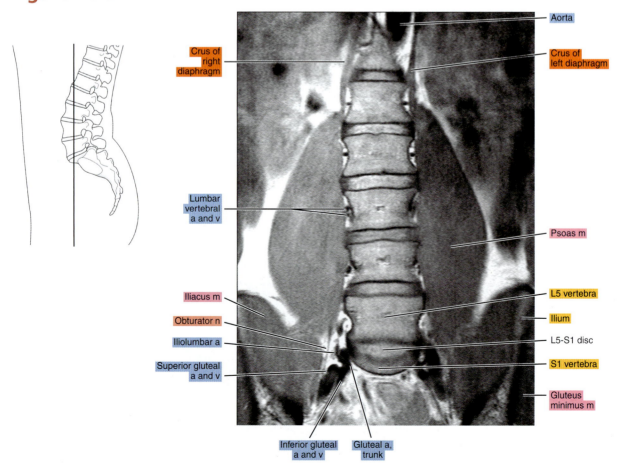

Aorta

Crus of right diaphragm

Crus of left diaphragm

Lumbar vertebral a and v

Psoas m

Iliacus m

L5 vertebra

Obturator n

Ilium

Iliolumbar a

L5-S1 disc

Superior gluteal a and v

S1 vertebra

Gluteus minimus m

Inferior gluteal a and v

Gluteal a, trunk

Figure 15.3.5

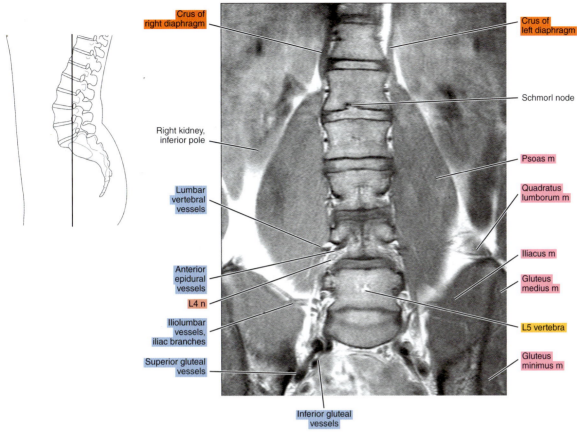

Crus of right diaphragm
Crus of left diaphragm
Schmorl node
Right kidney, inferior pole
Psoas m
Lumbar vertebral vessels
Quadratus lumborum m
Iliacus m
Anterior epidural vessels
Gluteus medius m
L4 n
Iliolumbar vessels, iliac branches
L5 vertebra
Superior gluteal vessels
Gluteus minimus m
Inferior gluteal vessels

Figure 15.3.6

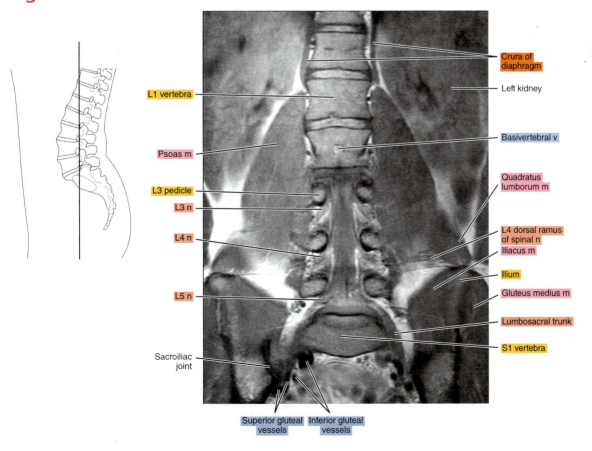

Crura of diaphragm
Left kidney
L1 vertebra
Basivertebral v
Psoas m
Quadratus lumborum m
L3 pedicle
L3 n
L4 dorsal ramus of spinal n
L4 n
Iliacus m
Ilium
Gluteus medius m
L5 n
Lumbosacral trunk
S1 vertebra
Sacroiliac joint
Superior gluteal vessels
Inferior gluteal vessels

Figure 15.3.7

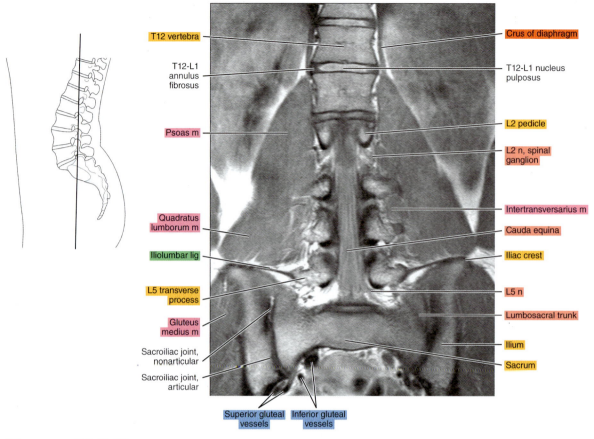

T12 vertebra
Crus of diaphragm
T12-L1 annulus fibrosus
T12-L1 nucleus pulposus
Psoas m
L2 pedicle
L2 n, spinal ganglion
Quadratus lumborum m
Intertransversarius m
Cauda equina
Iliolumbar lig
Iliac crest
L5 transverse process
L5 n
Gluteus medius m
Lumbosacral trunk
Sacroiliac joint, nonarticular
Ilium
Sacroiliac joint, articular
Sacrum
Superior gluteal vessels
Inferior gluteal vessels

Figure 15.3.8

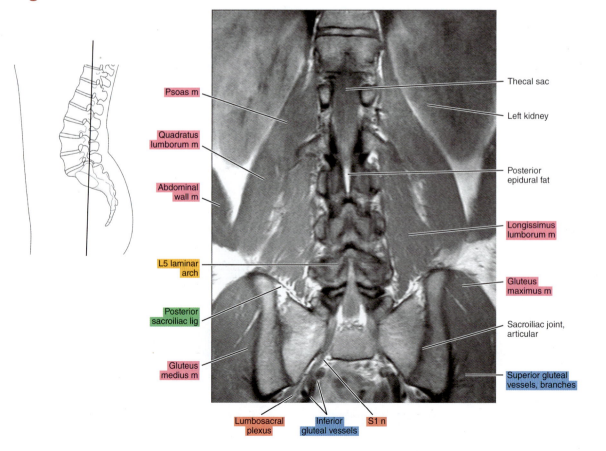

Psoas m
Thecal sac
Quadratus lumborum m
Left kidney
Abdominal wall m
Posterior epidural fat
Longissimus lumborum m
L5 laminar arch
Posterior sacroiliac lig
Gluteus maximus m
Sacroiliac joint, articular
Gluteus medius m
Superior gluteal vessels, branches
Lumbosacral plexus
Inferior gluteal vessels
S1 n

Figure 15.3.9

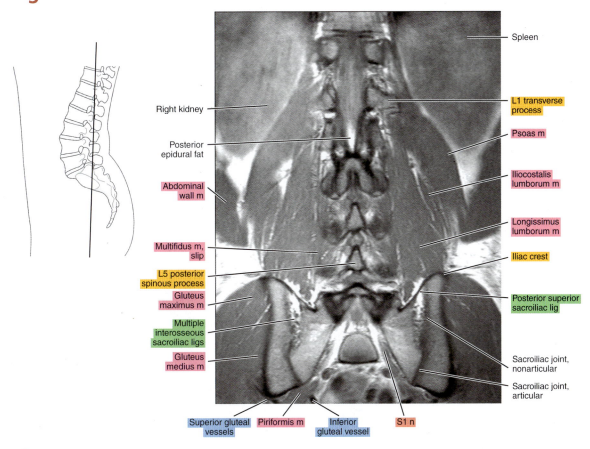

Spleen

Right kidney

Posterior epidural fat

Abdominal wall m

Multifidus m, slip

L5 posterior spinous process

Gluteus maximus m

Multiple interosseous sacroiliac ligs

Gluteus medius m

L1 transverse process

Psoas m

Iliocostalis lumborum m

Longissimus lumborum m

Iliac crest

Posterior superior sacroiliac lig

Sacroiliac joint, nonarticular

Sacroiliac joint, articular

Superior gluteal vessels

Piriformis m

Inferior gluteal vessel

S1 n

Figure 15.3.10

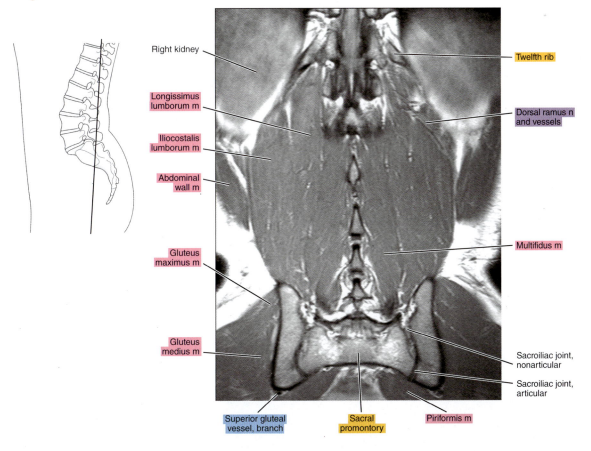

Right kidney

Longissimus lumborum m

Iliocostalis lumborum m

Abdominal wall m

Gluteus maximus m

Gluteus medius m

Twelfth rib

Dorsal ramus n and vessels

Multifidus m

Sacroiliac joint, nonarticular

Sacroiliac joint, articular

Superior gluteal vessel, branch

Sacral promontory

Piriformis m

Figure 15.3.11

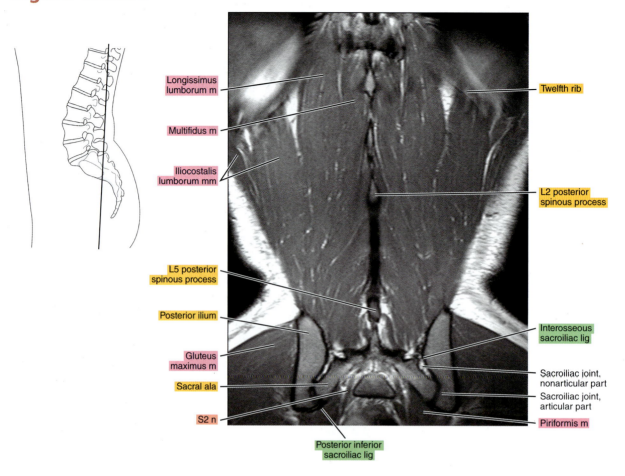

Longissimus lumborum m

Multifidus m

Iliocostalis lumborum mm

L5 posterior spinous process

Posterior ilium

Gluteus maximus m

Sacral ala

S2 n

Posterior inferior sacroiliac lig

Twelfth rib

L2 posterior spinous process

Interosseous sacroiliac lig

Sacroiliac joint, nonarticular part

Sacroiliac joint, articular part

Piriformis m

Section

V

Abdomen

Chapter

16

CT of the Abdomen

AXIAL
Figure 16.1.1

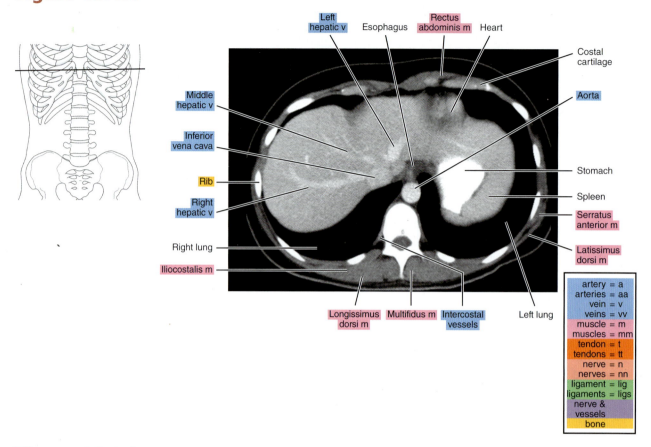

Left hepatic v — Esophagus — Rectus abdominis m — Heart — Costal cartilage

Middle hepatic v — Aorta

Inferior vena cava — Stomach

Rib — Spleen

Right hepatic v — Serratus anterior m

Right lung — Latissimus dorsi m

Iliocostalis m

Longissimus dorsi m — Multifidus m — Intercostal vessels — Left lung

artery	= a
arteries	= aa
vein	= v
veins	= vv
muscle	= m
muscles	= mm
tendon	= t
tendons	= tt
nerve	= n
nerves	= nn
ligament	= lig
ligaments	= ligs
nerve & vessels	
bone	

Figure 16.1.2

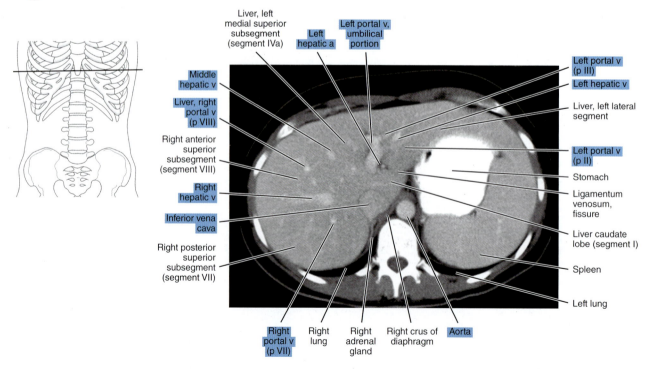

Liver, left medial superior subsegment (segment IVa) — Left hepatic a — Left portal v, umbilical portion

Middle hepatic v — Left portal v (p III)

Liver, right portal v (p VIII) — Left hepatic v

Right anterior superior subsegment (segment VIII) — Liver, left lateral segment

Right hepatic v — Left portal v (p II)

Inferior vena cava — Stomach

Right posterior superior subsegment (segment VII) — Ligamentum venosum, fissure

Liver caudate lobe (segment I)

Spleen

Left lung

Right portal v (p VII) — Right lung — Right adrenal gland — Right crus of diaphragm — Aorta

Figure 16.1.3

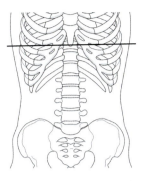

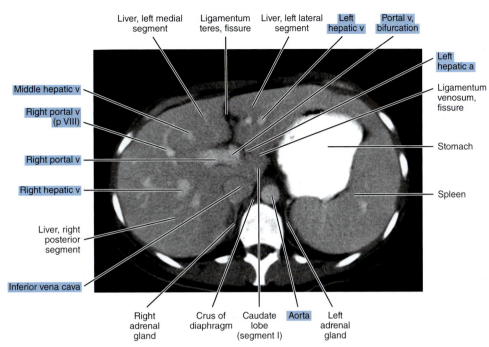

Liver, left medial segment · Ligamentum teres, fissure · Liver, left lateral segment · Left hepatic v · Portal v, bifurcation · Left hepatic a · Ligamentum venosum, fissure · Stomach · Spleen

Middle hepatic v · Right portal v (p VIII) · Right portal v · Right hepatic v · Liver, right posterior segment · Inferior vena cava

Right adrenal gland · Crus of diaphragm · Caudate lobe (segment I) · Aorta · Left adrenal gland

Figure 16.1.4

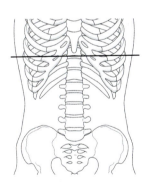

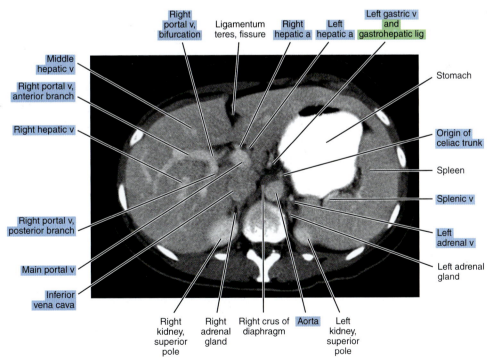

Right portal v, bifurcation · Ligamentum teres, fissure · Right hepatic a · Left hepatic a · Left gastric v and gastrohepatic lig

Middle hepatic v · Right portal v, anterior branch · Right hepatic v · Right portal v, posterior branch · Main portal v · Inferior vena cava

Stomach · Origin of celiac trunk · Spleen · Splenic v · Left adrenal v · Left adrenal gland

Right kidney, superior pole · Right adrenal gland · Right crus of diaphragm · Aorta · Left kidney, superior pole

Figure 16.1.5

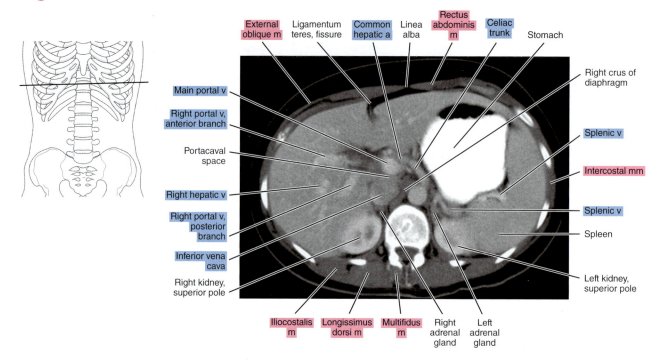

Figure 16.1.6

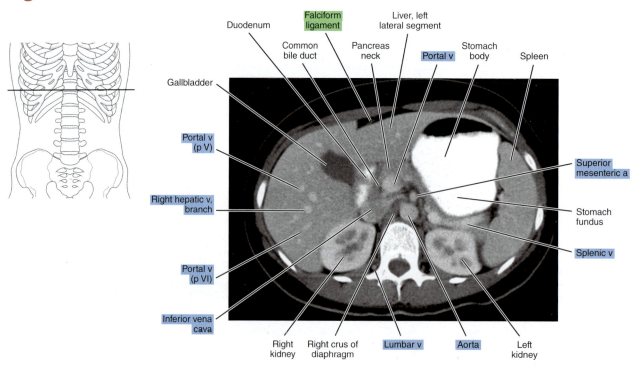

Figure 16.1.7

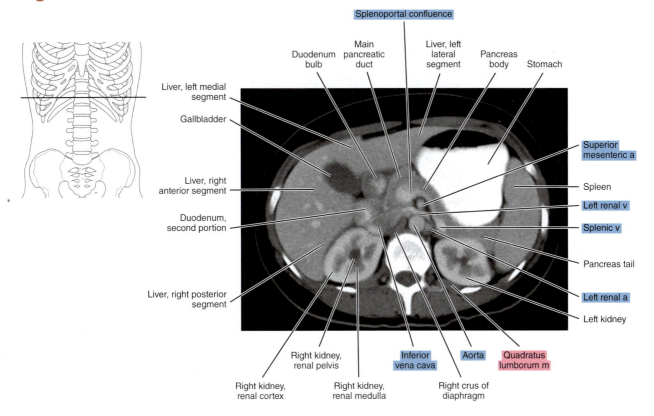

Splenoportal confluence

Main pancreatic duct

Duodenum bulb

Liver, left lateral segment

Pancreas body

Stomach

Liver, left medial segment

Gallbladder

Liver, right anterior segment

Duodenum, second portion

Liver, right posterior segment

Superior mesenteric a

Spleen

Left renal v

Splenic v

Pancreas tail

Left renal a

Left kidney

Right kidney, renal pelvis

Inferior vena cava

Aorta

Quadratus lumborum m

Right kidney, renal cortex

Right kidney, renal medulla

Right crus of diaphragm

Figure 16.1.8

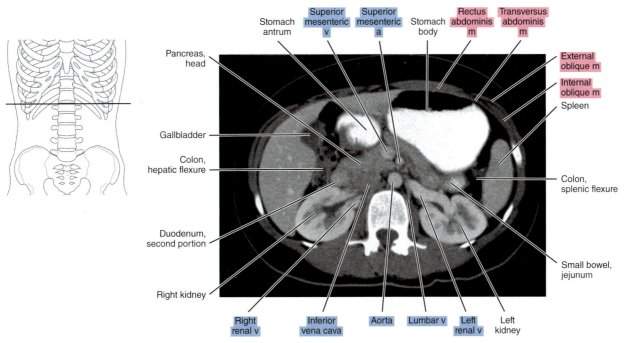

Stomach antrum

Superior mesenteric v

Superior mesenteric a

Stomach body

Rectus abdominis m

Transversus abdominis m

Pancreas, head

Gallbladder

Colon, hepatic flexure

Duodenum, second portion

Right kidney

External oblique m

Internal oblique m

Spleen

Colon, splenic flexure

Small bowel, jejunum

Right renal v

Inferior vena cava

Aorta

Lumbar v

Left renal v

Left kidney

Figure 16.1.9

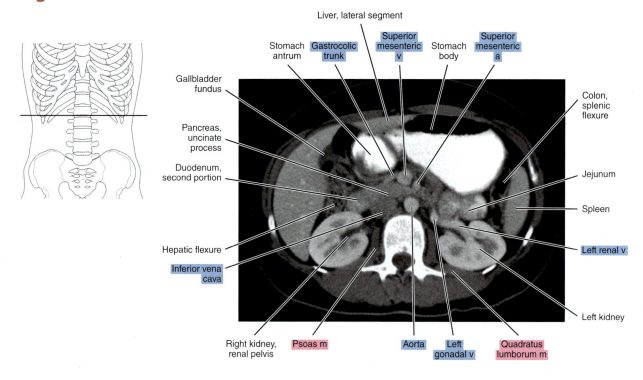

Liver, lateral segment

Stomach antrum   Gastrocolic trunk   Superior mesenteric v   Stomach body   Superior mesenteric a

Gallbladder fundus

Pancreas, uncinate process

Duodenum, second portion

Hepatic flexure

Inferior vena cava

Colon, splenic flexure

Jejunum

Spleen

Left renal v

Left kidney

Right kidney, renal pelvis   Psoas m   Aorta   Left gonadal v   Quadratus lumborum m

Figure 16.1.10

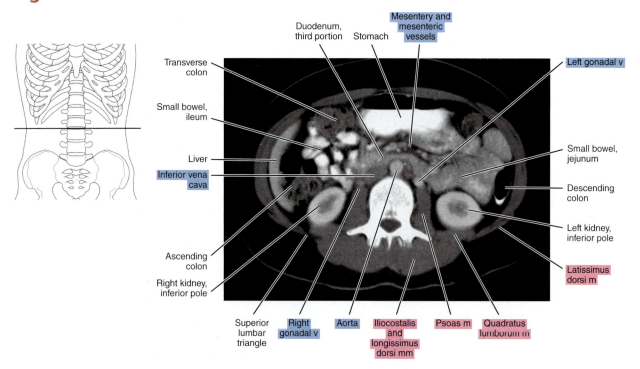

Duodenum, third portion   Stomach   Mesentery and mesenteric vessels

Transverse colon

Small bowel, ileum

Liver

Inferior vena cava

Ascending colon

Right kidney, inferior pole

Left gonadal v

Small bowel, jejunum

Descending colon

Left kidney, inferior pole

Latissimus dorsi m

Superior lumbar triangle   Right gonadal v   Aorta   Iliocostalis and longissimus dorsi mm   Psoas m   Quadratus lumborum m

Figure 16.1.11

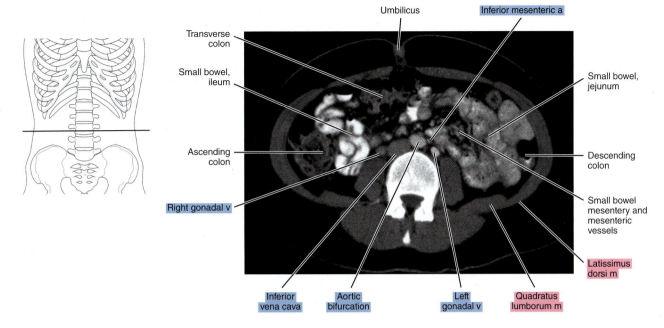

Umbilicus

Inferior mesenteric a

Transverse colon

Small bowel, ileum

Small bowel, jejunum

Ascending colon

Descending colon

Right gonadal v

Small bowel mesentery and mesenteric vessels

Latissimus dorsi m

Inferior vena cava

Aortic bifurcation

Left gonadal v

Quadratus lumborum m

Figure 16.1.12

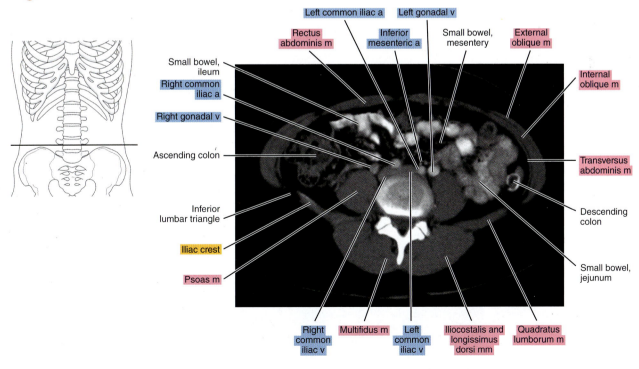

Left common iliac a

Left gonadal v

Rectus abdominis m

Inferior mesenteric a

Small bowel, mesentery

External oblique m

Small bowel, ileum

Internal oblique m

Right common iliac a

Right gonadal v

Ascending colon

Transversus abdominis m

Inferior lumbar triangle

Descending colon

Iliac crest

Psoas m

Small bowel, jejunum

Right common iliac v

Multifidus m

Left common iliac v

Iliocostalis and longissimus dorsi mm

Quadratus lumborum m

SAGITTAL
Figure 16.2.1

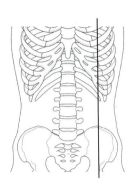

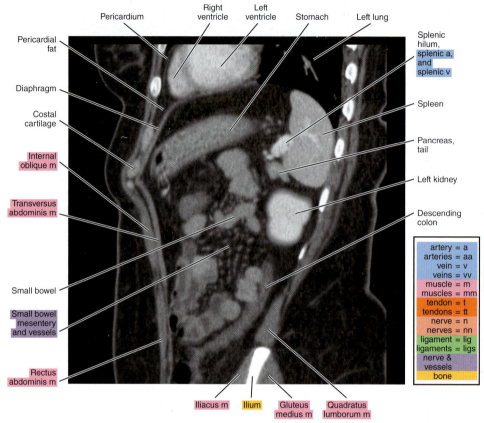

Pericardium

Right ventricle

Left ventricle

Stomach

Left lung

Splenic hilum, splenic a, and splenic v

Spleen

Pancreas, tail

Left kidney

Descending colon

Pericardial fat

Diaphragm

Costal cartilage

Internal oblique m

Transversus abdominis m

Small bowel

Small bowel mesentery and vessels

Rectus abdominis m

Iliacus m   Ilium   Gluteus medius m   Quadratus lumborum m

artery = a	
arteries = aa	
vein = v	
veins = vv	
muscle = m	
muscles = mm	
tendon = t	
tendons = tt	
nerve = n	
nerves = nn	
ligament = lig	
ligaments = ligs	
nerve & vessels	
bone	

Figure 16.2.2

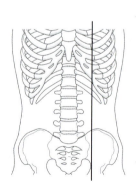

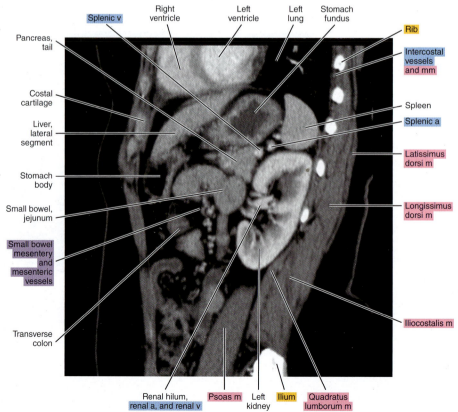

Splenic v

Right ventricle

Left ventricle

Left lung

Stomach fundus

Rib

Intercostal vessels and mm

Spleen

Splenic a

Latissimus dorsi m

Longissimus dorsi m

Iliocostalis m

Pancreas, tail

Costal cartilage

Liver, lateral segment

Stomach body

Small bowel, jejunum

Small bowel mesentery and mesenteric vessels

Transverse colon

Renal hilum, renal a, and renal v   Psoas m   Left kidney   Ilium   Quadratus lumborum m

Figure 16.2.3

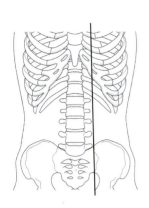

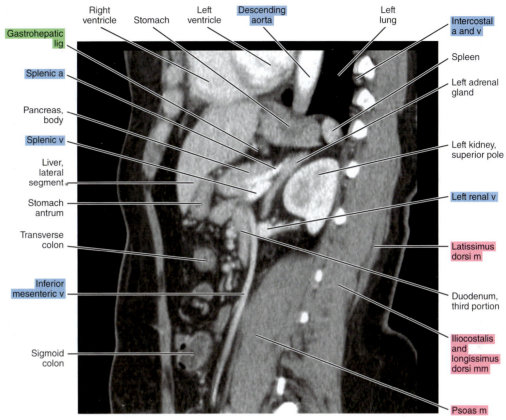

Right ventricle
Stomach
Left ventricle
Descending aorta
Left lung
Intercostal a and v
Spleen
Left adrenal gland
Left kidney, superior pole
Left renal v
Latissimus dorsi m
Duodenum, third portion
Iliocostalis and longissimus dorsi mm
Psoas m

Gastrohepatic lig
Splenic a
Pancreas, body
Splenic v
Liver, lateral segment
Stomach antrum
Transverse colon
Inferior mesenteric v
Sigmoid colon

Figure 16.2.4

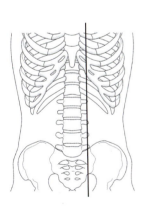

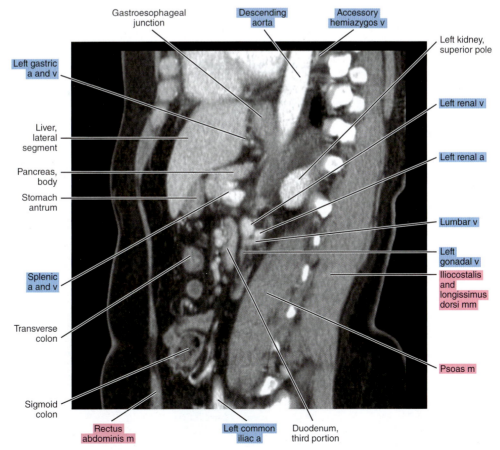

Gastroesophageal junction
Descending aorta
Accessory hemiazygos v
Left kidney, superior pole
Left renal v
Left renal a
Lumbar v
Left gonadal v
Iliocostalis and longissimus dorsi mm
Psoas m

Left gastric a and v
Liver, lateral segment
Pancreas, body
Stomach antrum
Splenic a and v
Transverse colon
Sigmoid colon

Rectus abdominis m
Left common iliac a
Duodenum, third portion

Figure 16.2.5

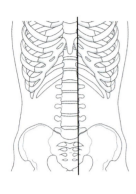

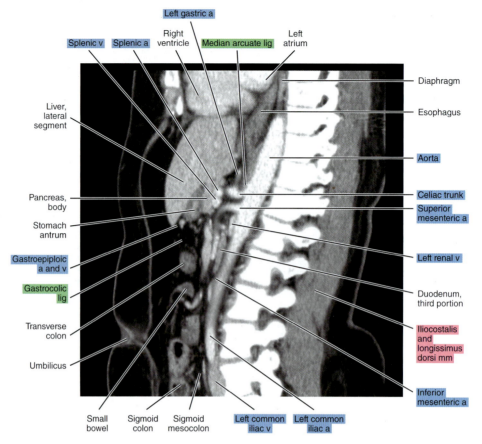

Left gastric a

Splenic v   Splenic a   Right ventricle   Median arcuate lig   Left atrium

Diaphragm

Esophagus

Liver, lateral segment

Aorta

Celiac trunk

Pancreas, body

Superior mesenteric a

Stomach antrum

Left renal v

Gastroepiploic a and v

Duodenum, third portion

Gastrocolic lig

Iliocostalis and longissimus dorsi mm

Transverse colon

Umbilicus

Inferior mesenteric a

Small bowel   Sigmoid colon   Sigmoid mesocolon   Left common iliac v   Left common iliac a

Figure 16.2.6

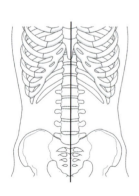

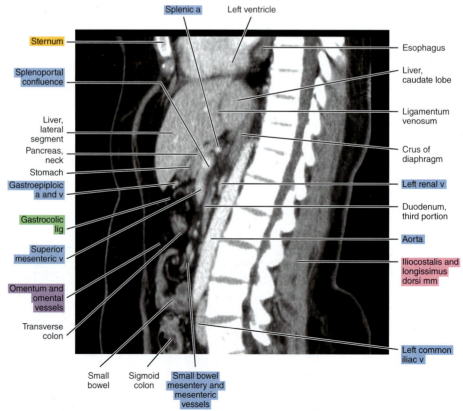

Splenic a   Left ventricle

Sternum

Esophagus

Splenoportal confluence

Liver, caudate lobe

Ligamentum venosum

Liver, lateral segment

Crus of diaphragm

Pancreas, neck

Stomach

Gastroepiploic a and v

Left renal v

Duodenum, third portion

Gastrocolic lig

Aorta

Superior mesenteric v

Iliocostalis and longissimus dorsi mm

Omentum and omental vessels

Transverse colon

Left common iliac v

Small bowel   Sigmoid colon   Small bowel mesentery and mesenteric vessels

Figure 16.2.7

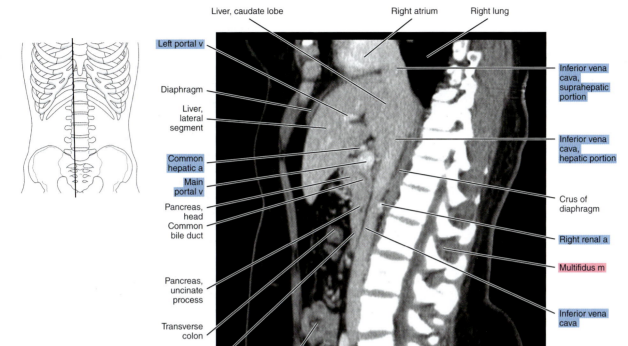

Liver, caudate lobe
Right atrium
Right lung
Left portal v
Diaphragm
Liver, lateral segment
Common hepatic a
Main portal v
Pancreas, head
Common bile duct
Pancreas, uncinate process
Transverse colon
Duodenum, third portion
Small bowel
Right common iliac a, bifurcation
Inferior vena cava, suprahepatic portion
Inferior vena cava, hepatic portion
Crus of diaphragm
Right renal a
Multifidus m
Inferior vena cava

Figure 16.2.8

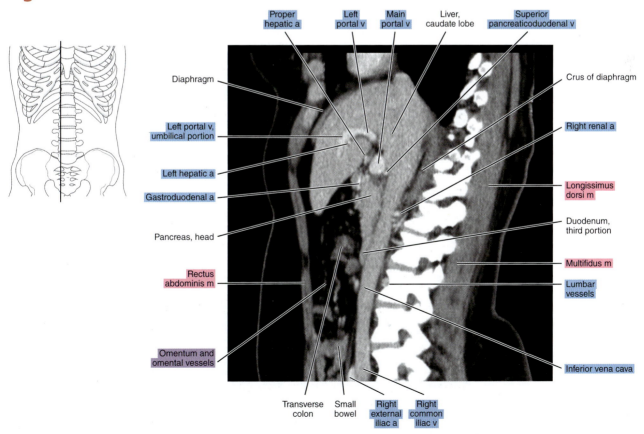

Proper hepatic a
Left portal v
Main portal v
Liver, caudate lobe
Superior pancreaticoduodenal v
Diaphragm
Left portal v, umbilical portion
Left hepatic a
Gastroduodenal a
Pancreas, head
Rectus abdominis m
Omentum and omental vessels
Transverse colon
Small bowel
Right external iliac a
Right common iliac v
Crus of diaphragm
Right renal a
Longissimus dorsi m
Duodenum, third portion
Multifidus m
Lumbar vessels
Inferior vena cava

Figure 16.2.9

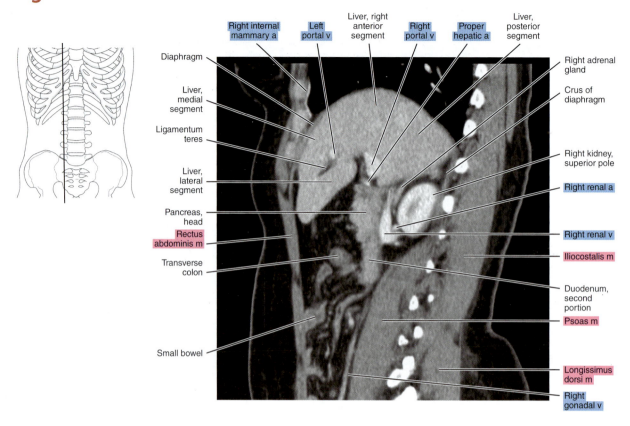

Right internal mammary a

Left portal v

Liver, right anterior segment

Right portal v

Proper hepatic a

Liver, posterior segment

Diaphragm

Liver, medial segment

Ligamentum teres

Liver, lateral segment

Pancreas, head

Rectus abdominis m

Transverse colon

Small bowel

Right adrenal gland

Crus of diaphragm

Right kidney, superior pole

Right renal a

Right renal v

Iliocostalis m

Duodenum, second portion

Psoas m

Longissimus dorsi m

Right gonadal v

Figure 16.2.10

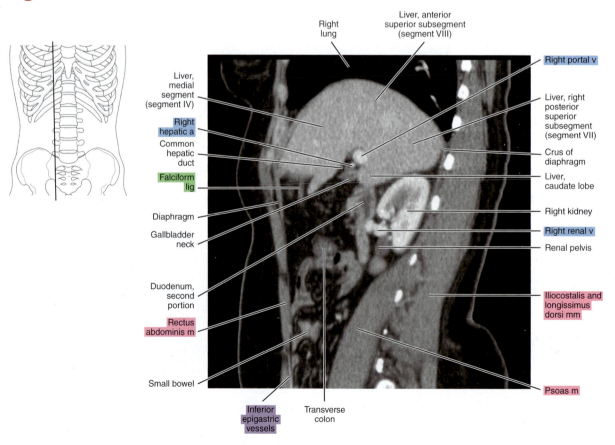

Right lung

Liver, anterior superior subsegment (segment VIII)

Right portal v

Liver, medial segment (segment IV)

Right hepatic a

Common hepatic duct

Falciform lig

Diaphragm

Gallbladder neck

Duodenum, second portion

Rectus abdominis m

Small bowel

Inferior epigastric vessels

Transverse colon

Liver, right posterior superior subsegment (segment VII)

Crus of diaphragm

Liver, caudate lobe

Right kidney

Right renal v

Renal pelvis

Iliocostalis and longissimus dorsi mm

Psoas m

Figure 16.2.11

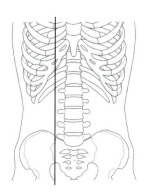

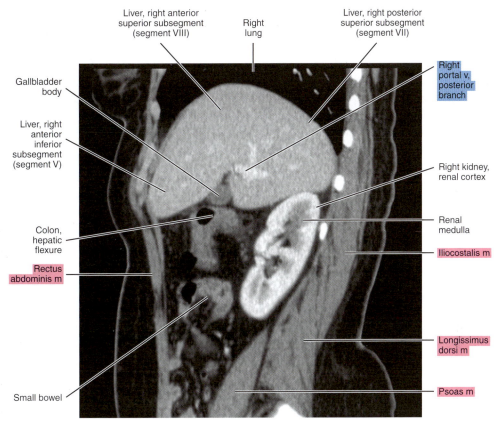

Liver, right anterior superior subsegment (segment VIII)

Right lung

Liver, right posterior superior subsegment (segment VII)

Right portal v, posterior branch

Gallbladder body

Liver, right anterior inferior subsegment (segment V)

Right kidney, renal cortex

Renal medulla

Colon, hepatic flexure

Iliocostalis m

Rectus abdominis m

Longissimus dorsi m

Small bowel

Psoas m

Figure 16.2.12

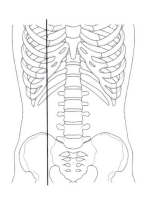

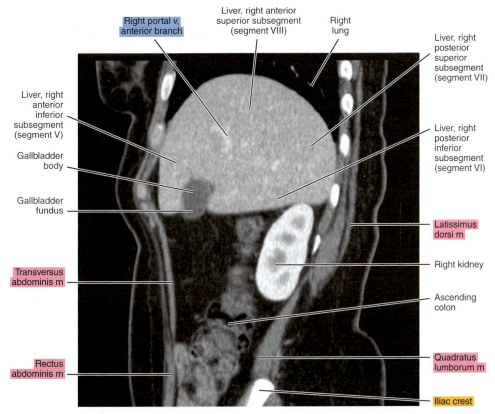

Right portal v, anterior branch

Liver, right anterior superior subsegment (segment VIII)

Right lung

Liver, right posterior superior subsegment (segment VII)

Liver, right anterior inferior subsegment (segment V)

Gallbladder body

Gallbladder fundus

Liver, right posterior inferior subsegment (segment VI)

Latissimus dorsi m

Right kidney

Transversus abdominis m

Ascending colon

Rectus abdominis m

Quadratus lumborum m

Iliac crest

CORONAL
Figure 16.3.1

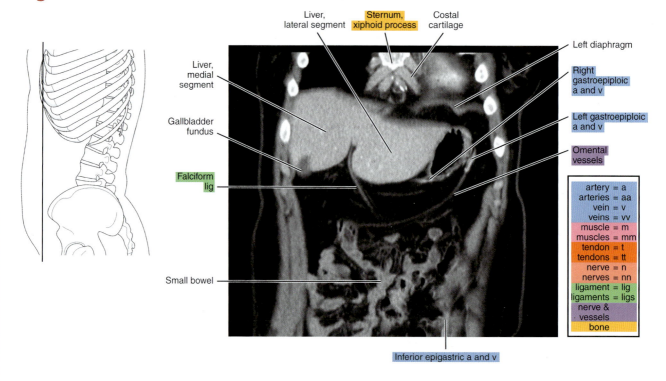

Liver, lateral segment
Sternum, xiphoid process
Costal cartilage
Liver, medial segment
Gallbladder fundus
Falciform lig
Small bowel
Left diaphragm
Right gastroepiploic a and v
Left gastroepiploic a and v
Omental vessels
Inferior epigastric a and v

artery = a	
arteries = aa	
vein = v	
veins = vv	
muscle = m	
muscles = mm	
tendon = t	
tendons = tt	
nerve = n	
nerves = nn	
ligament = lig	
ligaments = ligs	
nerve & vessels	
bone	

Figure 16.3.2

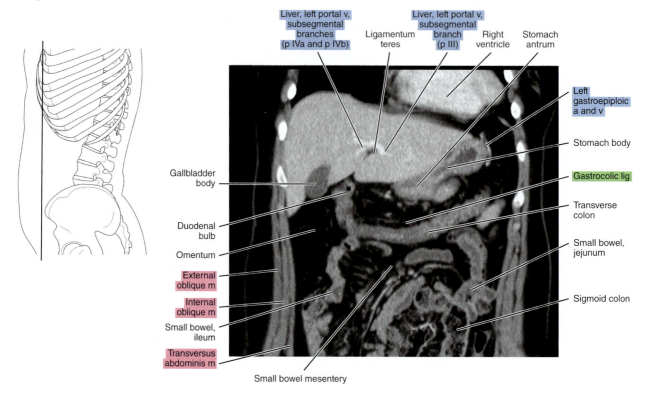

Liver, left portal v, subsegmental branches (p IVa and p IVb)
Ligamentum teres
Liver, left portal v, subsegmental branch (p III)
Right ventricle
Stomach antrum
Gallbladder body
Duodenal bulb
Omentum
External oblique m
Internal oblique m
Small bowel, ileum
Transversus abdominis m
Small bowel mesentery
Left gastroepiploic a and v
Stomach body
Gastrocolic lig
Transverse colon
Small bowel, jejunum
Sigmoid colon

Figure 16.3.3

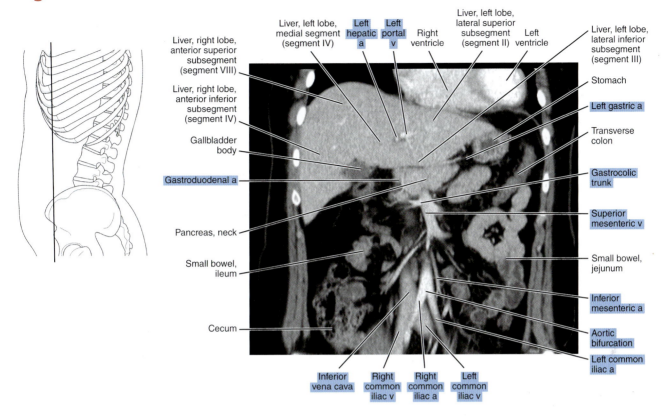

Liver, right lobe, anterior superior subsegment (segment VIII)
Liver, right lobe, anterior inferior subsegment (segment IV)
Gallbladder body
Gastroduodenal a
Pancreas, neck
Small bowel, ileum
Cecum

Liver, left lobe, medial segment (segment IV)
Left hepatic a
Left portal v
Right ventricle
Liver, left lobe, lateral superior subsegment (segment II)
Left ventricle
Liver, left lobe, lateral inferior subsegment (segment III)
Stomach
Left gastric a
Transverse colon
Gastrocolic trunk
Superior mesenteric v
Small bowel, jejunum
Inferior mesenteric a
Aortic bifurcation
Left common iliac a

Inferior vena cava
Right common iliac v
Right common iliac a
Left common iliac v

Figure 16.3.4

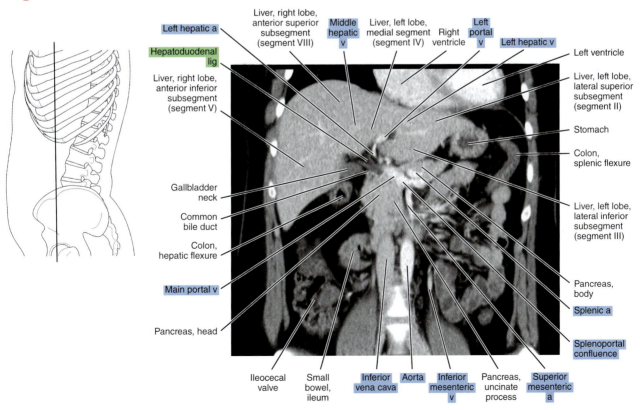

Left hepatic a
Hepatoduodenal lig
Liver, right lobe, anterior inferior subsegment (segment V)
Gallbladder neck
Common bile duct
Colon, hepatic flexure
Main portal v
Pancreas, head

Liver, right lobe, anterior superior subsegment (segment VIII)
Middle hepatic v
Liver, left lobe, medial segment (segment IV)
Right ventricle
Left portal v
Left hepatic v
Left ventricle
Liver, left lobe, lateral superior subsegment (segment II)
Stomach
Colon, splenic flexure
Liver, left lobe, lateral inferior subsegment (segment III)
Pancreas, body
Splenic a
Splenoportal confluence

Ileocecal valve
Small bowel, ileum
Inferior vena cava
Aorta
Inferior mesenteric v
Pancreas, uncinate process
Superior mesenteric a

Figure 16.3.5

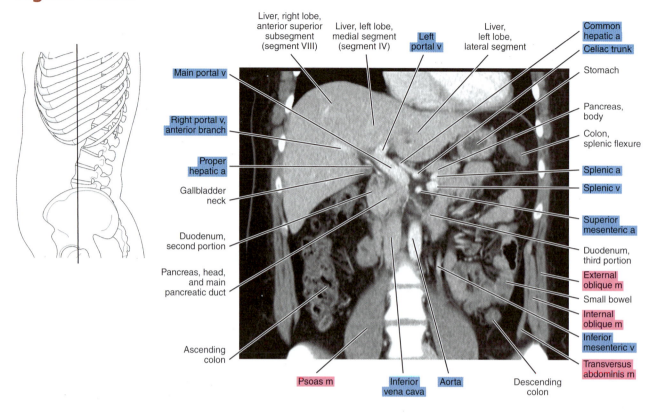

Liver, right lobe, anterior superior subsegment (segment VIII)
Liver, left lobe, medial segment (segment IV)
Left portal v
Liver, left lobe, lateral segment
Common hepatic a
Celiac trunk
Main portal v
Stomach
Pancreas, body
Right portal v, anterior branch
Colon, splenic flexure
Proper hepatic a
Splenic a
Splenic v
Gallbladder neck
Superior mesenteric a
Duodenum, second portion
Duodenum, third portion
Pancreas, head, and main pancreatic duct
External oblique m
Small bowel
Internal oblique m
Inferior mesenteric v
Ascending colon
Transversus abdominis m
Psoas m
Inferior vena cava
Aorta
Descending colon

Figure 16.3.6

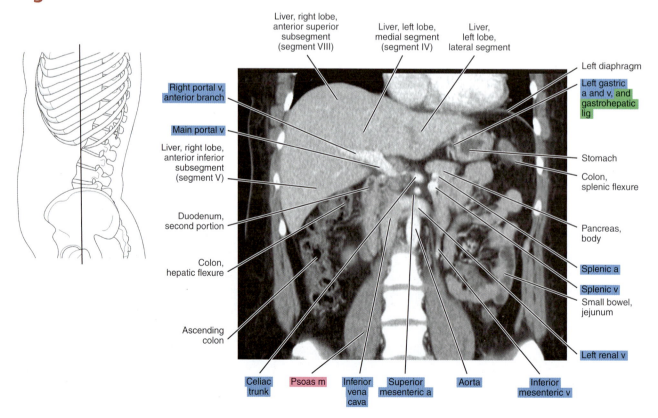

Liver, right lobe, anterior superior subsegment (segment VIII)
Liver, left lobe, medial segment (segment IV)
Liver, left lobe, lateral segment
Left diaphragm
Right portal v, anterior branch
Left gastric a and v, and gastrohepatic lig
Main portal v
Liver, right lobe, anterior inferior subsegment (segment V)
Stomach
Colon, splenic flexure
Duodenum, second portion
Pancreas, body
Colon, hepatic flexure
Splenic a
Splenic v
Small bowel, jejunum
Ascending colon
Left renal v
Celiac trunk
Psoas m
Inferior vena cava
Superior mesenteric a
Aorta
Inferior mesenteric v

Figure 16.3.7

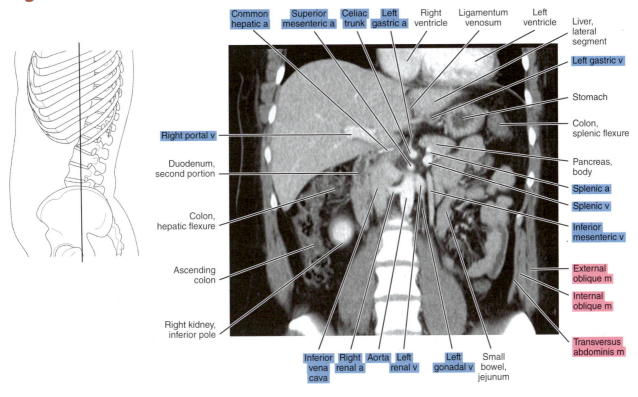

Common hepatic a — Superior mesenteric a — Celiac trunk — Left gastric a — Right ventricle — Ligamentum venosum — Left ventricle — Liver, lateral segment — Left gastric v — Stomach — Colon, splenic flexure — Pancreas, body — Splenic a — Splenic v — Inferior mesenteric v — External oblique m — Internal oblique m — Transversus abdominis m — Right portal v — Duodenum, second portion — Colon, hepatic flexure — Ascending colon — Right kidney, inferior pole — Inferior vena cava — Right renal a — Aorta — Left renal v — Left gonadal v — Small bowel, jejunum

Figure 16.3.8

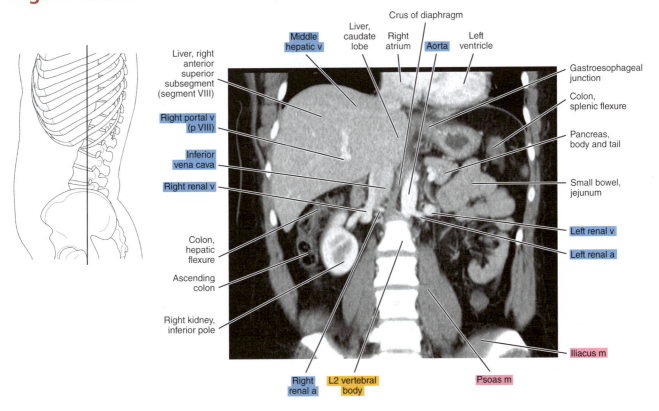

Middle hepatic v — Liver, caudate lobe — Crus of diaphragm — Right atrium — Aorta — Left ventricle — Gastroesophageal junction — Colon, splenic flexure — Pancreas, body and tail — Small bowel, jejunum — Left renal v — Left renal a — Iliacus m — Psoas m — L2 vertebral body — Right renal a — Right kidney, inferior pole — Ascending colon — Colon, hepatic flexure — Right renal v — Inferior vena cava — Right portal v (p VIII) — Liver, right anterior superior subsegment (segment VIII)

Figure 16.3.9

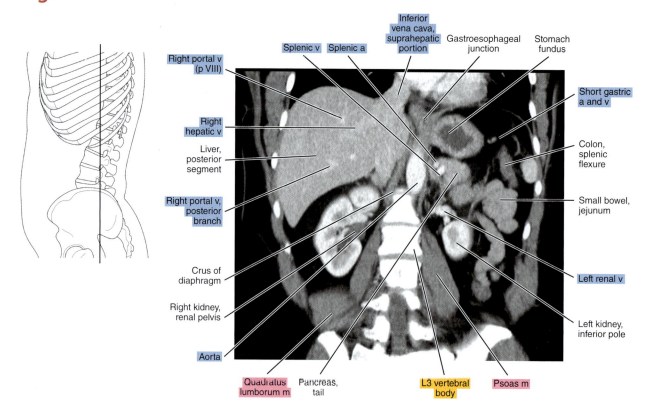

Right portal v (p VIII)
Splenic v
Splenic a
Inferior vena cava, suprahepatic portion
Gastroesophageal junction
Stomach fundus
Short gastric a and v
Right hepatic v
Liver, posterior segment
Colon, splenic flexure
Right portal v, posterior branch
Small bowel, jejunum
Crus of diaphragm
Left renal v
Right kidney, renal pelvis
Left kidney, inferior pole
Aorta
Quadratus lumborum m
Pancreas, tail
L3 vertebral body
Psoas m

Figure 16.3.10

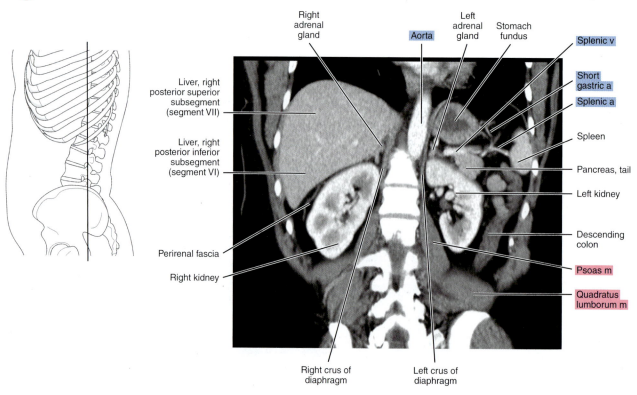

Right adrenal gland
Left adrenal gland
Aorta
Stomach fundus
Splenic v
Liver, right posterior superior subsegment (segment VII)
Short gastric a
Splenic a
Liver, right posterior inferior subsegment (segment VI)
Spleen
Pancreas, tail
Left kidney
Descending colon
Perirenal fascia
Psoas m
Right kidney
Quadratus lumborum m
Right crus of diaphragm
Left crus of diaphragm

Figure 16.3.11

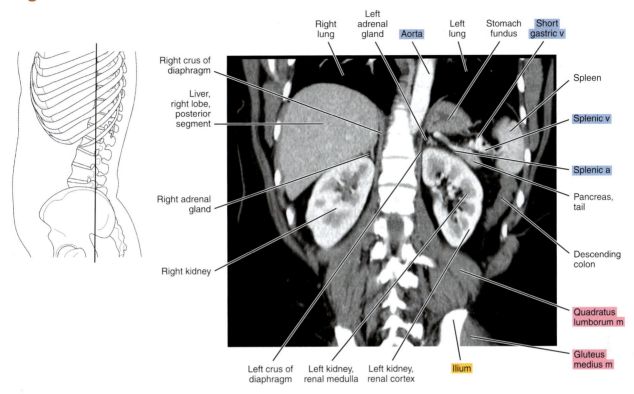

Right lung
Left adrenal gland
Aorta
Left lung
Stomach fundus
Short gastric v

Right crus of diaphragm

Liver, right lobe, posterior segment

Right adrenal gland

Right kidney

Spleen

Splenic v

Splenic a

Pancreas, tail

Descending colon

Quadratus lumborum m

Gluteus medius m

Left crus of diaphragm
Left kidney, renal medulla
Left kidney, renal cortex
Ilium

Figure 16.3.12

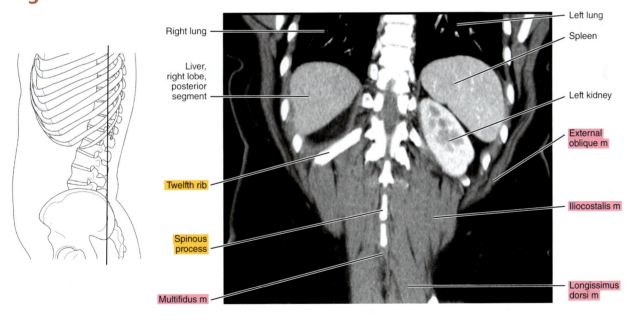

Right lung

Liver, right lobe, posterior segment

Twelfth rib

Spinous process

Multifidus m

Left lung

Spleen

Left kidney

External oblique m

Iliocostalis m

Longissimus dorsi m

Table 16-1. Muscles of the Abdominal Wall

MUSCLE	ORIGIN	INSERTION	NERVE SUPPLY
Rectus abdominis	Crest and symphysis of the pubis	Xiphoid process and fifth to seventh costal cartilages	Branches of the lower thoracic
External oblique (obliquus externus abdominis)	Fifth to 12th ribs	Anterior half of the iliac crest, inguinal ligament, and anterior layer of the sheath of the rectus abdominis	Ventral branches of the lower thoracic
Internal oblique (obliquus internus abdominis)	Tenth to 12th ribs and sheath of the rectus abdominis; some fibers from the inguinal ligament terminate in the falx inguinalis	Iliac fascia deep to the lateral part of the inguinal ligament, the anterior half of the iliac crest, and the lumbar fascia	Lower thoracic
Transversus abdominis	Seventh to 12th costal cartilages, lumbar fascia, iliac crest, and inguinal ligament	Xiphoid cartilage and linea alba and through the falx inguinalis, pubic tubercle, and pecten pubis	Lower thoracic

MRI of the Abdomen

AXIAL
Figure 17.1.1

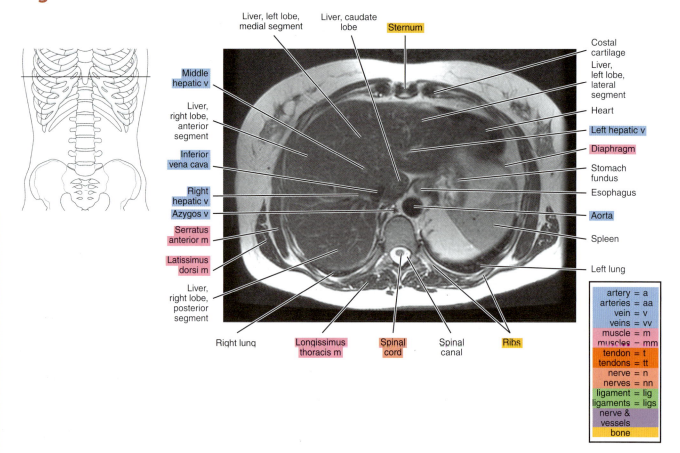

Liver, left lobe, medial segment
Liver, caudate lobe
Sternum
Costal cartilage
Liver, left lobe, lateral segment
Heart
Left hepatic v
Diaphragm
Stomach fundus
Esophagus
Aorta
Spleen
Left lung
Middle hepatic v
Liver, right lobe, anterior segment
Inferior vena cava
Right hepatic v
Azygos v
Serratus anterior m
Latissimus dorsi m
Liver, right lobe, posterior segment
Right lung
Longissimus thoracis m
Spinal cord
Spinal canal
Ribs

artery = a	
arteries = aa	
vein = v	
veins = vv	
muscle = m	
muscles = mm	
tendon = t	
tendons = tt	
nerve = n	
nerves = nn	
ligament = lig	
ligaments = ligs	
nerve & vessels	
bone	

Figure 17.1.2

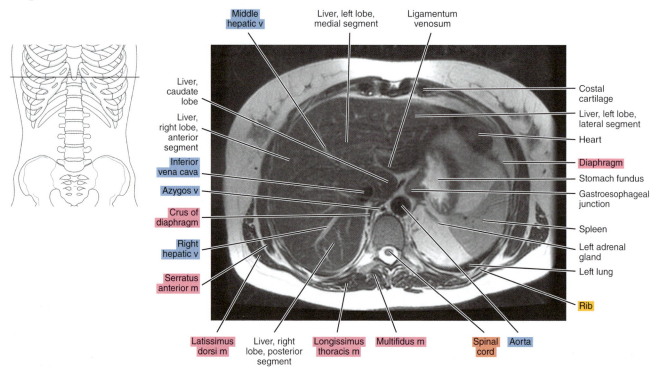

Middle hepatic v
Liver, left lobe, medial segment
Ligamentum venosum
Liver, caudate lobe
Liver, right lobe, anterior segment
Inferior vena cava
Azygos v
Crus of diaphragm
Right hepatic v
Serratus anterior m
Costal cartilage
Liver, left lobe, lateral segment
Heart
Diaphragm
Stomach fundus
Gastroesophageal junction
Spleen
Left adrenal gland
Left lung
Rib
Latissimus dorsi m
Liver, right lobe, posterior segment
Longissimus thoracis m
Multifidus m
Spinal cord
Aorta

Figure 17.1.3

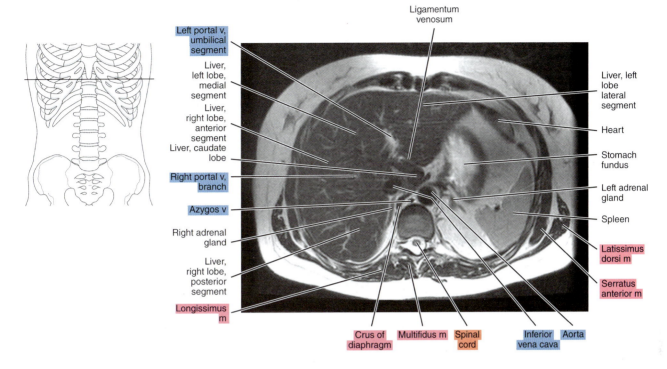

Ligamentum venosum

Left portal v, umbilical segment

Liver, left lobe, medial segment

Liver, right lobe, anterior segment

Liver, caudate lobe

Right portal v, branch

Azygos v

Right adrenal gland

Liver, right lobe, posterior segment

Longissimus m

Liver, left lobe lateral segment

Heart

Stomach fundus

Left adrenal gland

Spleen

Latissimus dorsi m

Serratus anterior m

Crus of diaphragm

Multifidus m

Spinal cord

Inferior vena cava

Aorta

Figure 17.1.4

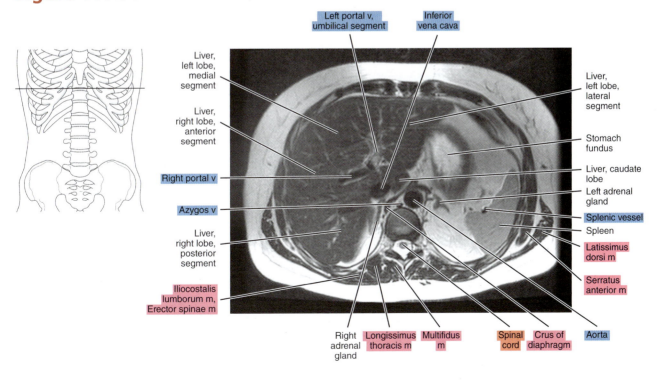

Left portal v, umbilical segment

Inferior vena cava

Liver, left lobe, medial segment

Liver, right lobe, anterior segment

Right portal v

Azygos v

Liver, right lobe, posterior segment

Iliocostalis lumborum m, Erector spinae m

Liver, left lobe, lateral segment

Stomach fundus

Liver, caudate lobe

Left adrenal gland

Splenic vessel

Spleen

Latissimus dorsi m

Serratus anterior m

Right adrenal gland

Longissimus thoracis m

Multifidus m

Spinal cord

Crus of diaphragm

Aorta

Figure 17.1.5

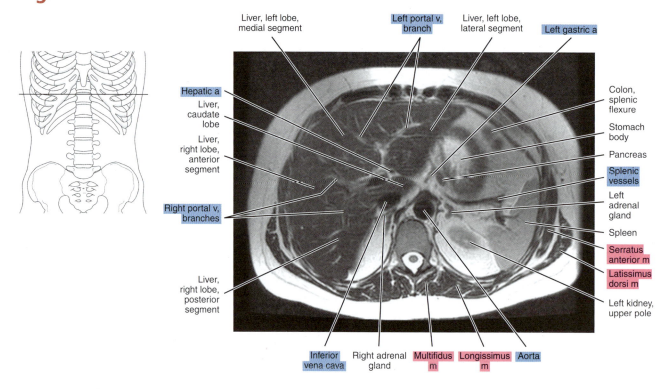

Liver, left lobe, medial segment

Left portal v, branch

Liver, left lobe, lateral segment

Left gastric a

Hepatic a

Liver, caudate lobe

Liver, right lobe, anterior segment

Right portal v, branches

Liver, right lobe, posterior segment

Colon, splenic flexure

Stomach body

Pancreas

Splenic vessels

Left adrenal gland

Spleen

Serratus anterior m

Latissimus dorsi m

Left kidney, upper pole

Inferior vena cava

Right adrenal gland

Multifidus m

Longissimus m

Aorta

Figure 17.1.6

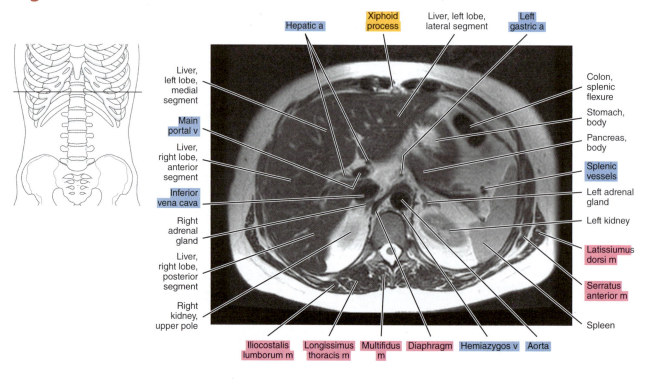

Hepatic a

Xiphoid process

Liver, left lobe, lateral segment

Left gastric a

Liver, left lobe, medial segment

Main portal v

Liver, right lobe, anterior segment

Inferior vena cava

Right adrenal gland

Liver, right lobe, posterior segment

Right kidney, upper pole

Colon, splenic flexure

Stomach, body

Pancreas, body

Splenic vessels

Left adrenal gland

Left kidney

Latissiumus dorsi m

Serratus anterior m

Spleen

Iliocostalis lumborum m

Longissimus thoracis m

Multifidus m

Diaphragm

Hemiazygos v

Aorta

Figure 17.1.7

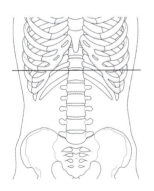

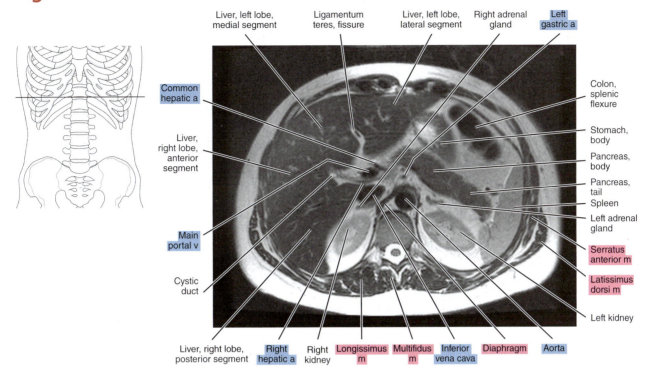

Liver, left lobe, medial segment

Ligamentum teres, fissure

Liver, left lobe, lateral segment

Right adrenal gland

Left gastric a

Common hepatic a

Colon, splenic flexure

Liver, right lobe, anterior segment

Stomach, body

Pancreas, body

Pancreas, tail

Spleen

Left adrenal gland

Main portal v

Serratus anterior m

Latissimus dorsi m

Cystic duct

Left kidney

Liver, right lobe, posterior segment

Right hepatic a

Right kidney

Longissimus m

Multifidus m

Inferior vena cava

Diaphragm

Aorta

Figure 17.1.8

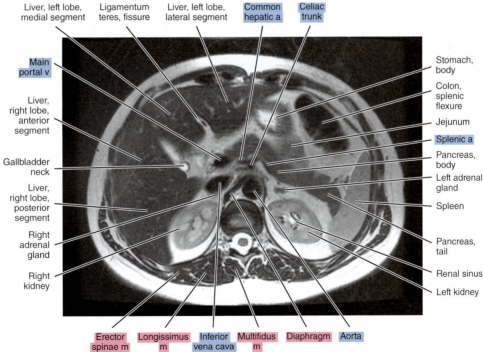

Liver, left lobe, medial segment

Ligamentum teres, fissure

Liver, left lobe, lateral segment

Common hepatic a

Celiac trunk

Main portal v

Stomach, body

Colon, splenic flexure

Jejunum

Liver, right lobe, anterior segment

Splenic a

Pancreas, body

Left adrenal gland

Gallblader neck

Spleen

Liver, right lobe, posterior segment

Right adrenal gland

Pancreas, tail

Renal sinus

Right kidney

Left kidney

Erector spinae m

Longissimus m

Inferior vena cava

Multifidus m

Diaphragm

Aorta

Figure 17.1.9

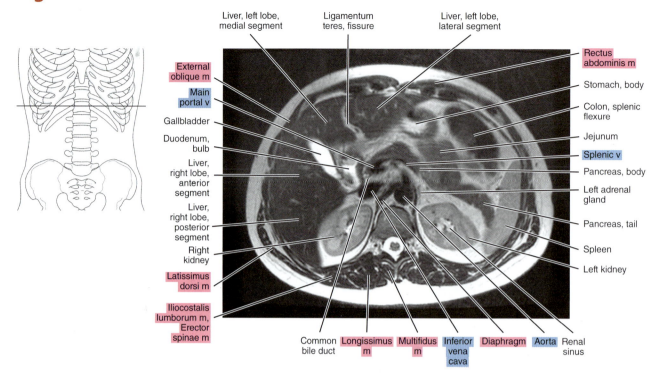

Liver, left lobe, medial segment
Ligamentum teres, fissure
Liver, left lobe, lateral segment
External oblique m
Main portal v
Gallbladder
Duodenum, bulb
Liver, right lobe, anterior segment
Liver, right lobe, posterior segment
Right kidney
Latissimus dorsi m
Iliocostalis lumborum m, Erector spinae m
Rectus abdominis m
Stomach, body
Colon, splenic flexure
Jejunum
Splenic v
Pancreas, body
Left adrenal gland
Pancreas, tail
Spleen
Left kidney
Common bile duct
Longissimus m
Multifidus m
Inferior vena cava
Diaphragm
Aorta
Renal sinus

Figure 17.1.10

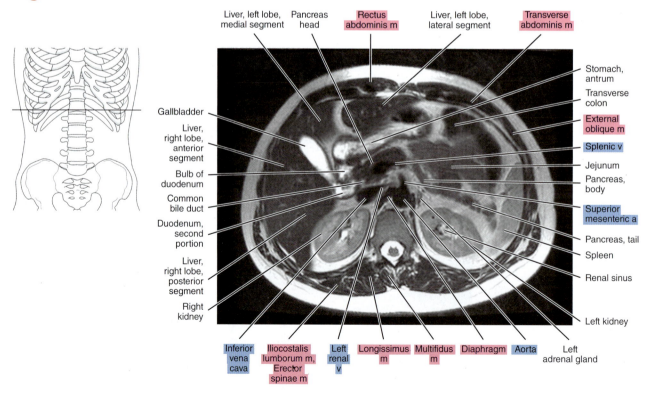

Liver, left lobe, medial segment
Pancreas head
Rectus abdominis m
Liver, left lobe, lateral segment
Transverse abdominis m
Gallbladder
Liver, right lobe, anterior segment
Bulb of duodenum
Common bile duct
Duodenum, second portion
Liver, right lobe, posterior segment
Right kidney
Stomach, antrum
Transverse colon
External oblique m
Splenic v
Jejunum
Pancreas, body
Superior mesenteric a
Pancreas, tail
Spleen
Renal sinus
Left kidney
Inferior vena cava
Iliocostalis lumborum m, Erector spinae m
Left renal v
Longissimus m
Multifidus m
Diaphragm
Aorta
Left adrenal gland

Figure 17.1.11

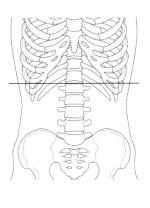

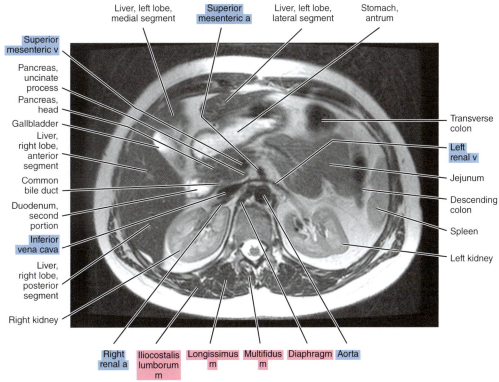

Liver, left lobe, medial segment
Superior mesenteric a
Liver, left lobe, lateral segment
Stomach, antrum
Superior mesenteric v
Pancreas, uncinate process
Pancreas, head
Gallbladder
Liver, right lobe, anterior segment
Common bile duct
Duodenum, second portion
Inferior vena cava
Liver, right lobe, posterior segment
Right kidney
Transverse colon
Left renal v
Jejunum
Descending colon
Spleen
Left kidney
Right renal a
Iliocostalis lumborum m
Longissimus m
Multifidus m
Diaphragm
Aorta

Figure 17.1.12

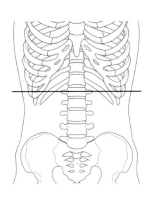

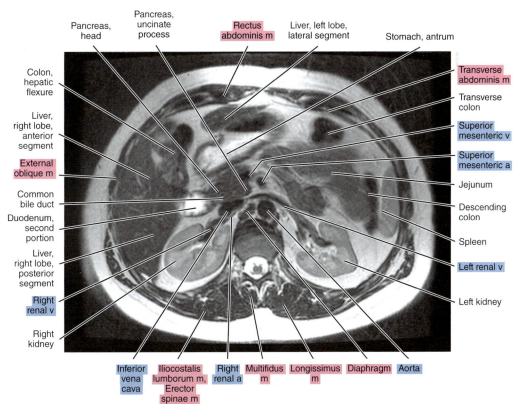

Pancreas, head
Pancreas, uncinate process
Rectus abdominis m
Liver, left lobe, lateral segment
Stomach, antrum
Colon, hepatic flexure
Liver, right lobe, anterior segment
External oblique m
Common bile duct
Duodenum, second portion
Liver, right lobe, posterior segment
Right renal v
Right kidney
Transverse abdominis m
Transverse colon
Superior mesenteric v
Superior mesenteric a
Jejunum
Descending colon
Spleen
Left renal v
Left kidney
Inferior vena cava
Iliocostalis lumborum m, Erector spinae m
Right renal a
Multifidus m
Longissimus m
Diaphragm
Aorta

Figure 17.1.13

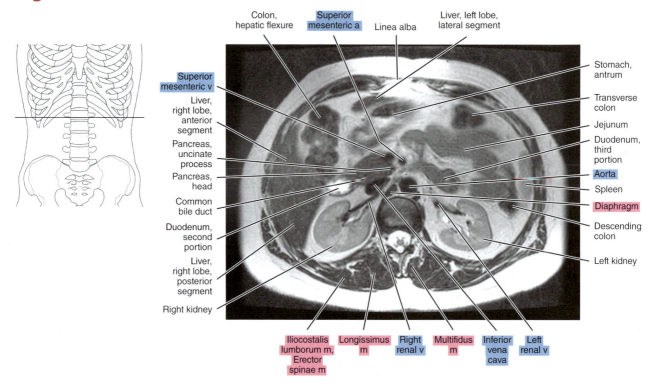

Colon, hepatic flexure
Superior mesenteric a
Linea alba
Liver, left lobe, lateral segment

Superior mesenteric v
Liver, right lobe, anterior segment
Pancreas, uncinate process
Pancreas, head
Common bile duct
Duodenum, second portion
Liver, right lobe, posterior segment
Right kidney

Stomach, antrum
Transverse colon
Jejunum
Duodenum, third portion
Aorta
Spleen
Diaphragm
Descending colon
Left kidney

Iliocostalis lumborum m, Erector spinae m
Longissimus m
Right renal v
Multifidus m
Inferior vena cava
Left renal v

Figure 17.1.14

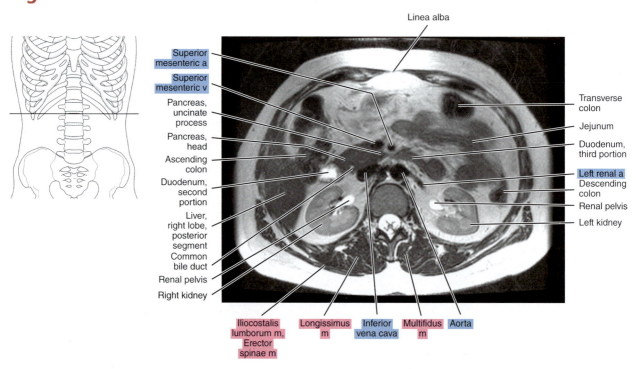

Linea alba

Superior mesenteric a
Superior mesenteric v
Pancreas, uncinate process
Pancreas, head
Ascending colon
Duodenum, second portion
Liver, right lobe, posterior segment
Common bile duct
Renal pelvis
Right kidney

Transverse colon
Jejunum
Duodenum, third portion
Left renal a
Descending colon
Renal pelvis
Left kidney

Iliocostalis lumborum m, Erector spinae m
Longissimus m
Inferior vena cava
Multifidus m
Aorta

Figure 17.1.15

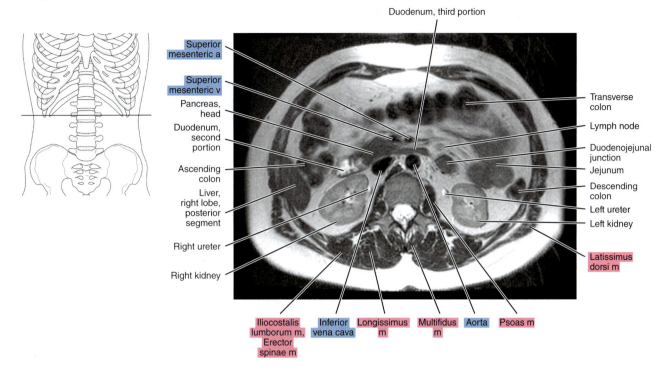

Duodenum, third portion

Superior mesenteric a

Superior mesenteric v

Pancreas, head

Duodenum, second portion

Ascending colon

Liver, right lobe, posterior segment

Right ureter

Right kidney

Transverse colon

Lymph node

Duodenojejunal junction

Jejunum

Descending colon

Left ureter

Left kidney

Latissimus dorsi m

Iliocostalis lumborum m, Erector spinae m

Inferior vena cava

Longissimus m

Multifidus m

Aorta

Psoas m

Figure 17.1.16

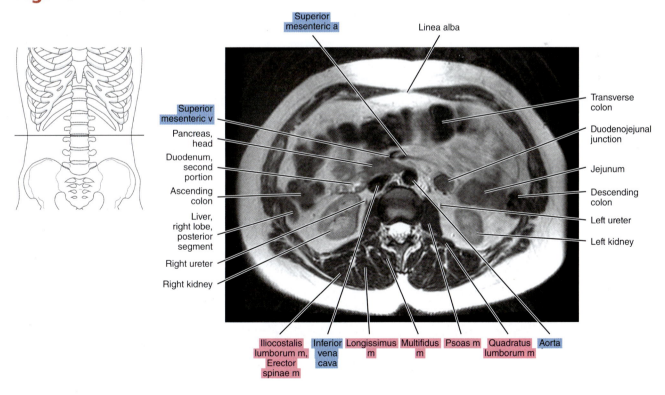

Superior mesenteric a

Linea alba

Superior mesenteric v

Pancreas, head

Duodenum, second portion

Ascending colon

Liver, right lobe, posterior segment

Right ureter

Right kidney

Transverse colon

Duodenojejunal junction

Jejunum

Descending colon

Left ureter

Left kidney

Iliocostalis lumborum m, Erector spinae m

Inferior vena cava

Longissimus m

Multifidus m

Psoas m

Quadratus lumborum m

Aorta

SAGITTAL
Figure 17.2.1

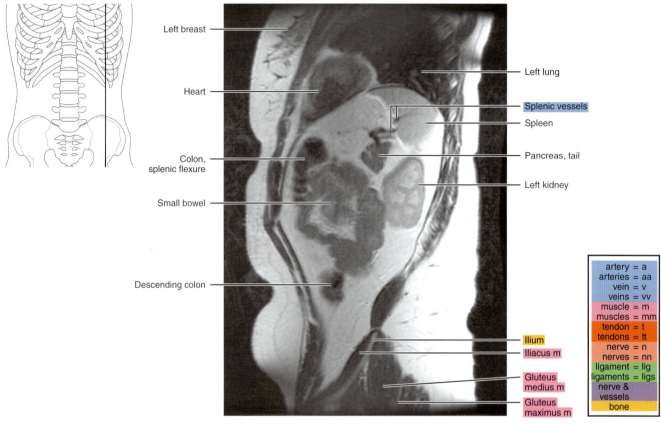

Left breast

Heart

Colon, splenic flexure

Small bowel

Descending colon

Left lung

Splenic vessels

Spleen

Pancreas, tail

Left kidney

Ilium

Iliacus m

Gluteus medius m

Gluteus maximus m

artery = a	
arteries = aa	
vein = v	
veins = vv	
muscle = m	
muscles = mm	
tendon = t	
tendons = tt	
nerve = n	
nerves = nn	
ligament = lig	
ligaments = ligs	
nerve & vessels	
bone	

Figure 17.2.2

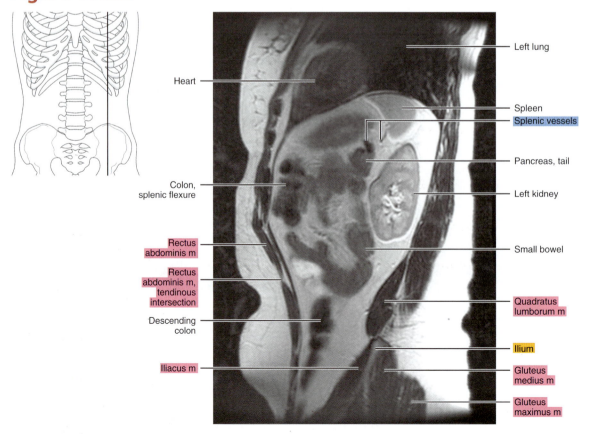

Heart

Colon, splenic flexure

Rectus abdominis m

Rectus abdominis m, tendinous intersection

Descending colon

Iliacus m

Left lung

Spleen

Splenic vessels

Pancreas, tail

Left kidney

Small bowel

Quadratus lumborum m

Ilium

Gluteus medius m

Gluteus maximus m

Figure 17.2.3

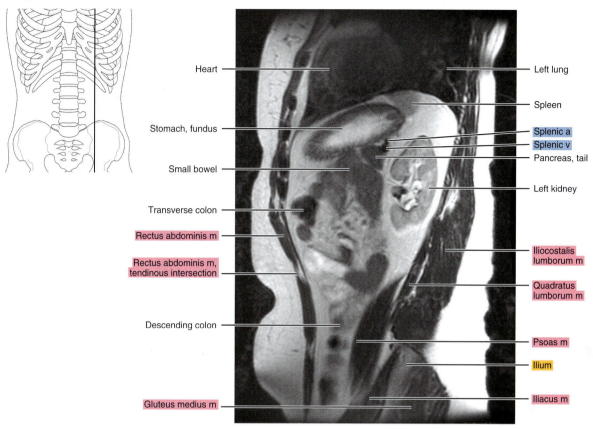

Heart
Left lung
Spleen
Stomach, fundus
Splenic a
Splenic v
Pancreas, tail
Small bowel
Left kidney
Transverse colon
Rectus abdominis m
Iliocostalis lumborum m
Rectus abdominis m, tendinous intersection
Quadratus lumborum m
Descending colon
Psoas m
Ilium
Gluteus medius m
Iliacus m

Figure 17.2.4

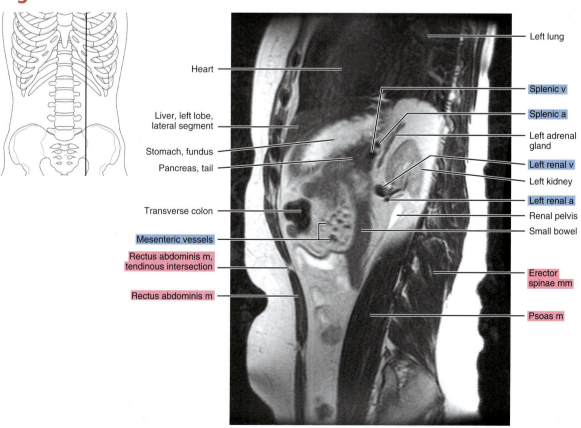

Left lung
Heart
Splenic v
Liver, left lobe, lateral segment
Splenic a
Stomach, fundus
Left adrenal gland
Pancreas, tail
Left renal v
Left kidney
Transverse colon
Left renal a
Renal pelvis
Mesenteric vessels
Small bowel
Rectus abdominis m, tendinous intersection
Erector spinae mm
Rectus abdominis m
Psoas m

Figure 17.2.5

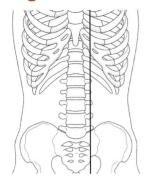

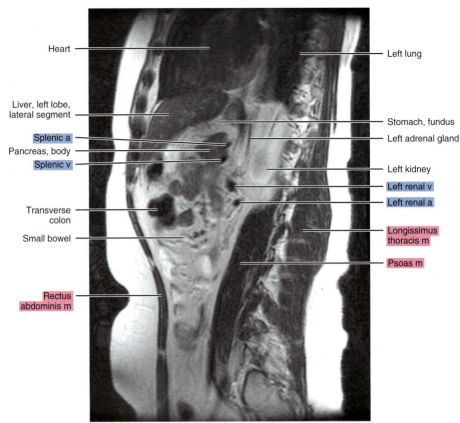

Heart

Liver, left lobe,
lateral segment

Splenic a

Pancreas, body

Splenic v

Transverse
colon

Small bowel

Rectus
abdominis m

Left lung

Stomach, fundus

Left adrenal gland

Left kidney

Left renal v

Left renal a

Longissimus
thoracis m

Psoas m

Figure 17.2.6

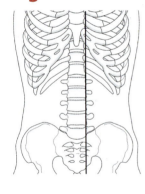

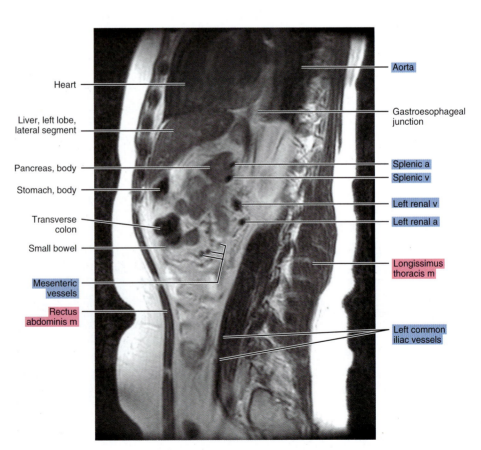

Heart

Liver, left lobe,
lateral segment

Pancreas, body

Stomach, body

Transverse
colon

Small bowel

Mesenteric
vessels

Rectus
abdominis m

Aorta

Gastroesophageal
junction

Splenic a

Splenic v

Left renal v

Left renal a

Longissimus
thoracis m

Left common
iliac vessels

Figure 17.2.7

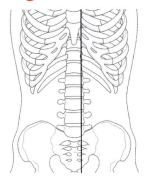

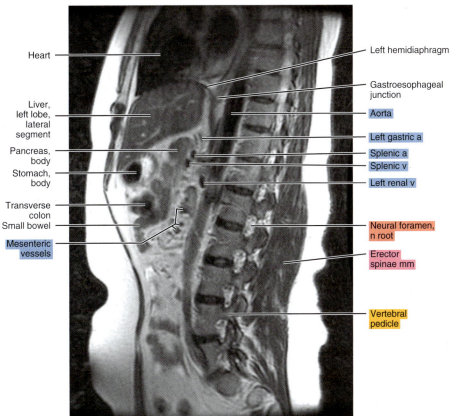

Heart

Liver, left lobe, lateral segment

Pancreas, body

Stomach, body

Transverse colon

Small bowel

Mesenteric vessels

Left hemidiaphragm

Gastroesophageal junction

Aorta

Left gastric a

Splenic a

Splenic v

Left renal v

Neural foramen, n root

Erector spinae mm

Vertebral pedicle

Figure 17.2.8

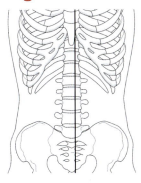

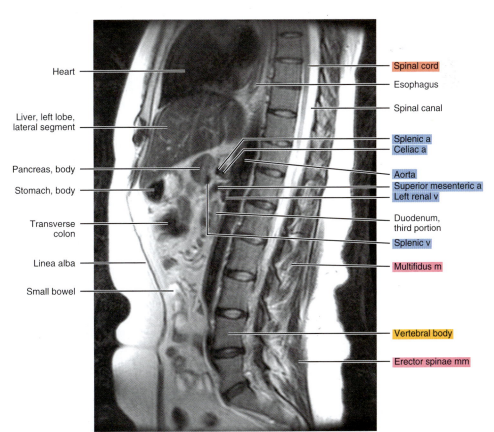

Heart

Liver, left lobe, lateral segment

Pancreas, body

Stomach, body

Transverse colon

Linea alba

Small bowel

Spinal cord

Esophagus

Spinal canal

Splenic a

Celiac a

Aorta

Superior mesenteric a

Left renal v

Duodenum, third portion

Splenic v

Multifidus m

Vertebral body

Erector spinae mm

Figure 17.2.9

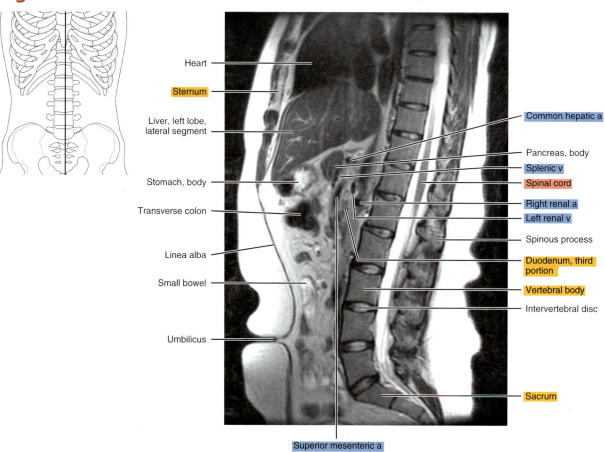

Heart

Sternum

Liver, left lobe, lateral segment

Stomach, body

Transverse colon

Linea alba

Small bowel

Umbilicus

Common hepatic a

Pancreas, body

Splenic v

Spinal cord

Right renal a

Left renal v

Spinous process

Duodenum, third portion

Vertebral body

Intervertebral disc

Sacrum

Superior mesenteric a

Figure 17.2.10

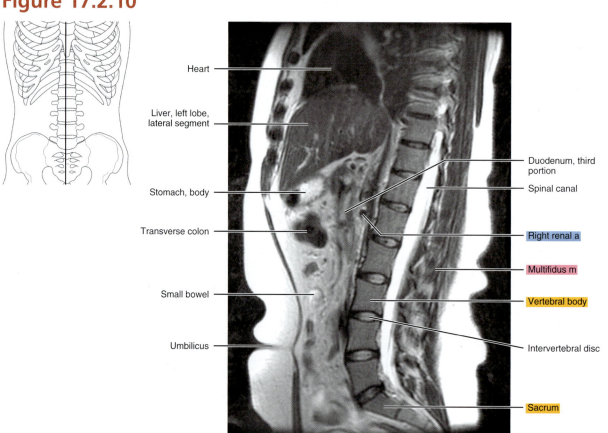

Heart

Liver, left lobe, lateral segment

Stomach, body

Transverse colon

Small bowel

Umbilicus

Duodenum, third portion

Spinal canal

Right renal a

Multifidus m

Vertebral body

Intervertebral disc

Sacrum

Figure 17.2.11

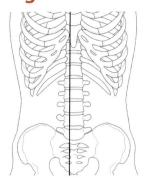

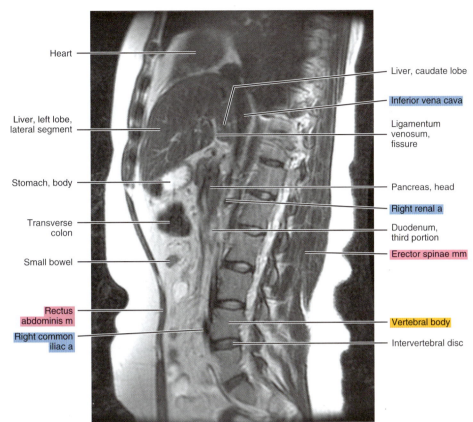

Heart

Liver, caudate lobe

Inferior vena cava

Liver, left lobe, lateral segment

Ligamentum venosum, fissure

Stomach, body

Pancreas, head

Right renal a

Transverse colon

Duodenum, third portion

Erector spinae mm

Small bowel

Rectus abdominis m

Vertebral body

Right common iliac a

Intervertebral disc

Figure 17.2.12

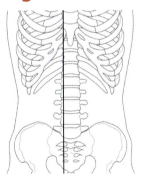

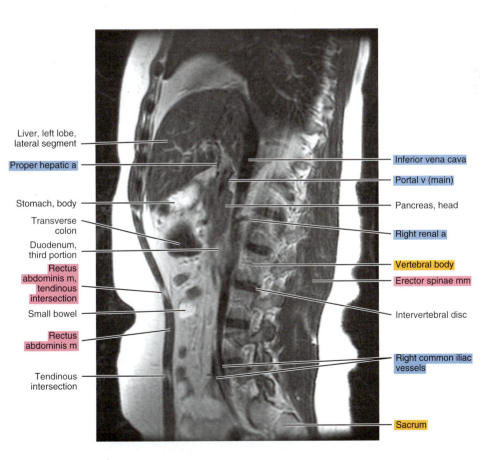

Liver, left lobe, lateral segment

Proper hepatic a

Inferior vena cava

Portal v (main)

Stomach, body

Pancreas, head

Transverse colon

Right renal a

Duodenum, third portion

Rectus abdominis m, tendinous intersection

Vertebral body

Erector spinae mm

Small bowel

Intervertebral disc

Rectus abdominis m

Right common iliac vessels

Tendinous intersection

Sacrum

Figure 17.2.13

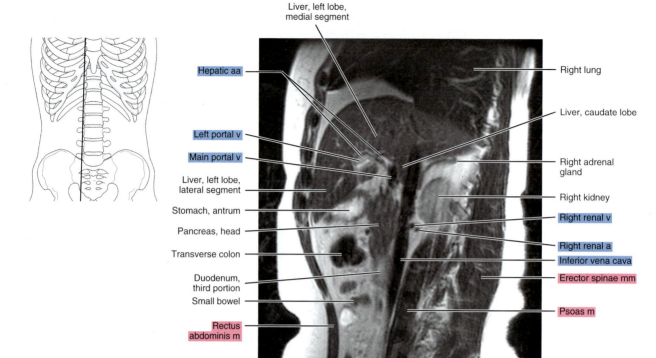

Liver, left lobe, medial segment

Hepatic aa

Left portal v

Main portal v

Liver, left lobe, lateral segment

Stomach, antrum

Pancreas, head

Transverse colon

Duodenum, third portion

Small bowel

Rectus abdominis m

Right lung

Liver, caudate lobe

Right adrenal gland

Right kidney

Right renal v

Right renal a

Inferior vena cava

Erector spinae mm

Psoas m

Sacrum

Figure 17.2.14

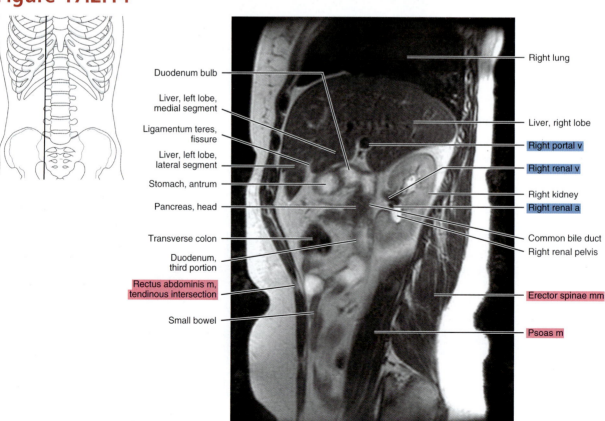

Duodenum bulb

Liver, left lobe, medial segment

Ligamentum teres, fissure

Liver, left lobe, lateral segment

Stomach, antrum

Pancreas, head

Transverse colon

Duodenum, third portion

Rectus abdominis m, tendinous intersection

Small bowel

Right lung

Liver, right lobe

Right portal v

Right renal v

Right kidney

Right renal a

Common bile duct

Right renal pelvis

Erector spinae mm

Psoas m

Figure 17.2.15

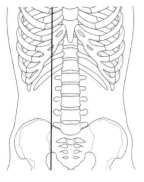

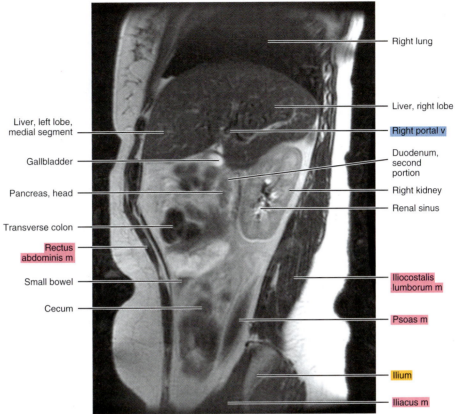

Liver, left lobe, medial segment

Gallbladder

Pancreas, head

Transverse colon

Rectus abdominis m

Small bowel

Cecum

Right lung

Liver, right lobe

Right portal v

Duodenum, second portion

Right kidney

Renal sinus

Iliocostalis lumborum m

Psoas m

Ilium

Iliacus m

Figure 17.2.16

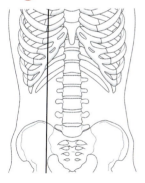

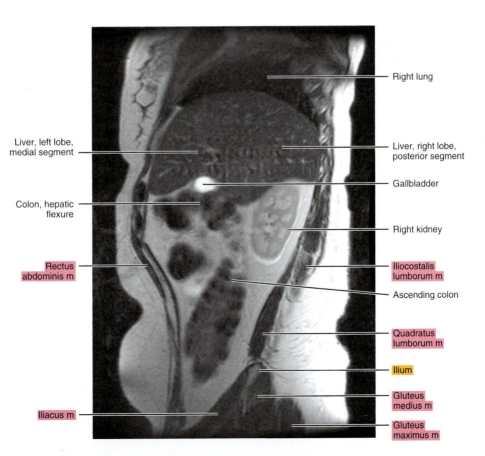

Liver, left lobe, medial segment

Colon, hepatic flexure

Rectus abdominis m

Iliacus m

Right lung

Liver, right lobe, posterior segment

Gallbladder

Right kidney

Iliocostalis lumborum m

Ascending colon

Quadratus lumborum m

Ilium

Gluteus medius m

Gluteus maximus m

CORONAL
Figure 17.3.1

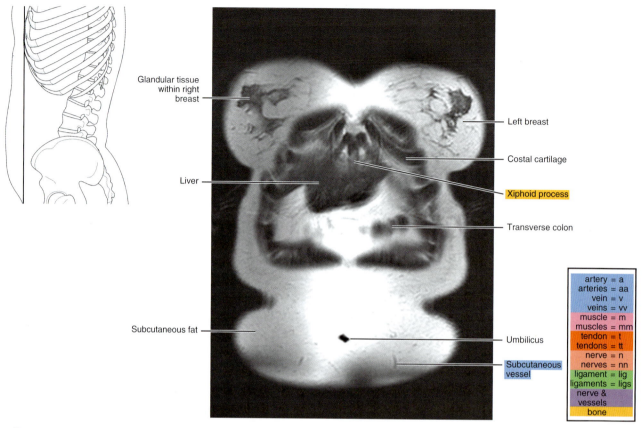

Glandular tissue within right breast

Left breast

Costal cartilage

Liver

Xiphoid process

Transverse colon

Subcutaneous fat

Umbilicus

Subcutaneous vessel

artery	= a
arteries	= aa
vein	= v
veins	= vv
muscle	= m
muscles	= mm
tendon	= t
tendons	= tt
nerve	= n
nerves	= nn
ligament	= lig
ligaments	= ligs
nerve & vessels	
bone	

Figure 17.3.2

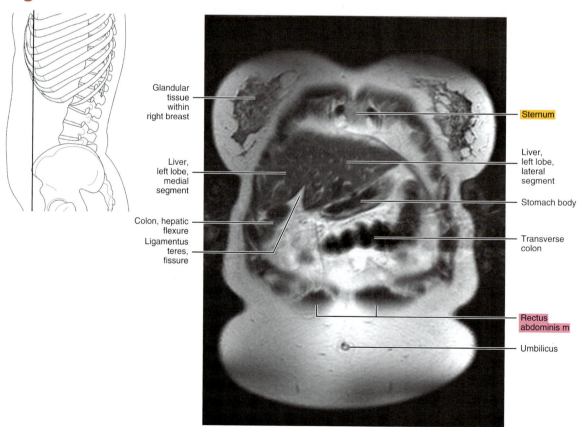

Glandular tissue within right breast

Sternum

Liver, left lobe, medial segment

Liver, left lobe, lateral segment

Stomach body

Colon, hepatic flexure

Ligamentus teres, fissure

Transverse colon

Rectus abdominis m

Umbilicus

Figure 17.3.3

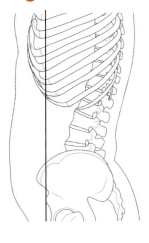

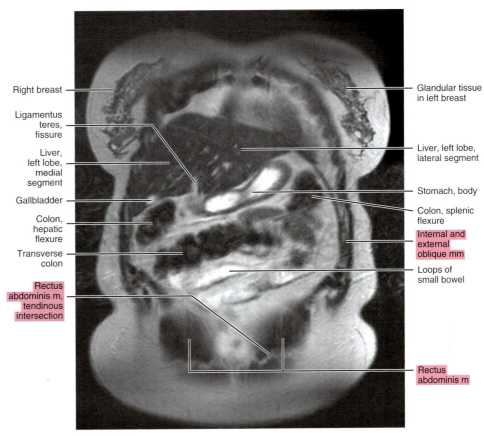

Right breast

Ligamentus teres, fissure

Liver, left lobe, medial segment

Gallbladder

Colon, hepatic flexure

Transverse colon

Rectus abdominis m, tendinous intersection

Glandular tissue in left breast

Liver, left lobe, lateral segment

Stomach, body

Colon, splenic flexure

Internal and external oblique mm

Loops of small bowel

Rectus abdominis m

Figure 17.3.4

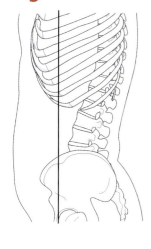

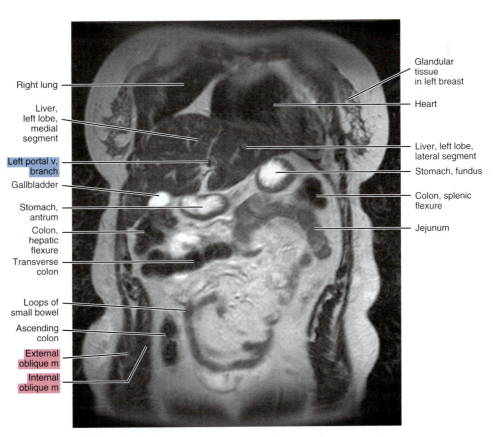

Right lung

Liver, left lobe, medial segment

Left portal v, branch

Gallbladder

Stomach, antrum

Colon, hepatic flexure

Transverse colon

Loops of small bowel

Ascending colon

External oblique m

Internal oblique m

Glandular tissue in left breast

Heart

Liver, left lobe, lateral segment

Stomach, fundus

Colon, splenic flexure

Jejunum

Figure 17.3.5

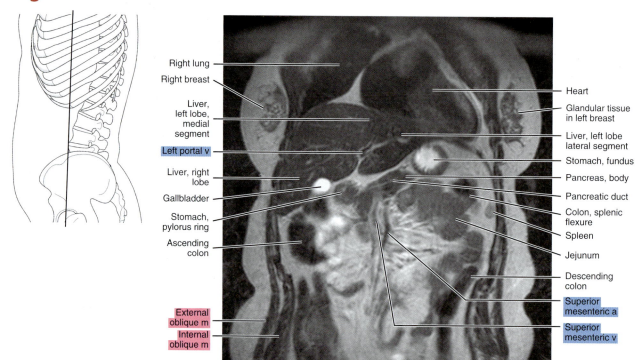

Right lung
Right breast
Liver, left lobe, medial segment
Left portal v
Liver, right lobe
Gallbladder
Stomach, pylorus ring
Ascending colon
External oblique m
Internal oblique m

Heart
Glandular tissue in left breast
Liver, left lobe lateral segment
Stomach, fundus
Pancreas, body
Pancreatic duct
Colon, splenic flexure
Spleen
Jejunum
Descending colon
Superior mesenteric a
Superior mesenteric v
Sigmoid colon

Figure 17.3.6

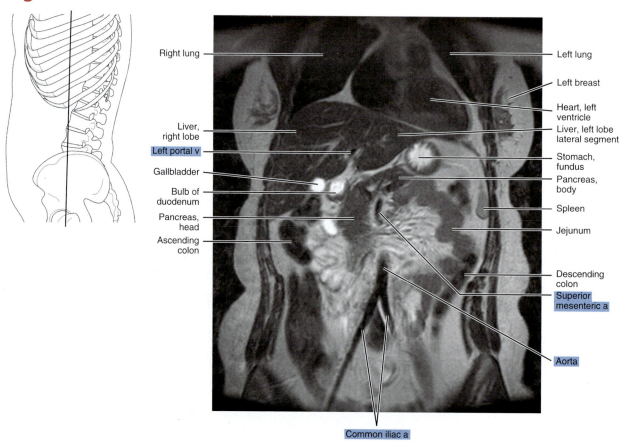

Right lung
Liver, right lobe
Left portal v
Gallbladder
Bulb of duodenum
Pancreas, head
Ascending colon

Left lung
Left breast
Heart, left ventricle
Liver, left lobe lateral segment
Stomach, fundus
Pancreas, body
Spleen
Jejunum
Descending colon
Superior mesenteric a
Aorta

Common iliac a

Figure 17.3.7

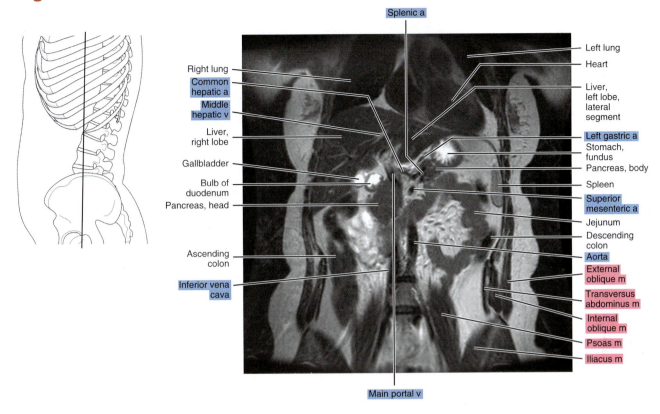

Splenic a

Right lung
Common hepatic a
Middle hepatic v
Liver, right lobe
Gallbladder
Bulb of duodenum
Pancreas, head
Ascending colon
Inferior vena cava

Left lung
Heart
Liver, left lobe, lateral segment
Left gastric a
Stomach, fundus
Pancreas, body
Spleen
Superior mesenteric a
Jejunum
Descending colon
Aorta
External oblique m
Transversus abdominus m
Internal oblique m
Psoas m
Iliacus m

Main portal v

Figure 17.3.8

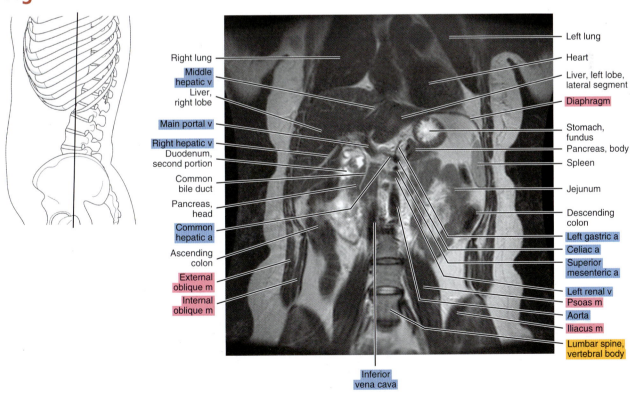

Right lung
Middle hepatic v
Liver, right lobe
Main portal v
Right hepatic v
Duodenum, second portion
Common bile duct
Pancreas, head
Common hepatic a
Ascending colon
External oblique m
Internal oblique m

Left lung
Heart
Liver, left lobe, lateral segment
Diaphragm
Stomach, fundus
Pancreas, body
Spleen
Jejunum
Descending colon
Left gastric a
Celiac a
Superior mesenteric a
Left renal v
Psoas m
Aorta
Iliacus m
Lumbar spine, vertebral body

Inferior vena cava

Figure 17.3.9

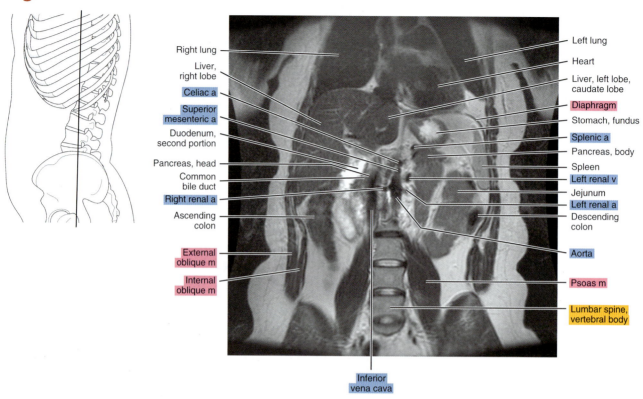

Right lung
Liver, right lobe
Celiac a
Superior mesenteric a
Duodenum, second portion
Pancreas, head
Common bile duct
Right renal a
Ascending colon
External oblique m
Internal oblique m

Left lung
Heart
Liver, left lobe, caudate lobe
Diaphragm
Stomach, fundus
Splenic a
Pancreas, body
Spleen
Left renal v
Jejunum
Left renal a
Descending colon
Aorta
Psoas m
Lumbar spine, vertebral body

Inferior vena cava

Figure 17.3.10

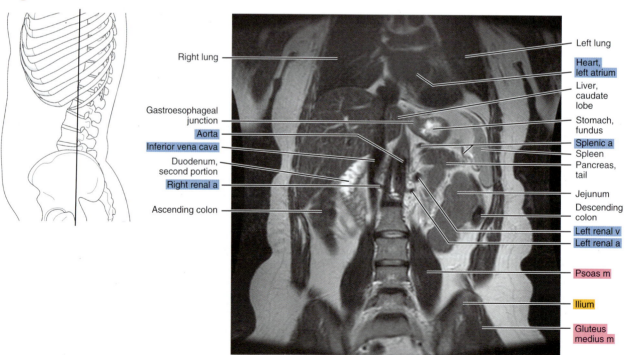

Right lung
Gastroesophageal junction
Aorta
Inferior vena cava
Duodenum, second portion
Right renal a
Ascending colon

Left lung
Heart, left atrium
Liver, caudate lobe
Stomach, fundus
Splenic a
Spleen
Pancreas, tail
Jejunum
Descending colon
Left renal v
Left renal a
Psoas m
Ilium
Gluteus medius m

Figure 17.3.11

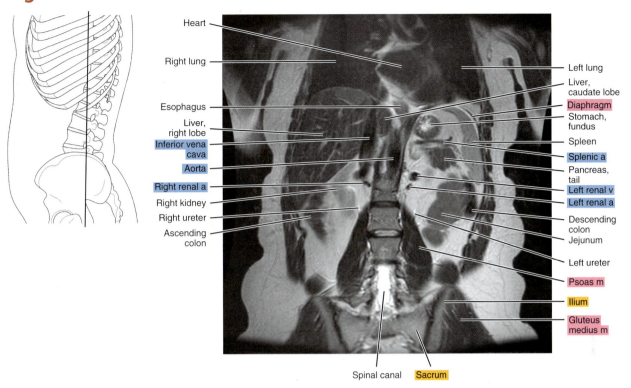

Heart
Right lung
Esophagus
Liver, right lobe
Inferior vena cava
Aorta
Right renal a
Right kidney
Right ureter
Ascending colon

Left lung
Liver, caudate lobe
Diaphragm
Stomach, fundus
Spleen
Splenic a
Pancreas, tail
Left renal v
Left renal a
Descending colon
Jejunum
Left ureter
Psoas m
Ilium
Gluteus medius m

Spinal canal   Sacrum

Figure 17.3.12

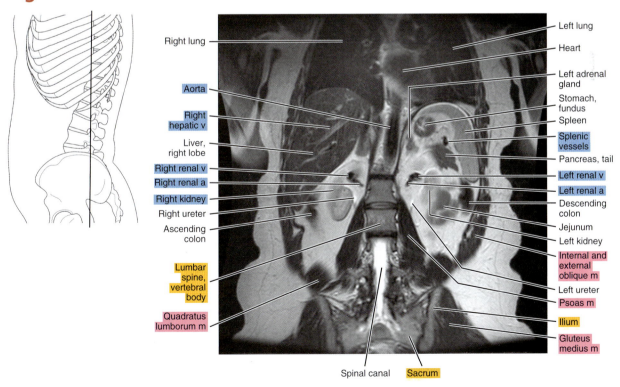

Right lung
Aorta
Right hepatic v
Liver, right lobe
Right renal v
Right renal a
Right kidney
Right ureter
Ascending colon
Lumbar spine, vertebral body
Quadratus lumborum m

Left lung
Heart
Left adrenal gland
Stomach, fundus
Spleen
Splenic vessels
Pancreas, tail
Left renal v
Left renal a
Descending colon
Jejunum
Left kidney
Internal and external oblique m
Left ureter
Psoas m
Ilium
Gluteus medius m

Spinal canal   Sacrum

Figure 17.3.13

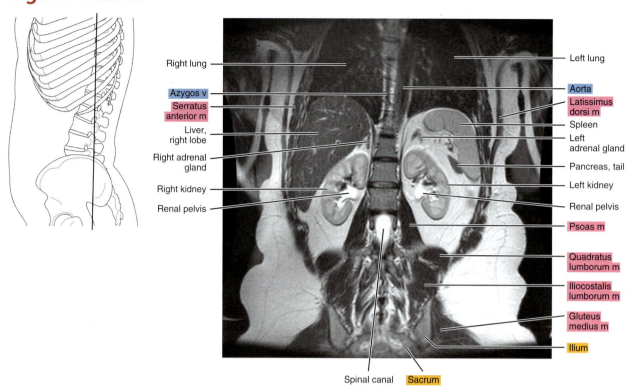

Right lung

Azygos v

Serratus anterior m

Liver, right lobe

Right adrenal gland

Right kidney

Renal pelvis

Left lung

Aorta

Latissimus dorsi m

Spleen

Left adrenal gland

Pancreas, tail

Left kidney

Renal pelvis

Psoas m

Quadratus lumborum m

Iliocostalis lumborum m

Gluteus medius m

Ilium

Spinal canal   Sacrum

Figure 17.3.14

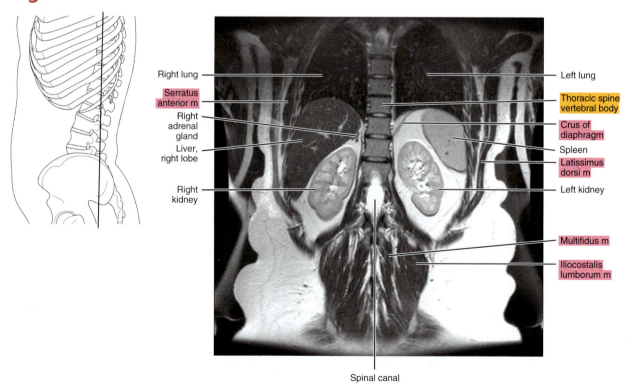

Right lung

Serratus anterior m

Right adrenal gland

Liver, right lobe

Right kidney

Left lung

Thoracic spine vertebral body

Crus of diaphragm

Spleen

Latissimus dorsi m

Left kidney

Multifidus m

Iliocostalis lumborum m

Spinal canal

Figure 17.3.15

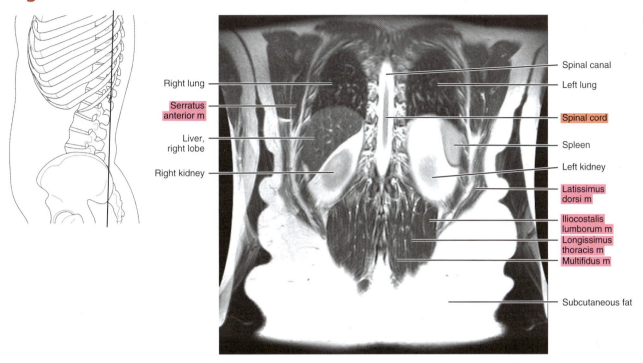

Right lung

Serratus anterior m

Liver, right lobe

Right kidney

Spinal canal

Left lung

Spinal cord

Spleen

Left kidney

Latissimus dorsi m

Iliocostalis lumborum m

Longissimus thoracis m

Multifidus m

Subcutaneous fat

Figure 17.3.16

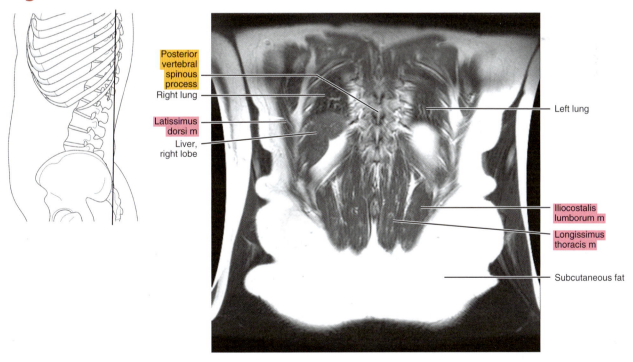

Posterior vertebral spinous process

Right lung

Latissimus dorsi m

Liver, right lobe

Left lung

Iliocostalis lumborum m

Longissimus thoracis m

Subcutaneous fat

Lower Extremity

Chapter 18

MRI of the Hip

AXIAL
Figure 18.1.1

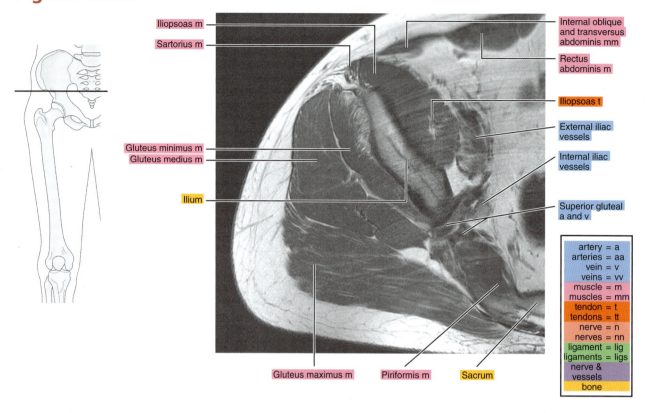

Iliopsoas m

Sartorius m

Gluteus minimus m

Gluteus medius m

Ilium

Internal oblique and transversus abdominis mm

Rectus abdominis m

Iliopsoas t

External iliac vessels

Internal iliac vessels

Superior gluteal a and v

Gluteus maximus m

Piriformis m

Sacrum

artery = a
arteries = aa
vein = v
veins = vv
muscle = m
muscles = mm
tendon = t
tendons = tt
nerve = n
nerves = nn
ligament = lig
ligaments = ligs
nerve & vessels
bone

Figure 18.1.2

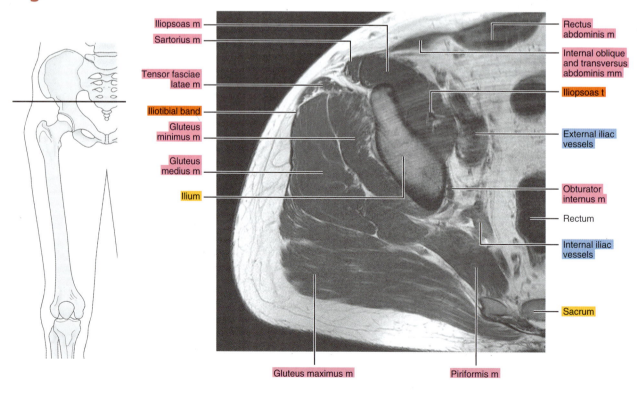

Iliopsoas m

Sartorius m

Tensor fasciae latae m

Iliotibial band

Gluteus minimus m

Gluteus medius m

Ilium

Rectus abdominis m

Internal oblique and transversus abdominis mm

Iliopsoas t

External iliac vessels

Obturator internus m

Rectum

Internal iliac vessels

Sacrum

Gluteus maximus m

Piriformis m

Figure 18.1.3

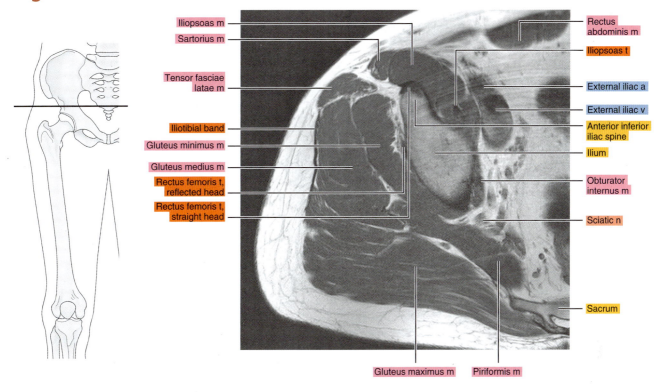

Iliopsoas m
Sartorius m
Tensor fasciae latae m
Iliotibial band
Gluteus minimus m
Rectus femoris t, reflected head
Rectus femoris t, straight head

Rectus abdominis m
Iliopsoas t
External iliac a
External iliac v
Anterior inferior iliac spine
Ilium
Obturator internus m
Sciatic n
Sacrum

Gluteus maximus m   Piriformis m

Figure 18.1.4

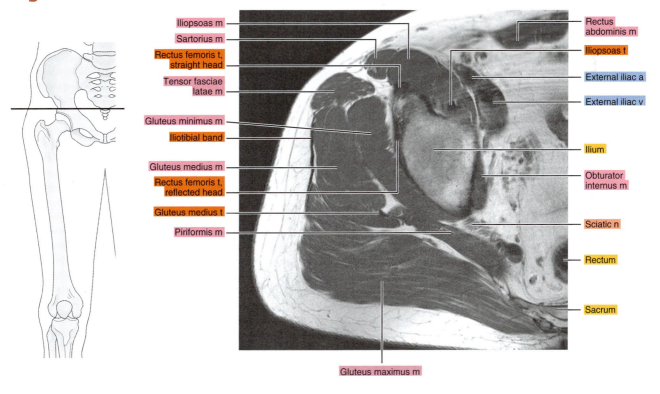

Iliopsoas m
Sartorius m
Rectus femoris t, straight head
Tensor fasciae latae m
Gluteus minimus m
Iliotibial band
Gluteus medius m
Rectus femoris t, reflected head
Gluteus medius t
Piriformis m

Rectus abdominis m
Iliopsoas t
External iliac a
External iliac v
Ilium
Obturator internus m
Sciatic n
Rectum
Sacrum

Gluteus maximus m

Figure 18.1.5

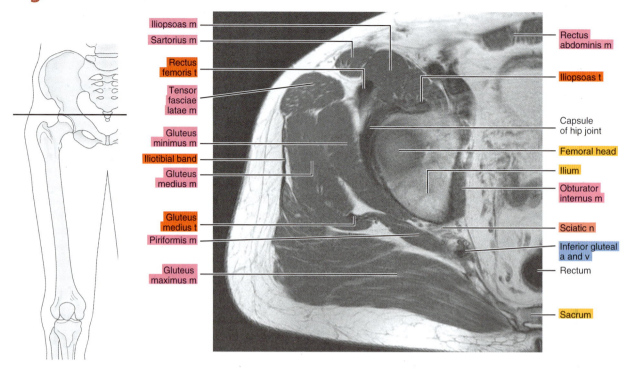

Iliopsoas m
Sartorius m
Rectus femoris t
Tensor fasciae latae m
Gluteus minimus m
Iliotibial band
Gluteus medius m
Gluteus medius t
Piriformis m
Gluteus maximus m

Rectus abdominis m
Iliopsoas t
Capsule of hip joint
Femoral head
Ilium
Obturator internus m
Sciatic n
Inferior gluteal a and v
Rectum
Sacrum

Figure 18.1.6

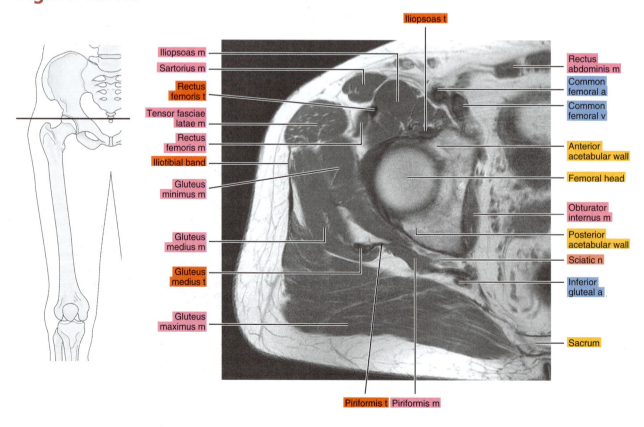

Iliopsoas t
Iliopsoas m
Sartorius m
Rectus femoris t
Tensor fasciae latae m
Rectus femoris m
Iliotibial band
Gluteus minimus m
Gluteus medius m
Gluteus medius t
Gluteus maximus m

Rectus abdominis m
Common femoral a
Common femoral v
Anterior acetabular wall
Femoral head
Obturator internus m
Posterior acetabular wall
Sciatic n
Inferior gluteal a
Sacrum

Piriformis t   Piriformis m

Figure 18.1.7

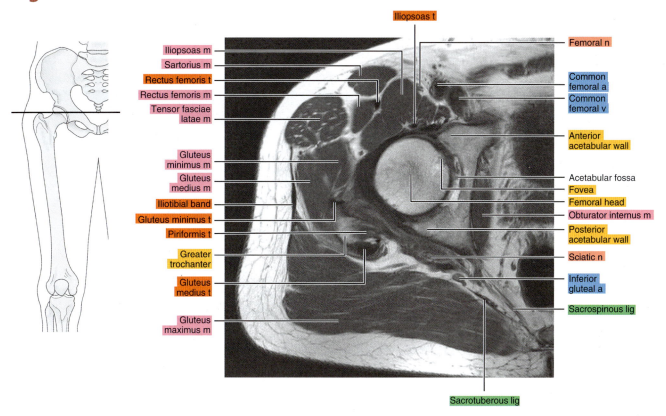

Iliopsoas t
Iliopsoas m
Sartorius m
Rectus femoris t
Rectus femoris m
Tensor fasciae latae m
Gluteus minimus m
Gluteus medius m
Iliotibial band
Gluteus minimus t
Piriformis t
Greater trochanter
Gluteus medius t
Gluteus maximus m
Femoral n
Common femoral a
Common femoral v
Anterior acetabular wall
Acetabular fossa
Fovea
Femoral head
Obturator internus m
Posterior acetabular wall
Sciatic n
Inferior gluteal a
Sacrospinous lig
Sacrotuberous lig

Figure 18.1.8

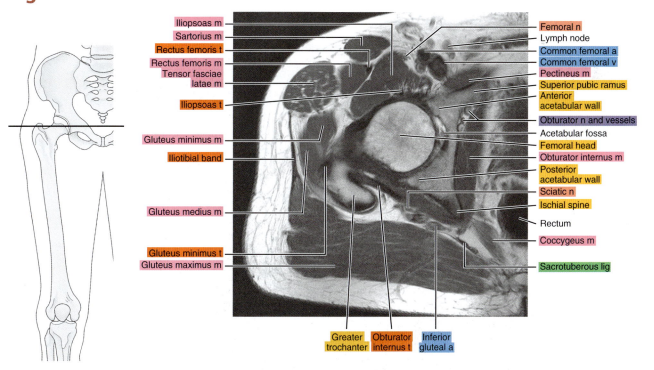

Iliopsoas m
Sartorius m
Rectus femoris t
Rectus femoris m
Tensor fasciae latae m
Iliopsoas t
Gluteus minimus m
Iliotibial band
Gluteus medius m
Gluteus minimus t
Gluteus maximus m
Femoral n
Lymph node
Common femoral a
Common femoral v
Pectineus m
Superior pubic ramus
Anterior acetabular wall
Obturator n and vessels
Acetabular fossa
Femoral head
Obturator internus m
Posterior acetabular wall
Sciatic n
Ischial spine
Rectum
Coccygeus m
Sacrotuberous lig
Greater trochanter
Obturator internus t
Inferior gluteal a

Figure 18.1.9

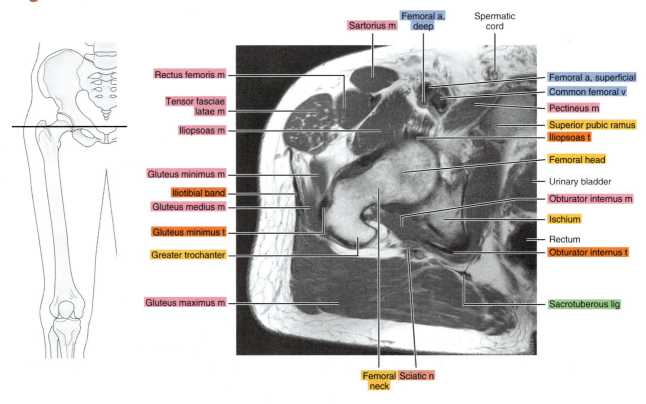

Sartorius m
Femoral a, deep
Spermatic cord
Rectus femoris m
Femoral a, superficial
Common femoral v
Tensor fasciae latae m
Pectineus m
Iliopsoas m
Superior pubic ramus
Iliopsoas t
Femoral head
Gluteus minimus m
Urinary bladder
Iliotibial band
Obturator internus m
Gluteus medius m
Ischium
Gluteus minimus t
Rectum
Greater trochanter
Obturator internus t
Gluteus maximus m
Sacrotuberous lig
Femoral neck
Sciatic n

Figure 18.1.10

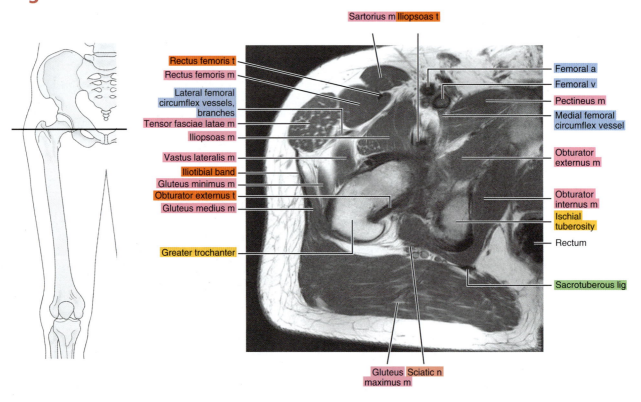

Sartorius m
Iliopsoas t
Rectus femoris t
Rectus femoris m
Femoral a
Femoral v
Lateral femoral circumflex vessels, branches
Pectineus m
Medial femoral circumflex vessel
Tensor fasciae latae m
Iliopsoas m
Vastus lateralis m
Obturator externus m
Iliotibial band
Gluteus minimus m
Obturator externus t
Obturator internus m
Gluteus medius m
Ischial tuberosity
Rectum
Greater trochanter
Sacrotuberous lig
Gluteus maximus m
Sciatic n

Figure 18.1.11

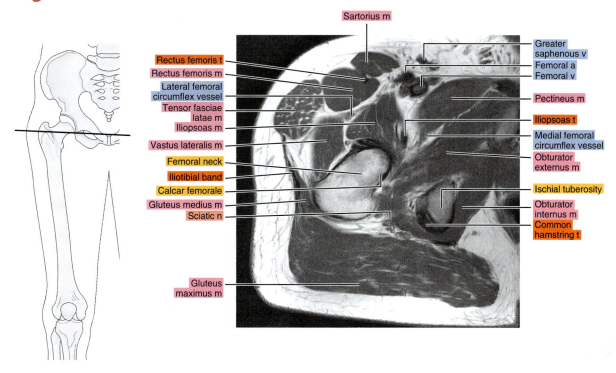

Figure 18.1.12

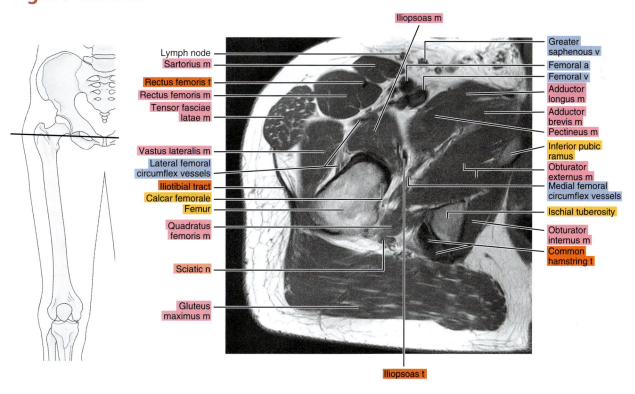

Figure 18.1.13

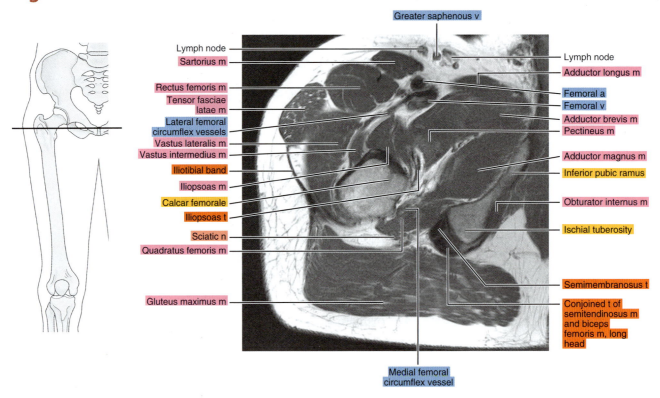

Greater saphenous v

Lymph node
Sartorius m

Rectus femoris m
Tensor fasciae latae m
Lateral femoral circumflex vessels
Vastus lateralis m
Vastus intermedius m
Iliotibial band
Iliopsoas m
Calcar femorale
Iliopsoas t
Sciatic n
Quadratus femoris m

Gluteus maximus m

Lymph node
Adductor longus m
Femoral a
Femoral v
Adductor brevis m
Pectineus m
Adductor magnus m
Inferior pubic ramus
Obturator internus m
Ischial tuberosity
Semimembranosus t
Conjoined t of semitendinosus m and biceps femoris m, long head

Medial femoral circumflex vessel

Figure 18.1.14

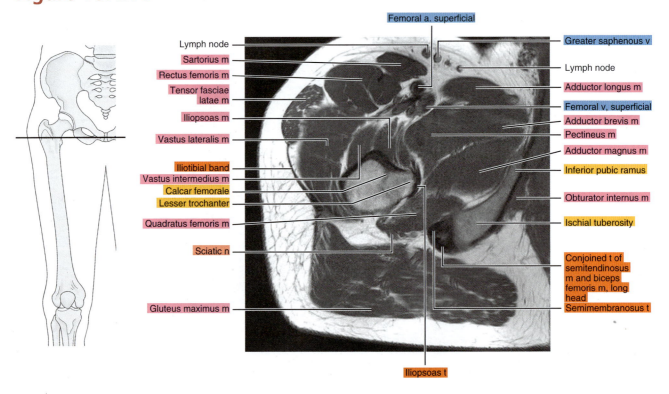

Femoral a. superficial

Lymph node
Sartorius m
Rectus femoris m
Tensor fasciae latae m
Iliopsoas m
Vastus lateralis m
Iliotibial band
Vastus intermedius m
Calcar femorale
Lesser trochanter
Quadratus femoris m
Sciatic n

Gluteus maximus m

Greater saphenous v
Lymph node
Adductor longus m
Femoral v, superficial
Adductor brevis m
Pectineus m
Adductor magnus m
Inferior pubic ramus
Obturator internus m
Ischial tuberosity
Conjoined t of semitendinosus m and biceps femoris m, long head
Semimembranosus t

Iliopsoas t

Figure 18.1.15

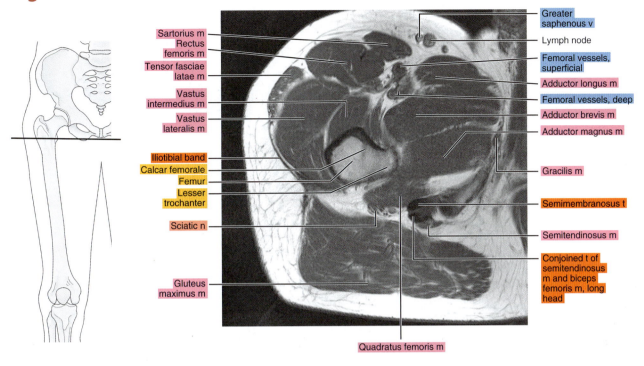

Sartorius m
Rectus femoris m
Tensor fasciae latae m
Vastus intermedius m
Vastus lateralis m
Iliotibial band
Calcar femorale
Femur
Lesser trochanter
Sciatic n
Gluteus maximus m

Greater saphenous v
Lymph node
Femoral vessels, superficial
Adductor longus m
Femoral vessels, deep
Adductor brevis m
Adductor magnus m
Gracilis m
Semimembranosus t
Semitendinosus m
Conjoined t of semitendinosus m and biceps femoris m, long head

Quadratus femoris m

Figure 18.1.16

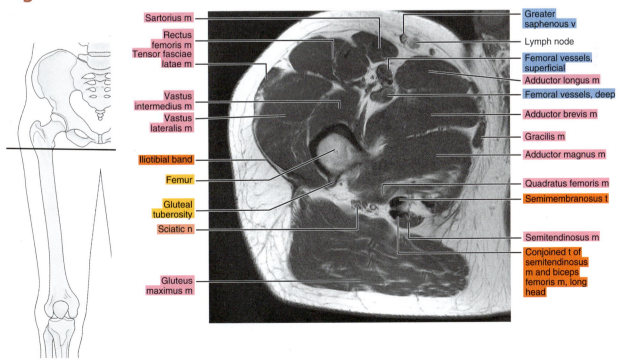

Sartorius m
Rectus femoris m
Tensor fasciae latae m
Vastus intermedius m
Vastus lateralis m
Iliotibial band
Femur
Gluteal tuberosity
Sciatic n
Gluteus maximus m

Greater saphenous v
Lymph node
Femoral vessels, superficial
Adductor longus m
Femoral vessels, deep
Adductor brevis m
Gracilis m
Adductor magnus m
Quadratus femoris m
Semimembranosus t
Semitendinosus m
Conjoined t of semitendinosus m and biceps femoris m, long head

Figure 18.1.17

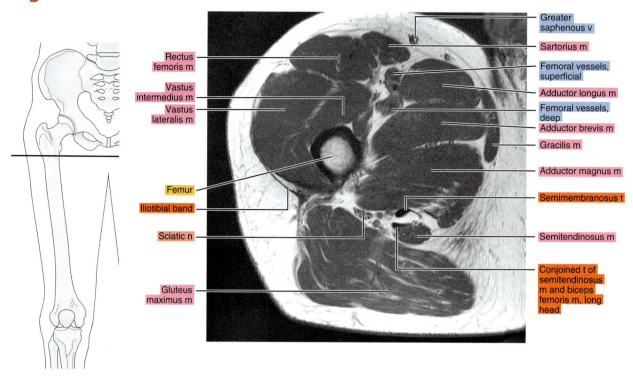

Rectus femoris m
Vastus intermedius m
Vastus lateralis m
Femur
Iliotibial band
Sciatic n
Gluteus maximus m

Greater saphenous v
Sartorius m
Femoral vessels, superficial
Adductor longus m
Femoral vessels, deep
Adductor brevis m
Gracilis m
Adductor magnus m
Semimembranosus t
Semitendinosus m
Conjoined t of semitendinosus m and biceps femoris m, long head

Figure 18.1.18

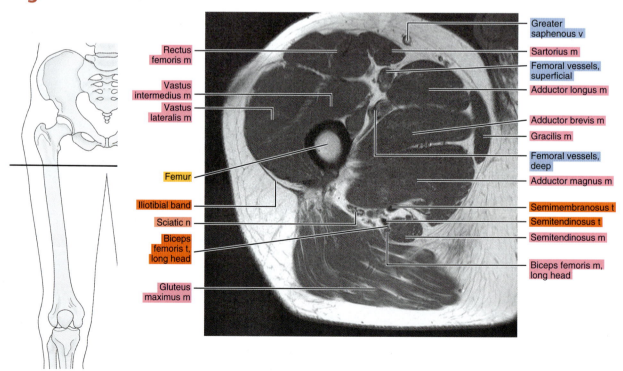

Rectus femoris m
Vastus intermedius m
Vastus lateralis m
Femur
Iliotibial band
Sciatic n
Biceps femoris t, long head
Gluteus maximus m

Greater saphenous v
Sartorius m
Femoral vessels, superficial
Adductor longus m
Adductor brevis m
Gracilis m
Femoral vessels, deep
Adductor magnus m
Semimembranosus t
Semitendinosus t
Semitendinosus m
Biceps femoris m, long head

SAGITTAL
Figure 18.2.1

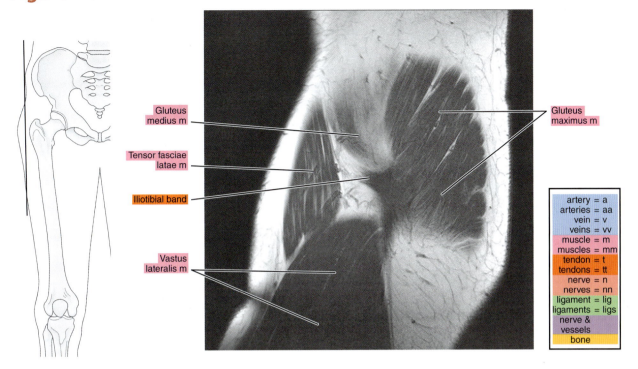

Gluteus medius m

Tensor fasciae latae m

Iliotibial band

Vastus lateralis m

Gluteus maximus m

artery = a	
arteries = aa	
vein = v	
veins = vv	
muscle = m	
muscles = mm	
tendon = t	
tendons = tt	
nerve = n	
nerves = nn	
ligament = lig	
ligaments = ligs	
nerve & vessels	
bone	

Figure 18.2.2

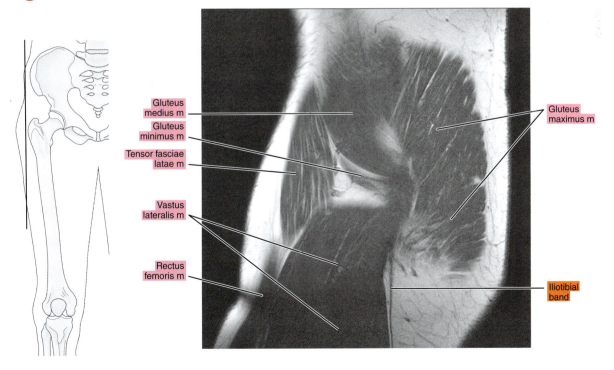

Gluteus medius m

Gluteus minimus m

Tensor fasciae latae m

Vastus lateralis m

Rectus femoris m

Gluteus maximus m

Iliotibial band

Figure 18.2.3

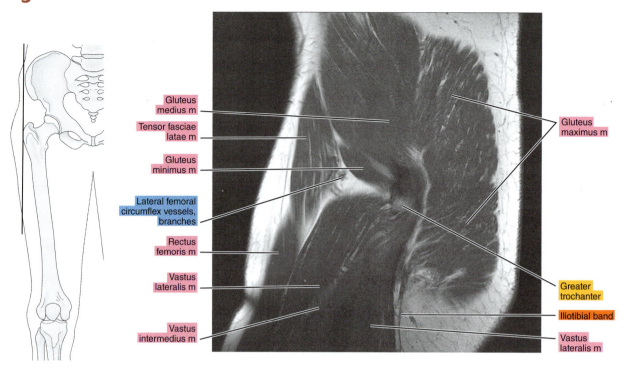

Gluteus medius m

Tensor fasciae latae m

Gluteus minimus m

Lateral femoral circumflex vessels, branches

Rectus femoris m

Vastus lateralis m

Vastus intermedius m

Gluteus maximus m

Greater trochanter

Iliotibial band

Vastus lateralis m

Figure 18.2.4

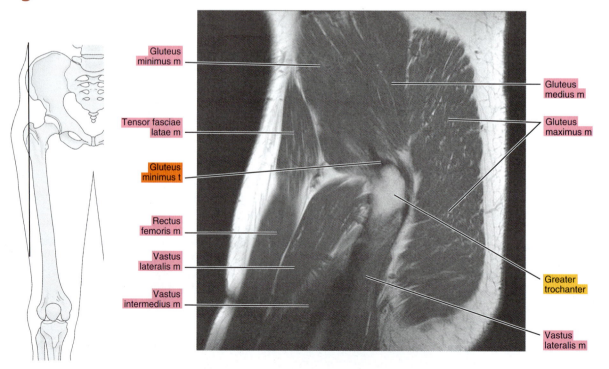

Gluteus minimus m

Tensor fasciae latae m

Gluteus minimus t

Rectus femoris m

Vastus lateralis m

Vastus intermedius m

Gluteus medius m

Gluteus maximus m

Greater trochanter

Vastus lateralis m

Figure 18.2.5

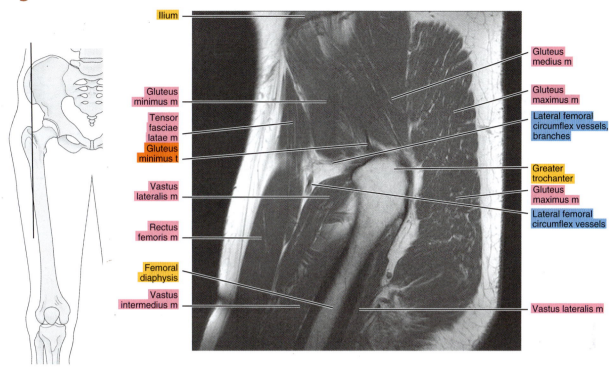

Ilium

Gluteus minimus m

Tensor fasciae latae m

Gluteus minimus t

Vastus lateralis m

Rectus femoris m

Femoral diaphysis

Vastus intermedius m

Gluteus medius m

Gluteus maximus m

Lateral femoral circumflex vessels, branches

Greater trochanter

Gluteus maximus m

Lateral femoral circumflex vessels

Vastus lateralis m

Figure 18.2.6

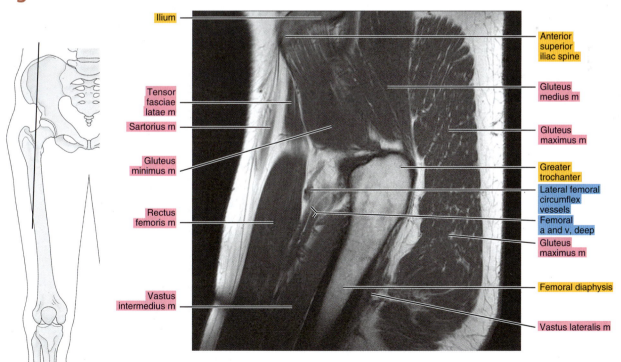

Ilium

Tensor fasciae latae m

Sartorius m

Gluteus minimus m

Rectus femoris m

Vastus intermedius m

Anterior superior iliac spine

Gluteus medius m

Gluteus maximus m

Greater trochanter

Lateral femoral circumflex vessels

Femoral a and v, deep

Gluteus maximus m

Femoral diaphysis

Vastus lateralis m

Figure 18.2.7

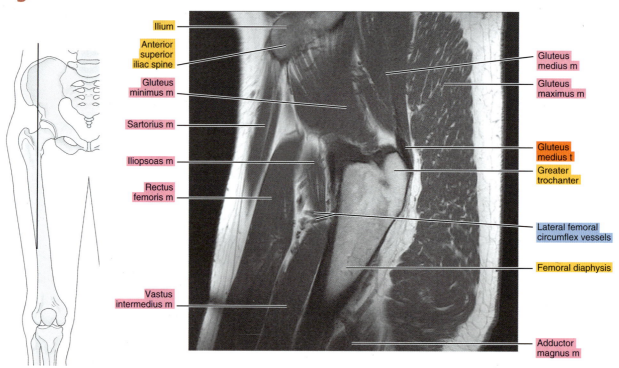

Ilium
Anterior superior iliac spine
Gluteus minimus m
Sartorius m
Iliopsoas m
Rectus femoris m
Vastus intermedius m

Gluteus medius m
Gluteus maximus m
Gluteus medius t
Greater trochanter
Lateral femoral circumflex vessels
Femoral diaphysis
Adductor magnus m

Figure 18.2.8

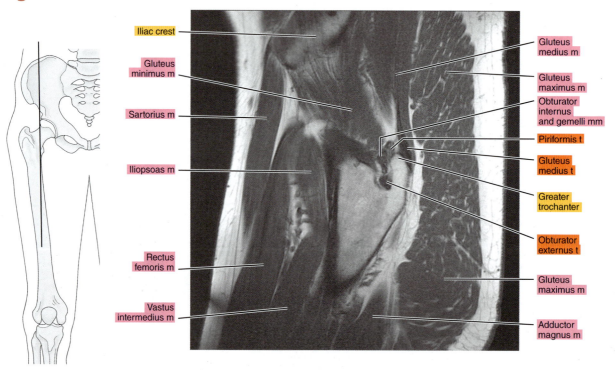

Iliac crest
Gluteus minimus m
Sartorius m
Iliopsoas m
Rectus femoris m
Vastus intermedius m

Gluteus medius m
Gluteus maximus m
Obturator internus and gemelli mm
Piriformis t
Gluteus medius t
Greater trochanter
Obturator externus t
Gluteus maximus m
Adductor magnus m

Figure 18.2.9

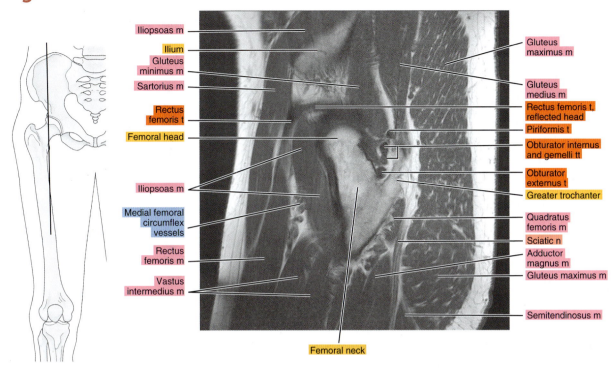

Iliopsoas m
Ilium
Gluteus minimus m
Sartorius m
Rectus femoris t
Femoral head
Iliopsoas m
Medial femoral circumflex vessels
Rectus femoris m
Vastus intermedius m

Gluteus maximus m
Gluteus medius m
Rectus femoris t, reflected head
Piriformis t
Obturator internus and gemelli tt
Obturator externus t
Greater trochanter
Quadratus femoris m
Sciatic n
Adductor magnus m
Gluteus maximus m
Semitendinosus m

Femoral neck

Figure 18.2.10

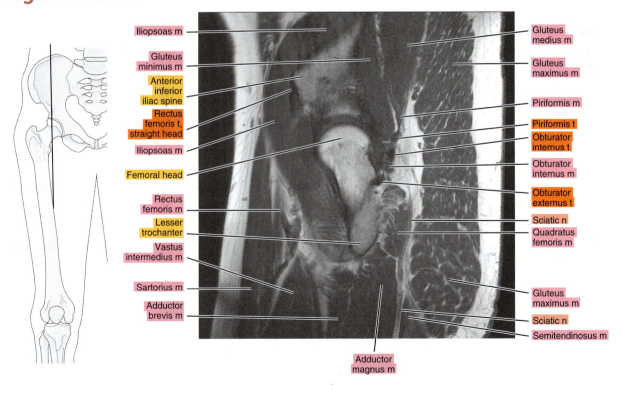

Iliopsoas m
Gluteus minimus m
Anterior inferior iliac spine
Rectus femoris t, straight head
Iliopsoas m
Femoral head
Rectus femoris m
Lesser trochanter
Vastus intermedius m
Sartorius m
Adductor brevis m

Gluteus medius m
Gluteus maximus m
Piriformis m
Piriformis t
Obturator internus t
Obturator internus m
Obturator externus t
Sciatic n
Quadratus femoris m
Gluteus maximus m
Sciatic n
Semitendinosus m

Adductor magnus m

Figure 18.2.11

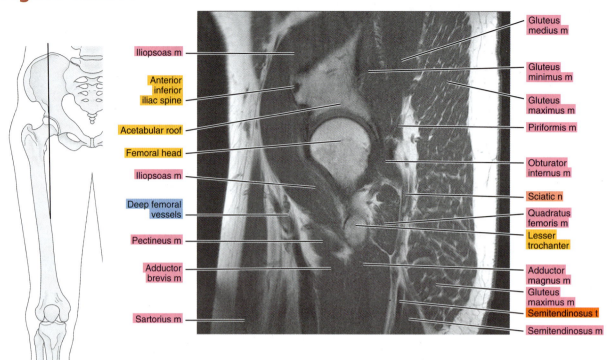

Iliopsoas m

Anterior inferior iliac spine

Acetabular roof

Femoral head

Iliopsoas m

Deep femoral vessels

Pectineus m

Adductor brevis m

Sartorius m

Gluteus medius m

Gluteus minimus m

Gluteus maximus m

Piriformis m

Obturator internus m

Sciatic n

Quadratus femoris m

Lesser trochanter

Adductor magnus m

Gluteus maximus m

Semitendinosus t

Semitendinosus m

Figure 18.2.12

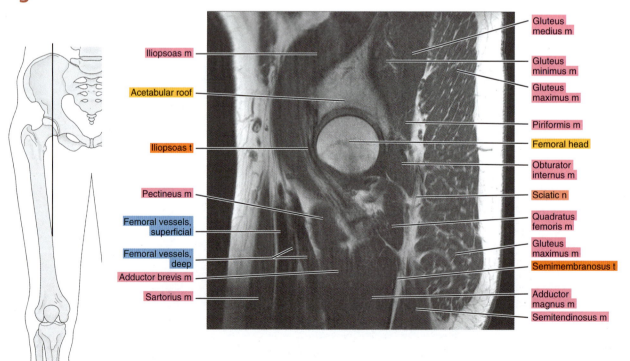

Iliopsoas m

Acetabular roof

Iliopsoas t

Pectineus m

Femoral vessels, superficial

Femoral vessels, deep

Adductor brevis m

Sartorius m

Gluteus medius m

Gluteus minimus m

Gluteus maximus m

Piriformis m

Femoral head

Obturator internus m

Sciatic n

Quadratus femoris m

Gluteus maximus m

Semimembranosus t

Adductor magnus m

Semitendinosus m

Figure 18.2.13

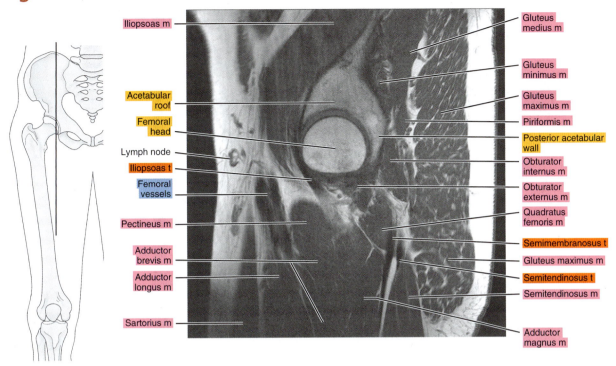

Iliopsoas m
Acetabular roof
Femoral head
Lymph node
Iliopsoas t
Femoral vessels
Pectineus m
Adductor brevis m
Adductor longus m
Sartorius m

Gluteus medius m
Gluteus minimus m
Gluteus maximus m
Piriformis m
Posterior acetabular wall
Obturator internus m
Obturator externus m
Quadratus femoris m
Semimembranosus t
Gluteus maximus m
Semitendinosus t
Semitendinosus m
Adductor magnus m

Figure 18.2.14

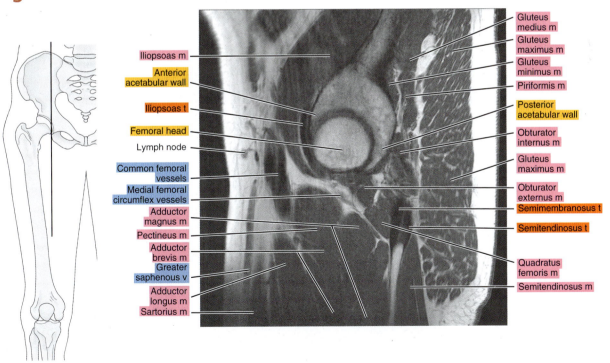

Iliopsoas m
Anterior acetabular wall
Iliopsoas t
Femoral head
Lymph node
Common femoral vessels
Medial femoral circumflex vessels
Adductor magnus m
Pectineus m
Adductor brevis m
Greater saphenous v
Adductor longus m
Sartorius m

Gluteus medius m
Gluteus maximus m
Gluteus minimus m
Piriformis m
Posterior acetabular wall
Obturator internus m
Gluteus maximus m
Obturator externus m
Semimembranosus t
Semitendinosus t
Quadratus femoris m
Semitendinosus m

Figure 18.2.15

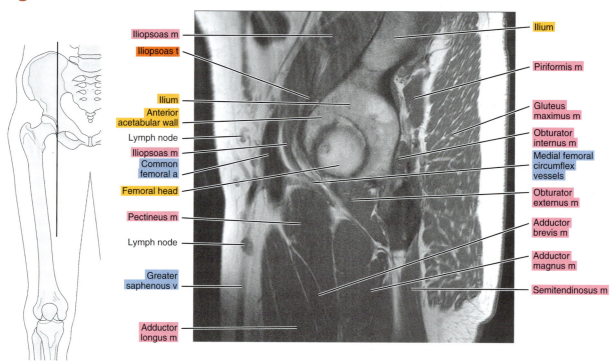

Iliopsoas m
Iliopsoas t
Ilium
Anterior acetabular wall
Lymph node
Iliopsoas m
Common femoral a
Femoral head
Pectineus m
Lymph node
Greater saphenous v
Adductor longus m

Ilium
Piriformis m
Gluteus maximus m
Obturator internus m
Medial femoral circumflex vessels
Obturator externus m
Adductor brevis m
Adductor magnus m
Semitendinosus m

Figure 18.2.16

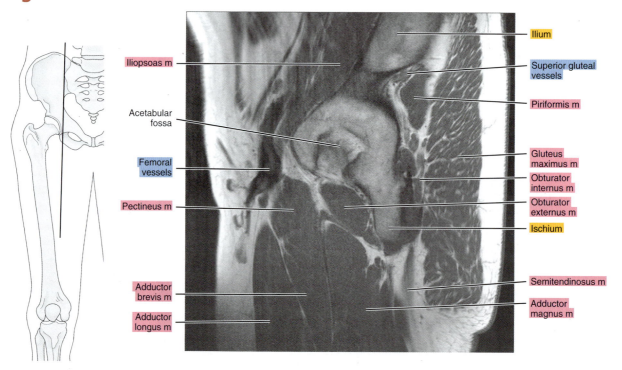

Iliopsoas m
Acetabular fossa
Femoral vessels
Pectineus m
Adductor brevis m
Adductor longus m

Ilium
Superior gluteal vessels
Piriformis m
Gluteus maximus m
Obturator internus m
Obturator externus m
Ischium
Semitendinosus m
Adductor magnus m

Figure 18.2.17

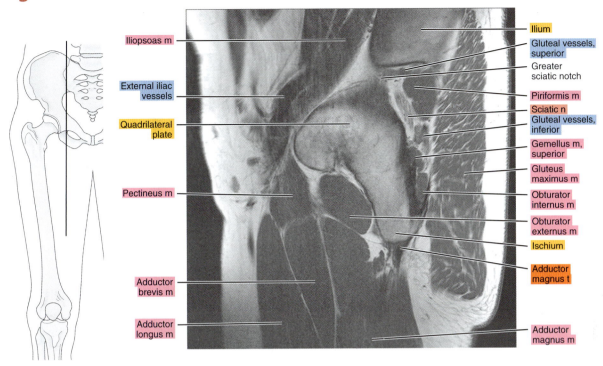

Iliopsoas m
External iliac vessels
Quadrilateral plate
Pectineus m
Adductor brevis m
Adductor longus m

Ilium
Gluteal vessels, superior
Greater sciatic notch
Piriformis m
Sciatic n
Gluteal vessels, inferior
Gemellus m, superior
Gluteus maximus m
Obturator internus m
Obturator externus m
Ischium
Adductor magnus t
Adductor magnus m

Figure 18.2.18

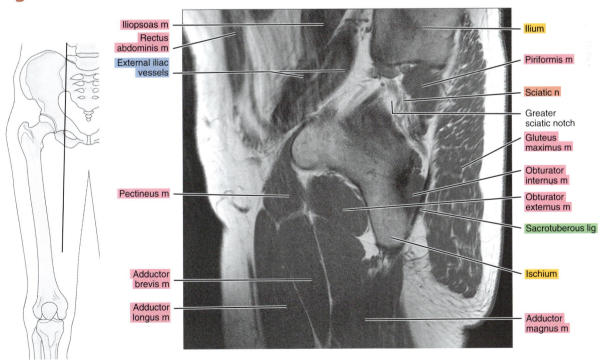

Iliopsoas m
Rectus abdominis m
External iliac vessels
Pectineus m
Adductor brevis m
Adductor longus m

Ilium
Piriformis m
Sciatic n
Greater sciatic notch
Gluteus maximus m
Obturator internus m
Obturator externus m
Sacrotuberous lig
Ischium
Adductor magnus m

Figure 18.2.19

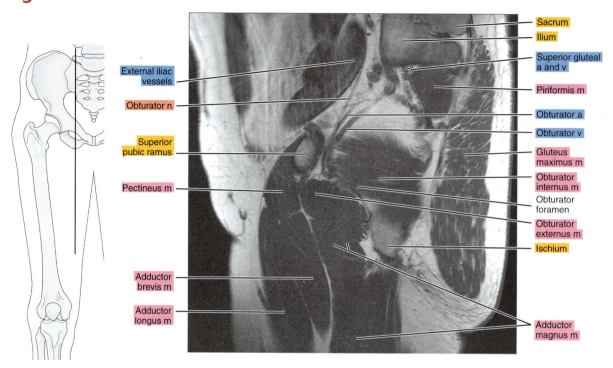

External iliac vessels

Obturator n

Superior pubic ramus

Pectineus m

Adductor brevis m

Adductor longus m

Sacrum

Ilium

Superior gluteal a and v

Piriformis m

Obturator a

Obturator v

Gluteus maximus m

Obturator internus m

Obturator foramen

Obturator externus m

Ischium

Adductor magnus m

CORONAL
Figure 18.3.1

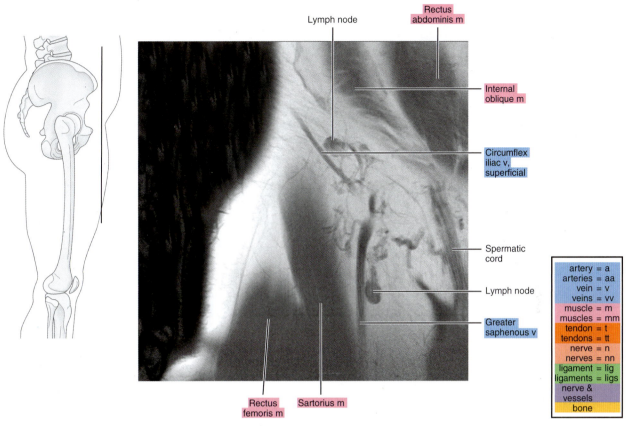

Lymph node

Rectus abdominis m

Internal oblique m

Circumflex iliac v, superficial

Spermatic cord

Lymph node

Greater saphenous v

Rectus femoris m

Sartorius m

artery = a	
arteries = aa	
vein = v	
veins = vv	
muscle = m	
muscles = mm	
tendon = t	
tendons = tt	
nerve = n	
nerves = nn	
ligament = lig	
ligaments = ligs	
nerve & vessels	
bone	

Figure 18.3.2

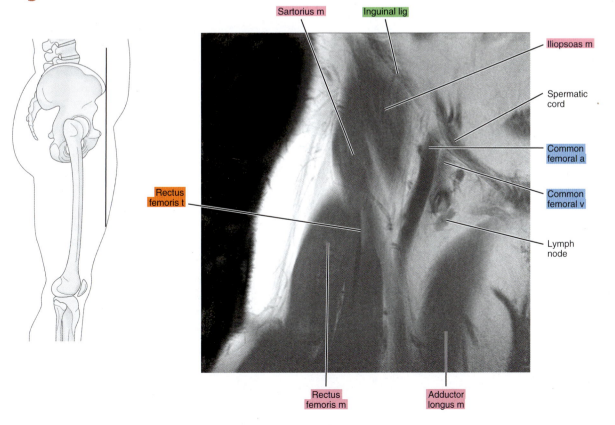

Sartorius m

Inguinal lig

Iliopsoas m

Spermatic cord

Common femoral a

Common femoral v

Lymph node

Rectus femoris t

Rectus femoris m

Adductor longus m

Figure 18.3.3

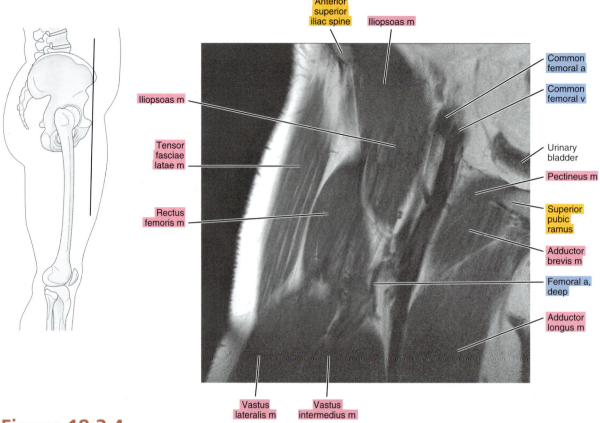

Figure 18.3.4

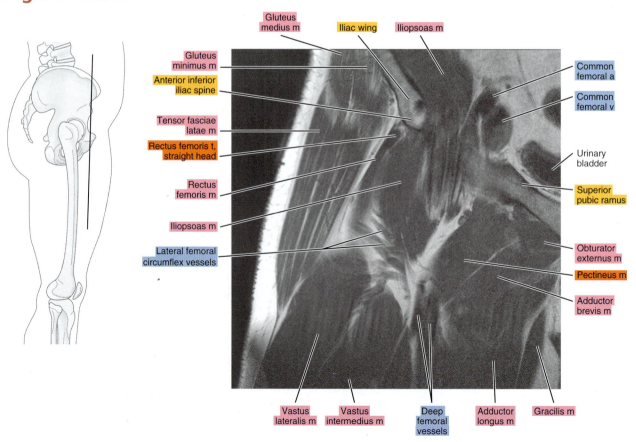

Figure 18.3.5

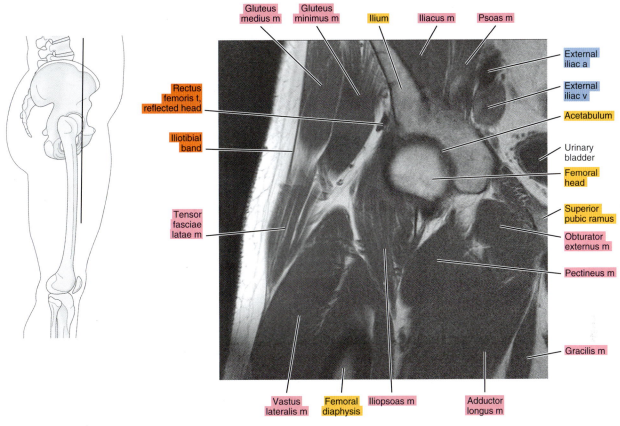

Gluteus medius m
Gluteus minimus m
Ilium
Iliacus m
Psoas m
External iliac a
External iliac v
Acetabulum
Urinary bladder
Femoral head
Superior pubic ramus
Obturator externus m
Pectineus m
Gracilis m
Rectus femoris t, reflected head
Iliotibial band
Tensor fasciae latae m
Vastus lateralis m
Femoral diaphysis
Iliopsoas m
Adductor longus m

Figure 18.3.6

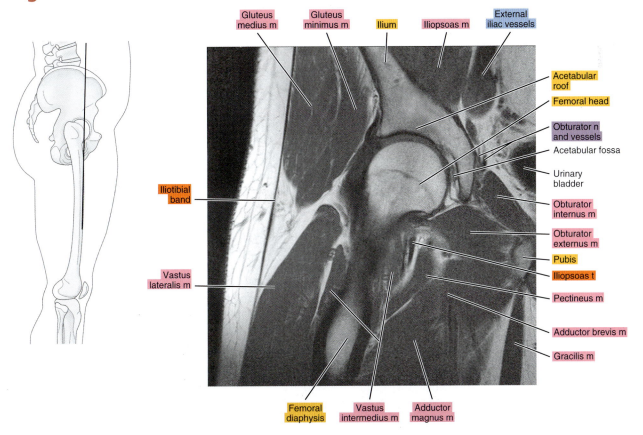

Gluteus medius m
Gluteus minimus m
Ilium
Iliopsoas m
External iliac vessels
Acetabular roof
Femoral head
Obturator n and vessels
Acetabular fossa
Urinary bladder
Obturator internus m
Obturator externus m
Pubis
Iliopsoas t
Pectineus m
Adductor brevis m
Gracilis m
Iliotibial band
Vastus lateralis m
Femoral diaphysis
Vastus intermedius m
Adductor magnus m

Figure 18.3.7

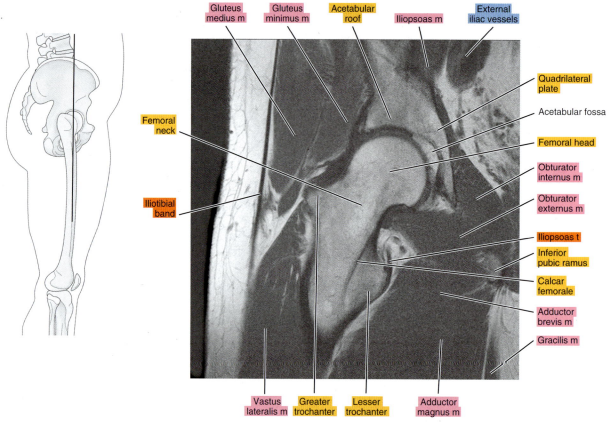

Gluteus medius m
Gluteus minimus m
Acetabular roof
Iliopsoas m
External iliac vessels
Quadrilateral plate
Acetabular fossa
Femoral neck
Femoral head
Obturator internus m
Obturator externus m
Iliotibial band
Iliopsoas t
Inferior pubic ramus
Calcar femorale
Adductor brevis m
Gracilis m
Vastus lateralis m
Greater trochanter
Lesser trochanter
Adductor magnus m

Figure 18.3.8

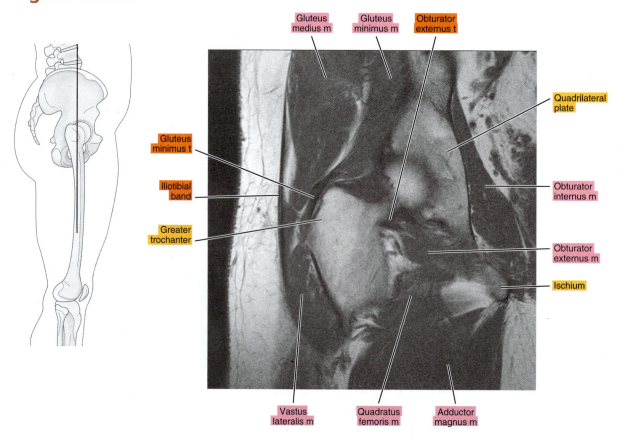

Gluteus medius m
Gluteus minimus m
Obturator externus t
Quadrilateral plate
Gluteus minimus t
Iliotibial band
Obturator internus m
Greater trochanter
Obturator externus m
Ischium
Vastus lateralis m
Quadratus femoris m
Adductor magnus m

Figure 18.3.9

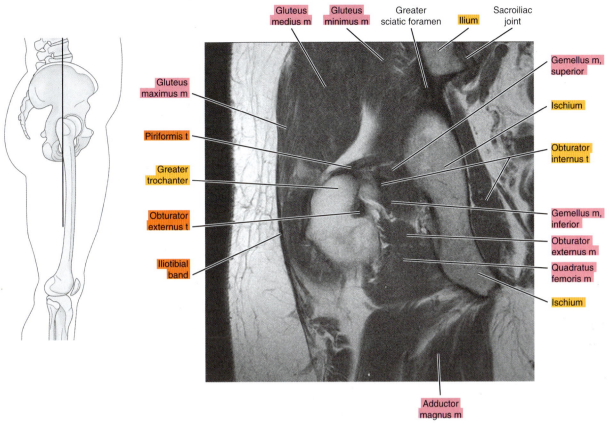

Gluteus medius m
Gluteus minimus m
Greater sciatic foramen
Ilium
Sacroiliac joint
Gemellus m, superior
Gluteus maximus m
Ischium
Piriformis t
Obturator internus t
Greater trochanter
Obturator externus t
Gemellus m, inferior
Obturator externus m
Iliotibial band
Quadratus femoris m
Ischium
Adductor magnus m

Figure 18.3.10

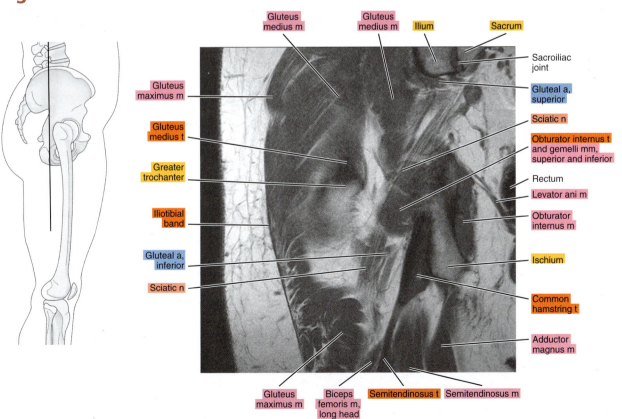

Gluteus medius m
Gluteus medius m
Ilium
Sacrum
Sacroiliac joint
Gluteus maximus m
Gluteal a, superior
Sciatic n
Gluteus medius t
Obturator internus t and gemelli mm, superior and inferior
Greater trochanter
Rectum
Levator ani m
Iliotibial band
Obturator internus m
Gluteal a, inferior
Ischium
Sciatic n
Common hamstring t
Adductor magnus m
Gluteus maximus m
Biceps femoris m, long head
Semitendinosus t
Semitendinosus m

Figure 18.3.11

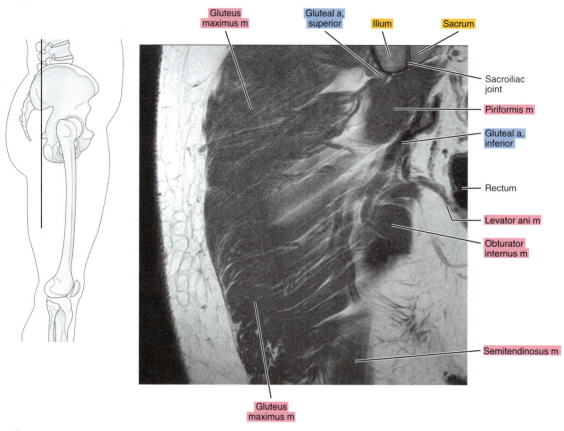

Gluteus maximus m

Gluteal a, superior

Ilium

Sacrum

Sacroiliac joint

Piriformis m

Gluteal a, inferior

Rectum

Levator ani m

Obturator internus m

Semitendinosus m

Gluteus maximus m

Figure 18.3.12

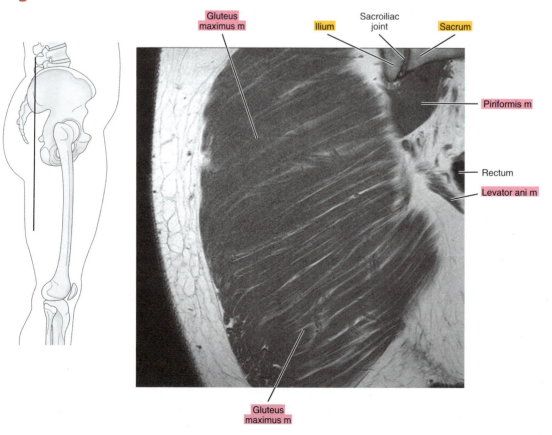

Gluteus maximus m

Ilium

Sacroiliac joint

Sacrum

Piriformis m

Rectum

Levator ani m

Gluteus maximus m

Figure 18.3.13

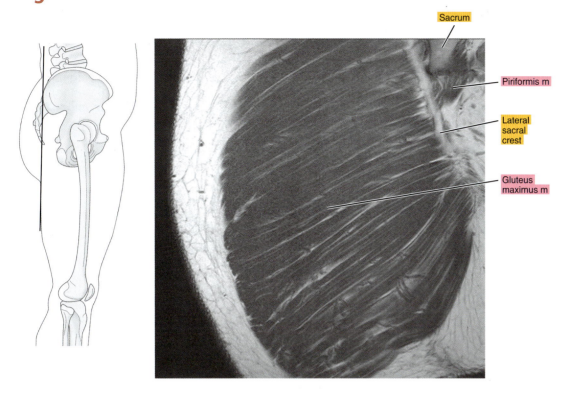

Sacrum

Piriformis m

Lateral
sacral
crest

Gluteus
maximus m

Table 18-1. Muscles of the Hip

MUSCLE	ORIGIN	INSERTION	NERVE SUPPLY
Obturator internus	Pelvic surface of the pubic rami near the obturator foramen, pelvic surface of the ischium between the foramen and the greater sciatic notch, deep surface of the obturator internus fascia, fibrous arch that surrounds the foramen for obturator vessels and nerve, most of the pelvic surface of the obturator membrane except the lower part	Medial side of the greater trochanter in front of the trochanteric fossa of the femur	Nerve to the obturator internus, from the lumbosacral trunk, and first and second sacral
Obturator externus	Lateral surface of the pubic and ischial rami, where they surround the obturator membrane, lateral surface of the obturator membrane	Trochanteric fossa	Obturator
Gemellus superior	Outer surface of the ischial spine and edge of the lesser sciatic notch	After union with the tendon of the obturator internus, inserts into the medial side of the greater trochanter in front of the trochanteric fossa	By a small nerve, branch of the nerve to obturator internus or branch of the nerve to the quadratus femoris
Gemellus inferior	Upper part of the inner border of the tuberosity of the ischium, sacrotuberous ligament, and edge of the lesser sciatic notch	By union with the tendon of the obturator internus or with the tendon onto the greater trochanter below the obturator internus muscle	By a small branch of the nerve to the quadratus femoris
Quadratus femoris	Upper part of the outer border of the tuberosity of the ischium	The inferior dorsal angle of the greater trochanter	Lumbosacral trunk and first sacral
Psoas major	By a series of thick fasciculi from the intervertebral discs and bodies between T12 and L5, from the bodies of L1 to L4, and from slender fascicles from the ventral surfaces of the transverse processes of the lumbar vertebrae	The lesser trochanter of the femur	Branches from L1 (often), L2, L3, and L4
Iliacus	Iliac crest, iliolumbar ligament, iliac fossa, anterior sacroiliac ligaments, often from the ala of the sacrum, and from the ventral border of the ilium between the two anterior spines	Lateral surface of the psoas tendon (above the inguinal ligament) onto the femur immediately distal to the lesser trochanter; the lateral portion arises from the ventral border of the ilium and is attached to the tendon of the rectus femoris and the capsule of the hip joint	Femoral and L1 to L4
Tensor fasciae latae	Anterior superior iliac spine and anterior part of the external lip of the iliac crest	Muscle fibers pass distally in a parallel array, unite with the tendon, and join the iliotibial tract about one-third of the way down the thigh	Superior gluteal
Gluteus medius	Ventral three-fourths of the iliac crest, outer surface of the ilium between the anterior and posterior gluteal lines, and from the investing fascia	Onto the posterosuperior angle and the external surface of the greater trochanter	Superior gluteal (L4, L5, and S1)

Table 18-1. Muscles of the Hip

MUSCLE	ORIGIN	INSERTION	NERVE SUPPLY
Piriformis	Lateral part of the ventral surface of S2, S3, and S4, posterior border of the greater sciatic notch, from the sacrotuberous ligament near the sacrum	Onto the anterior and inner parts of the upper border of the greater trochanter	S1 or S2 or from a loop between S1 and S2
Gluteus maximus	Dorsal fifth of the outer lip of the iliac crest, ilium dorsal to the posterior gluteal line, thoracolumbar fascia between the posterior superior spine of the ilium and the side of the sacrum, lateral parts of S4, S5, and coccygeal vertebrae, and from the back of the sacrotuberous ligament	Into the iliotibial tract, gluteal tuberosity of the femur, adjacent part of the tendinous origin of the vastus lateralis	Inferior gluteal by two branches from the sacral plexus (separately or as a united nerve)
Gluteus minimus	Outer surface of the ilium between the anterior and inferior gluteal lines, from the septum between the gluteus minimus and the gluteus medius near the anterior superior, iliac spine and the capsule of the hip joint	Onto the anterior border of the greater trochanter of the femur	Superior gluteal from a branch that supplies the tensor fasciae latae
Biceps femoris, long head	Medial facet on the posterior surface of the ischial tuberosity and sacrotuberous ligament	By a tendon that extends to the head of the fibula	Tibial part of the sciatic
Semitendinosus	Distal margin of the ischial tuberosity and from the tendon common to it and the long head of the biceps femoris	By a triangular tendinous expansion into the proximal part of the medial surface of the tibia behind and distal to the insertion of the gracilis	Sciatic or directly from the lumbosacral plexus by two nerves: from S1 and S2 and from L5 and S1
Semimembranosus	Lateral facet on the posterior surface of the ischial tuberosity	Posterior aspect of the medial tibial condyle	Sciatic branch (also supplies the adductor magnus)

Chapter 19

MR Arthrography of the Hip

AXIAL
Figure 19.1.1

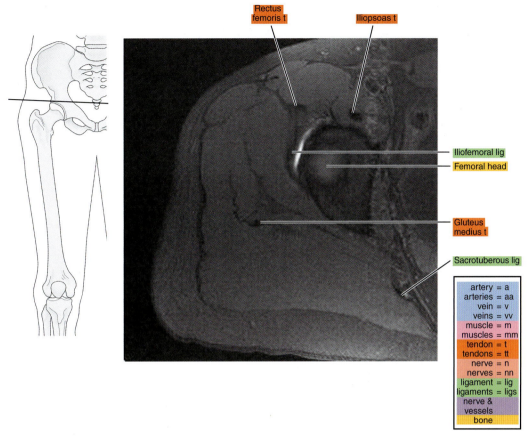

Rectus femoris t

Iliopsoas t

Iliofemoral lig

Femoral head

Gluteus medius t

Sacrotuberous lig

artery =	a
arteries =	aa
vein =	v
veins =	vv
muscle =	m
muscles =	mm
tendon =	t
tendons =	tt
nerve =	n
nerves =	nn
ligament =	lig
ligaments =	ligs
nerve & vessels	
bone	

Figure 19.1.2

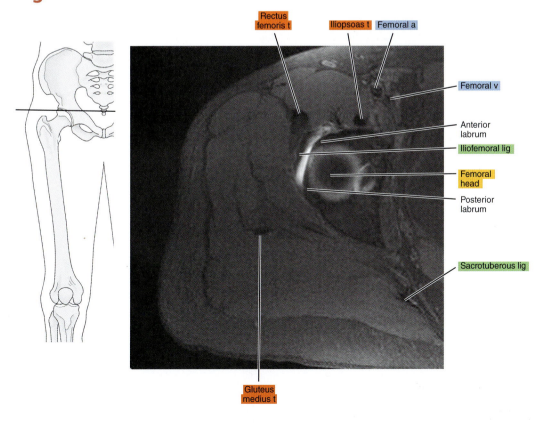

Rectus femoris t

Iliopsoas t

Femoral a

Femoral v

Anterior labrum

Iliofemoral lig

Femoral head

Posterior labrum

Sacrotuberous lig

Gluteus medius t

Figure 19.1.3

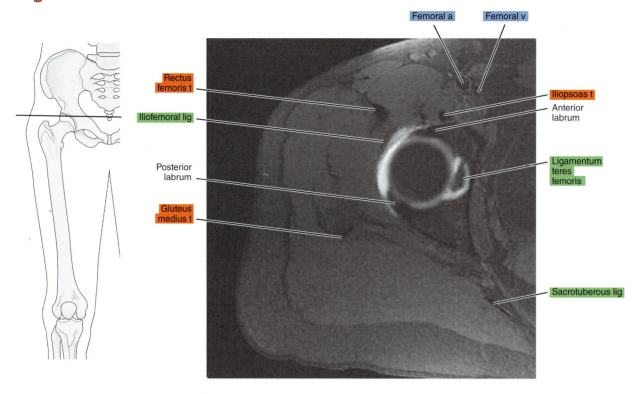

Figure 19.1.4

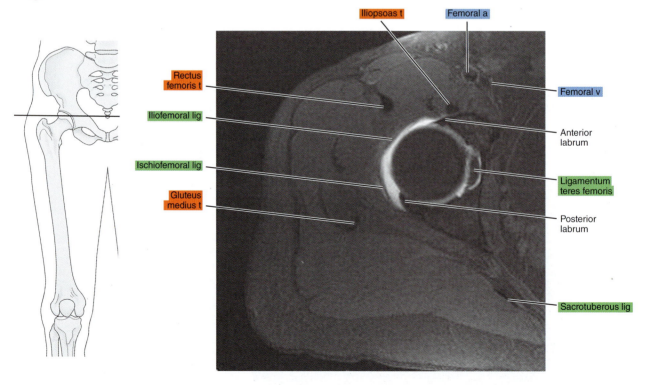

Figure 19.1.5

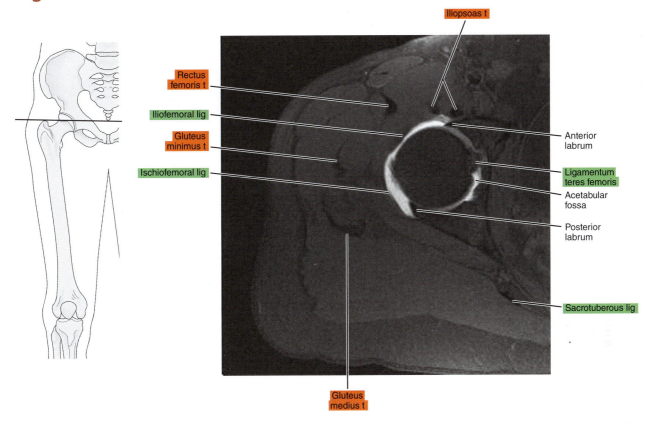

Iliopsoas t

Rectus
femoris t

Iliofemoral lig

Gluteus
minimus t

Ischiofemoral lig

Anterior
labrum

Ligamentum
teres femoris

Acetabular
fossa

Posterior
labrum

Sacrotuberous lig

Gluteus
medius t

Figure 19.1.6

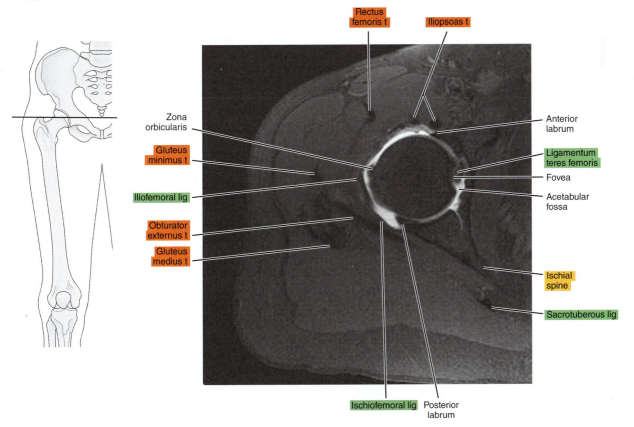

Rectus
femoris t

Iliopsoas t

Zona
orbicularis

Gluteus
minimus t

Iliofemoral lig

Obturator
externus t

Gluteus
medius t

Anterior
labrum

Ligamentum
teres femoris

Fovea

Acetabular
fossa

Ischial
spine

Sacrotuberous lig

Ischiofemoral lig   Posterior
labrum

Figure 19.1.7

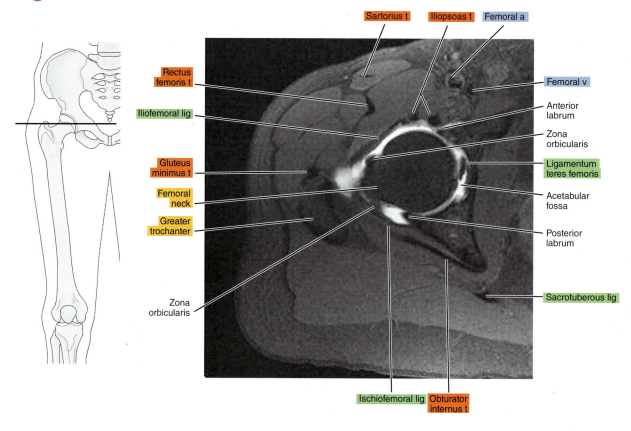

Sartorius t
Iliopsoas t
Femoral a
Rectus femoris t
Iliofemoral lig
Femoral v
Anterior labrum
Zona orbicularis
Gluteus minimus t
Ligamentum teres femoris
Femoral neck
Acetabular fossa
Greater trochanter
Posterior labrum
Zona orbicularis
Sacrotuberous lig
Ischiofemoral lig
Obturator internus t

Figure 19.1.8

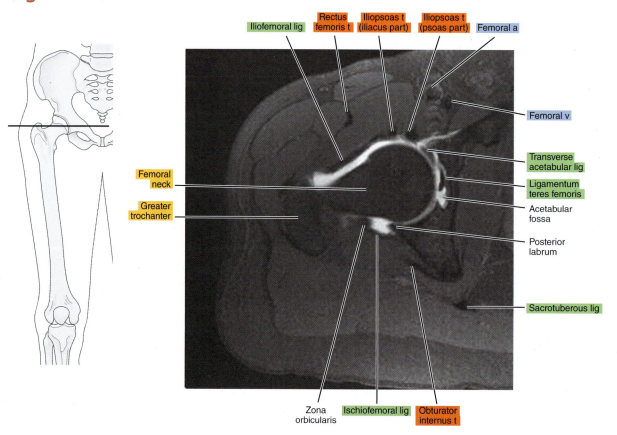

Iliofemoral lig
Rectus femoris t
Iliopsoas t (iliacus part)
Iliopsoas t (psoas part)
Femoral a
Femoral v
Femoral neck
Transverse acetabular lig
Ligamentum teres femoris
Acetabular fossa
Greater trochanter
Posterior labrum
Sacrotuberous lig
Zona orbicularis
Ischiofemoral lig
Obturator internus t

Figure 19.1.9

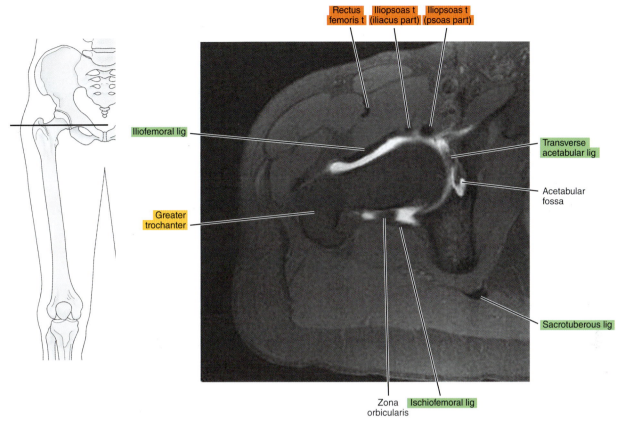

Rectus femoris t
Iliopsoas t (iliacus part)
Iliopsoas t (psoas part)
Iliofemoral lig
Transverse acetabular lig
Acetabular fossa
Greater trochanter
Sacrotuberous lig
Zona orbicularis
Ischiofemoral lig

Figure 19.1.10

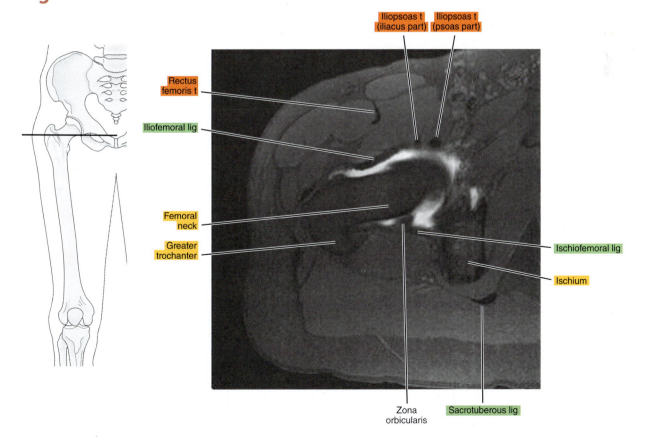

Iliopsoas t (iliacus part)
Iliopsoas t (psoas part)
Rectus femoris t
Iliofemoral lig
Femoral neck
Greater trochanter
Ischiofemoral lig
Ischium
Zona orbicularis
Sacrotuberous lig

Figure 19.1.11

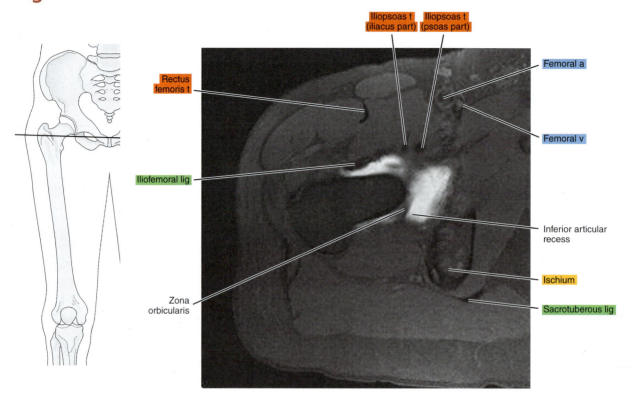

Figure 19.1.12

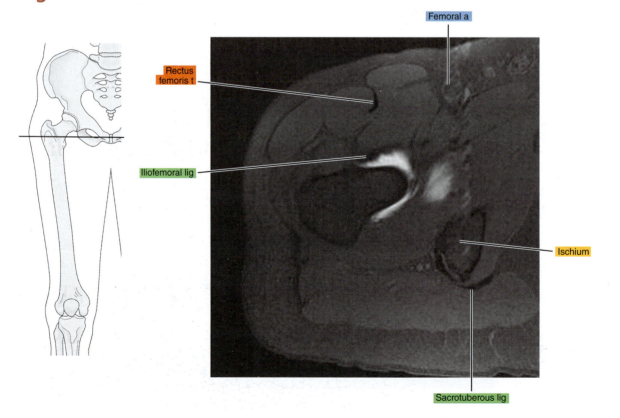

SAGITTAL
Figure 19.2.1

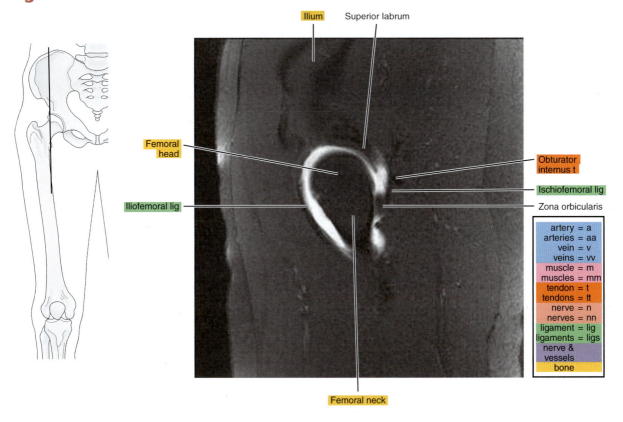

Ilium
Superior labrum
Femoral head
Obturator internus t
Ischiofemoral lig
Iliofemoral lig
Zona orbicularis
Femoral neck

artery = a
arteries = aa
vein = v
veins = vv
muscle = m
muscles = mm
tendon = t
tendons = tt
nerve = n
nerves = nn
ligament = lig
ligaments = ligs
nerve &
vessels
bone

Figure 19.2.2

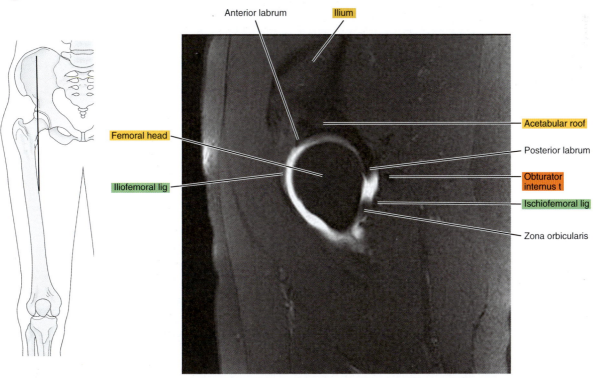

Anterior labrum
Ilium
Acetabular roof
Femoral head
Posterior labrum
Obturator internus t
Iliofemoral lig
Ischiofemoral lig
Zona orbicularis

Figure 19.2.3

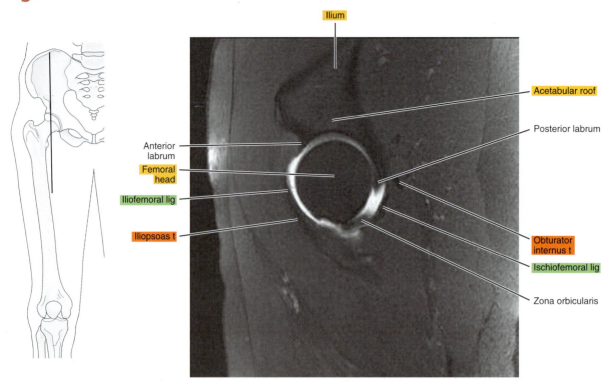

Ilium

Acetabular roof

Posterior labrum

Anterior labrum

Femoral head

Iliofemoral lig

Iliopsoas t

Obturator internus t

Ischiofemoral lig

Zona orbicularis

Figure 19.2.4

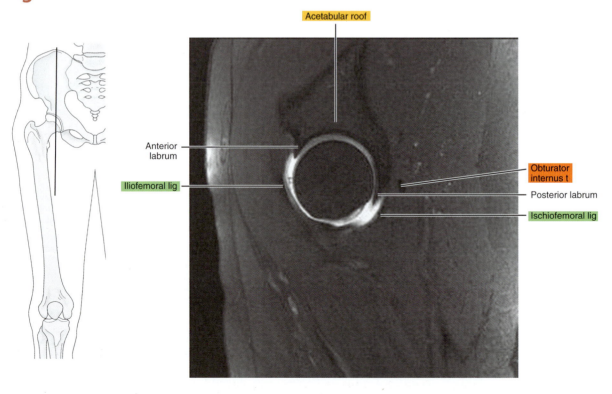

Acetabular roof

Anterior labrum

Iliofemoral lig

Obturator internus t

Posterior labrum

Ischiofemoral lig

Figure 19.2.5

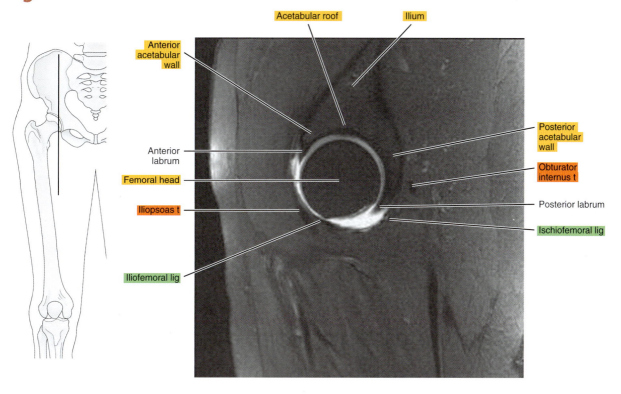

Figure 19.2.6

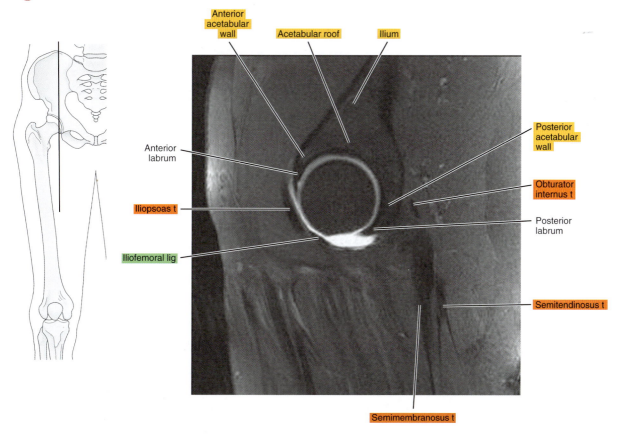

Figure 19.2.7

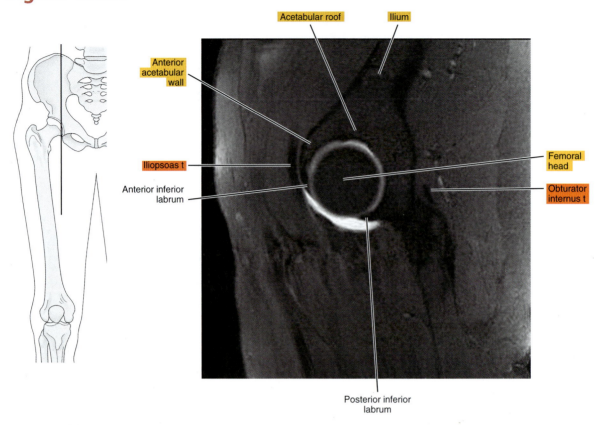

Acetabular roof — Ilium

Anterior acetabular wall

Iliopsoas t — Femoral head

Anterior inferior labrum — Obturator internus t

Posterior inferior labrum

Figure 19.2.8

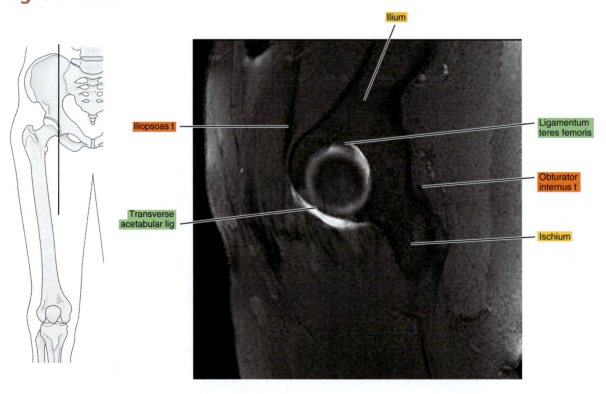

Ilium

Iliopsoas t — Ligamentum teres femoris

Transverse acetabular lig — Obturator internus t

Ischium

Figure 19.2.9

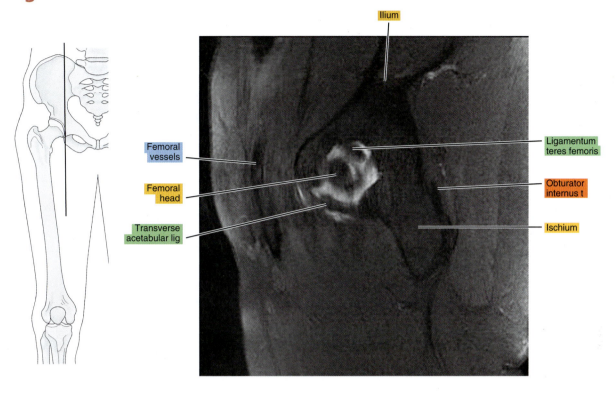

- Ilium
- Femoral vessels
- Femoral head
- Transverse acetabular lig
- Ligamentum teres femoris
- Obturator internus t
- Ischium

Figure 19.2.10

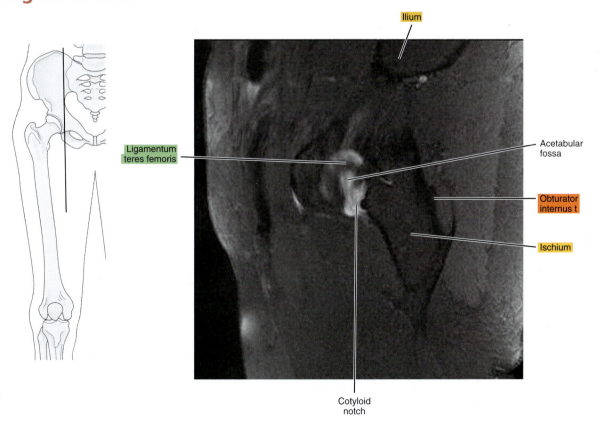

- Ilium
- Ligamentum teres femoris
- Acetabular fossa
- Obturator internus t
- Ischium
- Cotyloid notch

CORONAL
Figure 19.3.1

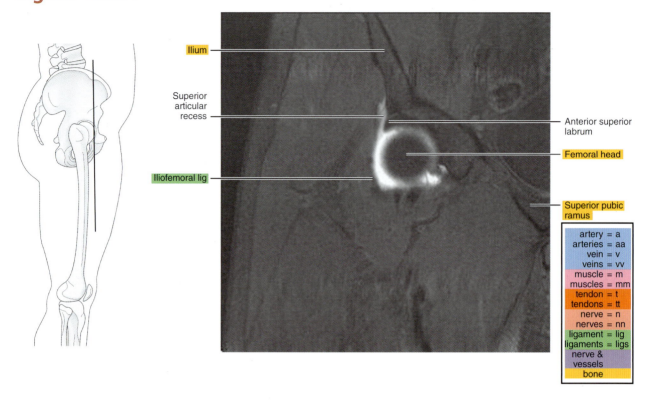

Ilium

Superior articular recess

Iliofemoral lig

Anterior superior labrum

Femoral head

Superior pubic ramus

artery =	a
arteries =	aa
vein =	v
veins =	vv
muscle =	m
muscles =	mm
tendon =	t
tendons =	tt
nerve =	n
nerves =	nn
ligament =	lig
ligaments =	ligs
nerve & vessels	
bone	

Figure 19.3.2

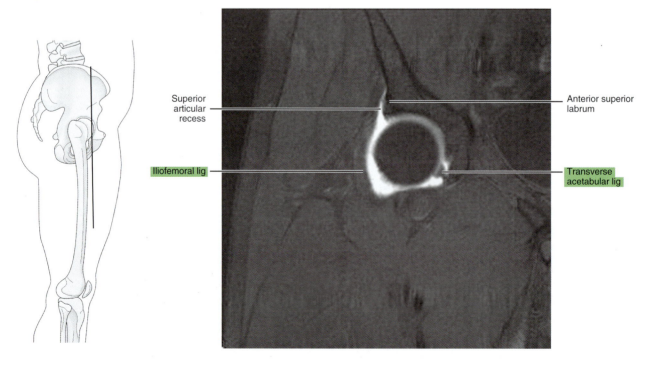

Superior articular recess

Iliofemoral lig

Anterior superior labrum

Transverse acetabular lig

Figure 19.3.3

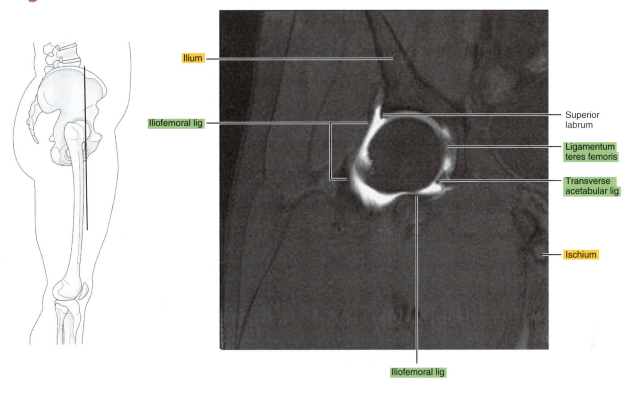

Ilium

Iliofemoral lig

Superior labrum

Ligamentum teres femoris

Transverse acetabular lig

Ischium

Iliofemoral lig

Figure 19.3.4

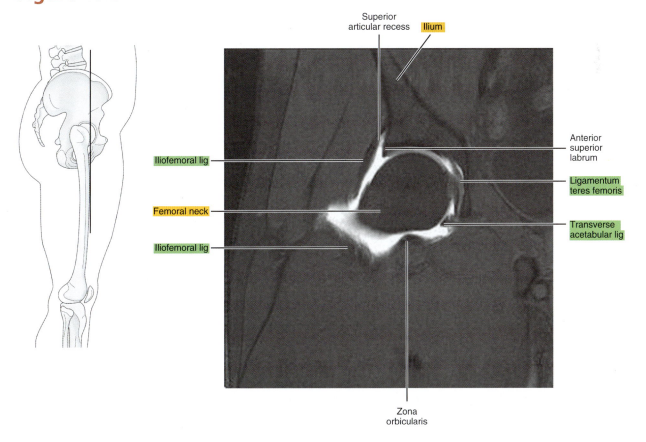

Superior articular recess   Ilium

Iliofemoral lig

Anterior superior labrum

Ligamentum teres femoris

Femoral neck

Transverse acetabular lig

Iliofemoral lig

Zona orbicularis

Figure 19.3.5

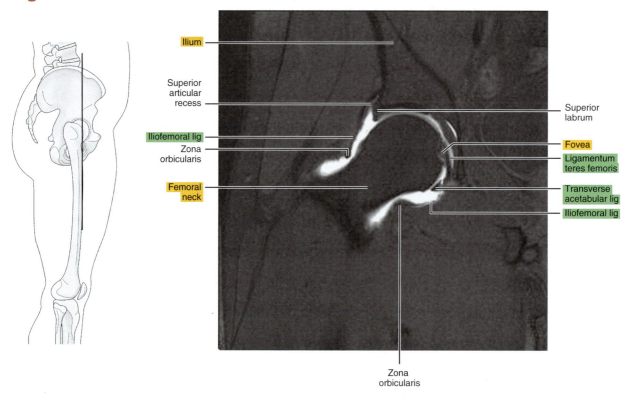

Ilium

Superior articular recess

Iliofemoral lig

Zona orbicularis

Femoral neck

Superior labrum

Fovea

Ligamentum teres femoris

Transverse acetabular lig

Iliofemoral lig

Zona orbicularis

Figure 19.3.6

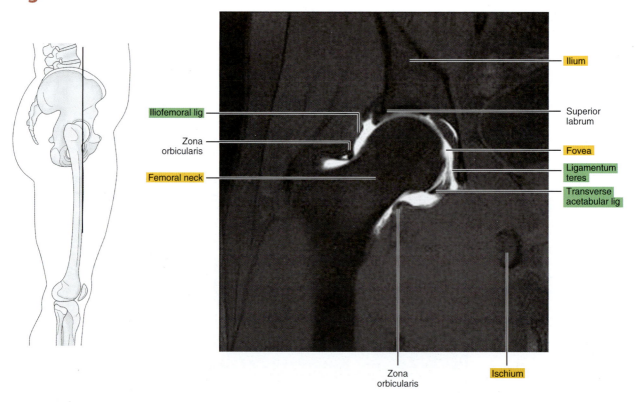

Iliofemoral lig

Zona orbicularis

Femoral neck

Ilium

Superior labrum

Fovea

Ligamentum teres

Transverse acetabular lig

Zona orbicularis

Ischium

Figure 19.3.7

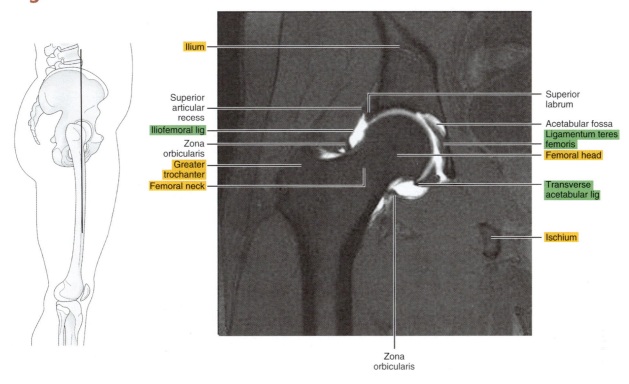

Ilium

Superior articular recess
Iliofemoral lig
Zona orbicularis
Greater trochanter
Femoral neck

Superior labrum
Acetabular fossa
Ligamentum teres femoris
Femoral head
Transverse acetabular lig
Ischium

Zona orbicularis

Figure 19.3.8

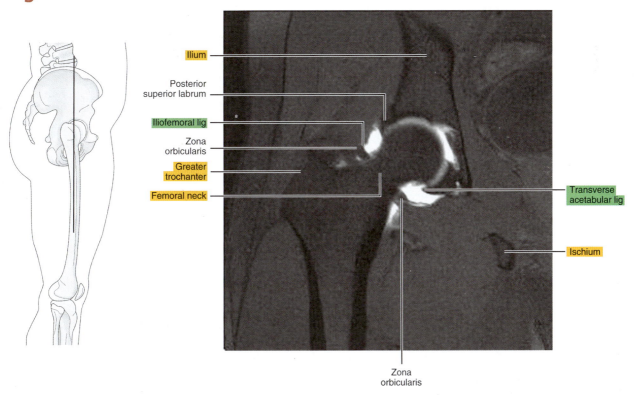

Ilium

Posterior superior labrum
Iliofemoral lig
Zona orbicularis
Greater trochanter
Femoral neck

Transverse acetabular lig
Ischium

Zona orbicularis

Figure 19.3.9

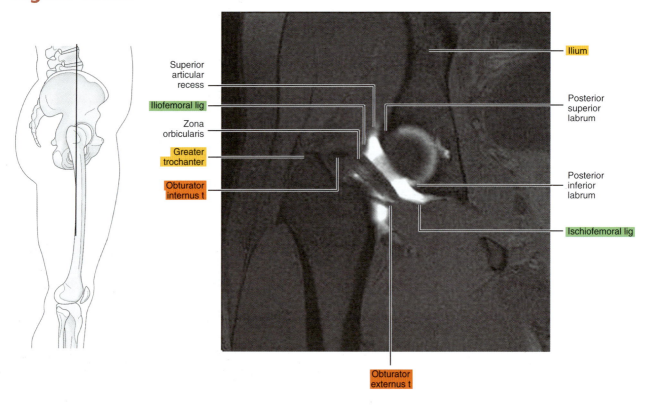

Superior articular recess
Iliofemoral lig
Zona orbicularis
Greater trochanter
Obturator internus t
Obturator externus t
Ilium
Posterior superior labrum
Posterior inferior labrum
Ischiofemoral lig

Figure 19.3.10

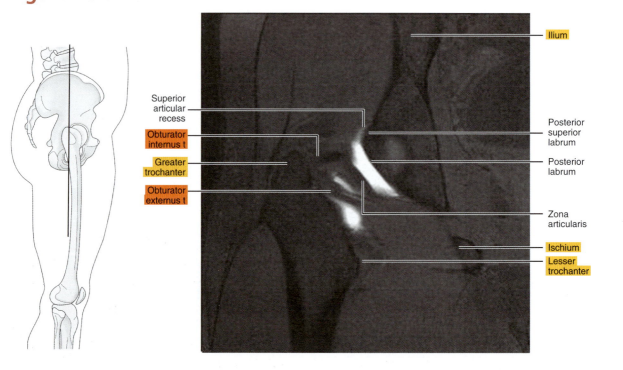

Superior articular recess
Obturator internus t
Greater trochanter
Obturator externus t
Ilium
Posterior superior labrum
Posterior labrum
Zona articularis
Ischium
Lesser trochanter

Chapter

20

MRI of the Thigh

AXIAL
Figure 20.1.1

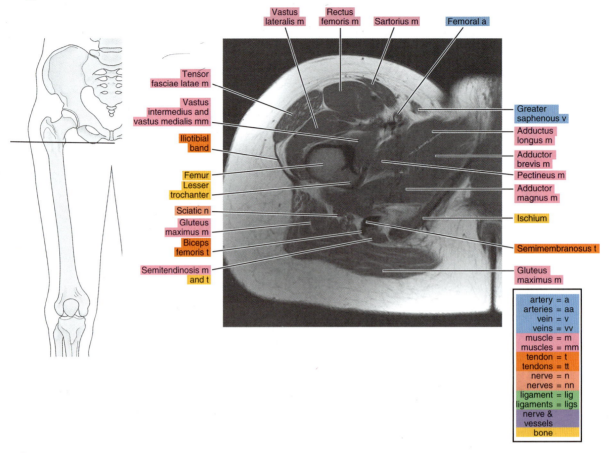

Vastus lateralis m
Rectus femoris m
Sartorius m
Femoral a

Tensor fasciae latae m
Vastus intermedius and vastus medialis mm
Iliotibial band
Femur
Lesser trochanter
Sciatic n
Gluteus maximus m
Biceps femoris t
Semitendinosis m and t

Greater saphenous v
Adductus longus m
Adductor brevis m
Pectineus m
Adductor magnus m
Ischium
Semimembranosus t
Gluteus maximus m

artery	= a
arteries	= aa
vein	= v
veins	= vv
muscle	= m
muscles	= mm
tendon	= t
tendons	= tt
nerve	= n
nerves	= nn
ligament	= lig
ligaments	= ligs
nerve & vessels	
bone	

Figure 20.1.2

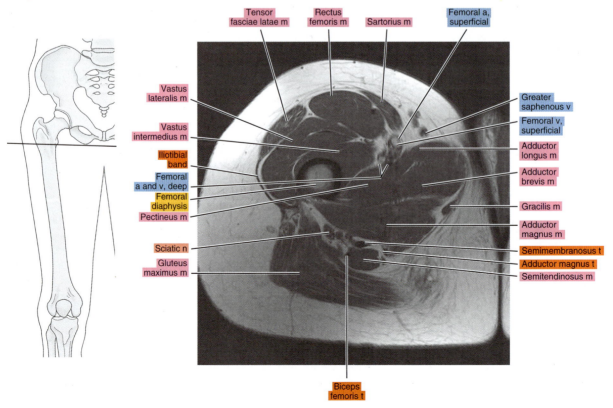

Tensor fasciae latae m
Rectus femoris m
Sartorius m
Femoral a, superficial

Vastus lateralis m
Vastus intermedius m
Iliotibial band
Femoral a and v, deep
Femoral diaphysis
Pectineus m
Sciatic n
Gluteus maximus m

Greater saphenous v
Femoral v, superficial
Adductor longus m
Adductor brevis m
Gracilis m
Adductor magnus m
Semimembranosus t
Adductor magnus t
Semitendinosus m

Biceps femoris t

Figure 20.1.3

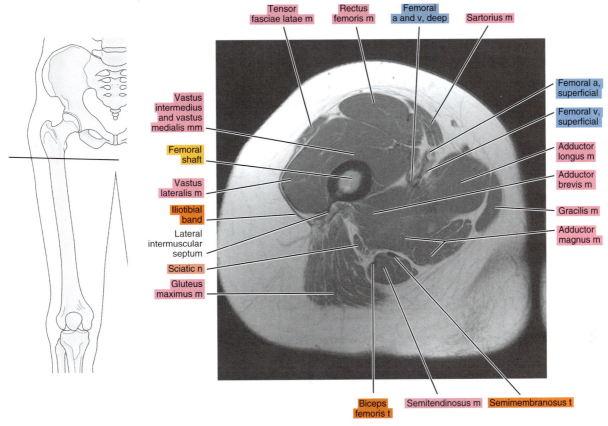

Tensor fasciae latae m

Rectus femoris m

Femoral a and v, deep

Sartorius m

Vastus intermedius and vastus medialis mm

Femoral shaft

Vastus lateralis m

Iliotibial band

Lateral intermuscular septum

Sciatic n

Gluteus maximus m

Femoral a, superficial

Femoral v, superficial

Adductor longus m

Adductor brevis m

Gracilis m

Adductor magnus m

Biceps femoris t

Semitendinosus m

Semimembranosus t

Figure 20.1.4

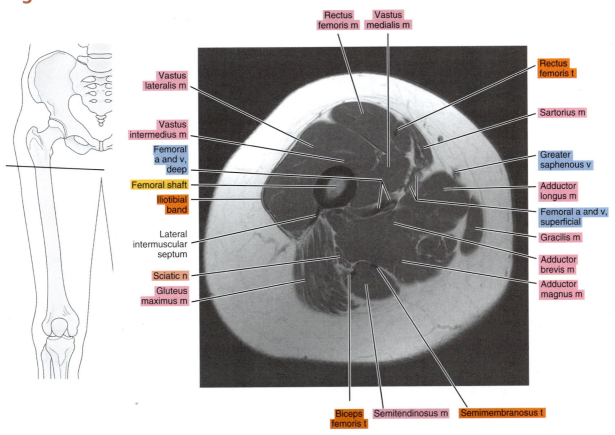

Rectus femoris m

Vastus medialis m

Vastus lateralis m

Vastus intermedius m

Femoral a and v, deep

Femoral shaft

Iliotibial band

Lateral intermuscular septum

Sciatic n

Gluteus maximus m

Rectus femoris t

Sartorius m

Greater saphenous v

Adductor longus m

Femoral a and v, superficial

Gracilis m

Adductor brevis m

Adductor magnus m

Biceps femoris t

Semitendinosus m

Semimembranosus t

Figure 20.1.5

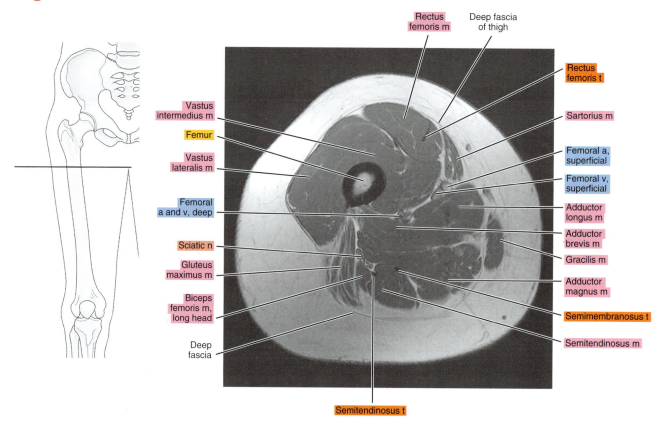

Rectus femoris m
Deep fascia of thigh
Rectus femoris t
Sartorius m
Femoral a, superficial
Femoral v, superficial
Adductor longus m
Adductor brevis m
Gracilis m
Adductor magnus m
Semimembranosus t
Semitendinosus m

Vastus intermedius m
Femur
Vastus lateralis m
Femoral a and v, deep
Sciatic n
Gluteus maximus m
Biceps femoris m, long head
Deep fascia

Semitendinosus t

Figure 20.1.6

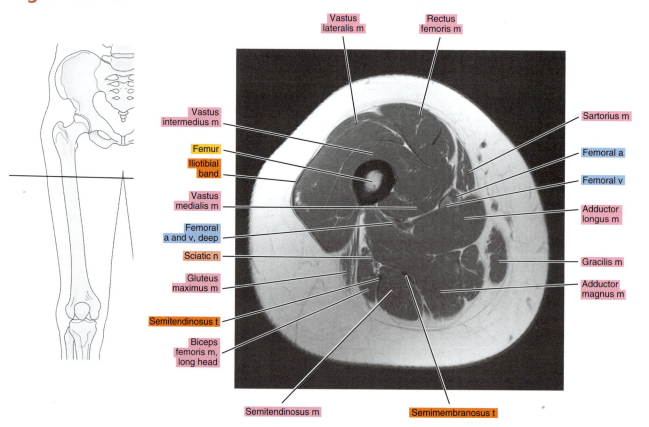

Vastus lateralis m
Rectus femoris m
Sartorius m
Femoral a
Femoral v
Adductor longus m
Gracilis m
Adductor magnus m

Vastus intermedius m
Femur
Iliotibial band
Vastus medialis m
Femoral a and v, deep
Sciatic n
Gluteus maximus m
Semitendinosus t
Biceps femoris m, long head

Semitendinosus m
Semimembranosus t

Figure 20.1.7

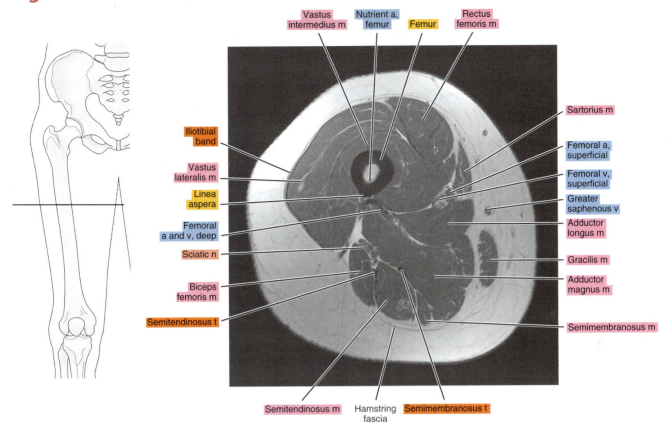

Vastus intermedius m
Nutrient a, femur
Femur
Rectus femoris m
Sartorius m
Femoral a, superficial
Femoral v, superficial
Greater saphenous v
Adductor longus m
Gracilis m
Adductor magnus m
Semimembranosus m
Iliotibial band
Vastus lateralis m
Linea aspera
Femoral a and v, deep
Sciatic n
Biceps femoris m
Semitendinosus t
Semitendinosus m
Hamstring fascia
Semimembranosus t

Figure 20.1.8

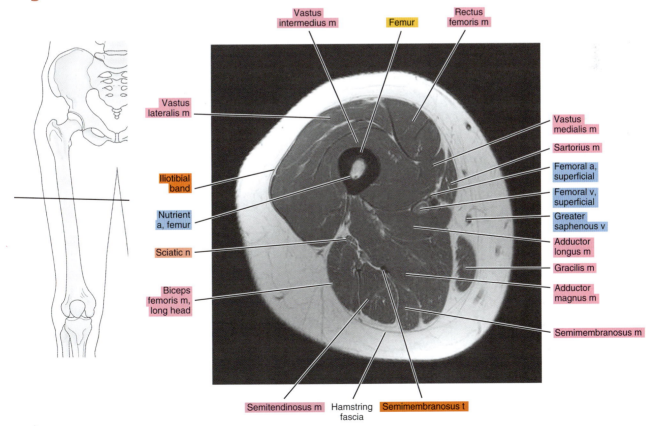

Vastus intermedius m
Femur
Rectus femoris m
Vastus lateralis m
Vastus medialis m
Sartorius m
Femoral a, superficial
Femoral v, superficial
Greater saphenous v
Adductor longus m
Gracilis m
Adductor magnus m
Semimembranosus m
Iliotibial band
Nutrient a, femur
Sciatic n
Biceps femoris m, long head
Semitendinosus m
Hamstring fascia
Semimembranosus t

Figure 20.1.9

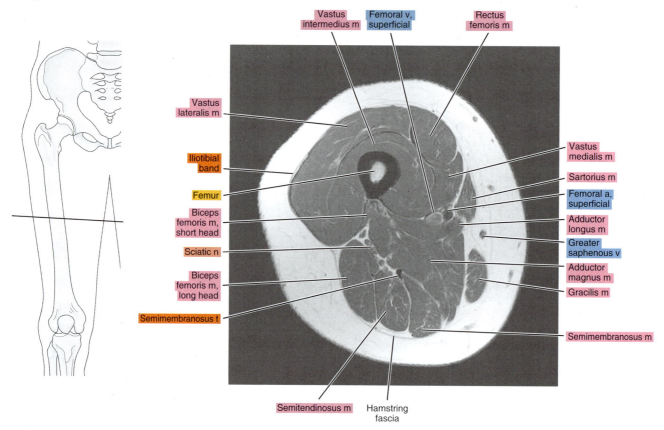

Vastus intermedius m

Femoral v, superficial

Rectus femoris m

Vastus lateralis m

Iliotibial band

Femur

Biceps femoris m, short head

Sciatic n

Biceps femoris m, long head

Semimembranosus t

Vastus medialis m

Sartorius m

Femoral a, superficial

Adductor longus m

Greater saphenous v

Adductor magnus m

Gracilis m

Semimembranosus m

Semitendinosus m

Hamstring fascia

Figure 20.1.10

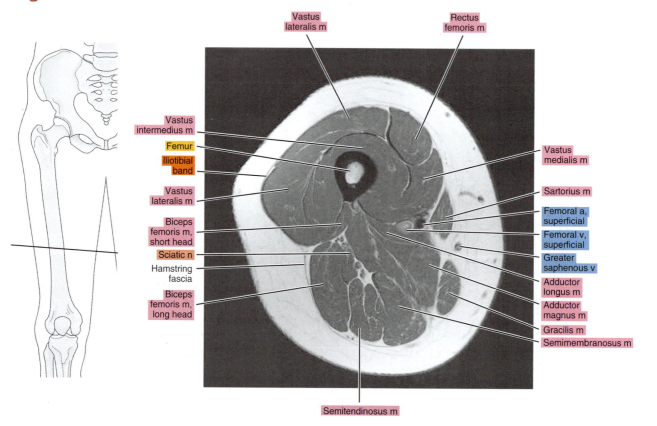

Vastus lateralis m

Rectus femoris m

Vastus intermedius m

Femur

Iliotibial band

Vastus lateralis m

Biceps femoris m, short head

Sciatic n

Hamstring fascia

Biceps femoris m, long head

Vastus medialis m

Sartorius m

Femoral a, superficial

Femoral v, superficial

Greater saphenous v

Adductor longus m

Adductor magnus m

Gracilis m

Semimembranosus m

Semitendinosus m

Figure 20.1.11

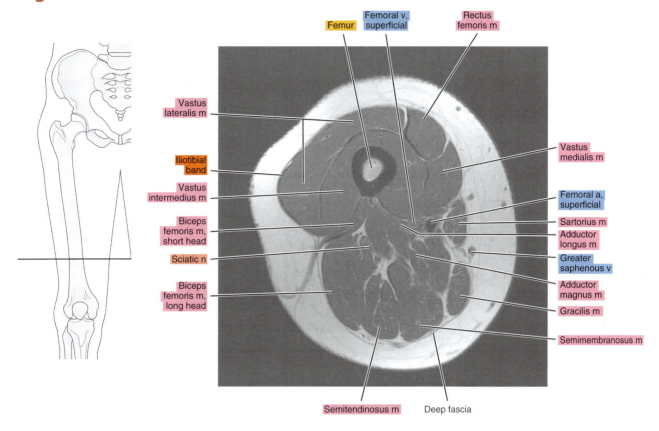

Femur

Femoral v, superficial

Rectus femoris m

Vastus lateralis m

Iliotibial band

Vastus intermedius m

Biceps femoris m, short head

Sciatic n

Biceps femoris m, long head

Vastus medialis m

Femoral a, superficial

Sartorius m

Adductor longus m

Greater saphenous v

Adductor magnus m

Gracilis m

Semimembranosus m

Semitendinosus m

Deep fascia

Figure 20.1.12

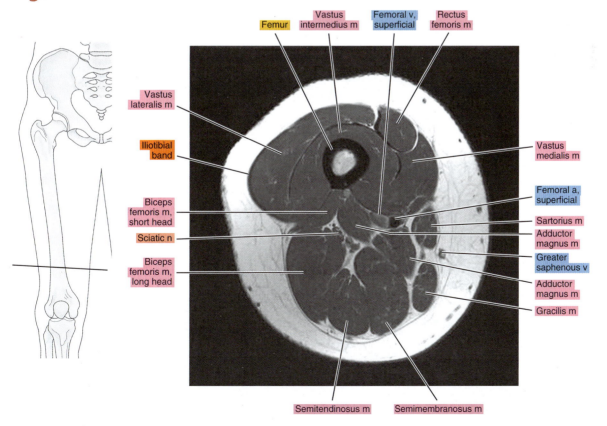

Femur

Vastus intermedius m

Femoral v, superficial

Rectus femoris m

Vastus lateralis m

Iliotibial band

Biceps femoris m, short head

Sciatic n

Biceps femoris m, long head

Vastus medialis m

Femoral a, superficial

Sartorius m

Adductor magnus m

Greater saphenous v

Adductor magnus m

Gracilis m

Semitendinosus m

Semimembranosus m

Figure 20.1.13

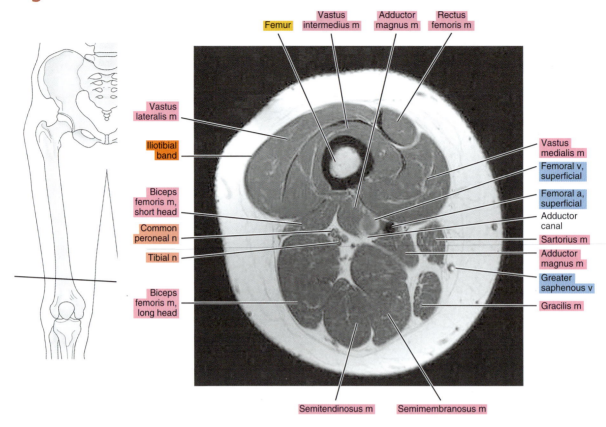

Femur — Vastus intermedius m — Adductor magnus m — Rectus femoris m

Vastus lateralis m

Iliotibial band

Biceps femoris m, short head

Common peroneal n

Tibial n

Biceps femoris m, long head

Vastus medialis m

Femoral v, superficial

Femoral a, superficial

Adductor canal

Sartorius m

Adductor magnus m

Greater saphenous v

Gracilis m

Semitendinosus m   Semimembranosus m

Figure 20.1.14

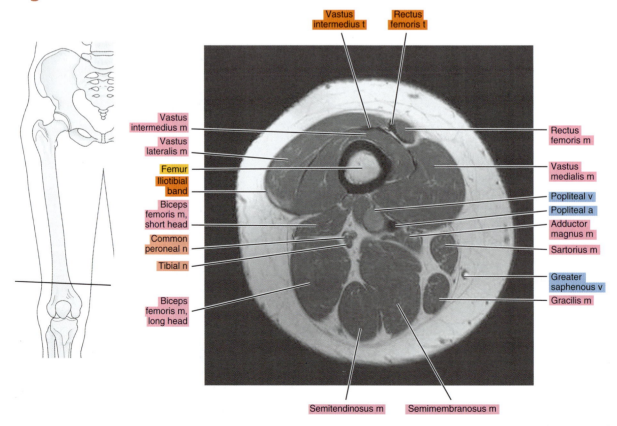

Vastus intermedius t   Rectus femoris t

Vastus intermedius m

Vastus lateralis m

Femur

Iliotibial band

Biceps femoris m, short head

Common peroneal n

Tibial n

Biceps femoris m, long head

Rectus femoris m

Vastus medialis m

Popliteal v

Popliteal a

Adductor magnus m

Sartorius m

Greater saphenous v

Gracilis m

Semitendinosus m   Semimembranosus m

Figure 20.1.15

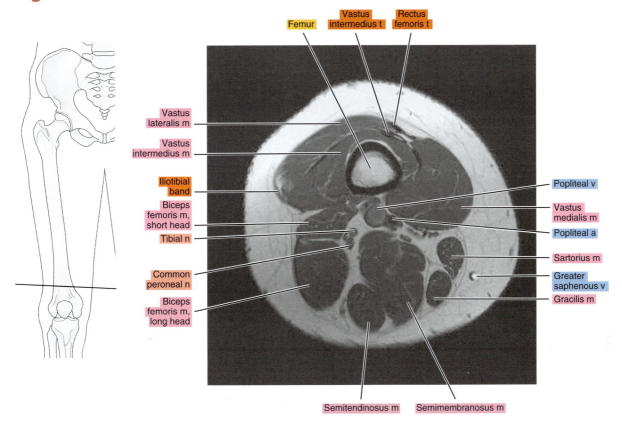

Figure 20.1.16

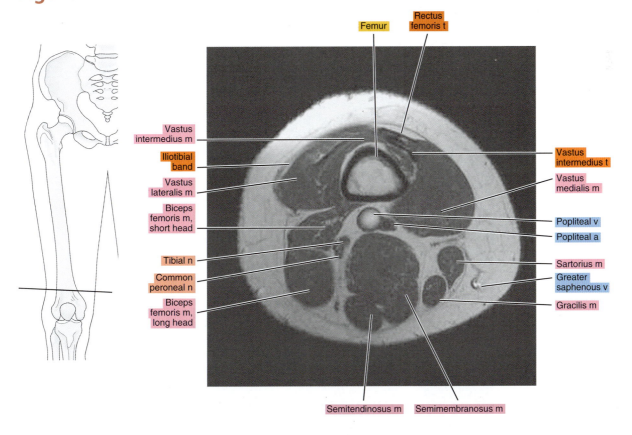

SAGITTAL
Figure 20.2.1

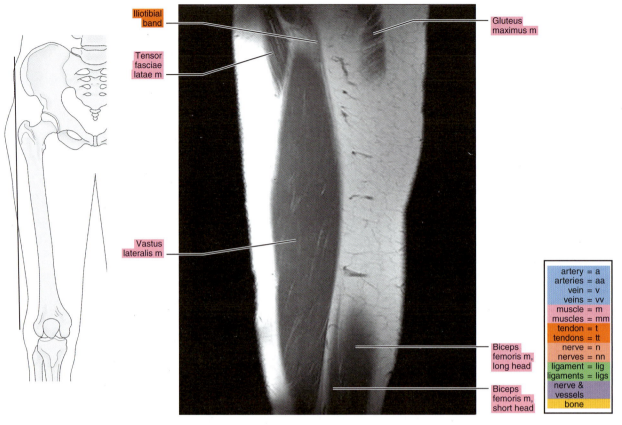

Iliotibial band

Tensor fasciae latae m

Vastus lateralis m

Gluteus maximus m

Biceps femoris m, long head

Biceps femoris m, short head

artery	= a
arteries	= aa
vein	= v
veins	= vv
muscle	= m
muscles	= mm
tendon	= t
tendons	= tt
nerve	= n
nerves	= nn
ligament	= lig
ligaments	= ligs
nerve & vessels	
bone	

Figure 20.2.2

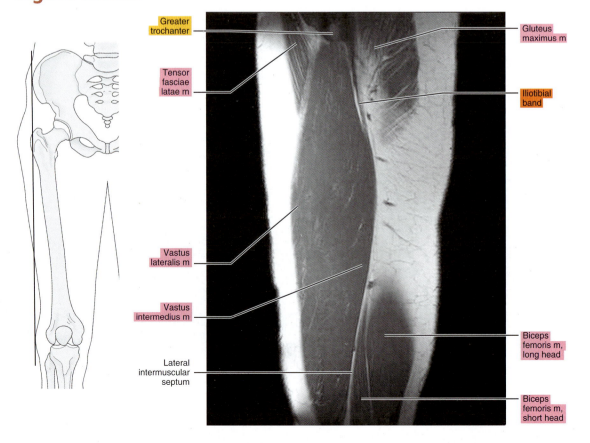

Greater trochanter

Tensor fasciae latae m

Vastus lateralis m

Vastus intermedius m

Lateral intermuscular septum

Gluteus maximus m

Iliotibial band

Biceps femoris m, long head

Biceps femoris m, short head

Figure 20.2.3

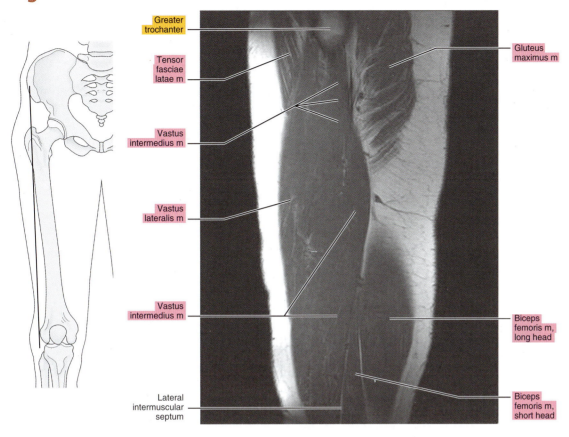

Greater trochanter

Tensor fasciae latae m

Vastus intermedius m

Vastus lateralis m

Vastus intermedius m

Lateral intermuscular septum

Gluteus maximus m

Biceps femoris m, long head

Biceps femoris m, short head

Figure 20.2.4

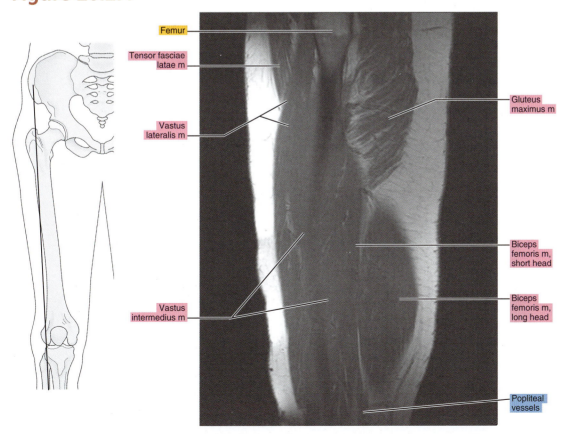

Femur

Tensor fasciae latae m

Vastus lateralis m

Vastus intermedius m

Gluteus maximus m

Biceps femoris m, short head

Biceps femoris m, long head

Popliteal vessels

Figure 20.2.5

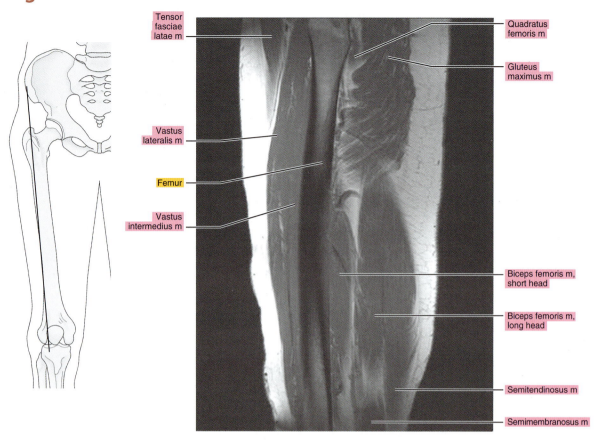

Tensor fasciae latae m

Quadratus femoris m

Gluteus maximus m

Vastus lateralis m

Femur

Vastus intermedius m

Biceps femoris m, short head

Biceps femoris m, long head

Semitendinosus m

Semimembranosus m

Figure 20.2.6

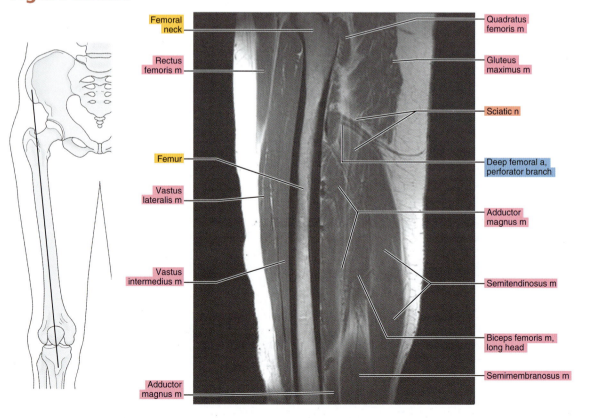

Femoral neck

Quadratus femoris m

Rectus femoris m

Gluteus maximus m

Sciatic n

Femur

Deep femoral a, perforator branch

Vastus lateralis m

Adductor magnus m

Vastus intermedius m

Semitendinosus m

Biceps femoris m, long head

Adductor magnus m

Semimembranosus m

Figure 20.2.7

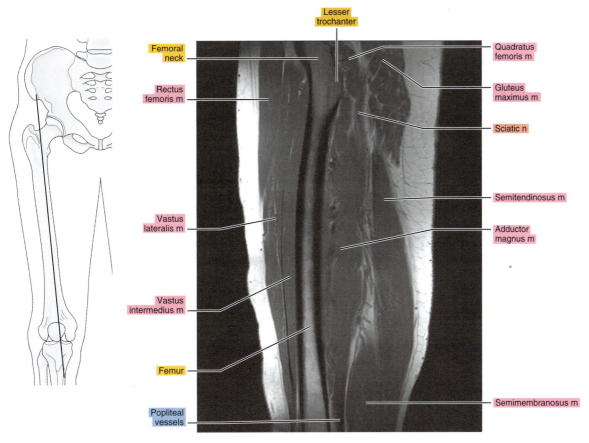

Lesser trochanter

Femoral neck

Quadratus femoris m

Rectus femoris m

Gluteus maximus m

Sciatic n

Semitendinosus m

Vastus lateralis m

Adductor magnus m

Vastus intermedius m

Femur

Semimembranosus m

Popliteal vessels

Figure 20.2.8

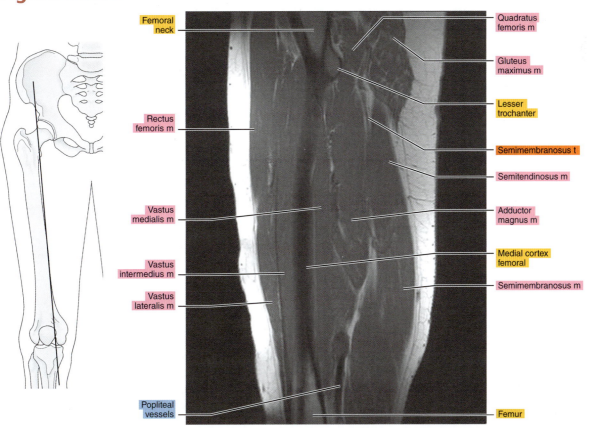

Femoral neck

Quadratus femoris m

Gluteus maximus m

Rectus femoris m

Lesser trochanter

Semimembranosus t

Semitendinosus m

Vastus medialis m

Adductor magnus m

Medial cortex femoral

Vastus intermedius m

Vastus lateralis m

Semimembranosus m

Popliteal vessels

Femur

Figure 20.2.9

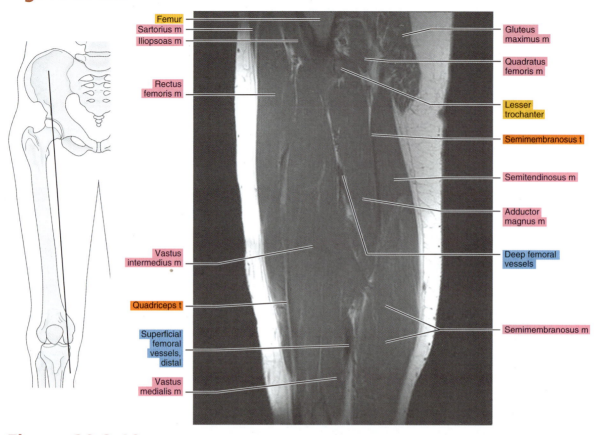

Femur
Sartorius m
Iliopsoas m

Rectus
femoris m

Vastus
intermedius m

Quadriceps t

Superficial
femoral
vessels,
distal

Vastus
medialis m

Gluteus
maximus m

Quadratus
femoris m

Lesser
trochanter

Semimembranosus t

Semitendinosus m

Adductor
magnus m

Deep femoral
vessels

Semimembranosus m

Figure 20.2.10

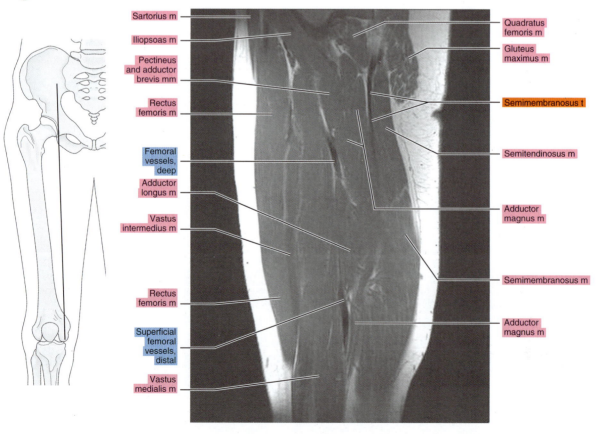

Sartorius m

Iliopsoas m

Pectineus
and adductor
brevis mm

Rectus
femoris m

Femoral
vessels,
deep

Adductor
longus m

Vastus
intermedius m

Rectus
femoris m

Superficial
femoral
vessels,
distal

Vastus
medialis m

Quadratus
femoris m

Gluteus
maximus m

Semimembranosus t

Semitendinosus m

Adductor
magnus m

Semimembranosus m

Adductor
magnus m

Figure 20.2.11

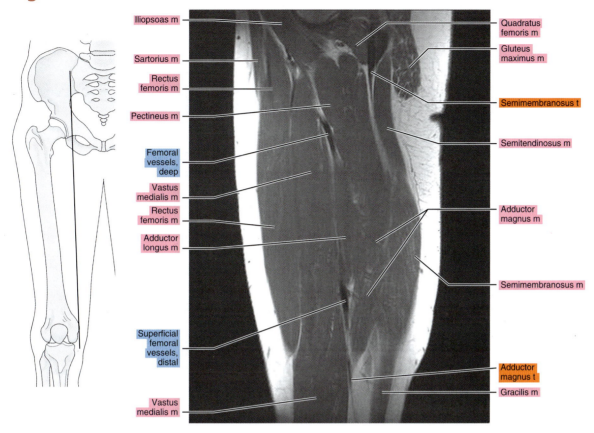

Iliopsoas m

Sartorius m

Rectus femoris m

Pectineus m

Femoral vessels, deep

Vastus medialis m

Rectus femoris m

Adductor longus m

Superficial femoral vessels, distal

Vastus medialis m

Quadratus femoris m

Gluteus maximus m

Semimembranosus t

Semitendinosus m

Adductor magnus m

Semimembranosus m

Adductor magnus t

Gracilis m

Figure 20.2.12

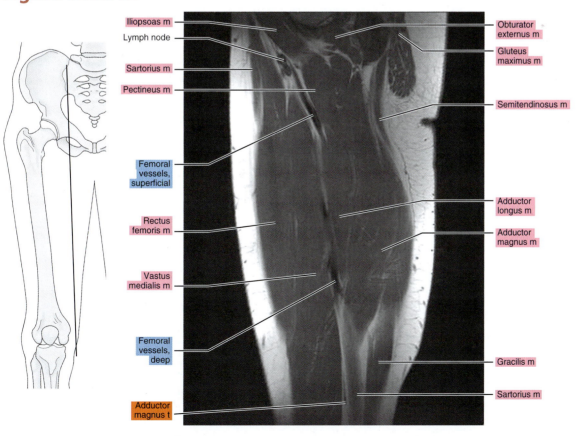

Iliopsoas m

Lymph node

Sartorius m

Pectineus m

Femoral vessels, superficial

Rectus femoris m

Vastus medialis m

Femoral vessels, deep

Adductor magnus t

Obturator externus m

Gluteus maximus m

Semitendinosus m

Adductor longus m

Adductor magnus m

Gracilis m

Sartorius m

Figure 20.2.13

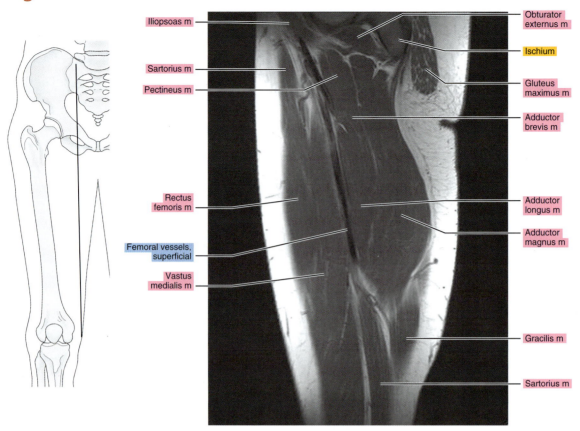

Iliopsoas m

Sartorius m

Pectineus m

Rectus femoris m

Femoral vessels, superficial

Vastus medialis m

Obturator externus m

Ischium

Gluteus maximus m

Adductor brevis m

Adductor longus m

Adductor magnus m

Gracilis m

Sartorius m

Figure 20.2.14

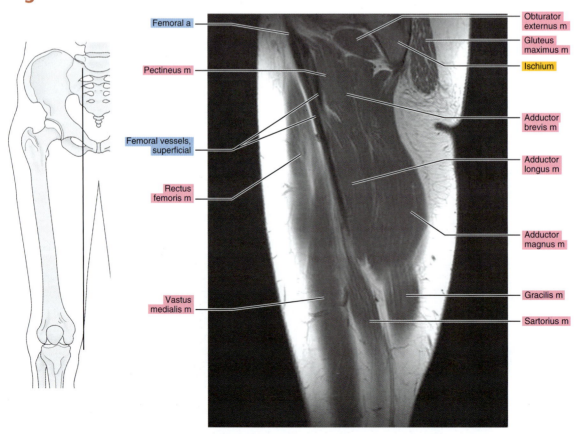

Femoral a

Pectineus m

Femoral vessels, superficial

Rectus femoris m

Vastus medialis m

Obturator externus m

Gluteus maximus m

Ischium

Adductor brevis m

Adductor longus m

Adductor magnus m

Gracilis m

Sartorius m

Figure 20.2.15

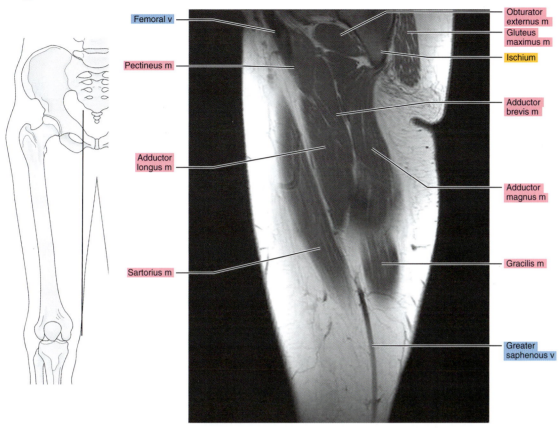

Femoral v — Obturator externus m
Pectineus m — Gluteus maximus m
— Ischium
Adductor longus m — Adductor brevis m
Sartorius m — Adductor magnus m
— Gracilis m
— Greater saphenous v

Figure 20.2.16

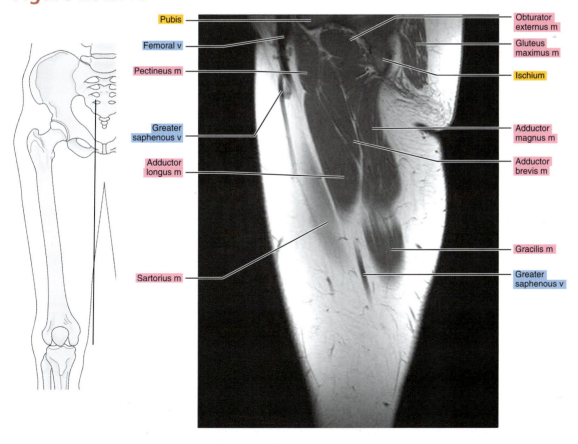

Pubis — Obturator externus m
Femoral v — Gluteus maximus m
Pectineus m — Ischium
Greater saphenous v — Adductor magnus m
Adductor longus m — Adductor brevis m
— Gracilis m
Sartorius m — Greater saphenous v

Figure 20.2.17

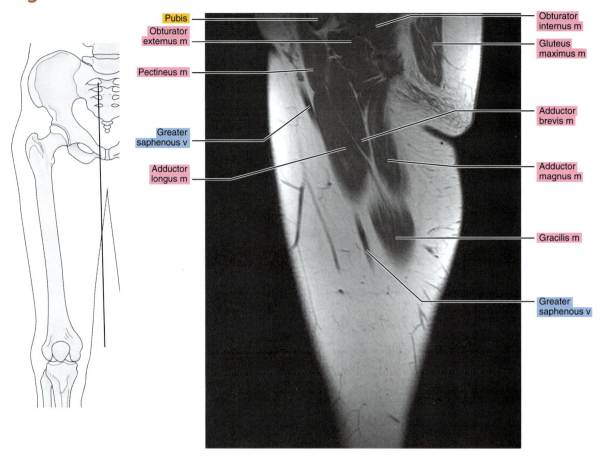

Pubis

Obturator externus m

Pectineus m

Greater saphenous v

Adductor longus m

Obturator internus m

Gluteus maximus m

Adductor brevis m

Adductor magnus m

Gracilis m

Greater saphenous v

CORONAL
Figure 20.3.1

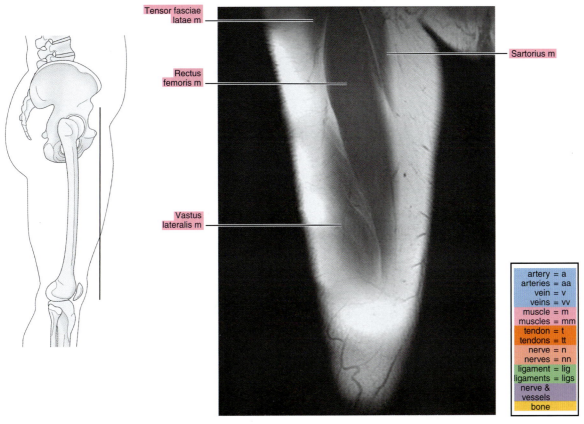

Tensor fasciae latae m

Rectus femoris m

Vastus lateralis m

Sartorius m

artery = a	
arteries = aa	
vein = v	
veins = vv	
muscle = m	
muscles = mm	
tendon = t	
tendons = tt	
nerve = n	
nerves = nn	
ligament = lig	
ligaments = ligs	
nerve & vessels	
bone	

Figure 20.3.2

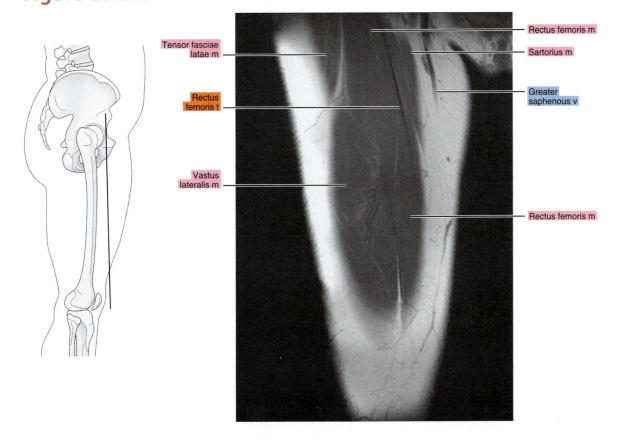

Tensor fasciae latae m

Rectus femoris t

Vastus lateralis m

Rectus femoris m

Sartorius m

Greater saphenous v

Rectus femoris m

Figure 20.3.3

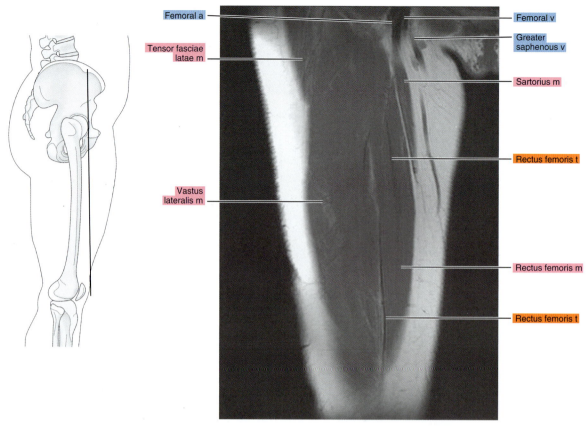

Femoral a

Tensor fasciae latae m

Vastus lateralis m

Femoral v

Greater saphenous v

Sartorius m

Rectus femoris t

Rectus femoris m

Rectus femoris t

Figure 20.3.4

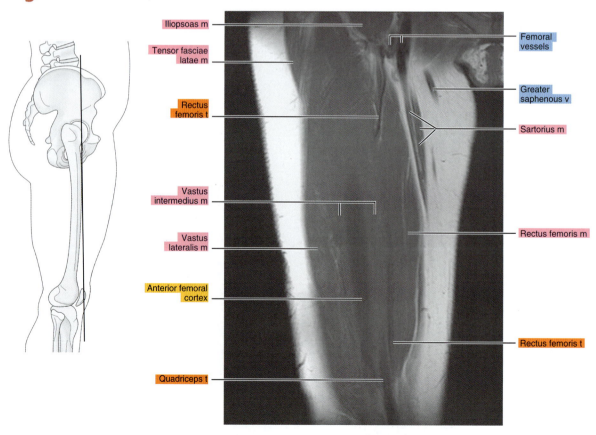

Iliopsoas m

Tensor fasciae latae m

Rectus femoris t

Vastus intermedius m

Vastus lateralis m

Anterior femoral cortex

Quadriceps t

Femoral vessels

Greater saphenous v

Sartorius m

Rectus femoris m

Rectus femoris t

Figure 20.3.5

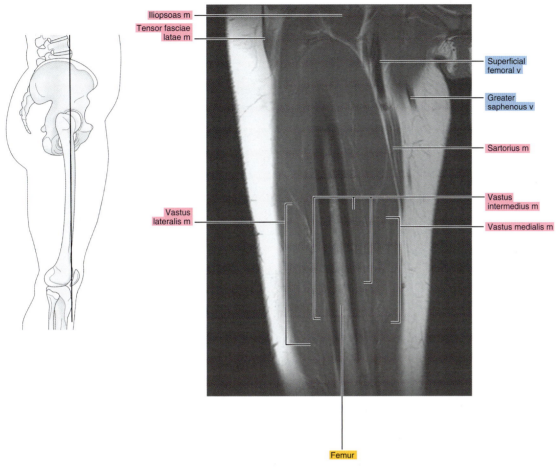

Iliopsoas m
Tensor fasciae latae m
Superficial femoral v
Greater saphenous v
Sartorius m
Vastus lateralis m
Vastus intermedius m
Vastus medialis m
Femur

Figure 20.3.6

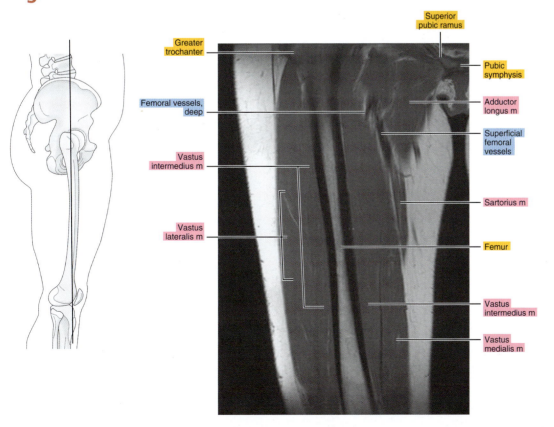

Superior pubic ramus
Greater trochanter
Pubic symphysis
Femoral vessels, deep
Adductor longus m
Superficial femoral vessels
Vastus intermedius m
Vastus lateralis m
Sartorius m
Femur
Vastus intermedius m
Vastus medialis m

Figure 20.3.7

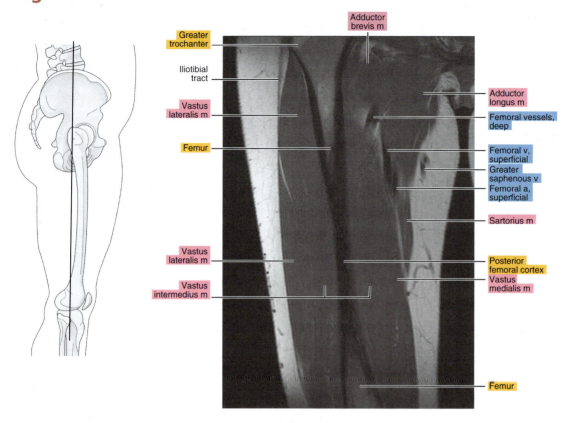

Greater trochanter
Iliotibial tract
Vastus lateralis m
Femur
Vastus lateralis m
Vastus intermedius m
Adductor brevis m
Adductor longus m
Femoral vessels, deep
Femoral v, superficial
Greater saphenous v
Femoral a, superficial
Sartorius m
Posterior femoral cortex
Vastus medialis m
Femur

Figure 20.3.8

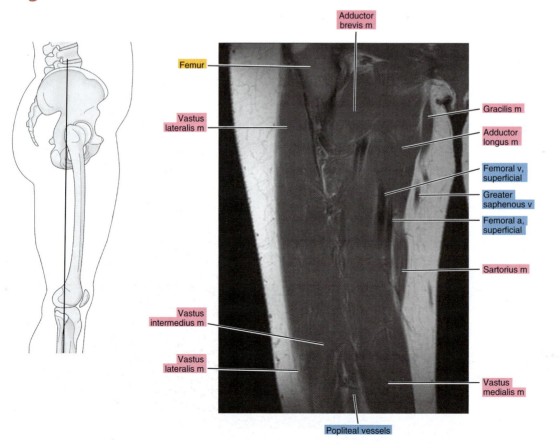

Femur
Vastus lateralis m
Vastus intermedius m
Vastus lateralis m
Adductor brevis m
Gracilis m
Adductor longus m
Femoral v, superficial
Greater saphenous v
Femoral a, superficial
Sartorius m
Vastus medialis m
Popliteal vessels

Figure 20.3.9

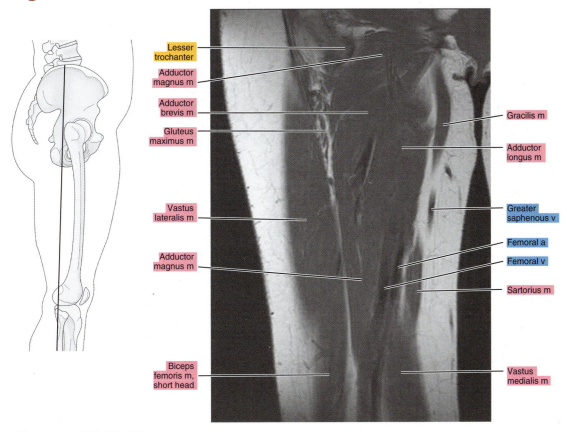

Lesser trochanter
Adductor magnus m
Adductor brevis m
Gluteus maximus m
Vastus lateralis m
Adductor magnus m
Biceps femoris m, short head

Gracilis m
Adductor longus m
Greater saphenous v
Femoral a
Femoral v
Sartorius m
Vastus medialis m

Figure 20.3.10

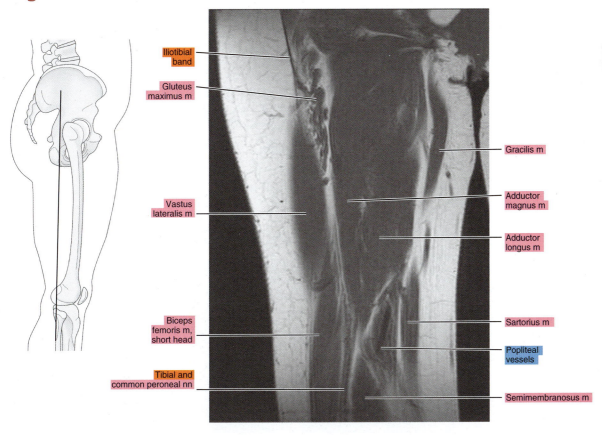

Iliotibial band
Gluteus maximus m
Vastus lateralis m
Biceps femoris m, short head
Tibial and common peroneal nn

Gracilis m
Adductor magnus m
Adductor longus m
Sartorius m
Popliteal vessels
Semimembranosus m

Figure 20.3.11

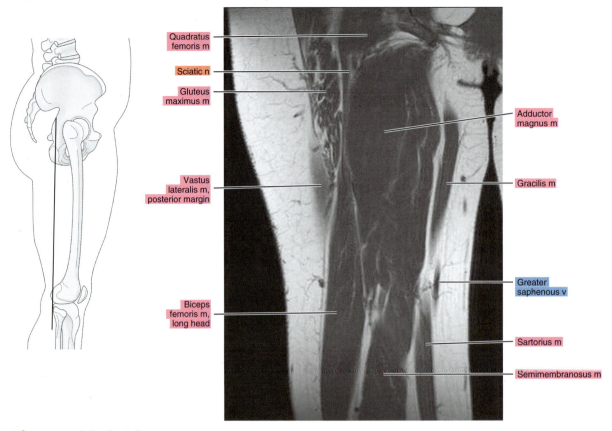

Quadratus femoris m
Sciatic n
Gluteus maximus m
Vastus lateralis m, posterior margin
Biceps femoris m, long head
Adductor magnus m
Gracilis m
Greater saphenous v
Sartorius m
Semimembranosus m

Figure 20.3.12

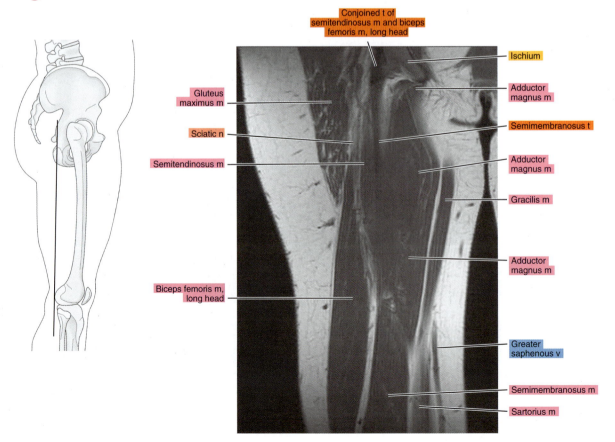

Conjoined t of semitendinosus m and biceps femoris m, long head
Gluteus maximus m
Sciatic n
Semitendinosus m
Biceps femoris m, long head
Ischium
Adductor magnus m
Semimembranosus t
Adductor magnus m
Gracilis m
Adductor magnus m
Greater saphenous v
Semimembranosus m
Sartorius m

Figure 20.3.13

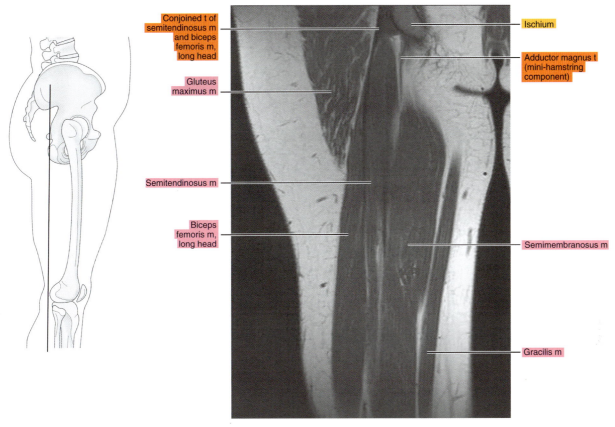

- Conjoined t of semitendinosus m and biceps femoris m, long head
- Ischium
- Gluteus maximus m
- Adductor magnus t (mini-hamstring component)
- Semitendinosus m
- Biceps femoris m, long head
- Semimembranosus m
- Gracilis m

Figure 20.3.14

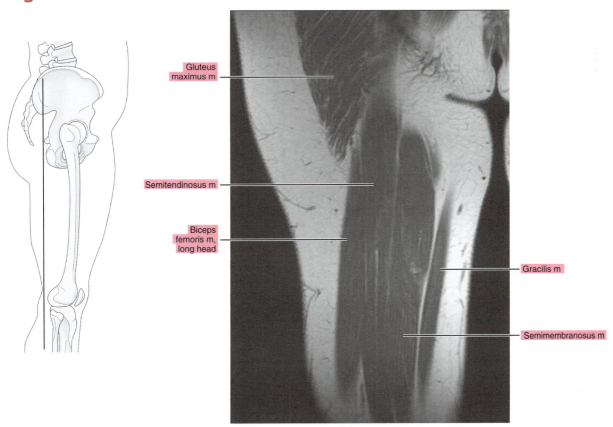

- Gluteus maximus m
- Semitendinosus m
- Biceps femoris m, long head
- Gracilis m
- Semimembranosus m

Figure 20.3.15

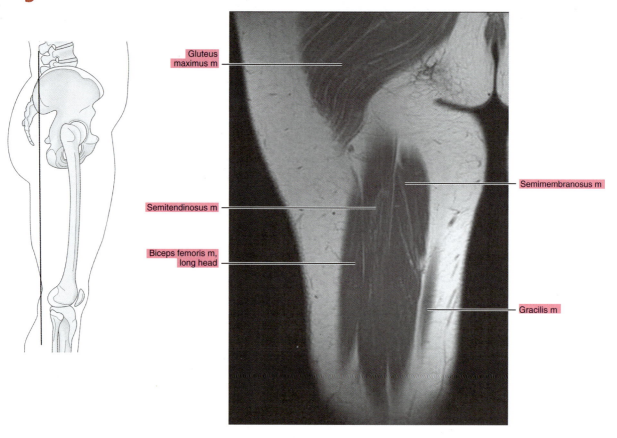

Gluteus maximus m

Semimembranosus m

Semitendinosus m

Biceps femoris m, long head

Gracilis m

Table 20-1. Muscles of the Thigh

MUSCLE	ORIGIN	INSERTION	NERVE SUPPLY
Sartorius	Anterior superior iliac spine and the adjacent area below	Medial surface of the tibia; near the tuberosity and neighboring fascia	Femoral
Rectus femoris	Straight head: anterior inferior iliac spine; reflected head: posterosuperior surface of the rim of the acetabulum	Through the patellar ligament to the tibial tuberosity	Femoral
Vastus lateralis	Shaft of the femur along the anteroinferior margin of the greater trochanter, above the gluteal tuberosity, and the upper half of the linea aspera	Proximal border of the patella, front of the lateral condyle of the tibia, and fascia of the leg	Femoral
Vastus medialis	Medial lip of the linea aspera and the distal half of the intertrochanteric line, and the aponeurosis of the tendons of insertion of the adductor muscles	Upper two-thirds of the medial margin and proximal margin of the patella, medial condyle of the tibia, and investing deep fascia of the leg with the tendons of vastus intermedius, lateralis, and rectus, and through the patellar ligament onto the front of the tibial tuberosity	Femoral
Vastus	Distal half of the lateral margin of the linea aspera and its lateral bifurcation and from the anterolateral part of the shaft of the femur	Proximal margin and deep surface of the patella, aponeurosis of the vastus lateralis, medially and laterally to the tendons of the vastus medialis and lateralis, to the patellar ligament and onto the tibial tuberosity	Femoral
Gracilis	Medial margin of inferior ramus of the pubis and the pubic end of the inferior ramus of the ischium	By an expanded tendinous process onto the tibia below the medial condyle	Anterior division of the obturator
Pectineus	Pectineal line, pectineal fascia, and anterior margin of the obturator sulcus, and from the pubofemoral ligament	Upper half of the pectineal line behind the lesser trochanter	Femoral, also from the accessory obturator and/or obturator
Adductor longus	Pubic tubercle to symphysis pubis	Middle third of the linea aspera	Anterior division of the obturator; also, occasionally, branch from the femoral
Adductor brevis	Medial part of the outer surface of the inferior ramus of the pubis	Distal two-thirds of the pectineal line and the upper one-third of the linea aspera	Anterior (or posterior) branch of the obturator
Adductor magnus	Inferior ramus of the pubis	Medial side of the gluteal ridge and the superior part of the linea aspera by a tendon from the distal three-fourths of the linea aspera and the adductor tubercle at the distal end of the medial supracondylar ridge	Posterior branch of the obturator and a branch from the sciatic
Biceps femoris	From the lateral lip of the linea aspera of the femur, from the middle of the shaft to the bifurcation of the linea aspera proximal two-thirds of the supracondylar ridge, and lateral intermuscular septum	Head of the fibula in front of the apex, partially onto the lateral condyle of the tibia, and into the fascia of the leg	Peroneal part of the sciatic

Chapter

21

MRI of the Knee

AXIAL
Figure 21.1.1

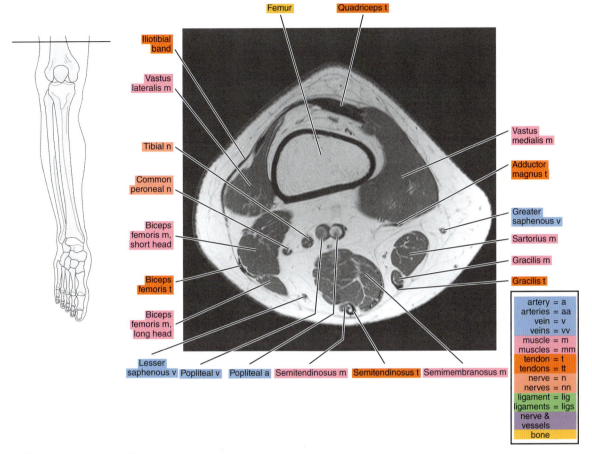

Femur Quadriceps t

Iliotibial band

Vastus lateralis m

Tibial n

Common peroneal n

Biceps femoris m, short head

Biceps femoris t

Biceps femoris m, long head

Vastus medialis m

Adductor magnus t

Greater saphenous v

Sartorius m

Gracilis m

Gracilis t

Lesser saphenous v Popliteal v Popliteal a Semitendinosus m Semitendinosus t Semimembranosus m

artery	= a
arteries	= aa
vein	= v
veins	= vv
muscle	= m
muscles	= mm
tendon	= t
tendons	= tt
nerve	= n
nerves	= nn
ligament	= lig
ligaments	= ligs
nerve & vessels	
bone	

Figure 21.1.2

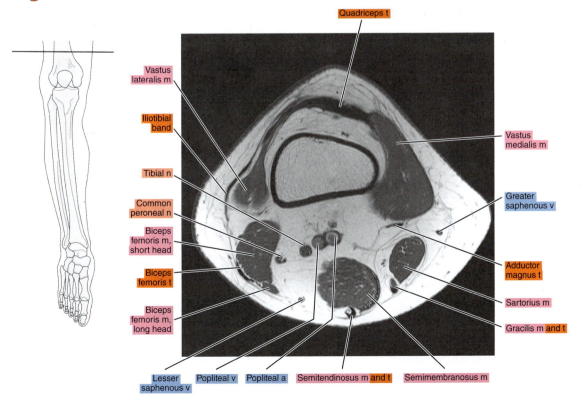

Quadriceps t

Vastus lateralis m

Iliotibial band

Tibial n

Common peroneal n

Biceps femoris m, short head

Biceps femoris t

Biceps femoris m, long head

Vastus medialis m

Greater saphenous v

Adductor magnus t

Sartorius m

Gracilis m and t

Lesser saphenous v Popliteal v Popliteal a Semitendinosus m and t Semimembranosus m

Figure 21.1.3

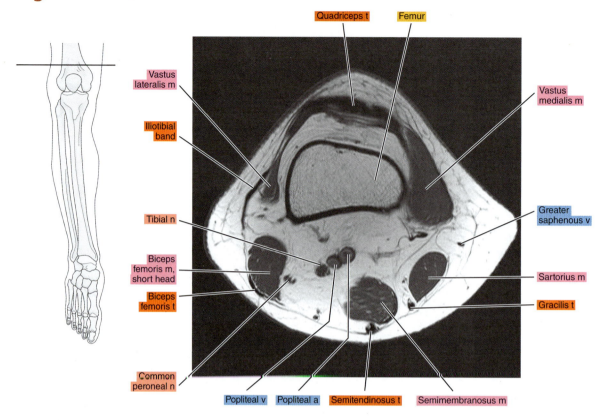

Quadriceps t — Femur

Vastus lateralis m

Iliotibial band

Tibial n

Biceps femoris m, short head

Biceps femoris t

Common peroneal n

Vastus medialis m

Greater saphenous v

Sartorius m

Gracilis t

Popliteal v — Popliteal a — Semitendinosus t — Semimembranosus m

Figure 21.1.4

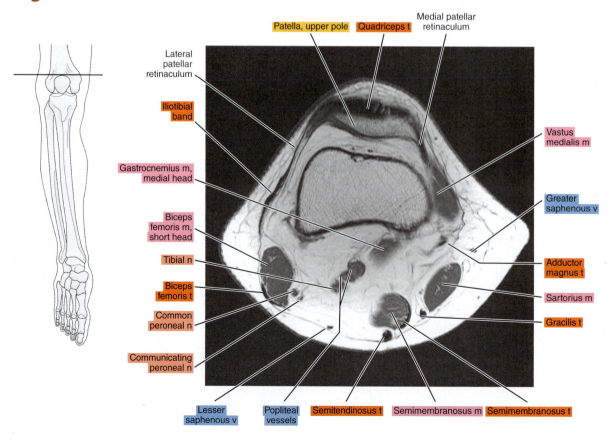

Patella, upper pole — Quadriceps t — Medial patellar retinaculum

Lateral patellar retinaculum

Iliotibial band

Gastrocnemius m, medial head

Biceps femoris m, short head

Tibial n

Biceps femoris t

Common peroneal n

Communicating peroneal n

Vastus medialis m

Greater saphenous v

Adductor magnus t

Sartorius m

Gracilis t

Lesser saphenous v — Popliteal vessels — Semitendinosus t — Semimembranosus m — Semimembranosus t

Figure 21.1.5

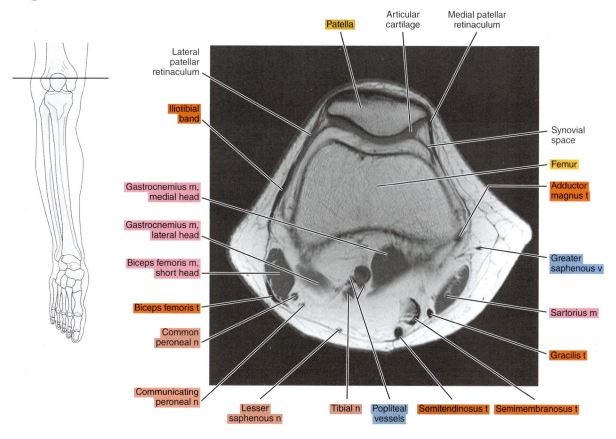

Lateral patellar retinaculum

Patella

Articular cartilage

Medial patellar retinaculum

Iliotibial band

Gastrocnemius m, medial head

Gastrocnemius m, lateral head

Biceps femoris m, short head

Biceps femoris t

Common peroneal n

Communicating peroneal n

Synovial space

Femur

Adductor magnus t

Greater saphenous v

Sartorius m

Gracilis t

Lesser saphenous n

Tibial n

Popliteal vessels

Semitendinosus t

Semimembranosus t

Figure 21.1.6

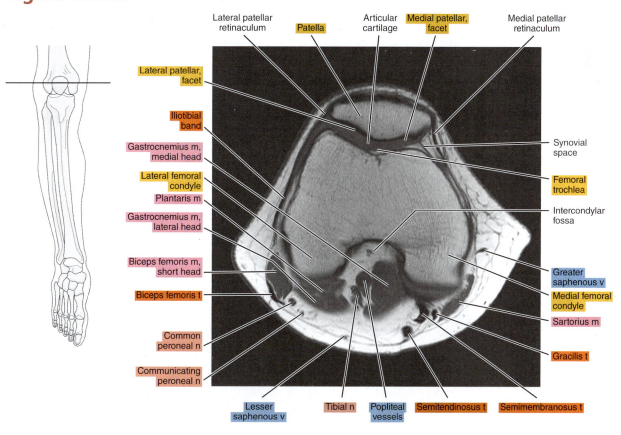

Lateral patellar retinaculum

Patella

Articular cartilage

Medial patellar, facet

Medial patellar retinaculum

Lateral patellar, facet

Iliotibial band

Gastrocnemius m, medial head

Lateral femoral condyle

Plantaris m

Gastrocnemius m, lateral head

Biceps femoris m, short head

Biceps femoris t

Common peroneal n

Communicating peroneal n

Synovial space

Femoral trochlea

Intercondylar fossa

Greater saphenous v

Medial femoral condyle

Sartorius m

Gracilis t

Lesser saphenous v

Tibial n

Popliteal vessels

Semitendinosus t

Semimembranosus t

Figure 21.1.7

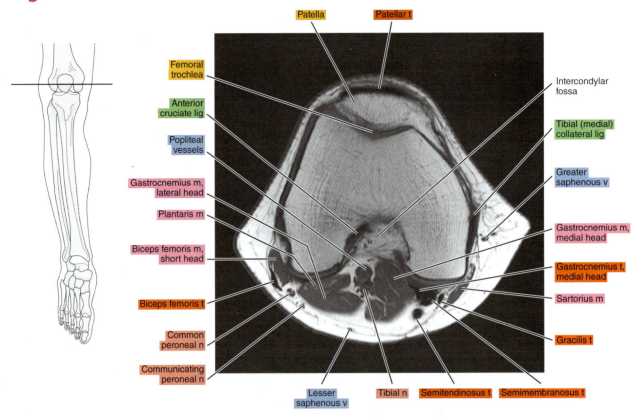

Patella — Patellar t

Femoral trochlea

Anterior cruciate lig

Popliteal vessels

Gastrocnemius m, lateral head

Plantaris m

Biceps femoris m, short head

Biceps femoris t

Common peroneal n

Communicating peroneal n

Intercondylar fossa

Tibial (medial) collateral lig

Greater saphenous v

Gastrocnemius m, medial head

Gastrocnemius t, medial head

Sartorius m

Gracilis t

Lesser saphenous v — Tibial n — Semitendinosus t — Semimembranosus t

Figure 21.1.8

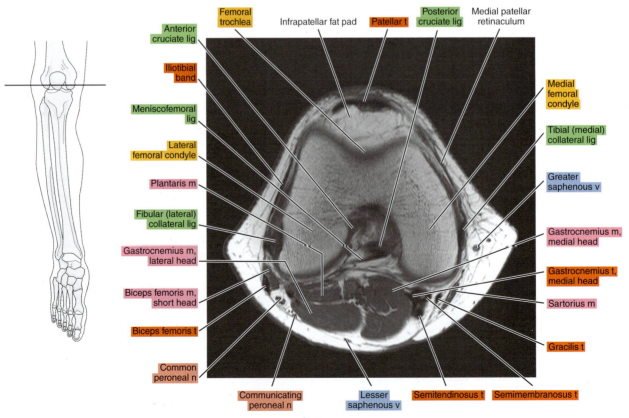

Anterior cruciate lig

Femoral trochlea

Infrapatellar fat pad — Patellar t — Posterior cruciate lig — Medial patellar retinaculum

Iliotibial band

Meniscofemoral lig

Lateral femoral condyle

Plantaris m

Fibular (lateral) collateral lig

Gastrocnemius m, lateral head

Biceps femoris m, short head

Biceps femoris t

Common peroneal n

Medial femoral condyle

Tibial (medial) collateral lig

Greater saphenous v

Gastrocnemius m, medial head

Gastrocnemius t, medial head

Sartorius m

Gracilis t

Communicating peroneal n — Lesser saphenous v — Semitendinosus t — Semimembranosus t

Figure 21.1.9

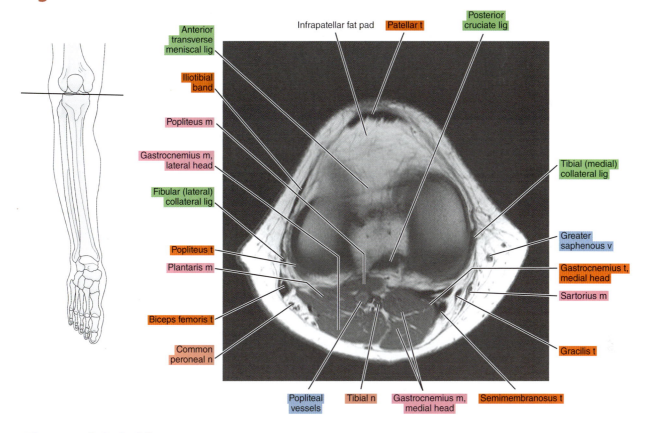

- Anterior transverse meniscal lig
- Iliotibial band
- Popliteus m
- Gastrocnemius m, lateral head
- Fibular (lateral) collateral lig
- Popliteus t
- Plantaris m
- Biceps femoris t
- Common peroneal n
- Infrapatellar fat pad
- Patellar t
- Posterior cruciate lig
- Tibial (medial) collateral lig
- Greater saphenous v
- Gastrocnemius t, medial head
- Sartorius m
- Gracilis t
- Popliteal vessels
- Tibial n
- Gastrocnemius m, medial head
- Semimembranosus t

Figure 21.1.10

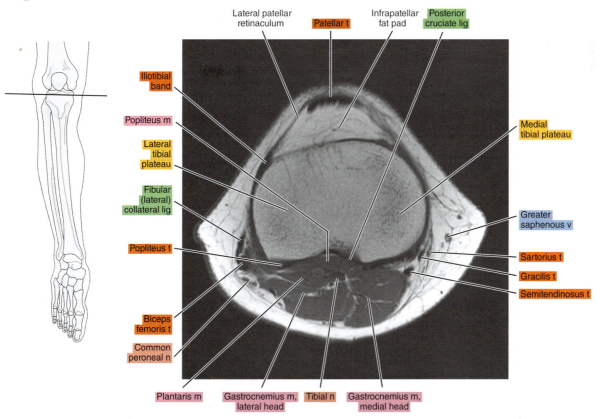

- Lateral patellar retinaculum
- Patellar t
- Infrapatellar fat pad
- Posterior cruciate lig
- Iliotibial band
- Popliteus m
- Lateral tibial plateau
- Fibular (lateral) collateral lig
- Popliteus t
- Biceps femoris t
- Common peroneal n
- Medial tibial plateau
- Greater saphenous v
- Sartorius t
- Gracilis t
- Semitendinosus t
- Plantaris m
- Gastrocnemius m, lateral head
- Tibial n
- Gastrocnemius m, medial head

Figure 21.1.11

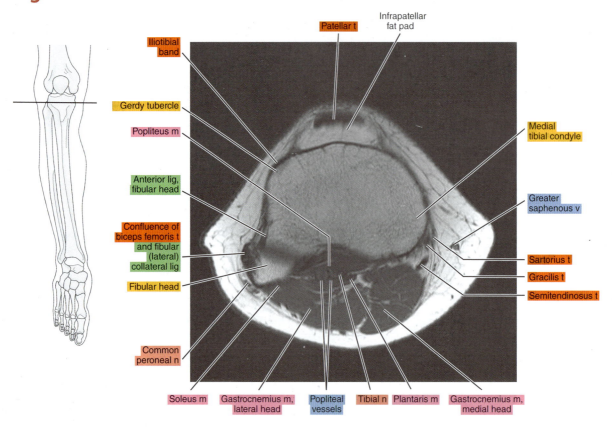

Infrapatellar fat pad

Patellar t

Iliotibial band

Gerdy tubercle

Popliteus m

Anterior lig, fibular head

Confluence of biceps femoris t and fibular (lateral) collateral lig

Fibular head

Common peroneal n

Medial tibial condyle

Greater saphenous v

Sartorius t

Gracilis t

Semitendinosus t

Soleus m

Gastrocnemius m, lateral head

Popliteal vessels

Tibial n

Plantaris m

Gastrocnemius m, medial head

Figure 21.1.12

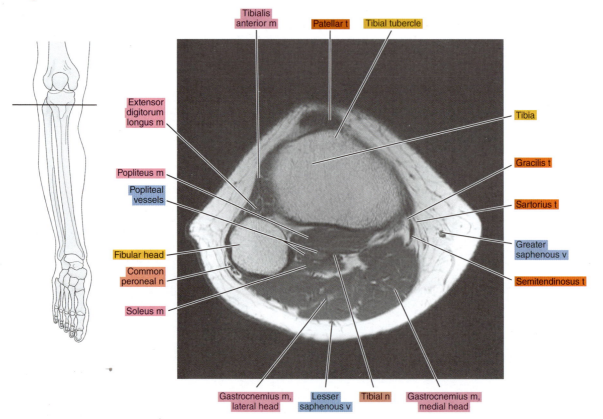

Tibialis anterior m

Patellar t

Tibial tubercle

Extensor digitorum longus m

Popliteus m

Popliteal vessels

Fibular head

Common peroneal n

Soleus m

Tibia

Gracilis t

Sartorius t

Greater saphenous v

Semitendinosus t

Gastrocnemius m, lateral head

Lesser saphenous v

Tibial n

Gastrocnemius m, medial head

Figure 21.1.13

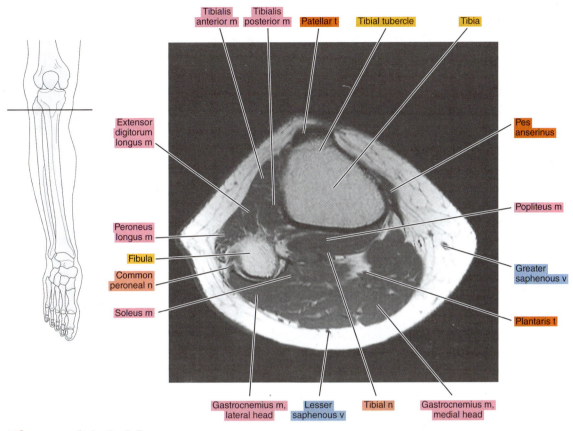

Tibialis anterior m
Tibialis posterior m
Patellar t
Tibial tubercle
Tibia
Extensor digitorum longus m
Pes anserinus
Peroneus longus m
Popliteus m
Fibula
Common peroneal n
Greater saphenous v
Soleus m
Plantaris t
Gastrocnemius m, lateral head
Lesser saphenous v
Tibial n
Gastrocnemius m, medial head

Figure 21.1.14

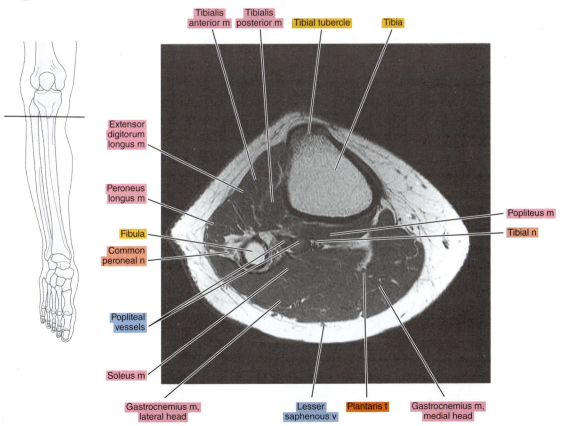

Tibialis anterior m
Tibialis posterior m
Tibial tubercle
Tibia
Extensor digitorum longus m
Peroneus longus m
Popliteus m
Fibula
Tibial n
Common peroneal n
Popliteal vessels
Soleus m
Gastrocnemius m, lateral head
Lesser saphenous v
Plantaris t
Gastrocnemius m, medial head

SAGITTAL
Figure 21.2.1

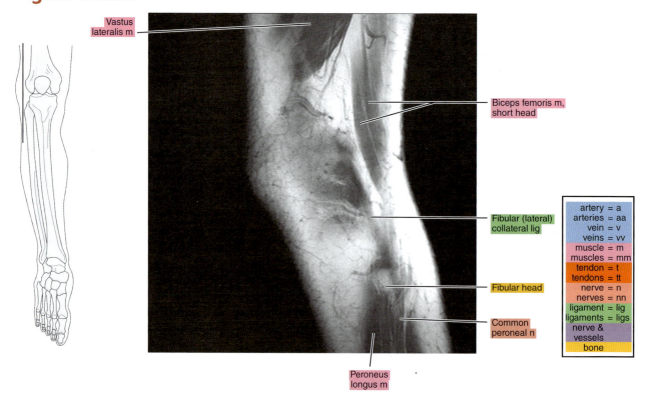

Vastus lateralis m

Biceps femoris m, short head

Fibular (lateral) collateral lig

Fibular head

Common peroneal n

Peroneus longus m

artery = a
arteries = aa
vein = v
veins = vv
muscle = m
muscles = mm
tendon = t
tendons = tt
nerve = n
nerves = nn
ligament = lig
ligaments = ligs
nerve & vessels
bone

Figure 21.2.2

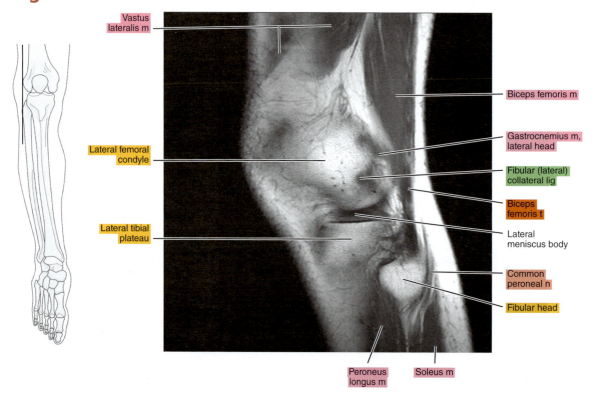

Vastus lateralis m

Lateral femoral condyle

Lateral tibial plateau

Biceps femoris m

Gastrocnemius m, lateral head

Fibular (lateral) collateral lig

Biceps femoris t

Lateral meniscus body

Common peroneal n

Fibular head

Peroneus longus m

Soleus m

Figure 21.2.3

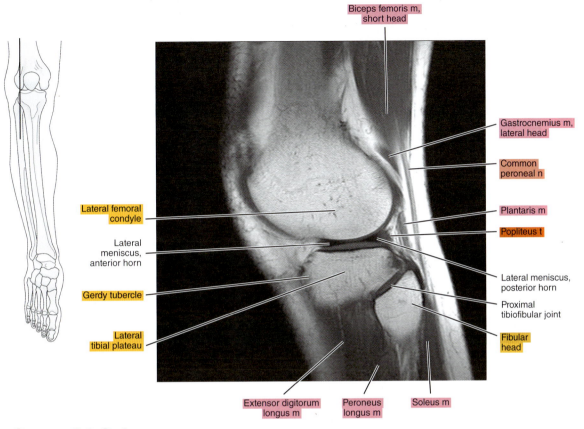

Biceps femoris m, short head

Gastrocnemius m, lateral head

Common peroneal n

Lateral femoral condyle

Plantaris m

Popliteus t

Lateral meniscus, anterior horn

Gerdy tubercle

Lateral meniscus, posterior horn

Proximal tibiofibular joint

Fibular head

Lateral tibial plateau

Extensor digitorum longus m

Peroneus longus m

Soleus m

Figure 21.2.4

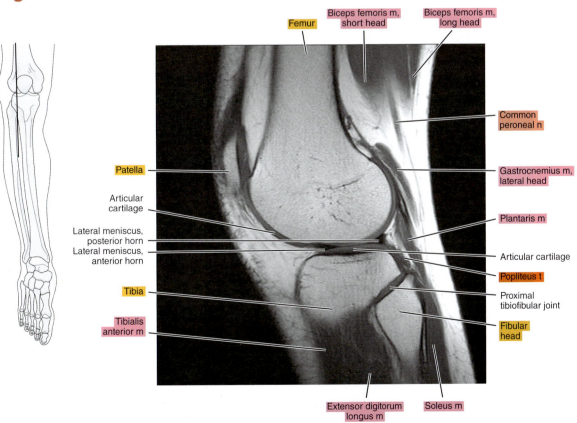

Femur

Biceps femoris m, short head

Biceps femoris m, long head

Common peroneal n

Patella

Gastrocnemius m, lateral head

Articular cartilage

Plantaris m

Lateral meniscus, posterior horn

Lateral meniscus, anterior horn

Articular cartilage

Popliteus t

Tibia

Proximal tibiofibular joint

Tibialis anterior m

Fibular head

Extensor digitorum longus m

Soleus m

Figure 21.2.5

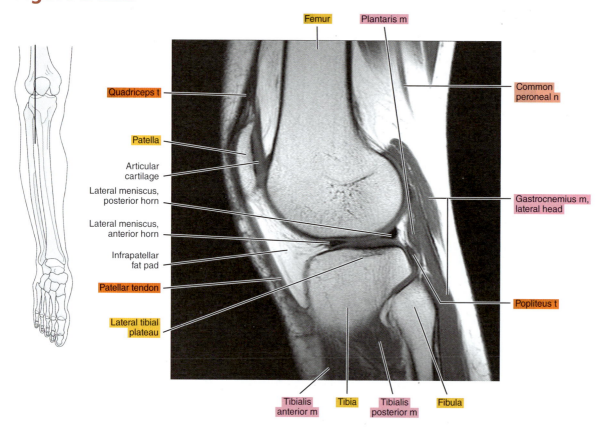

Femur

Plantaris m

Quadriceps t

Common peroneal n

Patella

Articular cartilage

Lateral meniscus, posterior horn

Gastrocnemius m, lateral head

Lateral meniscus, anterior horn

Infrapatellar fat pad

Patellar tendon

Popliteus t

Lateral tibial plateau

Tibialis anterior m

Tibia

Tibialis posterior m

Fibula

Figure 21.2.6

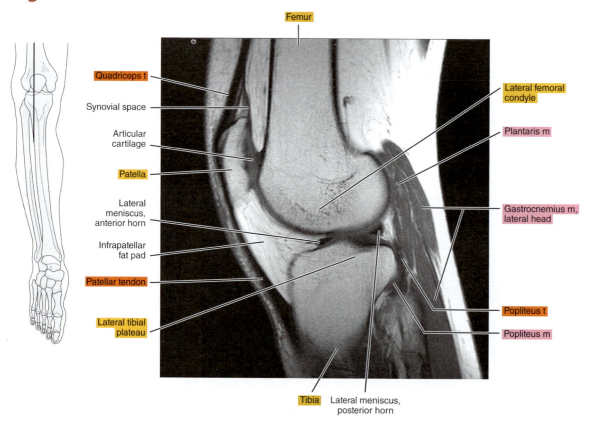

Femur

Quadriceps t

Lateral femoral condyle

Synovial space

Articular cartilage

Plantaris m

Patella

Lateral meniscus, anterior horn

Gastrocnemius m, lateral head

Infrapatellar fat pad

Patellar tendon

Popliteus t

Lateral tibial plateau

Popliteus m

Tibia Lateral meniscus, posterior horn

Figure 21.2.7

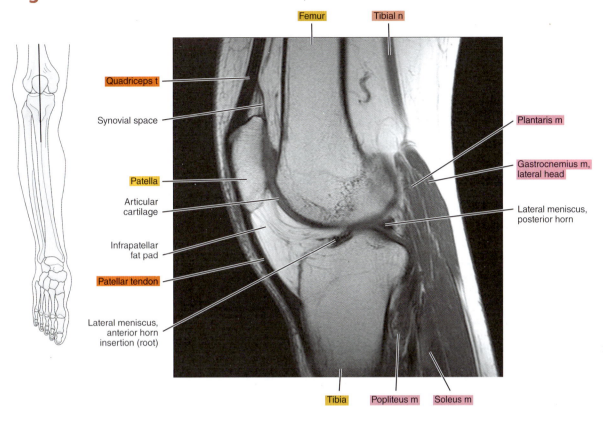

Femur | Tibial n
Quadriceps t
Synovial space
Plantaris m
Gastrocnemius m, lateral head
Patella
Articular cartilage
Lateral meniscus, posterior horn
Infrapatellar fat pad
Patellar tendon
Lateral meniscus, anterior horn insertion (root)
Tibia | Popliteus m | Soleus m

Figure 21.2.8

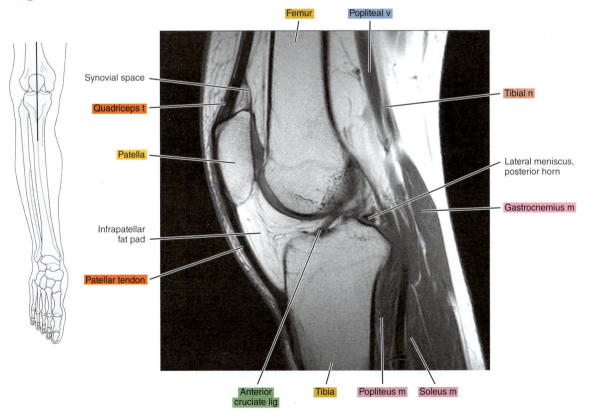

Femur | Popliteal v
Synovial space
Quadriceps t
Tibial n
Patella
Lateral meniscus, posterior horn
Gastrocnemius m
Infrapatellar fat pad
Patellar tendon
Anterior cruciate lig | Tibia | Popliteus m | Soleus m

Figure 21.2.9

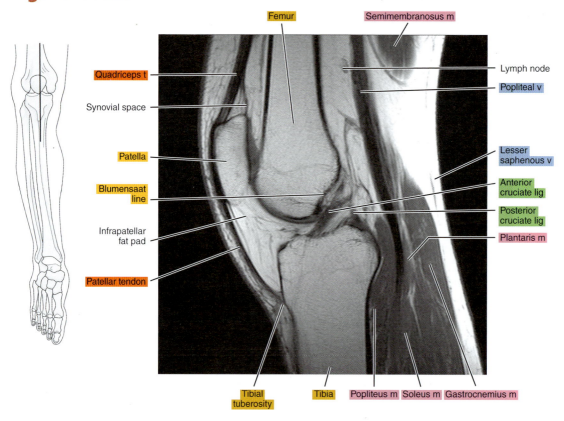

Femur
Semimembranosus m
Quadriceps t
Synovial space
Patella
Blumensaat line
Infrapatellar fat pad
Patellar tendon
Tibial tuberosity
Tibia
Popliteus m
Soleus m
Gastrocnemius m
Lymph node
Popliteal v
Lesser saphenous v
Anterior cruciate lig
Posterior cruciate lig
Plantaris m

Figure 21.2.10

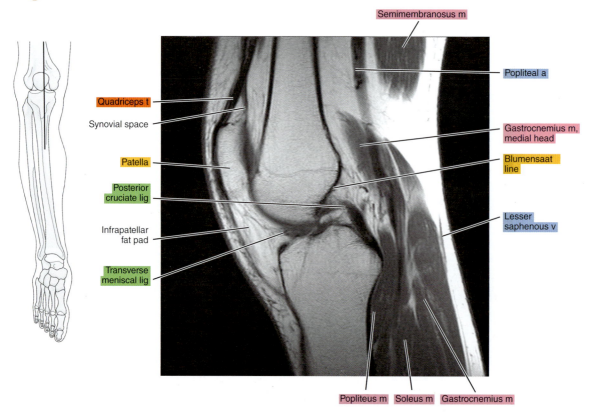

Semimembranosus m
Quadriceps t
Synovial space
Patella
Posterior cruciate lig
Infrapatellar fat pad
Transverse meniscal lig
Popliteus m
Soleus m
Gastrocnemius m
Popliteal a
Gastrocnemius m, medial head
Blumensaat line
Lesser saphenous v

Figure 21.2.11

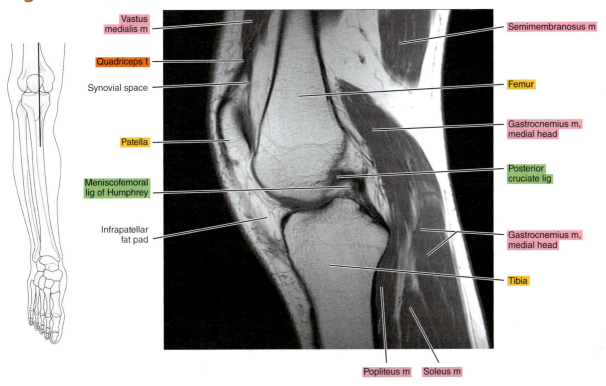

Vastus medialis m

Quadriceps t

Synovial space

Patella

Meniscofemoral lig of Humphrey

Infrapatellar fat pad

Semimembranosus m

Femur

Gastrocnemius m, medial head

Posterior cruciate lig

Gastrocnemius m, medial head

Tibia

Popliteus m   Soleus m

Figure 21.2.12

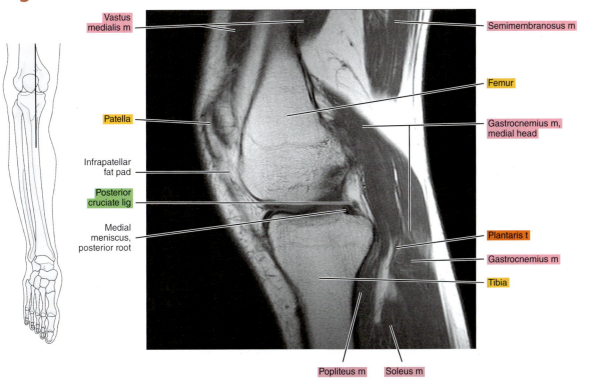

Vastus medialis m

Patella

Infrapatellar fat pad

Posterior cruciate lig

Medial meniscus, posterior root

Semimembranosus m

Femur

Gastrocnemius m, medial head

Plantaris t

Gastrocnemius m

Tibia

Popliteus m   Soleus m

Figure 21.2.13

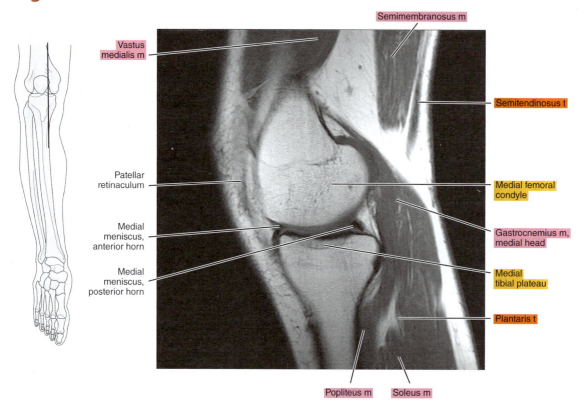

Semimembranosus m

Vastus medialis m

Semitendinosus t

Patellar retinaculum

Medial femoral condyle

Medial meniscus, anterior horn

Gastrocnemius m, medial head

Medial meniscus, posterior horn

Medial tibial plateau

Plantaris t

Popliteus m   Soleus m

Figure 21.2.14

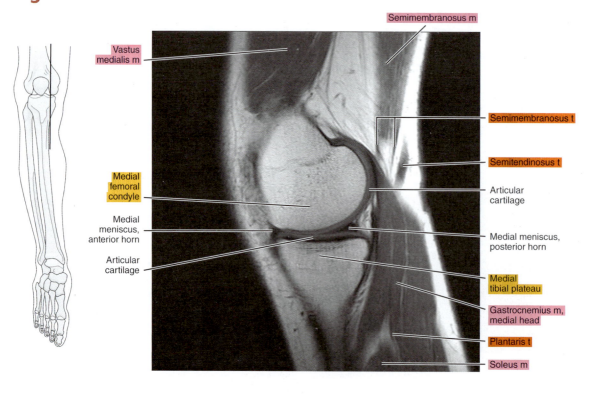

Semimembranosus m

Vastus medialis m

Semimembranosus t

Semitendinosus t

Medial femoral condyle

Articular cartilage

Medial meniscus, anterior horn

Medial meniscus, posterior horn

Articular cartilage

Medial tibial plateau

Gastrocnemius m, medial head

Plantaris t

Soleus m

Figure 21.2.15

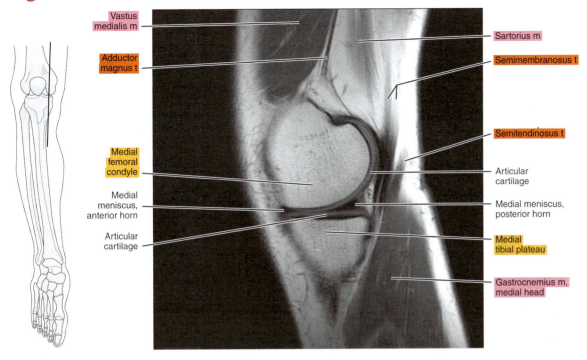

Vastus medialis m

Adductor magnus t

Medial femoral condyle

Medial meniscus, anterior horn

Articular cartilage

Sartorius m

Semimembranosus t

Semitendinosus t

Articular cartilage

Medial meniscus, posterior horn

Medial tibial plateau

Gastrocnemius m, medial head

Figure 21.2.16

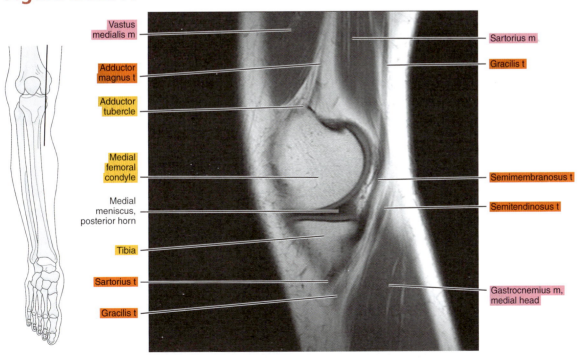

Vastus medialis m

Adductor magnus t

Adductor tubercle

Medial femoral condyle

Medial meniscus, posterior horn

Tibia

Sartorius t

Gracilis t

Sartorius m

Gracilis t

Semimembranosus t

Semitendinosus t

Gastrocnemius m, medial head

Figure 21.2.17

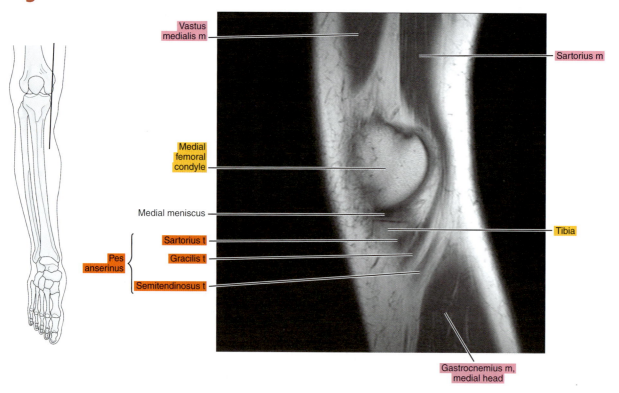

Vastus medialis m

Sartorius m

Medial femoral condyle

Medial meniscus

Pes anserinus
- Sartorius t
- Gracilis t
- Semitendinosus t

Tibia

Gastrocnemius m, medial head

CORONAL
Figure 21.3.1

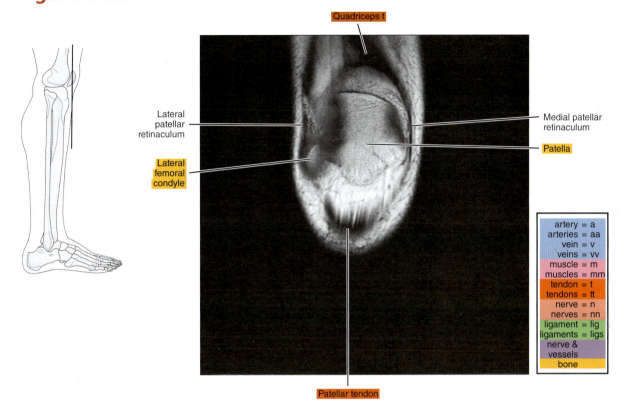

Quadriceps t

Lateral patellar retinaculum

Medial patellar retinaculum

Patella

Lateral femoral condyle

artery = a	
arteries = aa	
vein = v	
veins = vv	
muscle = m	
muscles = mm	
tendon = t	
tendons = tt	
nerve = n	
nerves = nn	
ligament = lig	
ligaments = ligs	
nerve & vessels	
bone	

Patellar tendon

Figure 21.3.2

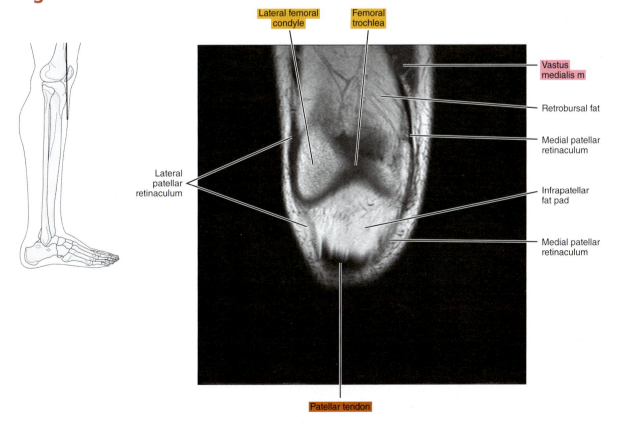

Lateral femoral condyle

Femoral trochlea

Vastus medialis m

Retrobursal fat

Medial patellar retinaculum

Lateral patellar retinaculum

Infrapatellar fat pad

Medial patellar retinaculum

Patellar tendon

Figure 21.3.3

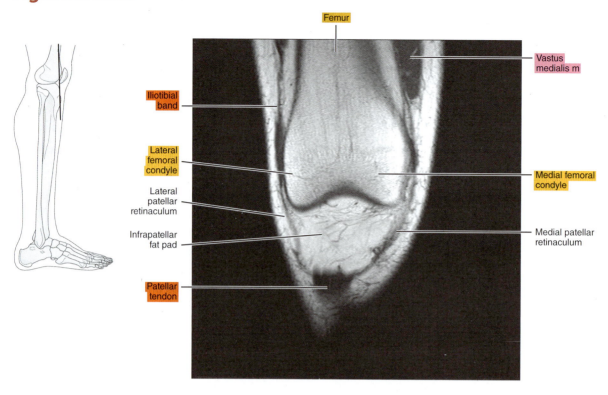

Femur

Vastus medialis m

Iliotibial band

Lateral femoral condyle

Medial femoral condyle

Lateral patellar retinaculum

Infrapatellar fat pad

Medial patellar retinaculum

Patellar tendon

Figure 21.3.4

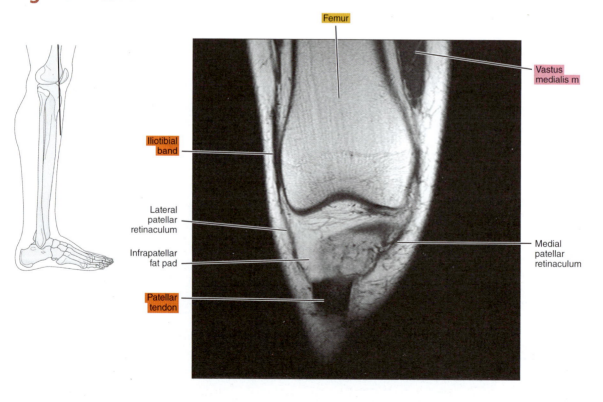

Femur

Vastus medialis m

Iliotibial band

Lateral patellar retinaculum

Infrapatellar fat pad

Medial patellar retinaculum

Patellar tendon

Figure 21.3.5

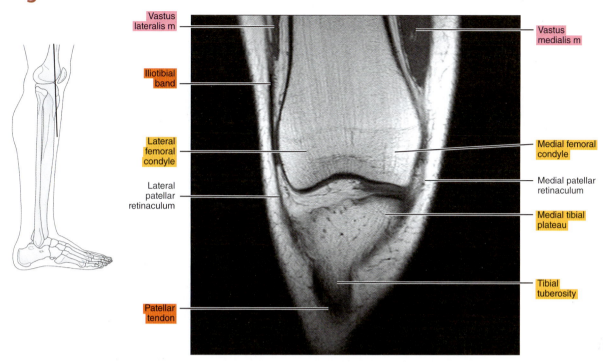

Vastus lateralis m

Iliotibial band

Lateral femoral condyle

Lateral patellar retinaculum

Patellar tendon

Vastus medialis m

Medial femoral condyle

Medial patellar retinaculum

Medial tibial plateau

Tibial tuberosity

Figure 21.3.6

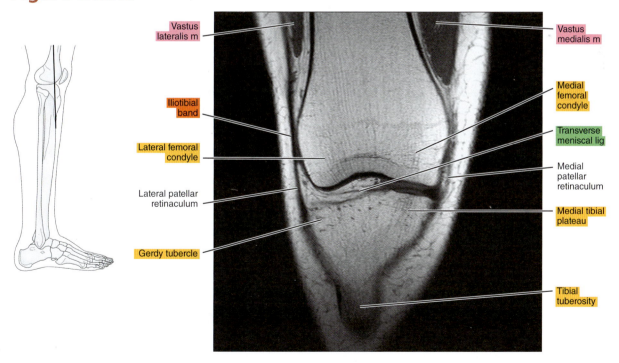

Vastus lateralis m

Iliotibial band

Lateral femoral condyle

Lateral patellar retinaculum

Gerdy tubercle

Vastus medialis m

Medial femoral condyle

Transverse meniscal lig

Medial patellar retinaculum

Medial tibial plateau

Tibial tuberosity

Figure 21.3.7

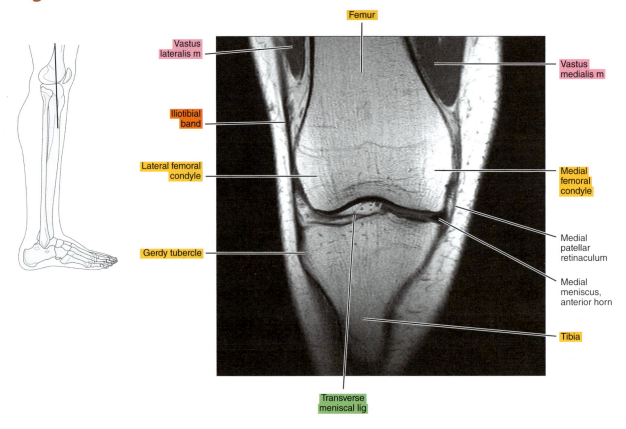

- Femur
- Vastus lateralis m
- Vastus medialis m
- Iliotibial band
- Lateral femoral condyle
- Medial femoral condyle
- Medial patellar retinaculum
- Gerdy tubercle
- Medial meniscus, anterior horn
- Tibia
- Transverse meniscal lig

Figure 21.3.8

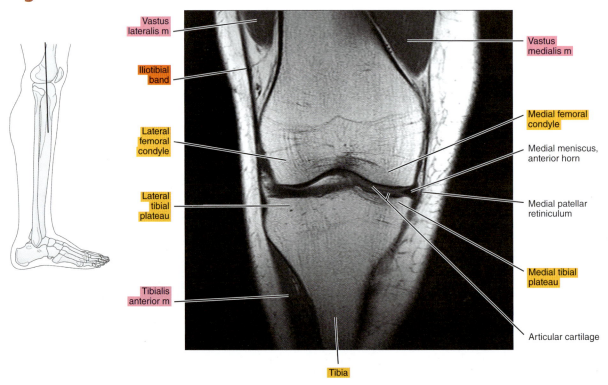

- Vastus lateralis m
- Vastus medialis m
- Iliotibial band
- Medial femoral condyle
- Lateral femoral condyle
- Medial meniscus, anterior horn
- Lateral tibial plateau
- Medial patellar retiniculum
- Tibialis anterior m
- Medial tibial plateau
- Articular cartilage
- Tibia

Figure 21.3.9

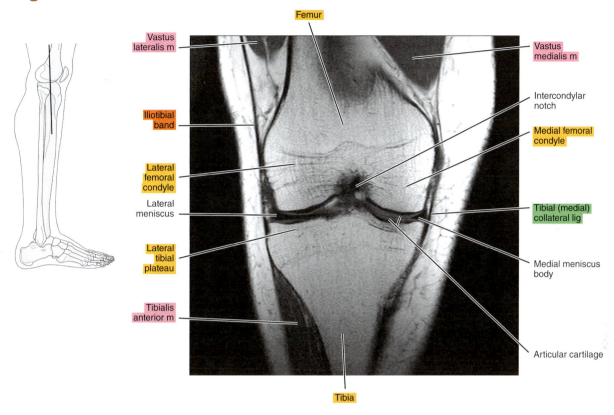

- Femur
- Vastus lateralis m
- Vastus medialis m
- Iliotibial band
- Intercondylar notch
- Medial femoral condyle
- Lateral femoral condyle
- Lateral meniscus
- Tibial (medial) collateral lig
- Lateral tibial plateau
- Medial meniscus body
- Tibialis anterior m
- Articular cartilage
- Tibia

Figure 21.3.10

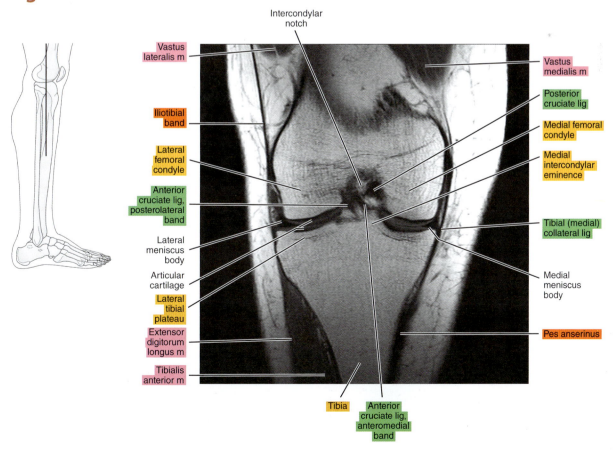

- Intercondylar notch
- Vastus lateralis m
- Vastus medialis m
- Iliotibial band
- Posterior cruciate lig
- Lateral femoral condyle
- Medial femoral condyle
- Anterior cruciate lig, posterolateral band
- Medial intercondylar eminence
- Lateral meniscus body
- Tibial (medial) collateral lig
- Articular cartilage
- Lateral tibial plateau
- Medial meniscus body
- Extensor digitorum longus m
- Pes anserinus
- Tibialis anterior m
- Tibia
- Anterior cruciate lig, anteromedial band

Figure 21.3.11

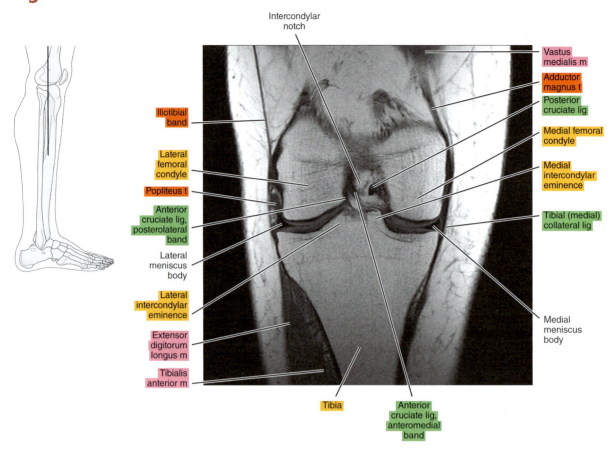

Intercondylar notch

Vastus medialis m

Adductor magnus t

Posterior cruciate lig

Medial femoral condyle

Medial intercondylar eminence

Tibial (medial) collateral lig

Medial meniscus body

Iliotibial band

Lateral femoral condyle

Popliteus t

Anterior cruciate lig, posterolateral band

Lateral meniscus body

Lateral intercondylar eminence

Extensor digitorum longus m

Tibialis anterior m

Tibia

Anterior cruciate lig, anteromedial band

Figure 21.3.12

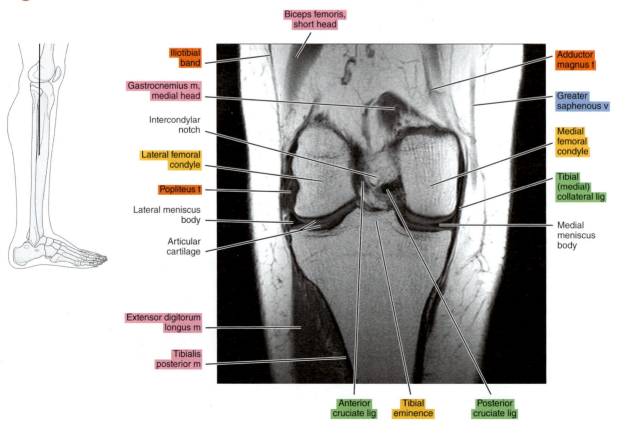

Biceps femoris, short head

Iliotibial band

Gastrocnemius m, medial head

Intercondylar notch

Lateral femoral condyle

Popliteus t

Lateral meniscus body

Articular cartilage

Extensor digitorum longus m

Tibialis posterior m

Adductor magnus t

Greater saphenous v

Medial femoral condyle

Tibial (medial) collateral lig

Medial meniscus body

Anterior cruciate lig

Tibial eminence

Posterior cruciate lig

Figure 21.3.13

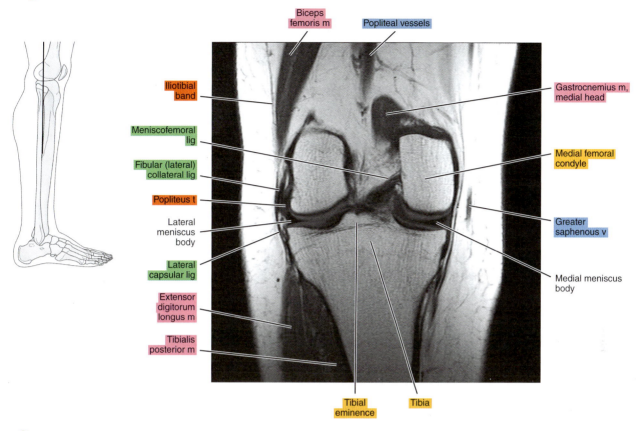

Biceps femoris m

Popliteal vessels

Iliotibial band

Meniscofemoral lig

Fibular (lateral) collateral lig

Popliteus t

Lateral meniscus body

Lateral capsular lig

Extensor digitorum longus m

Tibialis posterior m

Gastrocnemius m, medial head

Medial femoral condyle

Greater saphenous v

Medial meniscus body

Tibial eminence

Tibia

Figure 21.3.14

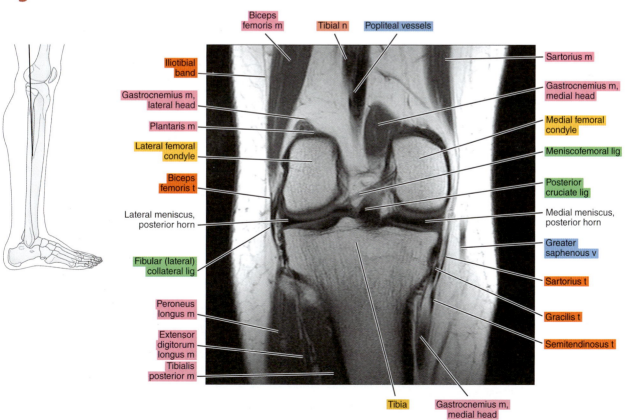

Biceps femoris m

Tibial n

Popliteal vessels

Iliotibial band

Gastrocnemius m, lateral head

Plantaris m

Lateral femoral condyle

Biceps femoris t

Lateral meniscus, posterior horn

Fibular (lateral) collateral lig

Peroneus longus m

Extensor digitorum longus m

Tibialis posterior m

Sartorius m

Gastrocnemius m, medial head

Medial femoral condyle

Meniscofemoral lig

Posterior cruciate lig

Medial meniscus, posterior horn

Greater saphenous v

Sartorius t

Gracilis t

Semitendinosus t

Tibia

Gastrocnemius m, medial head

Figure 21.3.15

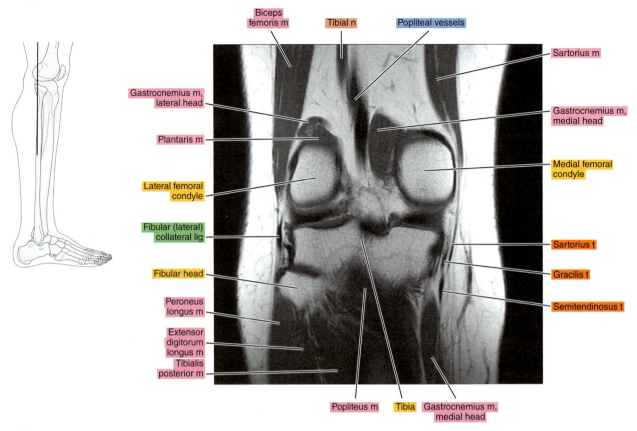

Biceps femoris m

Tibial n

Popliteal vessels

Sartorius m

Gastrocnemius m, lateral head

Gastrocnemius m, medial head

Plantaris m

Medial femoral condyle

Lateral femoral condyle

Fibular (lateral) collateral lig

Sartorius t

Fibular head

Gracilis t

Peroneus longus m

Semitendinosus t

Extensor digitorum longus m

Tibialis posterior m

Popliteus m

Tibia

Gastrocnemius m, medial head

Figure 21.3.16

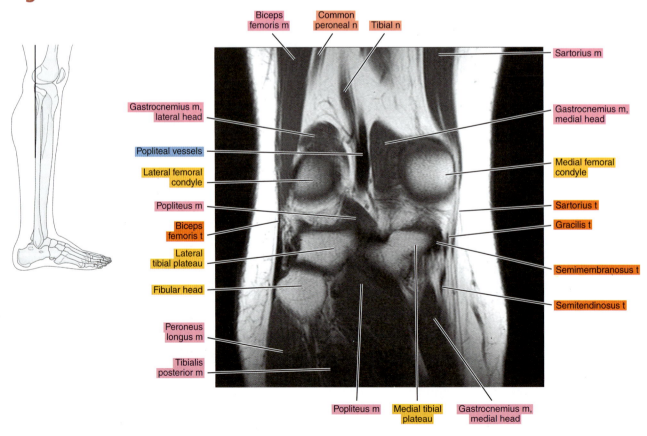

Biceps femoris m

Common peroneal n

Tibial n

Sartorius m

Gastrocnemius m, lateral head

Gastrocnemius m, medial head

Popliteal vessels

Medial femoral condyle

Lateral femoral condyle

Popliteus m

Sartorius t

Biceps femoris t

Gracilis t

Lateral tibial plateau

Fibular head

Semimembranosus t

Peroneus longus m

Semitendinosus t

Tibialis posterior m

Popliteus m

Medial tibial plateau

Gastrocnemius m, medial head

Figure 21.3.17

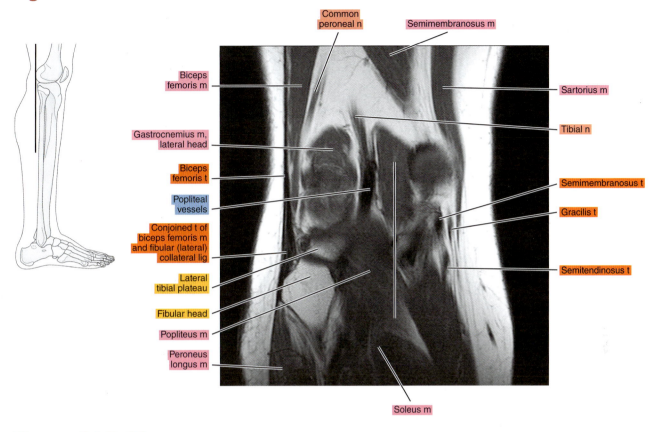

Common peroneal n

Semimembranosus m

Biceps femoris m

Sartorius m

Gastrocnemius m, lateral head

Tibial n

Biceps femoris t

Popliteal vessels

Semimembranosus t

Gracilis t

Conjoined t of biceps femoris m and fibular (lateral) collateral lig

Lateral tibial plateau

Semitendinosus t

Fibular head

Popliteus m

Peroneus longus m

Soleus m

Figure 21.3.18

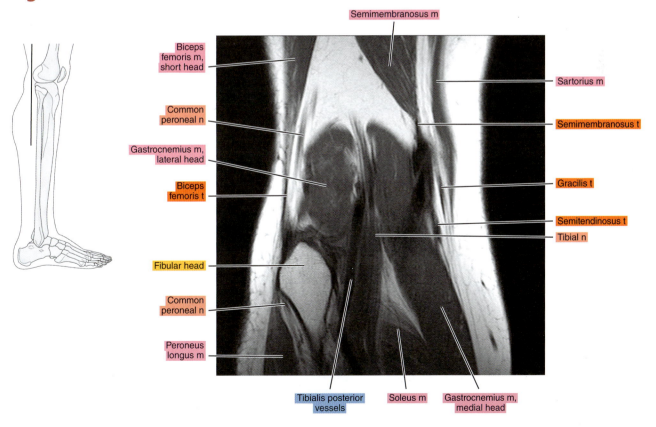

Semimembranosus m

Biceps femoris m, short head

Sartorius m

Common peroneal n

Semimembranosus t

Gastrocnemius m, lateral head

Biceps femoris t

Gracilis t

Semitendinosus t

Tibial n

Fibular head

Common peroneal n

Peroneus longus m

Tibialis posterior vessels

Soleus m

Gastrocnemius m, medial head

Figure 21.3.19

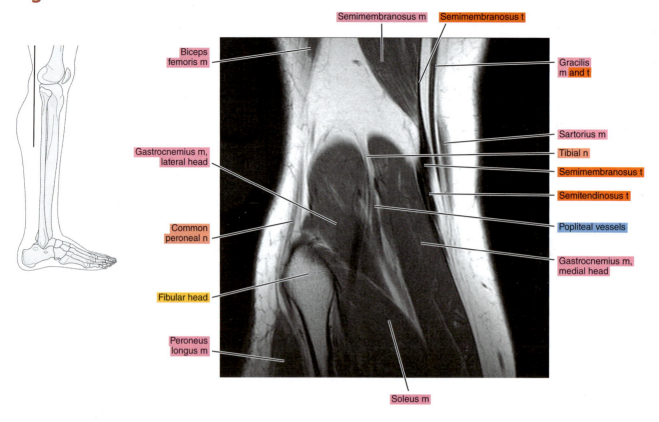

Semimembranosus m

Semimembranosus t

Biceps femoris m

Gracilis m and t

Gastrocnemius m, lateral head

Sartorius m

Tibial n

Semimembranosus t

Semitendinosus t

Common peroneal n

Popliteal vessels

Gastrocnemius m, medial head

Fibular head

Peroneus longus m

Soleus m

Chapter

22

MRI of the Leg

AXIAL
Figure 22.1.1

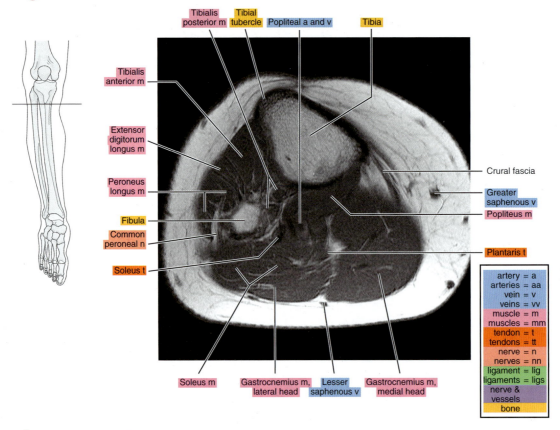

Tibialis posterior m | Tibial tubercle | Popliteal a and v | Tibia

Tibialis anterior m

Extensor digitorum longus m

Peroneus longus m

Fibula

Common peroneal n

Soleus t

Crural fascia

Greater saphenous v

Popliteus m

Plantaris t

Soleus m | Gastrocnemius m, lateral head | Lesser saphenous v | Gastrocnemius m, medial head

artery = a
arteries = aa
vein = v
veins = vv
muscle = m
muscles = mm
tendon = t
tendons = tt
nerve = n
nerves = nn
ligament = lig
ligaments = ligs
nerve & vessels
bone

Figure 22.1.2

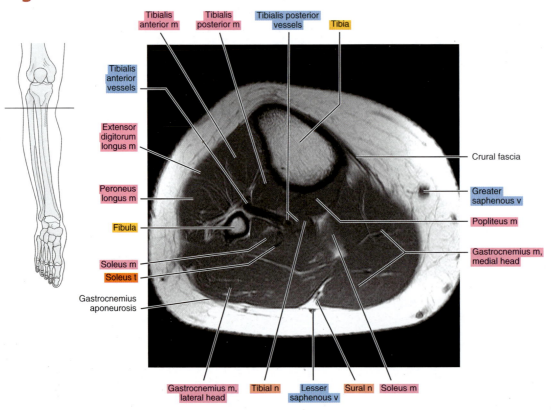

Tibialis anterior m | Tibialis posterior m | Tibialis posterior vessels | Tibia

Tibialis anterior vessels

Extensor digitorum longus m

Peroneus longus m

Fibula

Soleus m

Soleus t

Gastrocnemius aponeurosis

Crural fascia

Greater saphenous v

Popliteus m

Gastrocnemius m, medial head

Gastrocnemius m, lateral head | Tibial n | Lesser saphenous v | Sural n | Soleus m

Figure 22.1.3

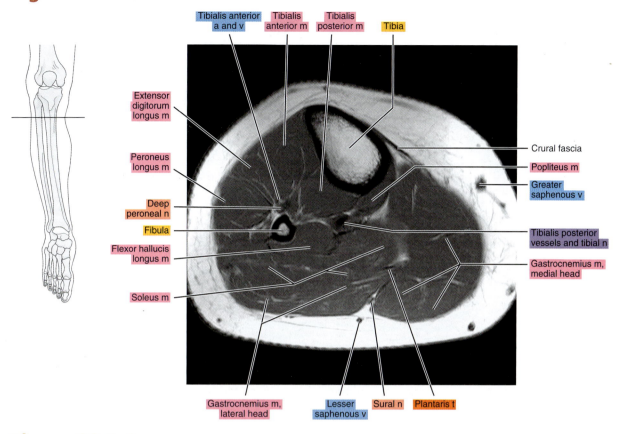

Tibialis anterior a and v

Tibialis anterior m

Tibialis posterior m

Tibia

Extensor digitorum longus m

Peroneus longus m

Deep peroneal n

Fibula

Flexor hallucis longus m

Soleus m

Crural fascia

Popliteus m

Greater saphenous v

Tibialis posterior vessels and tibial n

Gastrocnemius m, medial head

Gastrocnemius m, lateral head

Lesser saphenous v

Sural n

Plantaris t

Figure 22.1.4

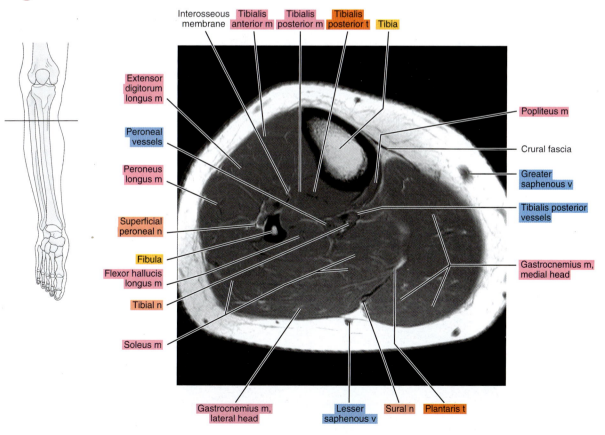

Interosseous membrane

Tibialis anterior m

Tibialis posterior m

Tibialis posterior t

Tibia

Extensor digitorum longus m

Peroneal vessels

Peroneus longus m

Superficial peroneal n

Fibula

Flexor hallucis longus m

Tibial n

Soleus m

Popliteus m

Crural fascia

Greater saphenous v

Tibialis posterior vessels

Gastrocnemius m, medial head

Gastrocnemius m, lateral head

Lesser saphenous v

Sural n

Plantaris t

Figure 22.1.5

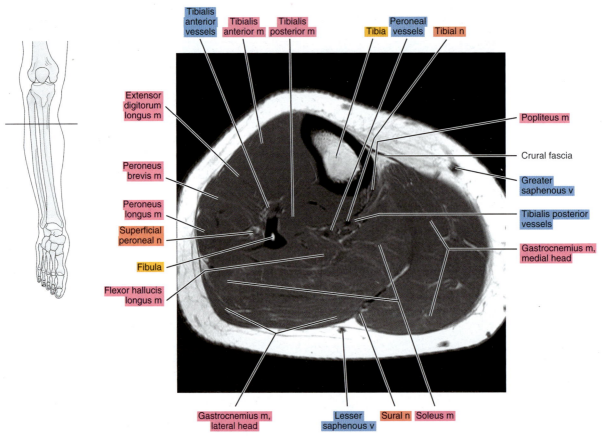

Tibialis anterior vessels
Tibialis anterior m
Tibialis posterior m
Tibia
Peroneal vessels
Tibial n

Extensor digitorum longus m
Peroneus brevis m
Peroneus longus m
Superficial peroneal n
Fibula
Flexor hallucis longus m

Popliteus m
Crural fascia
Greater saphenous v
Tibialis posterior vessels
Gastrocnemius m, medial head

Gastrocnemius m, lateral head
Lesser saphenous v
Sural n
Soleus m

Figure 22.1.6

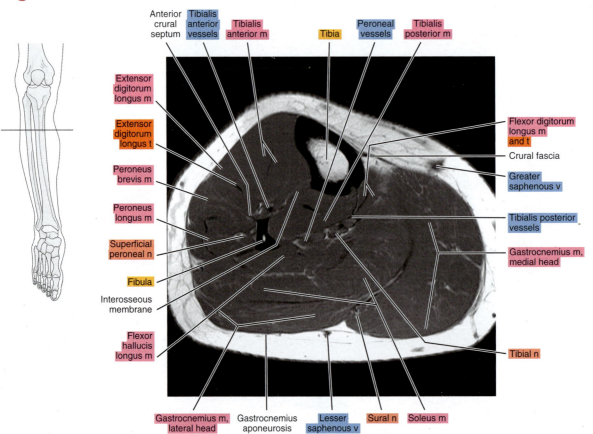

Anterior crural septum
Tibialis anterior vessels
Tibialis anterior m
Tibia
Peroneal vessels
Tibialis posterior m

Extensor digitorum longus m
Extensor digitorum longus t
Peroneus brevis m
Peroneus longus m
Superficial peroneal n
Fibula
Interosseous membrane
Flexor hallucis longus m

Flexor digitorum longus m and t
Crural fascia
Greater saphenous v
Tibialis posterior vessels
Gastrocnemius m, medial head
Tibial n

Gastrocnemius m, lateral head
Gastrocnemius aponeurosis
Lesser saphenous v
Sural n
Soleus m

Figure 22.1.7

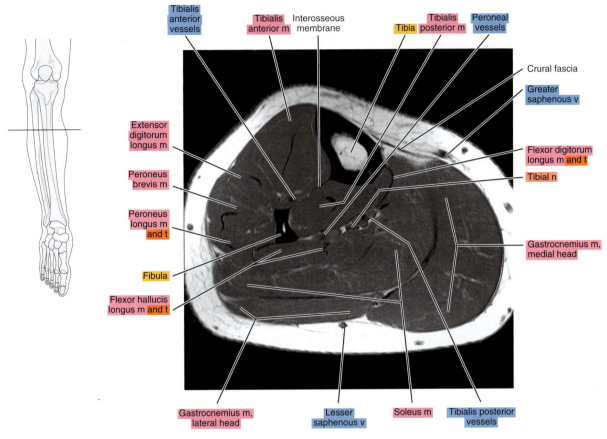

Tibialis anterior vessels

Tibialis anterior m

Interosseous membrane

Tibia

Tibialis posterior m

Peroneal vessels

Crural fascia

Greater saphenous v

Extensor digitorum longus m

Peroneus brevis m

Peroneus longus m and t

Fibula

Flexor hallucis longus m and t

Flexor digitorum longus m and t

Tibial n

Gastrocnemius m, medial head

Gastrocnemius m, lateral head

Lesser saphenous v

Soleus m

Tibialis posterior vessels

Figure 22.1.8

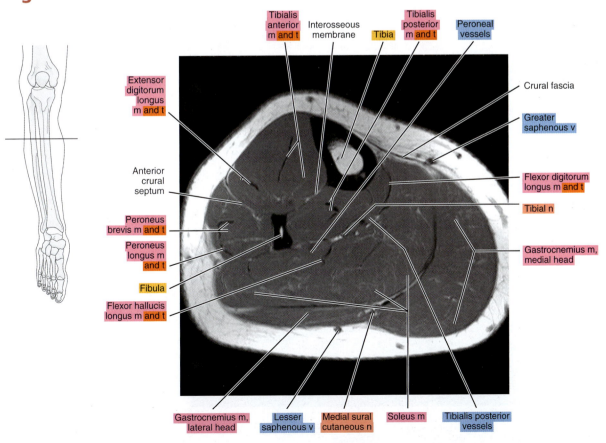

Tibialis anterior m and t

Interosseous membrane

Tibia

Tibialis posterior m and t

Peroneal vessels

Crural fascia

Extensor digitorum longus m and t

Greater saphenous v

Anterior crural septum

Peroneus brevis m and t

Peroneus longus m and t

Fibula

Flexor hallucis longus m and t

Flexor digitorum longus m and t

Tibial n

Gastrocnemius m, medial head

Gastrocnemius m, lateral head

Lesser saphenous v

Medial sural cutaneous n

Soleus m

Tibialis posterior vessels

Figure 22.1.9

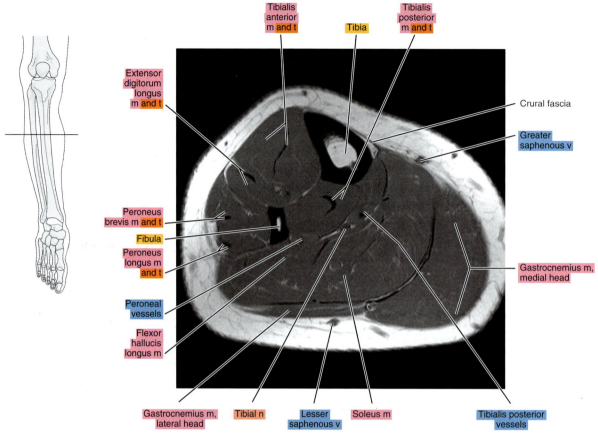

Tibialis anterior m and t
Tibia
Tibialis posterior m and t
Extensor digitorum longus m and t
Crural fascia
Greater saphenous v
Peroneus brevis m and t
Fibula
Peroneus longus m and t
Peroneal vessels
Flexor hallucis longus m
Gastrocnemius m, medial head
Gastrocnemius m, lateral head
Tibial n
Lesser saphenous v
Soleus m
Tibialis posterior vessels

Figure 22.1.10

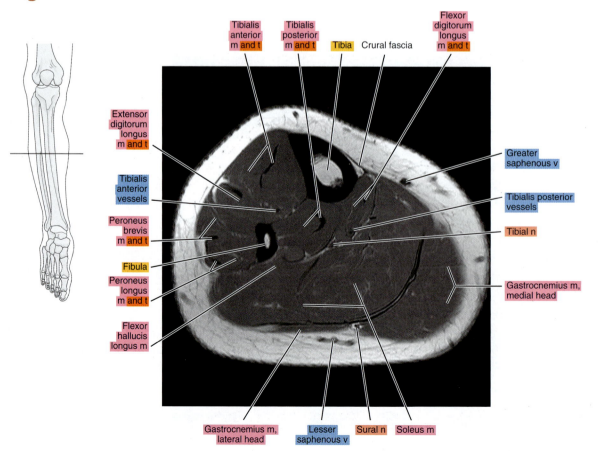

Tibialis anterior m and t
Tibialis posterior m and t
Tibia
Crural fascia
Flexor digitorum longus m and t
Extensor digitorum longus m and t
Greater saphenous v
Tibialis anterior vessels
Tibialis posterior vessels
Peroneus brevis m and t
Tibial n
Fibula
Peroneus longus m and t
Gastrocnemius m, medial head
Flexor hallucis longus m
Gastrocnemius m, lateral head
Lesser saphenous v
Sural n
Soleus m

Figure 22.1.11

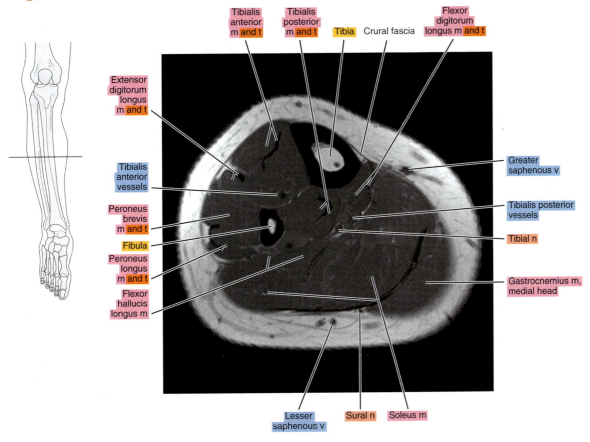

Tibialis anterior m and t

Tibialis posterior m and t

Tibia

Crural fascia

Flexor digitorum longus m and t

Extensor digitorum longus m and t

Tibialis anterior vessels

Peroneus brevis m and t

Fibula

Peroneus longus m and t

Flexor hallucis longus m

Greater saphenous v

Tibialis posterior vessels

Tibial n

Gastrocnemius m, medial head

Lesser saphenous v

Sural n

Soleus m

Figure 22.1.12

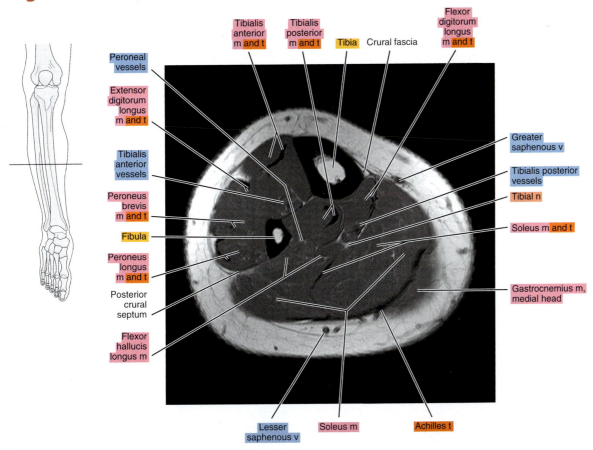

Tibialis anterior m and t

Tibialis posterior m and t

Tibia

Crural fascia

Flexor digitorum longus m and t

Peroneal vessels

Extensor digitorum longus m and t

Tibialis anterior vessels

Peroneus brevis m and t

Fibula

Peroneus longus m and t

Posterior crural septum

Flexor hallucis longus m

Greater saphenous v

Tibialis posterior vessels

Tibial n

Soleus m and t

Gastrocnemius m, medial head

Lesser saphenous v

Soleus m

Achilles t

Figure 22.1.13

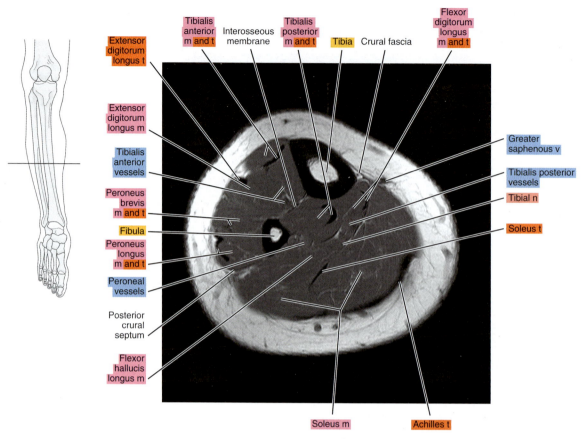

Extensor digitorum longus t

Extensor digitorum longus m

Tibialis anterior vessels

Peroneus brevis m and t

Fibula

Peroneus longus m and t

Peroneal vessels

Posterior crural septum

Flexor hallucis longus m

Tibialis anterior m and t

Interosseous membrane

Tibialis posterior m and t

Tibia

Crural fascia

Flexor digitorum longus m and t

Greater saphenous v

Tibialis posterior vessels

Tibial n

Soleus t

Soleus m

Achilles t

Figure 22.1.14

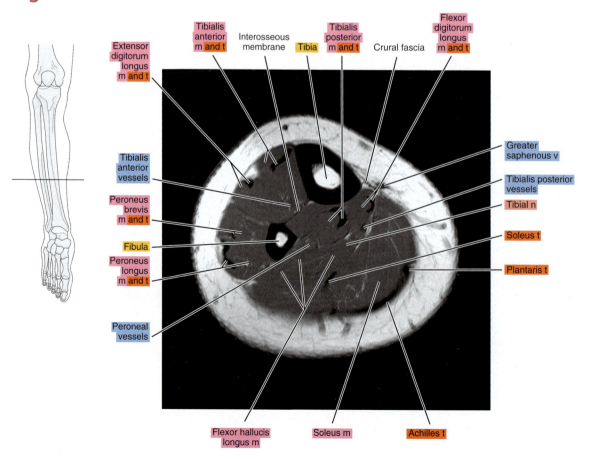

Extensor digitorum longus m and t

Tibialis anterior vessels

Peroneus brevis m and t

Fibula

Peroneus longus m and t

Peroneal vessels

Tibialis anterior m and t

Interosseous membrane

Tibia

Tibialis posterior m and t

Crural fascia

Flexor digitorum longus m and t

Greater saphenous v

Tibialis posterior vessels

Tibial n

Soleus t

Plantaris t

Flexor hallucis longus m

Soleus m

Achilles t

Figure 22.1.15

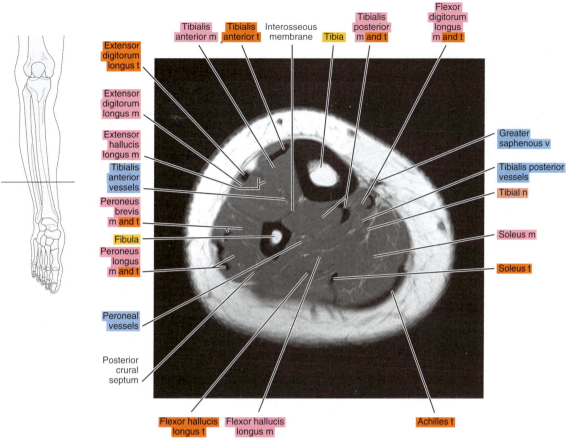

Extensor digitorum longus t

Extensor digitorum longus m

Extensor hallucis longus m

Tibialis anterior vessels

Peroneus brevis m and t

Fibula

Peroneus longus m and t

Peroneal vessels

Posterior crural septum

Tibialis anterior m

Tibialis anterior t

Interosseous membrane

Tibia

Tibialis posterior m and t

Flexor digitorum longus m and t

Greater saphenous v

Tibialis posterior vessels

Tibial n

Soleus m

Soleus t

Flexor hallucis longus t

Flexor hallucis longus m

Achilles t

Figure 22.1.16

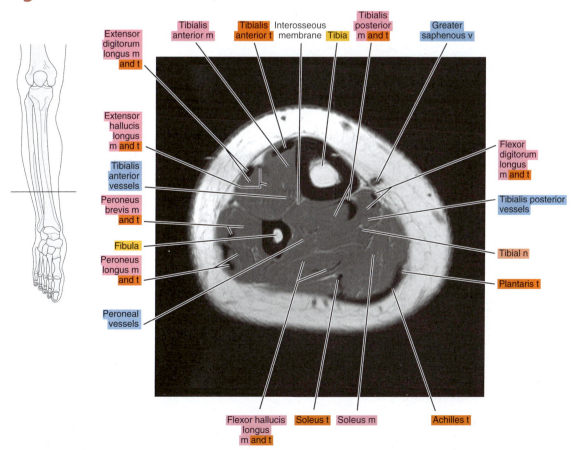

Extensor digitorum longus m and t

Extensor hallucis longus m and t

Tibialis anterior vessels

Peroneus brevis m and t

Fibula

Peroneus longus m and t

Peroneal vessels

Tibialis anterior m

Tibialis anterior t

Interosseous membrane

Tibia

Tibialis posterior m and t

Greater saphenous v

Flexor digitorum longus m and t

Tibialis posterior vessels

Tibial n

Plantaris t

Flexor hallucis longus m and t

Soleus t

Soleus m

Achilles t

Figure 22.1.17

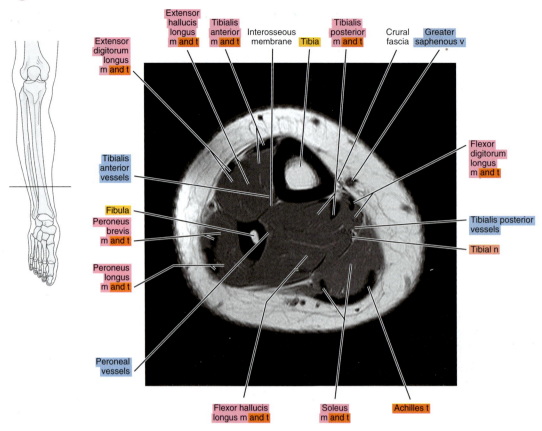

Extensor hallucis longus m and t
Tibialis anterior m and t
Interosseous membrane
Tibia
Tibialis posterior m and t
Crural fascia
Greater saphenous v
Extensor digitorum longus m and t
Tibialis anterior vessels
Fibula
Peroneus brevis m and t
Peroneus longus m and t
Peroneal vessels
Flexor digitorum longus m and t
Tibialis posterior vessels
Tibial n
Flexor hallucis longus m and t
Soleus m and t
Achilles t

Figure 22.1.18

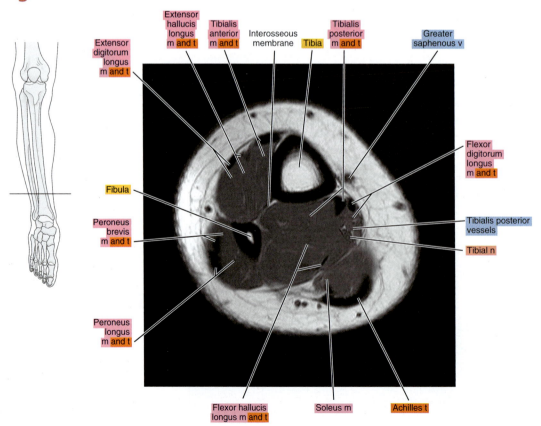

Extensor hallucis longus m and t
Tibialis anterior m and t
Interosseous membrane
Tibia
Tibialis posterior m and t
Greater saphenous v
Extensor digitorum longus m and t
Fibula
Peroneus brevis m and t
Peroneus longus m and t
Flexor digitorum longus m and t
Tibialis posterior vessels
Tibial n
Flexor hallucis longus m and t
Soleus m
Achilles t

Figure 22.1.19

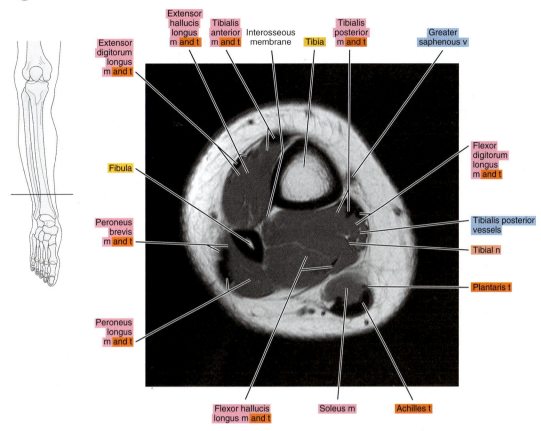

Extensor digitorum longus m and t · Extensor hallucis longus m and t · Tibialis anterior m and t · Interosseous membrane · Tibia · Tibialis posterior m and t · Greater saphenous v · Flexor digitorum longus m and t · Fibula · Tibialis posterior vessels · Tibial n · Peroneus brevis m and t · Plantaris t · Peroneus longus m and t · Flexor hallucis longus m and t · Soleus m · Achilles t

Figure 22.1.20

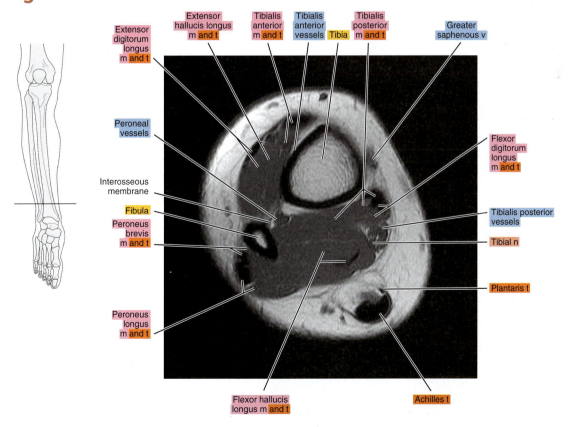

Extensor digitorum longus m and t · Extensor hallucis longus m and t · Tibialis anterior m and t · Tibialis anterior vessels · Tibia · Tibialis posterior m and t · Greater saphenous v · Peroneal vessels · Flexor digitorum longus m and t · Interosseous membrane · Fibula · Tibialis posterior vessels · Peroneus brevis m and t · Tibial n · Plantaris t · Peroneus longus m and t · Flexor hallucis longus m and t · Achilles t

SAGITTAL
Figure 22.2.1

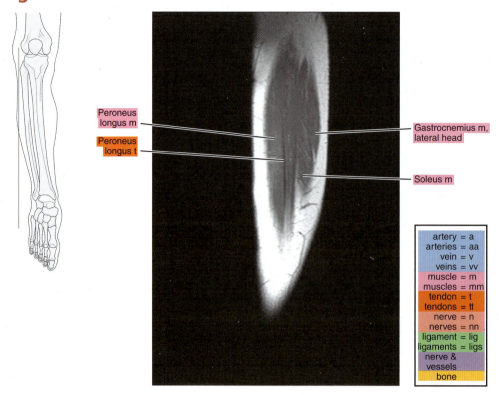

Peroneus longus m

Peroneus longus t

Gastrocnemius m, lateral head

Soleus m

artery	= a
arteries	= aa
vein	= v
veins	= vv
muscle	= m
muscles	= mm
tendon	= t
tendons	= tt
nerve	= n
nerves	= nn
ligament	= lig
ligaments	= ligs
nerve & vessels	
bone	

Figure 22.2.2

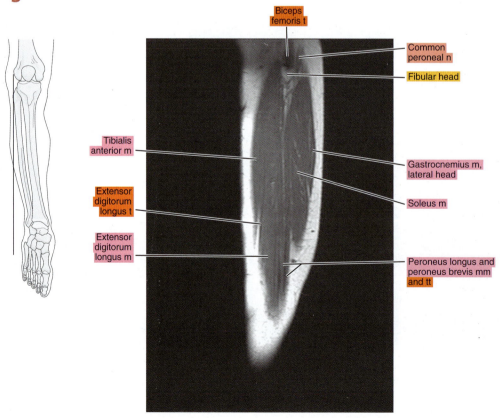

Biceps femoris t

Common peroneal n

Fibular head

Tibialis anterior m

Gastrocnemius m, lateral head

Extensor digitorum longus t

Soleus m

Extensor digitorum longus m

Peroneus longus and peroneus brevis mm and tt

Figure 22.2.3

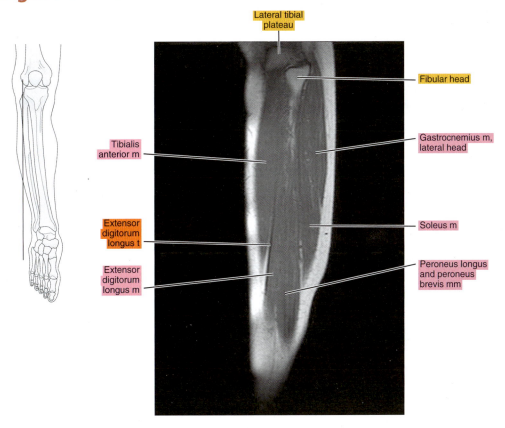

Lateral tibial plateau

Fibular head

Tibialis anterior m

Gastrocnemius m, lateral head

Extensor digitorum longus t

Soleus m

Extensor digitorum longus m

Peroneus longus and peroneus brevis mm

Figure 22.2.4

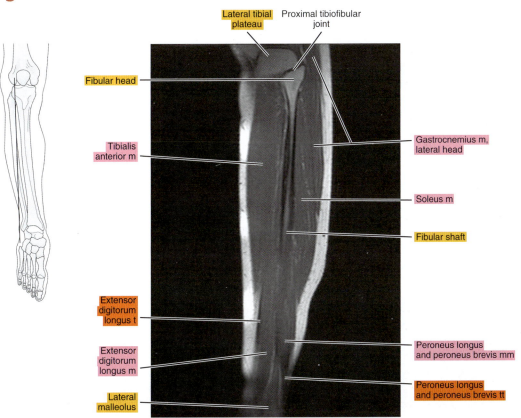

Lateral tibial plateau

Proximal tibiofibular joint

Fibular head

Tibialis anterior m

Gastrocnemius m, lateral head

Soleus m

Fibular shaft

Extensor digitorum longus t

Extensor digitorum longus m

Peroneus longus and peroneus brevis mm

Peroneus longus and peroneus brevis tt

Lateral malleolus

Figure 22.2.5

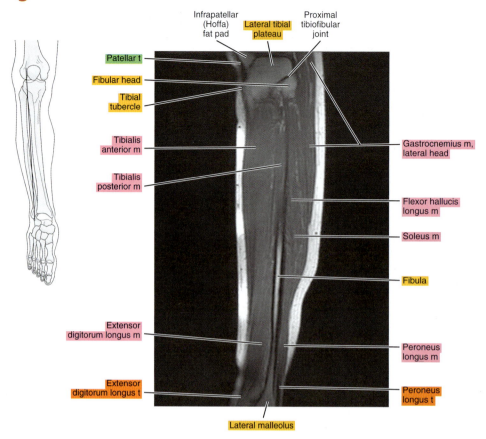

Infrapatellar (Hoffa) fat pad

Lateral tibial plateau

Proximal tibiofibular joint

Patellar t

Fibular head

Tibial tubercle

Tibialis anterior m

Tibialis posterior m

Gastrocnemius m, lateral head

Flexor hallucis longus m

Soleus m

Fibula

Extensor digitorum longus m

Extensor digitorum longus t

Peroneus longus m

Peroneus longus t

Lateral malleolus

Figure 22.2.6

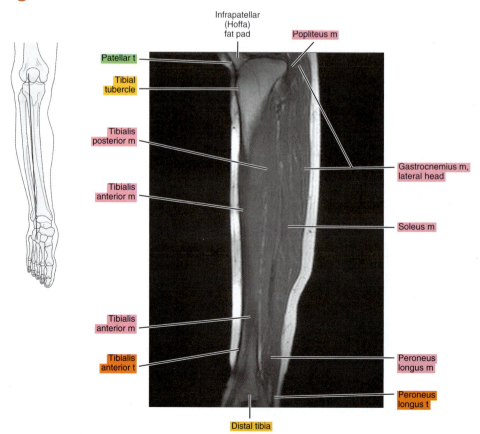

Infrapatellar (Hoffa) fat pad

Popliteus m

Patellar t

Tibial tubercle

Tibialis posterior m

Tibialis anterior m

Gastrocnemius m, lateral head

Soleus m

Tibialis anterior m

Tibialis anterior t

Peroneus longus m

Peroneus longus t

Distal tibia

Figure 22.2.7

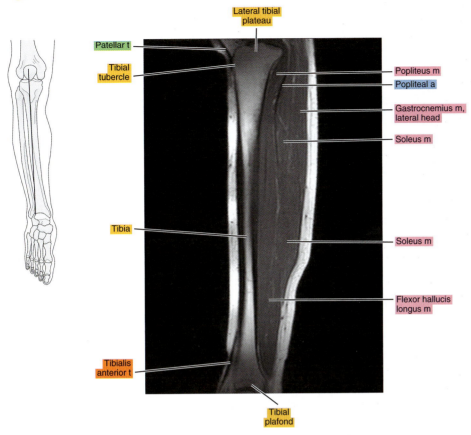

Lateral tibial plateau

Patellar t

Tibial tubercle

Popliteus m

Popliteal a

Gastrocnemius m, lateral head

Soleus m

Tibia

Soleus m

Flexor hallucis longus m

Tibialis anterior t

Tibial plafond

Figure 22.2.8

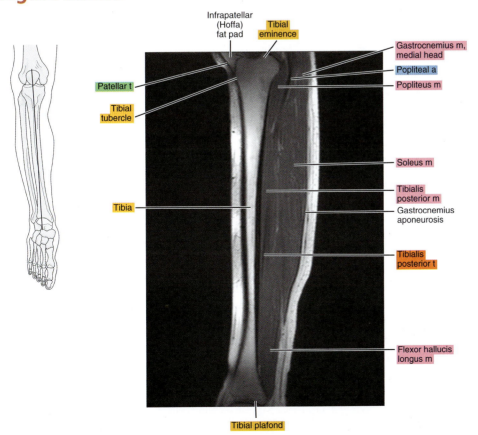

Infrapatellar (Hoffa) fat pad

Tibial eminence

Gastrocnemius m, medial head

Popliteal a

Patellar t

Popliteus m

Tibial tubercle

Soleus m

Tibialis posterior m

Gastrocnemius aponeurosis

Tibia

Tibialis posterior t

Flexor hallucis longus m

Tibial plafond

Figure 22.2.9

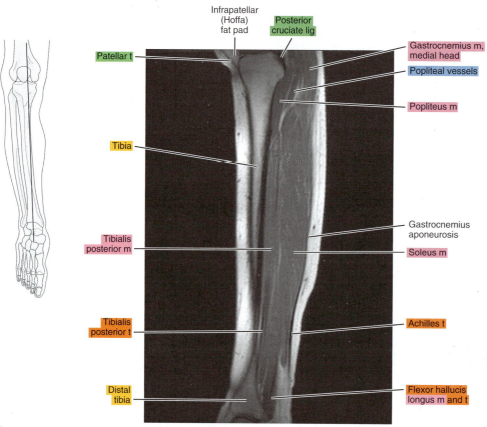

Infrapatellar (Hoffa) fat pad

Posterior cruciate lig

Patellar t

Gastrocnemius m, medial head

Popliteal vessels

Popliteus m

Tibia

Gastrocnemius aponeurosis

Tibialis posterior m

Soleus m

Tibialis posterior t

Achilles t

Distal tibia

Flexor hallucis longus m and t

Figure 22.2.10

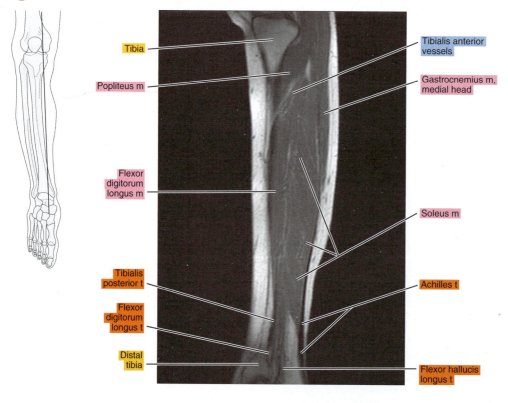

Tibia

Tibialis anterior vessels

Popliteus m

Gastrocnemius m, medial head

Flexor digitorum longus m

Soleus m

Tibialis posterior t

Achilles t

Flexor digitorum longus t

Distal tibia

Flexor hallucis longus t

Figure 22.2.11

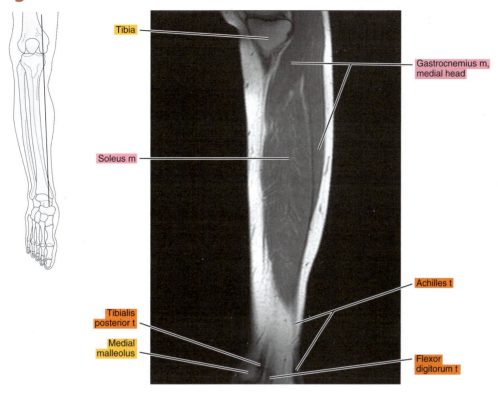

Tibia

Gastrocnemius m, medial head

Soleus m

Achilles t

Tibialis posterior t

Medial malleolus

Flexor digitorum t

Figure 22.2.12

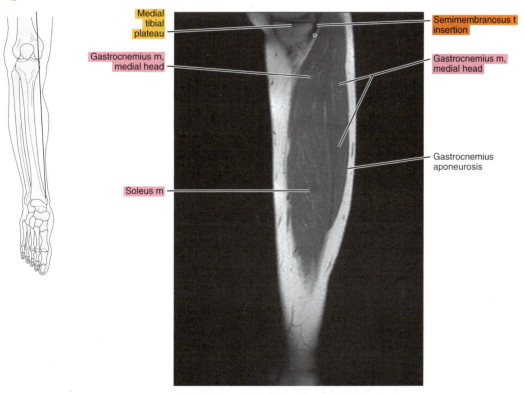

Medial tibial plateau

Semimembranosus t insertion

Gastrocnemius m, medial head

Gastrocnemius m, medial head

Gastrocnemius aponeurosis

Soleus m

Figure 22.2.13

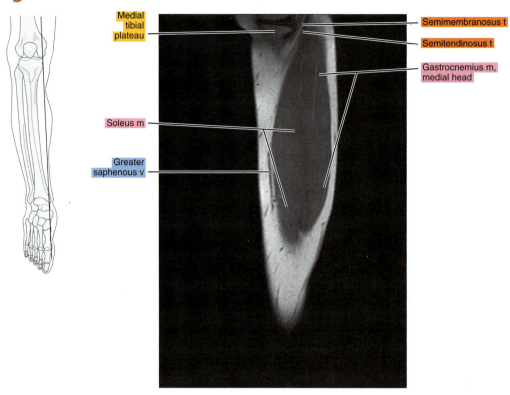

Medial tibial plateau

Semimembranosus t

Semitendinosus t

Gastrocnemius m, medial head

Soleus m

Greater saphenous v

Figure 22.2.14

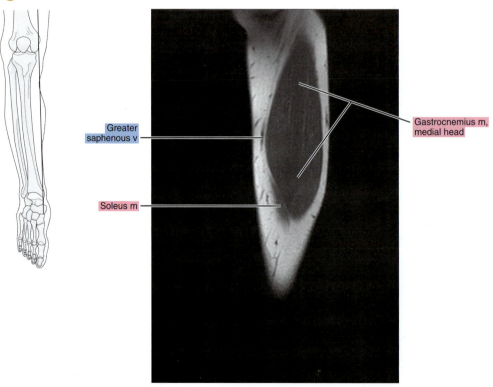

Greater saphenous v

Gastrocnemius m, medial head

Soleus m

Figure 22.2.15

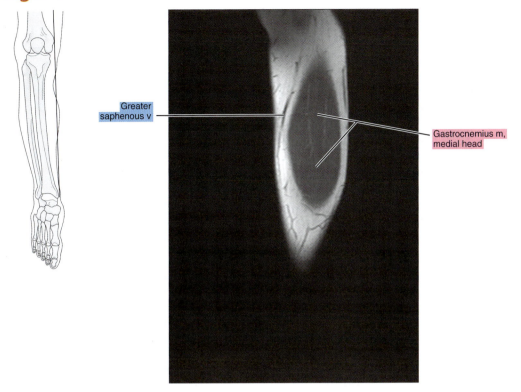

Greater saphenous v

Gastrocnemius m, medial head

CORONAL
Figure 22.3.1

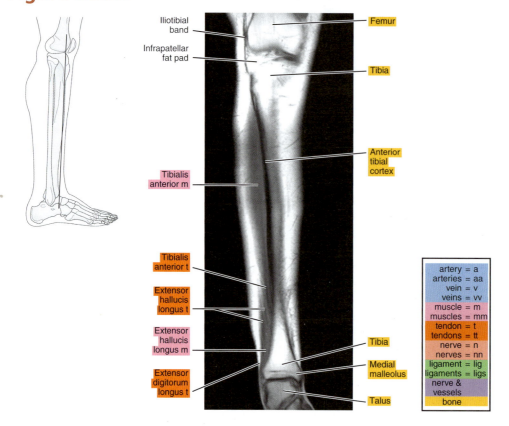

Iliotibial band

Infrapatellar fat pad

Tibialis anterior m

Tibialis anterior t

Extensor hallucis longus t

Extensor hallucis longus m

Extensor digitorum longus t

Femur

Tibia

Anterior tibial cortex

Tibia

Medial malleolus

Talus

artery	= a
arteries	= aa
vein	= v
veins	= vv
muscle	= m
muscles	= mm
tendon	= t
tendons	= tt
nerve	= n
nerves	= nn
ligament	= lig
ligaments	= ligs
nerve & vessels	
bone	

Figure 22.3.2

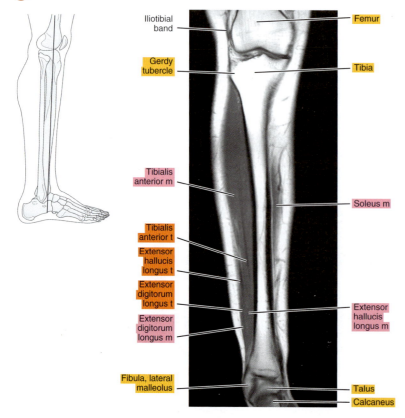

Iliotibial band

Gerdy tubercle

Tibialis anterior m

Tibialis anterior t

Extensor hallucis longus t

Extensor digitorum longus t

Extensor digitorum longus m

Fibula, lateral malleolus

Femur

Tibia

Soleus m

Extensor hallucis longus m

Talus

Calcaneus

Figure 22.3.3

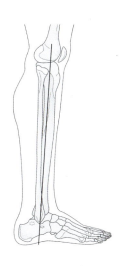

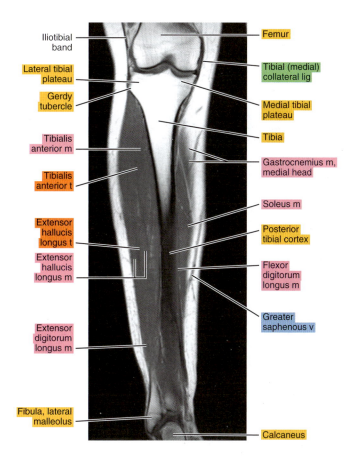

Iliotibial band

Femur

Lateral tibial plateau

Tibial (medial) collateral lig

Gerdy tubercle

Medial tibial plateau

Tibialis anterior m

Tibia

Tibialis anterior t

Gastrocnemius m, medial head

Extensor hallucis longus t

Soleus m

Extensor hallucis longus m

Posterior tibial cortex

Flexor digitorum longus m

Extensor digitorum longus m

Greater saphenous v

Fibula, lateral malleolus

Calcaneus

Figure 22.3.4

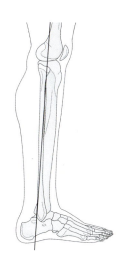

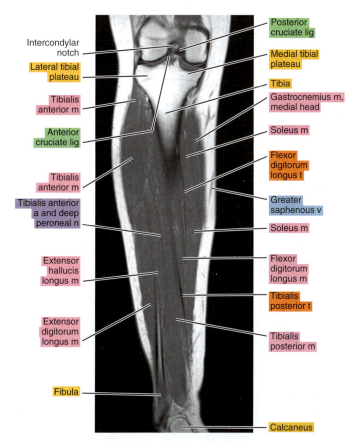

Intercondylar notch

Posterior cruciate lig

Lateral tibial plateau

Medial tibial plateau

Tibialis anterior m

Tibia

Gastrocnemius m, medial head

Anterior cruciate lig

Soleus m

Flexor digitorum longus t

Tibialis anterior m

Greater saphenous v

Tibialis anterior a and deep peroneal n

Soleus m

Extensor hallucis longus m

Flexor digitorum longus m

Tibialis posterior t

Extensor digitorum longus m

Tibialis posterior m

Fibula

Calcaneus

Figure 22.3.5

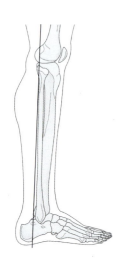

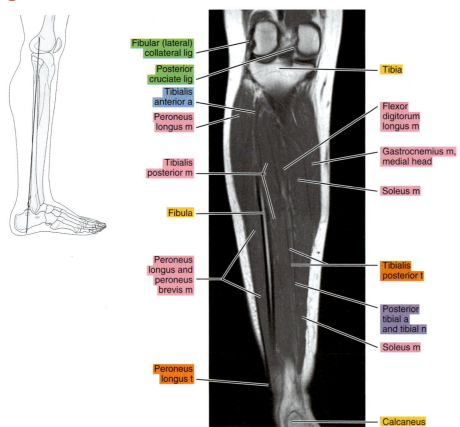

Fibular (lateral) collateral lig

Posterior cruciate lig

Tibialis anterior a

Peroneus longus m

Tibialis posterior m

Fibula

Peroneus longus and peroneus brevis m

Peroneus longus t

Tibia

Flexor digitorum longus m

Gastrocnemius m, medial head

Soleus m

Tibialis posterior t

Posterior tibial a and tibial n

Soleus m

Calcaneus

Figure 22.3.6

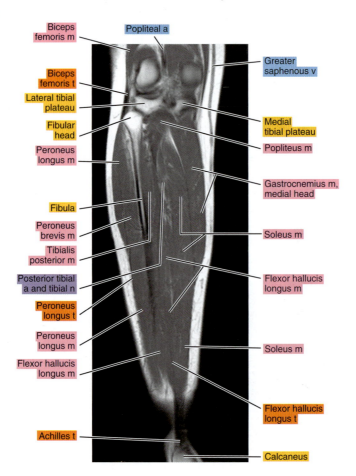

Biceps femoris m

Biceps femoris t

Lateral tibial plateau

Fibular head

Peroneus longus m

Fibula

Peroneus brevis m

Tibialis posterior m

Posterior tibial a and tibial n

Peroneus longus t

Peroneus longus m

Flexor hallucis longus m

Achilles t

Popliteal a

Greater saphenous v

Medial tibial plateau

Popliteus m

Gastrocnemius m, medial head

Soleus m

Flexor hallucis longus m

Soleus m

Flexor hallucis longus t

Calcaneus

Figure 22.3.7

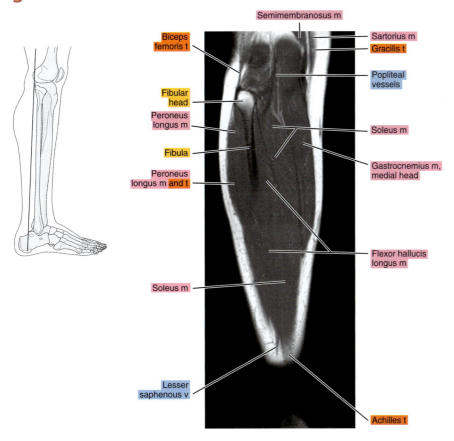

Semimembranosus m

Biceps femoris t

Sartorius m

Gracilis t

Popliteal vessels

Fibular head

Peroneus longus m

Soleus m

Fibula

Gastrocnemius m, medial head

Peroneus longus m and t

Flexor hallucis longus m

Soleus m

Lesser saphenous v

Achilles t

Figure 22.3.8

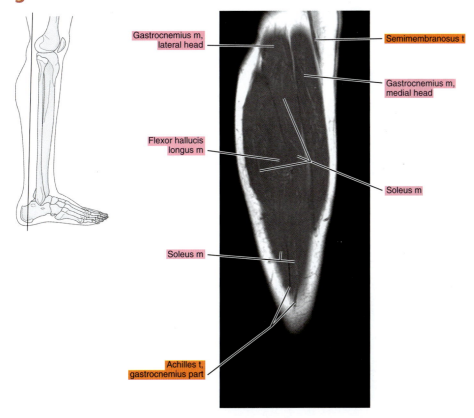

Gastrocnemius m, lateral head

Semimembranosus t

Gastrocnemius m, medial head

Flexor hallucis longus m

Soleus m

Soleus m

Achilles t, gastrocnemius part

Figure 22.3.9

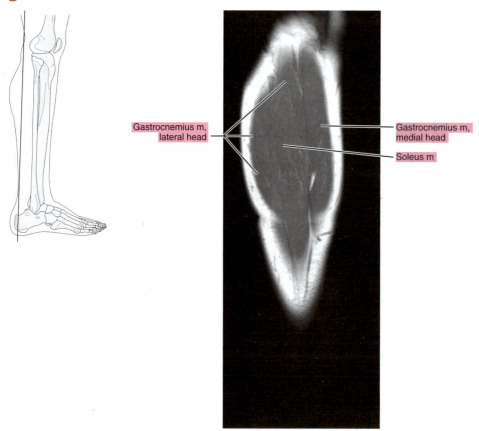

Gastrocnemius m, lateral head

Gastrocnemius m, medial head

Soleus m

Figure 22.3.10

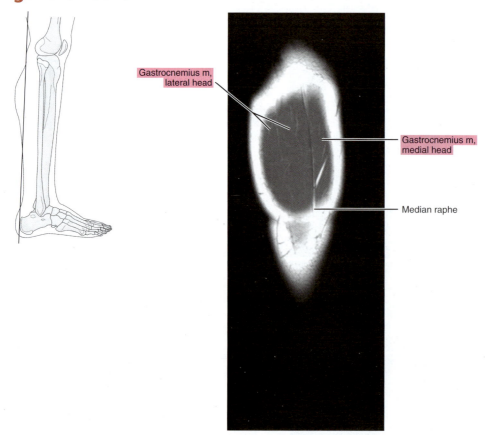

Gastrocnemius m, lateral head

Gastrocnemius m, medial head

Median raphe

Figure 22.3.11

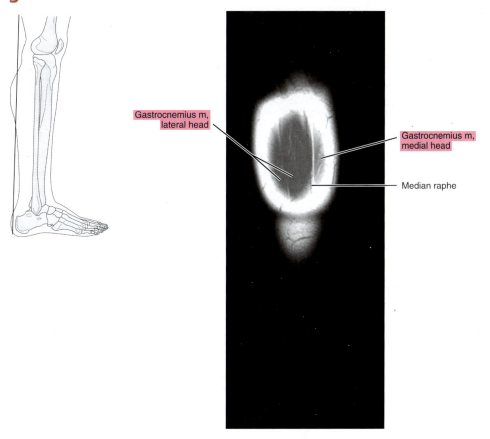

Gastrocnemius m, lateral head

Gastrocnemius m, medial head

Median raphe

Table 22-1. Muscles of the Leg

MUSCLE	ORIGIN	INSERTION	NERVE SUPPLY
Tibialis anterior	Distal part of the lateral condyle of the tibia, lateral surface of the proximal half of the shaft of the tibia, adjacent interosseous membrane, overlying fascia near the condyle of the tibia, and intermuscular septum between it and the extensor digitorum longus	Medial surface of the first cuneiform and the base of the first metatarsal.	Branch from the common peroneal and another from the deep peroneal
Extensor digitorum longus	Lateral condyle of the tibia, anterior crest of the fibula intermuscular membrane between it and the tibialis anterior, lateral margin of the interosseous membrane, the septum between it and the peroneus longus, and fascia of the leg near the tibial origin	Each tendon, located on the dorsal surface of the toe to which it goes, divides into three fasciculi: the intermediate, attached to the dorsum of the base of the middle phalanx, and two lateral, which converge to the dorsum of the base on the distal phalanx. The margins of each tendon are bound to the sides of the back of the proximal phalanx.	By two branches of the deep peroneal
Peroneus tertius	Distal one-third of the anterior surface of the fibula, neighboring interosseous membrane, and anterior intermuscular septum	Onto the base of the fifth metatarsal and often onto the base of the fourth.	The more distal nerve to the extensor digitorum supplies this muscle (deep peroneal)
Extensor hallucis longus	Middle half of the anterior surface of the fibula near the interosseous crest and distal half of the interosseous membrane	At the base of the dorsal aspect of the great toe.	Deep peroneal
Peroneus longus	Proximal two-thirds of the lateral surface of the fibula	Inferior surface of the first cuneiform and on the adjacent part of the inferolateral border and the base of the first metatarsal.	Usually, the common peroneal, sometimes partially by superficial peroneal
Peroneus brevis	Middle one-third of the lateral surface of the fibula, from the septum that separates it from the anterior and posterior groups of muscles	Dorsal aspect of the tuberosity of the fifth metatarsal.	Superficial peroneal or a branch to peroneus longus
Popliteus	Facet at the anterior end of the groove on the lateral aspect of the femoral condyle	Proximal lip of the popliteal line of the tibia and the shaft of the tibia proximal to this line.	Tibial: a branch that arises independently or with the nerve to the posterior tibial muscle
Flexor digitorum longus	Popliteal line, medial side of the second quarter of the dorsal surface of the tibia, fibrous septum between the muscle and the tibialis fascia posterior, and covering its proximal extremity	Onto the bases of the terminal phalanges of the second to fourth toes.	Tibial: in company with nerves to other muscles of this group

Table 22-1. Muscles of the Leg

MUSCLE	ORIGIN	INSERTION	NERVE SUPPLY
Flexor hallucis longus	Distal two-thirds of the posterior surface of the fibula, the septa between it and the tibialis posterior, and peroneal muscles	Onto the base of the terminal phalanx of the great toe.	Tibial: often in company with the nerve to the flexor digitorum longus or other muscles of this group
Tibialis posterior	Lateral half of the popliteal line and lateral half of the middle one-third of the posterior surface of the tibia, medial side of the head and part of the body of the fibula next to the interosseous membrane in the proximal two-thirds, the entire proximal and lateral portion of the lateral part of the posterior surface of the interosseous membrane, and the septum between its proximal portion and the long flexor muscles	The tendon divides into two parts: the deep part becomes attached primarily to the tubercle of the navicular bone and usually to the first cuneiform; the superficial part attaches to the third cuneiform and the base of the fourth metatarsal, and also, in part, to the second cuneiform, to the capsule of the naviculocuneiform joint, to the sulcus of the cuboid, and usually also to the origin of the short flexor of the big toe and base of the second metatarsal; slip may extend to other structures.	Tibial: in company with nerves to other muscles of this group
	Medial head: posterior surface of the medial condyle of the femur above the articular surface; lateral head: a facet on the proximal part of the posterolateral surface of the lateral condyle of the femur	Via the Achilles tendon onto the posterior surface of the calcaneus.	Sciatic, tibial part
Soleus	By a fibular head from the back of the head and the proximal one-third of the posterior surface of the shaft of the fibula; intermuscular septum between it and the peroneus longus, by a tibial head from the popliteal line and the middle one-third of the medial border of the tibia	Via the calcaneal tendon onto the posterior surface of the calcaneus.	Sciatic, tibial part
Plantaris	Distal part of the lateral line of the bifurcation of the linea aspera, in close association with the lateral head of the gastrocnemius	Via a flat narrow tendon running along the medial edge of the Achilles tendon to the posterior surface of the calcaneus.	Sciatic, tibial part

Chapter 23

MRI of the Ankle

AXIAL
Figure 23.1.1

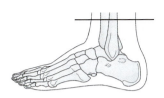

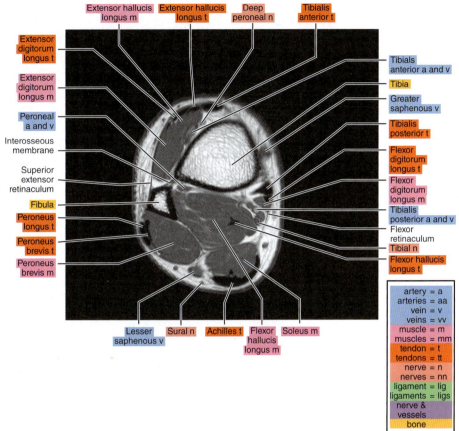

Extensor hallucis longus m

Extensor hallucis longus t

Deep peroneal n

Tibialis anterior t

Extensor digitorum longus t

Extensor digitorum longus m

Peroneal a and v

Interosseous membrane

Superior extensor retinaculum

Fibula

Peroneus longus t

Peroneus brevis t

Peroneus brevis m

Tibials anterior a and v

Tibia

Greater saphenous v

Tibialis posterior t

Flexor digitorum longus t

Flexor digitorum longus m

Tibialis posterior a and v

Flexor retinaculum

Tibial n

Flexor hallucis longus t

Lesser saphenous v

Sural n

Achilles t

Flexor hallucis longus m

Soleus m

artery = a	
arteries = aa	
vein = v	
veins = vv	
muscle = m	
muscles = mm	
tendon = t	
tendons = tt	
nerve = n	
nerves = nn	
ligament = lig	
ligaments = ligs	
nerve & vessels	
bone	

Figure 23.1.2

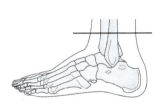

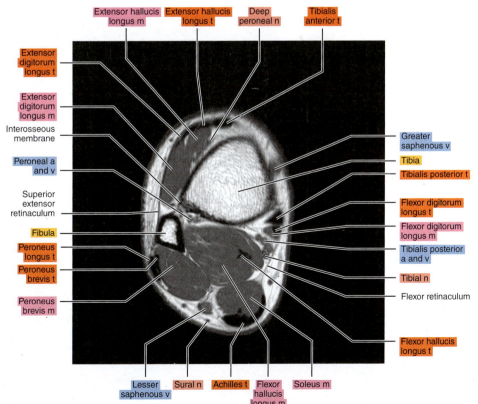

Extensor hallucis longus m

Extensor hallucis longus t

Deep peroneal n

Tibialis anterior t

Extensor digitorum longus t

Extensor digitorum longus m

Interosseous membrane

Peroneal a and v

Superior extensor retinaculum

Fibula

Peroneus longus t

Peroneus brevis t

Peroneus brevis m

Greater saphenous v

Tibia

Tibialis posterior t

Flexor digitorum longus t

Flexor digitorum longus m

Tibialis posterior a and v

Tibial n

Flexor retinaculum

Flexor hallucis longus t

Lesser saphenous v

Sural n

Achilles t

Flexor hallucis longus m

Soleus m

Figure 23.1.3

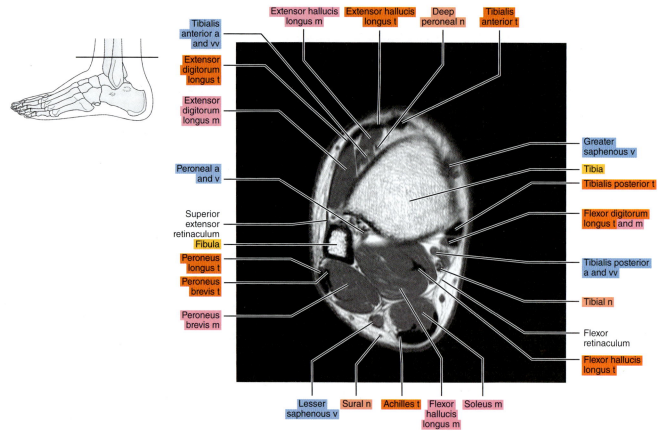

Figure 23.1.4

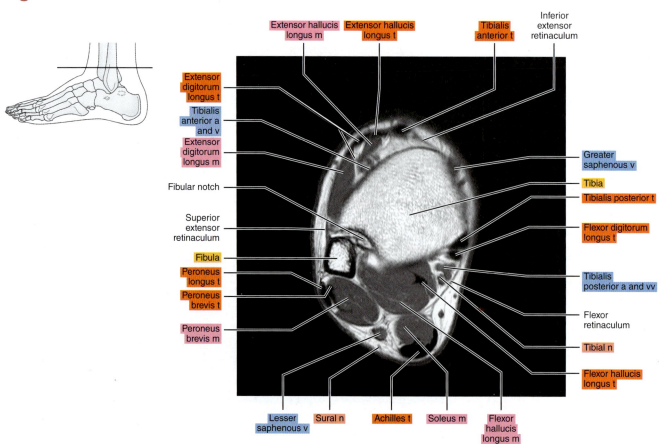

Figure 23.1.5

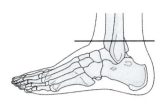

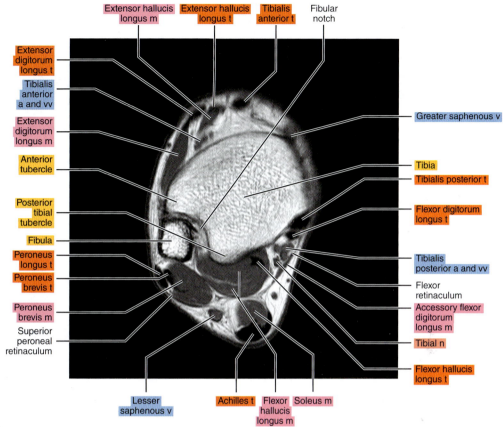

Extensor hallucis longus m
Extensor hallucis longus t
Tibialis anterior t
Fibular notch
Extensor digitorum longus t
Tibialis anterior a and vv
Extensor digitorum longus m
Anterior tubercle
Posterior tibial tubercle
Fibula
Peroneus longus t
Peroneus brevis t
Peroneus brevis m
Superior peroneal retinaculum
Greater saphenous v
Tibia
Tibialis posterior t
Flexor digitorum longus t
Tibialis posterior a and vv
Flexor retinaculum
Accessory flexor digitorum longus m
Tibial n
Flexor hallucis longus t
Lesser saphenous v
Achilles t
Flexor hallucis longus m
Soleus m

Figure 23.1.6

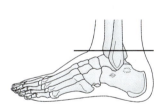

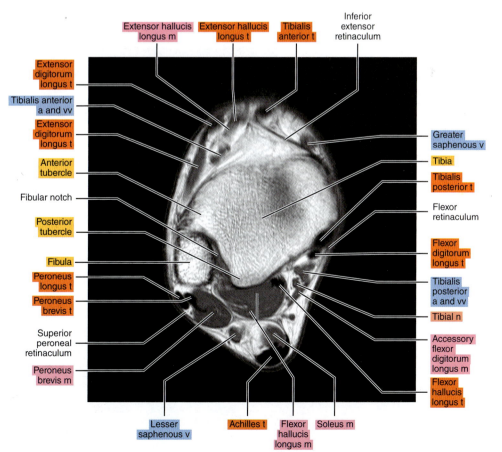

Extensor hallucis longus m
Extensor hallucis longus t
Tibialis anterior t
Inferior extensor retinaculum
Extensor digitorum longus t
Tibialis anterior a and vv
Extensor digitorum longus t
Anterior tubercle
Fibular notch
Posterior tubercle
Fibula
Peroneus longus t
Peroneus brevis t
Superior peroneal retinaculum
Peroneus brevis m
Greater saphenous v
Tibia
Tibialis posterior t
Flexor retinaculum
Flexor digitorum longus t
Tibialis posterior a and vv
Tibial n
Accessory flexor digitorum longus m
Flexor hallucis longus t
Lesser saphenous v
Achilles t
Flexor hallucis longus m
Soleus m

Figure 23.1.7

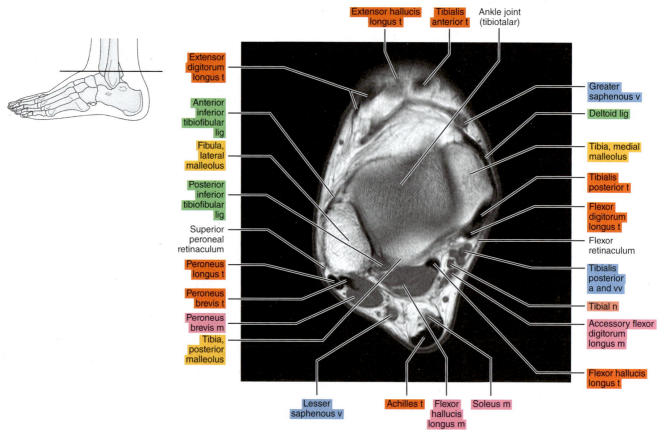

Extensor hallucis longus t

Tibialis anterior t

Ankle joint (tibiotalar)

Extensor digitorum longus t

Anterior inferior tibiofibular lig

Fibula, lateral malleolus

Posterior inferior tibiofibular lig

Superior peroneal retinaculum

Peroneus longus t

Peroneus brevis t

Peroneus brevis m

Tibia, posterior malleolus

Greater saphenous v

Deltoid lig

Tibia, medial malleolus

Tibialis posterior t

Flexor digitorum longus t

Flexor retinaculum

Tibialis posterior a and vv

Tibial n

Accessory flexor digitorum longus m

Flexor hallucis longus t

Lesser saphenous v

Achilles t

Flexor hallucis longus m

Soleus m

Figure 23.1.8

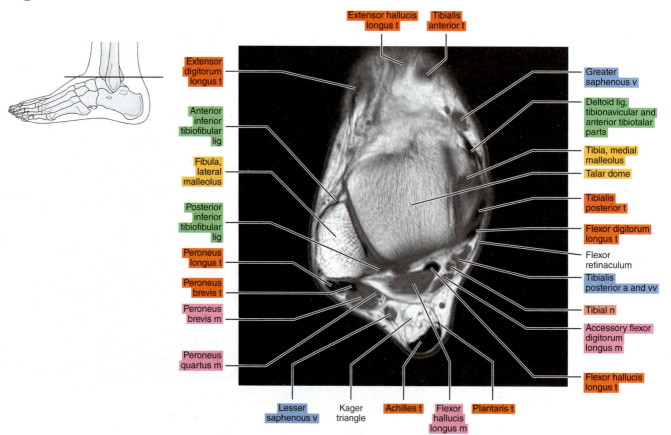

Extensor hallucis longus t

Tibialis anterior t

Extensor digitorum longus t

Anterior inferior tibiofibular lig

Fibula, lateral malleolus

Posterior inferior tibiofibular lig

Peroneus longus t

Peroneus brevis t

Peroneus brevis m

Peroneus quartus m

Greater saphenous v

Deltoid lig, tibionavicular and anterior tibiotalar parts

Tibia, medial malleolus

Talar dome

Tibialis posterior t

Flexor digitorum longus t

Flexor retinaculum

Tibialis posterior a and vv

Tibial n

Accessory flexor digitorum longus m

Flexor hallucis longus t

Lesser saphenous v

Kager triangle

Achilles t

Flexor hallucis longus m

Plantaris t

Figure 23.1.9

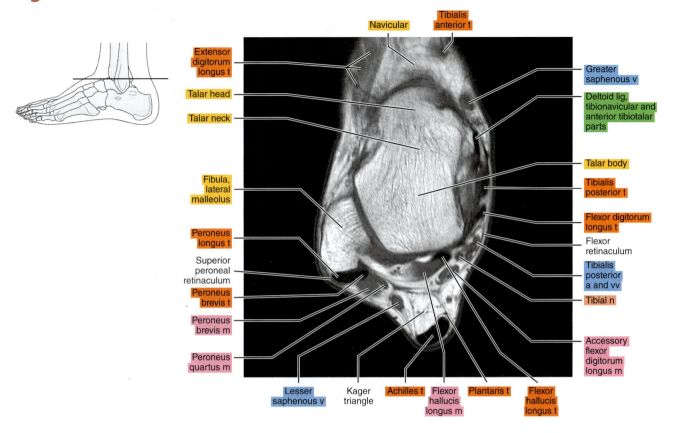

Extensor digitorum longus t
Navicular
Tibialis anterior t
Greater saphenous v
Deltoid lig, tibionavicular and anterior tibiotalar parts
Talar head
Talar neck
Talar body
Tibialis posterior t
Fibula, lateral malleolus
Flexor digitorum longus t
Flexor retinaculum
Peroneus longus t
Tibialis posterior a and vv
Superior peroneal retinaculum
Tibial n
Peroneus brevis t
Peroneus brevis m
Accessory flexor digitorum longus m
Peroneus quartus m
Lesser saphenous v
Kager triangle
Achilles t
Flexor hallucis longus m
Plantaris t
Flexor hallucis longus t

Figure 23.1.10

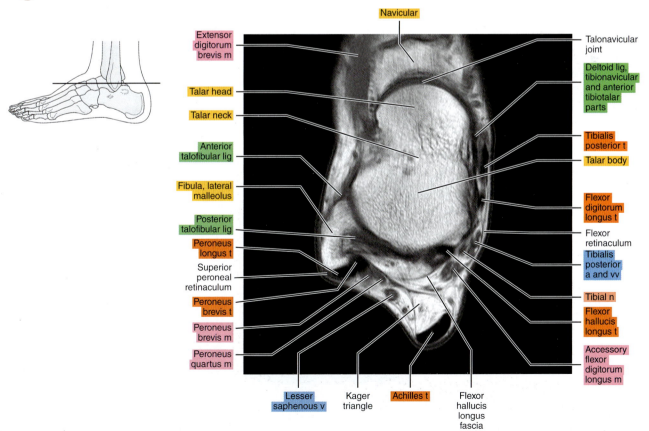

Extensor digitorum brevis m
Navicular
Talonavicular joint
Deltoid lig, tibionavicular and anterior tibiotalar parts
Talar head
Talar neck
Tibialis posterior t
Anterior talofibular lig
Talar body
Fibula, lateral malleolus
Flexor digitorum longus t
Posterior talofibular lig
Flexor retinaculum
Peroneus longus t
Tibialis posterior a and vv
Superior peroneal retinaculum
Tibial n
Peroneus brevis t
Flexor hallucis longus t
Peroneus brevis m
Accessory flexor digitorum longus m
Peroneus quartus m
Lesser saphenous v
Kager triangle
Achilles t
Flexor hallucis longus fascia

Figure 23.1.11

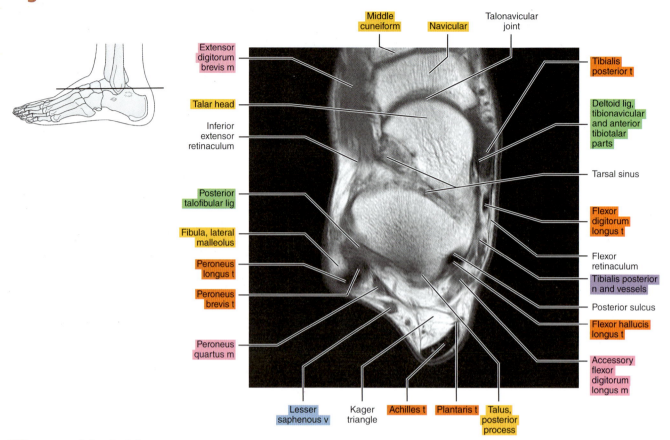

Extensor digitorum brevis m
Middle cuneiform
Navicular
Talonavicular joint
Tibialis posterior t
Talar head
Deltoid lig, tibionavicular and anterior tibiotalar parts
Inferior extensor retinaculum
Tarsal sinus
Posterior talofibular lig
Flexor digitorum longus t
Fibula, lateral malleolus
Flexor retinaculum
Peroneus longus t
Tibialis posterior n and vessels
Peroneus brevis t
Posterior sulcus
Flexor hallucis longus t
Peroneus quartus m
Accessory flexor digitorum longus m
Lesser saphenous v
Kager triangle
Achilles t
Plantaris t
Talus, posterior process

Figure 23.1.12

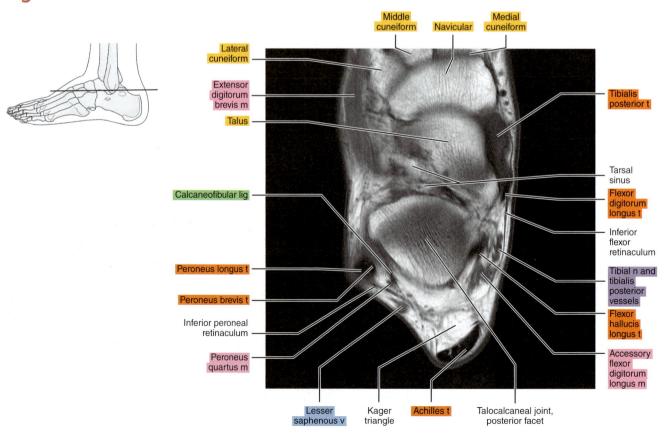

Lateral cuneiform
Middle cuneiform
Navicular
Medial cuneiform
Extensor digitorum brevis m
Tibialis posterior t
Talus
Tarsal sinus
Calcaneofibular lig
Flexor digitorum longus t
Inferior flexor retinaculum
Peroneus longus t
Tibial n and tibialis posterior vessels
Peroneus brevis t
Flexor hallucis longus t
Inferior peroneal retinaculum
Accessory flexor digitorum longus m
Peroneus quartus m
Lesser saphenous v
Kager triangle
Achilles t
Talocalcaneal joint, posterior facet

Figure 23.1.13

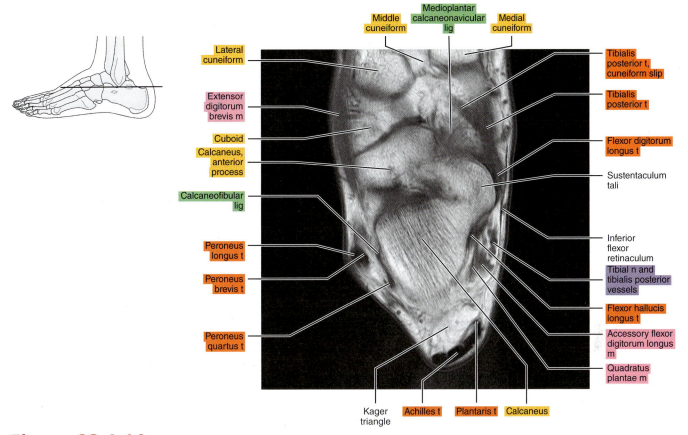

Lateral cuneiform

Extensor digitorum brevis m

Cuboid

Calcaneus, anterior process

Calcaneofibular lig

Peroneus longus t

Peroneus brevis t

Peroneus quartus t

Middle cuneiform

Medioplantar calcaneonavicular lig

Medial cuneiform

Tibialis posterior t, cuneiform slip

Tibialis posterior t

Flexor digitorum longus t

Sustentaculum tali

Inferior flexor retinaculum

Tibial n and tibialis posterior vessels

Flexor hallucis longus t

Accessory flexor digitorum longus m

Quadratus plantae m

Kager triangle

Achilles t

Plantaris t

Calcaneus

Figure 23.1.14

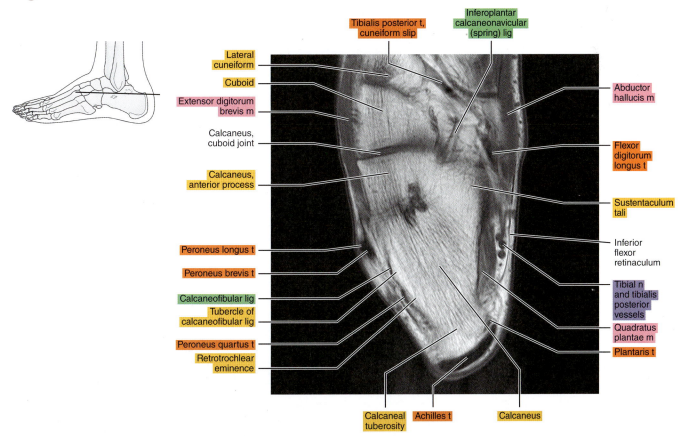

Tibialis posterior t, cuneiform slip

Inferoplantar calcaneonavicular (spring) lig

Lateral cuneiform

Cuboid

Extensor digitorum brevis m

Calcaneus, cuboid joint

Calcaneus, anterior process

Peroneus longus t

Peroneus brevis t

Calcaneofibular lig

Tubercle of calcaneofibular lig

Peroneus quartus t

Retrotrochlear eminence

Abductor hallucis m

Flexor digitorum longus t

Sustentaculum tali

Inferior flexor retinaculum

Tibial n and tibialis posterior vessels

Quadratus plantae m

Plantaris t

Calcaneal tuberosity

Achilles t

Calcaneus

Figure 23.1.15

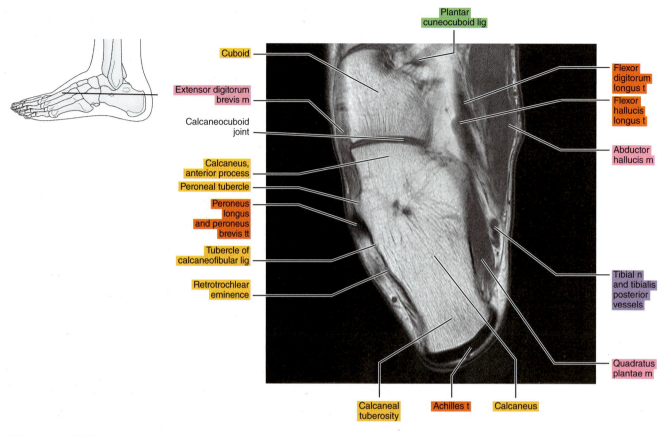

Plantar cuneocuboid lig

Cuboid

Extensor digitorum brevis m

Calcaneocuboid joint

Calcaneus, anterior process

Peroneal tubercle

Peroneus longus and peroneus brevis tt

Tubercle of calcaneofibular lig

Retrotrochlear eminence

Flexor digitorum longus t

Flexor hallucis longus t

Abductor hallucis m

Tibial n and tibialis posterior vessels

Quadratus plantae m

Calcaneal tuberosity

Achilles t

Calcaneus

Figure 23.1.16

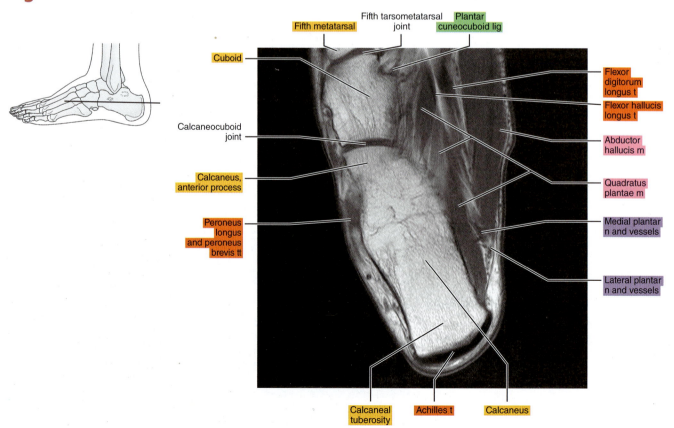

Fifth tarsometatarsal joint

Fifth metatarsal

Plantar cuneocuboid lig

Cuboid

Calcaneocuboid joint

Calcaneus, anterior process

Peroneus longus and peroneus brevis tt

Flexor digitorum longus t

Flexor hallucis longus t

Abductor hallucis m

Quadratus plantae m

Medial plantar n and vessels

Lateral plantar n and vessels

Calcaneal tuberosity

Achilles t

Calcaneus

Figure 23.1.17

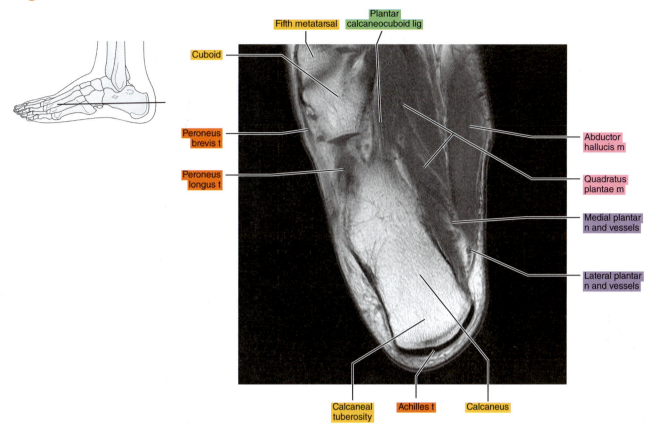

Fifth metatarsal

Plantar calcaneocuboid lig

Cuboid

Peroneus brevis t

Peroneus longus t

Abductor hallucis m

Quadratus plantae m

Medial plantar n and vessels

Lateral plantar n and vessels

Calcaneal tuberosity

Achilles t

Calcaneus

Figure 23.1.18

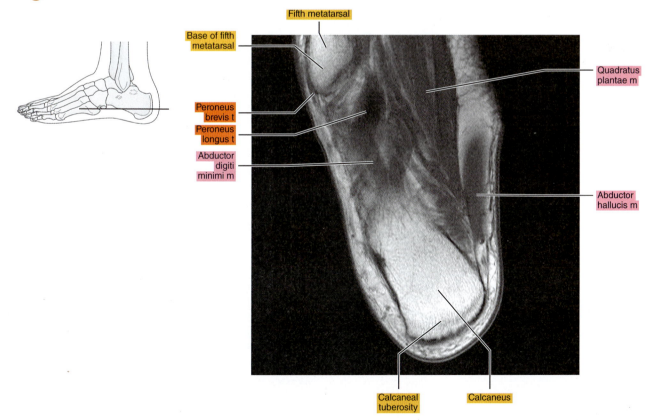

Fifth metatarsal

Base of fifth metatarsal

Quadratus plantae m

Peroneus brevis t

Peroneus longus t

Abductor digiti minimi m

Abductor hallucis m

Calcaneal tuberosity

Calcaneus

Figure 23.1.19

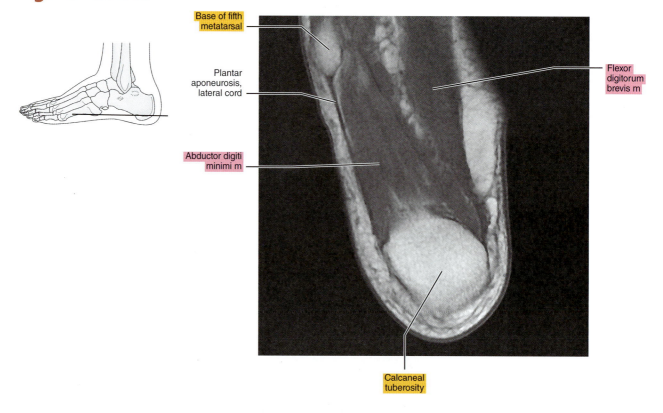

Base of fifth metatarsal

Plantar aponeurosis, lateral cord

Abductor digiti minimi m

Flexor digitorum brevis m

Calcaneal tuberosity

Figure 23.1.20

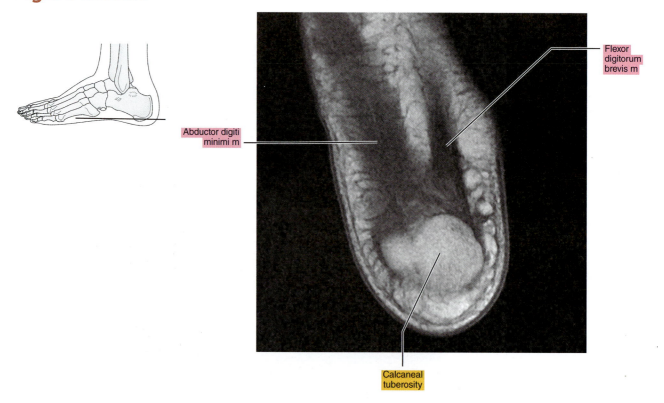

Abductor digiti minimi m

Flexor digitorum brevis m

Calcaneal tuberosity

OBLIQUE AXIAL
Figure 23.2.1

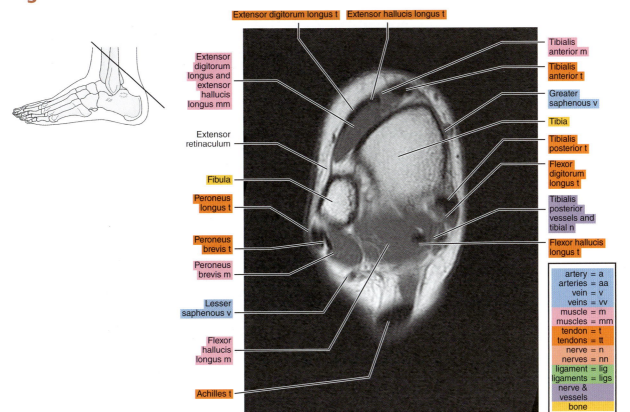

Extensor digitorum longus t

Extensor hallucis longus t

Extensor digitorum longus and extensor hallucis longus mm

Extensor retinaculum

Fibula

Peroneus longus t

Peroneus brevis t

Peroneus brevis m

Lesser saphenous v

Flexor hallucis longus m

Achilles t

Tibialis anterior m

Tibialis anterior t

Greater saphenous v

Tibia

Tibialis posterior t

Flexor digitorum longus t

Tibialis posterior vessels and tibial n

Flexor hallucis longus t

artery = a
arteries = aa
vein = v
veins = vv
muscle = m
muscles = mm
tendon = t
tendons = tt
nerve = n
nerves = nn
ligament = lig
ligaments = ligs
nerve & vessels
bone

Figure 23.2.2

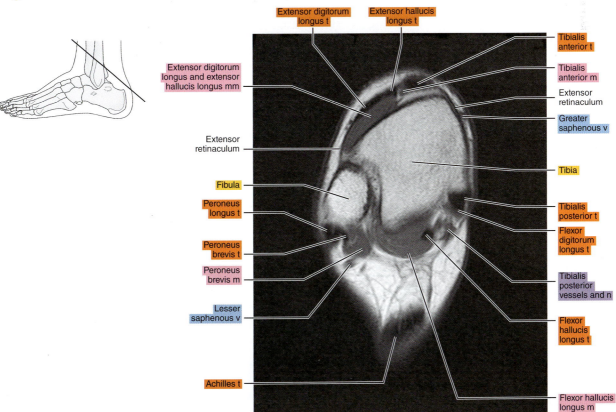

Extensor digitorum longus t

Extensor hallucis longus t

Extensor digitorum longus and extensor hallucis longus mm

Extensor retinaculum

Fibula

Peroneus longus t

Peroneus brevis t

Peroneus brevis m

Lesser saphenous v

Achilles t

Tibialis anterior t

Tibialis anterior m

Extensor retinaculum

Greater saphenous v

Tibia

Tibialis posterior t

Flexor digitorum longus t

Tibialis posterior vessels and n

Flexor hallucis longus t

Flexor hallucis longus m

Figure 23.2.3

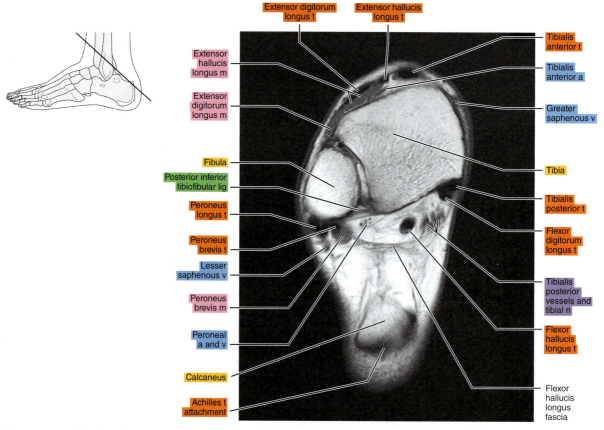

Extensor digitorum longus t
Extensor hallucis longus t
Tibialis anterior t
Tibialis anterior a
Greater saphenous v
Extensor hallucis longus m
Extensor digitorum longus m
Tibia
Fibula
Posterior inferior tibiofibular lig
Tibialis posterior t
Peroneus longus t
Flexor digitorum longus t
Peroneus brevis t
Lesser saphenous v
Tibialis posterior vessels and tibial n
Peroneus brevis m
Flexor hallucis longus t
Peroneal a and v
Calcaneus
Flexor hallucis longus fascia
Achilles t attachment

Figure 23.2.4

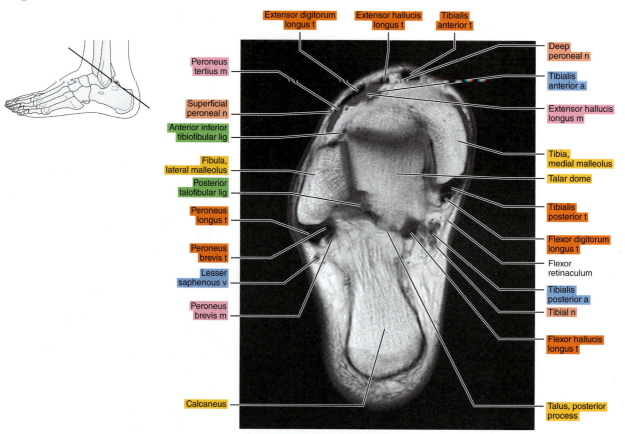

Extensor digitorum longus t
Extensor hallucis longus t
Tibialis anterior t
Deep peroneal n
Peroneus tertius m
Tibialis anterior a
Superficial peroneal n
Extensor hallucis longus m
Anterior inferior tibiofibular lig
Tibia, medial malleolus
Fibula, lateral malleolus
Talar dome
Posterior talofibular lig
Tibialis posterior t
Peroneus longus t
Flexor digitorum longus t
Peroneus brevis t
Flexor retinaculum
Lesser saphenous v
Tibialis posterior a
Peroneus brevis m
Tibial n
Flexor hallucis longus t
Calcaneus
Talus, posterior process

Figure 23.2.5

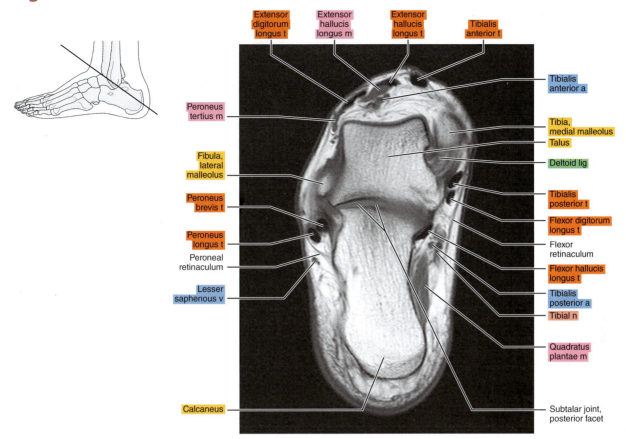

Extensor digitorum longus t
Extensor hallucis longus m
Extensor hallucis longus t
Tibialis anterior t
Tibialis anterior a
Peroneus tertius m
Tibia, medial malleolus
Talus
Deltoid lig
Fibula, lateral malleolus
Tibialis posterior t
Flexor digitorum longus t
Peroneus brevis t
Flexor retinaculum
Peroneus longus t
Flexor hallucis longus t
Peroneal retinaculum
Tibialis posterior a
Lesser saphenous v
Tibial n
Quadratus plantae m
Calcaneus
Subtalar joint, posterior facet

Figure 23.2.6

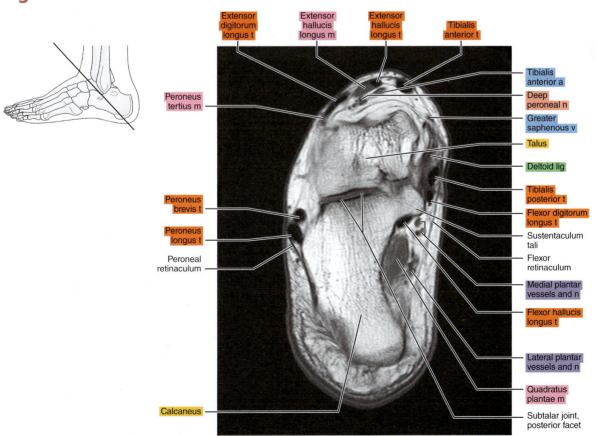

Extensor digitorum longus t
Extensor hallucis longus m
Extensor hallucis longus t
Tibialis anterior t
Tibialis anterior a
Deep peroneal n
Peroneus tertius m
Greater saphenous v
Talus
Deltoid lig
Tibialis posterior t
Flexor digitorum longus t
Peroneus brevis t
Sustentaculum tali
Peroneus longus t
Flexor retinaculum
Peroneal retinaculum
Medial plantar vessels and n
Flexor hallucis longus t
Lateral plantar vessels and n
Quadratus plantae m
Calcaneus
Subtalar joint, posterior facet

Figure 23.2.7

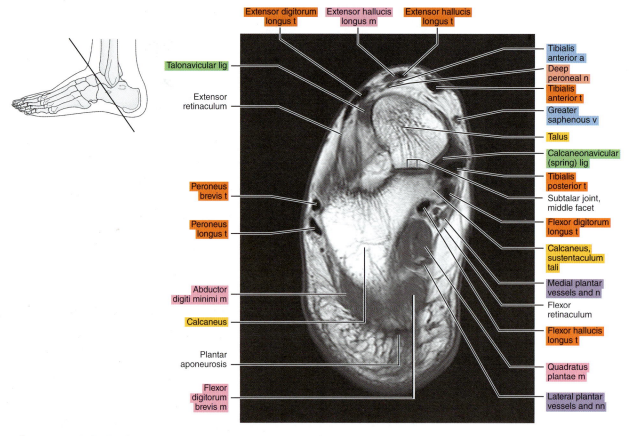

Extensor digitorum longus t
Extensor hallucis longus m
Extensor hallucis longus t
Tibialis anterior a
Deep peroneal n
Tibialis anterior t
Greater saphenous v
Talus
Calcaneonavicular (spring) lig
Tibialis posterior t
Subtalar joint, middle facet
Flexor digitorum longus t
Calcaneus, sustentaculum tali
Medial plantar vessels and n
Flexor retinaculum
Flexor hallucis longus t
Quadratus plantae m
Lateral plantar vessels and nn

Talonavicular lig
Extensor retinaculum
Peroneus brevis t
Peroneus longus t
Abductor digiti minimi m
Calcaneus
Plantar aponeurosis
Flexor digitorum brevis m

Figure 23.2.8

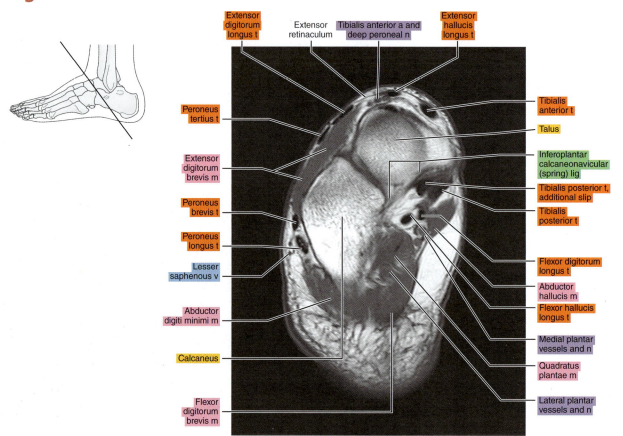

Extensor digitorum longus t
Extensor retinaculum
Tibialis anterior a and deep peroneal n
Extensor hallucis longus t
Tibialis anterior t
Talus
Inferoplantar calcaneonavicular (spring) lig
Tibialis posterior t, additional slip
Tibialis posterior t
Flexor digitorum longus t
Abductor hallucis m
Flexor hallucis longus t
Medial plantar vessels and n
Quadratus plantae m
Lateral plantar vessels and n

Peroneus tertius t
Extensor digitorum brevis m
Peroneus brevis t
Peroneus longus t
Lesser saphenous v
Abductor digiti minimi m
Calcaneus
Flexor digitorum brevis m

Figure 23.2.9

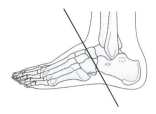

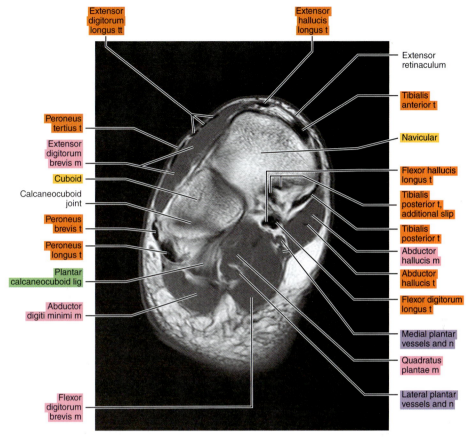

Extensor digitorum longus tt

Extensor hallucis longus t

Extensor retinaculum

Peroneus tertius t

Extensor digitorum brevis m

Cuboid

Calcaneocuboid joint

Peroneus brevis t

Peroneus longus t

Plantar calcaneocuboid lig

Abductor digiti minimi m

Flexor digitorum brevis m

Tibialis anterior t

Navicular

Flexor hallucis longus t

Tibialis posterior t, additional slip

Tibialis posterior t

Abductor hallucis m

Abductor hallucis t

Flexor digitorum longus t

Medial plantar vessels and n

Quadratus plantae m

Lateral plantar vessels and n

Figure 23.2.10

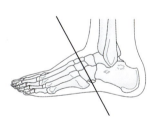

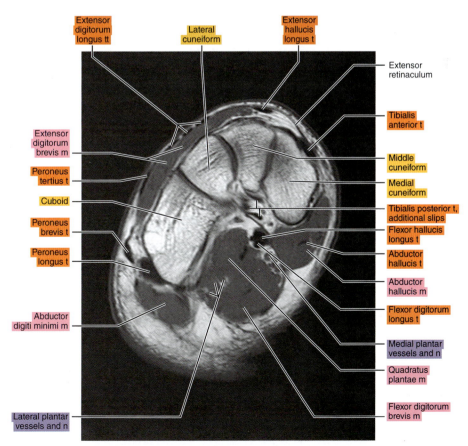

Extensor digitorum longus tt

Lateral cuneiform

Extensor hallucis longus t

Extensor retinaculum

Extensor digitorum brevis m

Peroneus tertius t

Cuboid

Peroneus brevis t

Peroneus longus t

Abductor digiti minimi m

Lateral plantar vessels and n

Tibialis anterior t

Middle cuneiform

Medial cuneiform

Tibialis posterior t, additional slips

Flexor hallucis longus t

Abductor hallucis t

Abductor hallucis m

Flexor digitorum longus t

Medial plantar vessels and n

Quadratus plantae m

Flexor digitorum brevis m

Figure 23.2.11

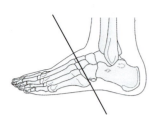

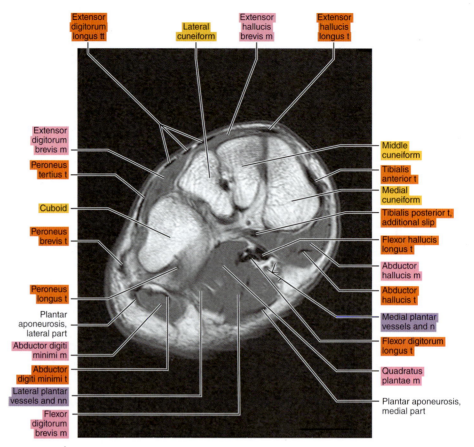

SAGITTAL
Figure 23.3.1

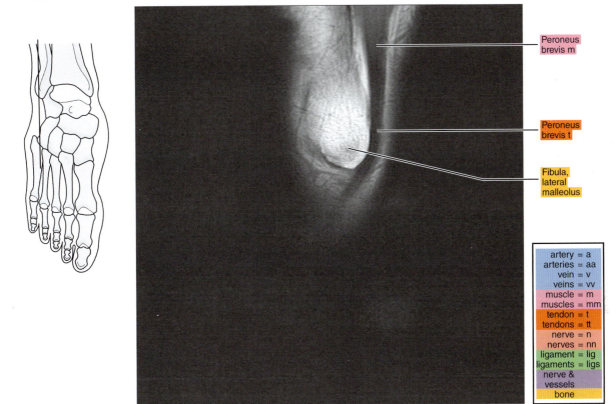

Peroneus brevis m

Peroneus brevis t

Fibula, lateral malleolus

artery = a	
arteries = aa	
vein = v	
veins = vv	
muscle = m	
muscles = mm	
tendon = t	
tendons = tt	
nerve = n	
nerves = nn	
ligament = lig	
ligaments = ligs	
nerve & vessels	
bone	

Figure 23.3.2

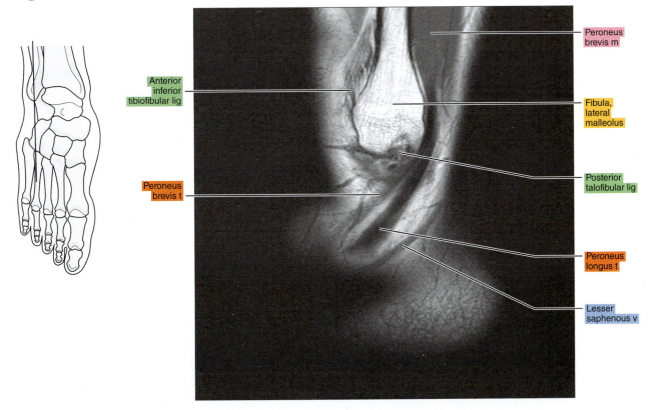

Anterior inferior tibiofibular lig

Peroneus brevis t

Peroneus brevis m

Fibula, lateral malleolus

Posterior talofibular lig

Peroneus longus t

Lesser saphenous v

Figure 23.3.3

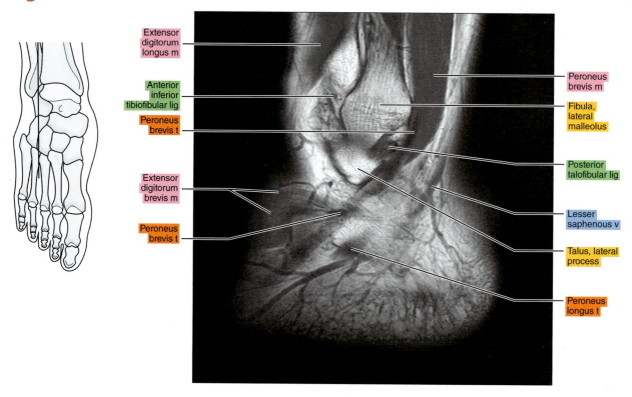

Extensor digitorum longus m

Anterior inferior tibiofibular lig

Peroneus brevis t

Extensor digitorum brevis m

Peroneus brevis t

Peroneus brevis m

Fibula, lateral malleolus

Posterior talofibular lig

Lesser saphenous v

Talus, lateral process

Peroneus longus t

Figure 23.3.4

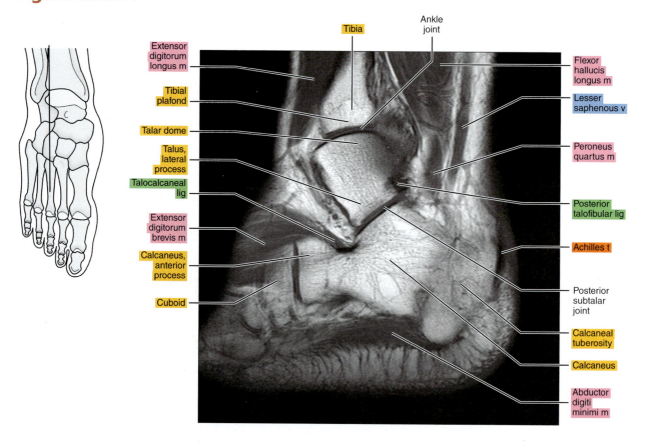

Tibia

Ankle joint

Extensor digitorum longus m

Tibial plafond

Talar dome

Talus, lateral process

Talocalcaneal lig

Extensor digitorum brevis m

Calcaneus, anterior process

Cuboid

Flexor hallucis longus m

Lesser saphenous v

Peroneus quartus m

Posterior talofibular lig

Achilles t

Posterior subtalar joint

Calcaneal tuberosity

Calcaneus

Abductor digiti minimi m

Figure 23.3.5

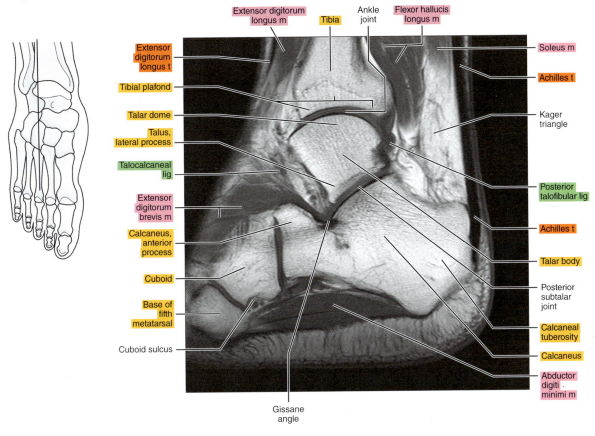

Extensor digitorum longus m
Tibia
Ankle joint
Flexor hallucis longus m
Soleus m
Achilles t
Extensor digitorum longus t
Tibial plafond
Talar dome
Talus, lateral process
Talocalcaneal lig
Extensor digitorum brevis m
Calcaneus, anterior process
Cuboid
Base of fifth metatarsal
Cuboid sulcus
Kager triangle
Posterior talofibular lig
Achilles t
Talar body
Posterior subtalar joint
Calcaneal tuberosity
Calcaneus
Abductor digiti minimi m
Gissane angle

Figure 23.3.6

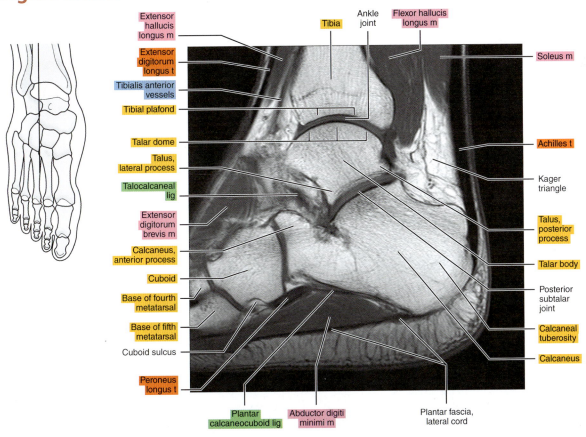

Extensor hallucis longus m
Tibia
Ankle joint
Flexor hallucis longus m
Extensor digitorum longus t
Tibialis anterior vessels
Tibial plafond
Talar dome
Talus, lateral process
Talocalcaneal lig
Extensor digitorum brevis m
Calcaneus, anterior process
Cuboid
Base of fourth metatarsal
Base of fifth metatarsal
Cuboid sulcus
Peroneus longus t
Soleus m
Achilles t
Kager triangle
Talus, posterior process
Talar body
Posterior subtalar joint
Calcaneal tuberosity
Calcaneus
Plantar calcaneocuboid lig
Abductor digiti minimi m
Plantar fascia, lateral cord

Figure 23.3.7

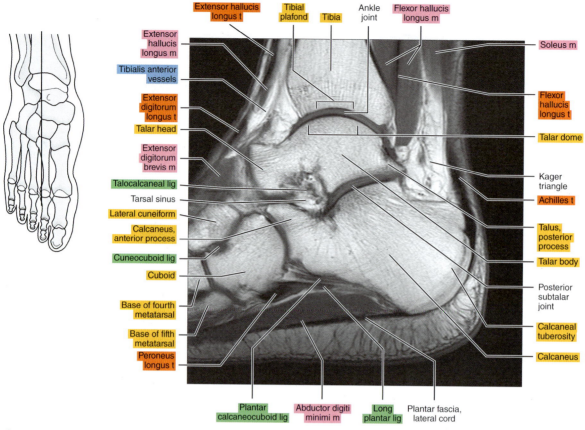

Extensor hallucis longus t — Tibial plafond — Tibia — Ankle joint — Flexor hallucis longus m

Extensor hallucis longus m
Tibialis anterior vessels
Extensor digitorum longus t
Talar head
Extensor digitorum brevis m
Talocalcaneal lig
Tarsal sinus
Lateral cuneiform
Calcaneus, anterior process
Cuneocuboid lig
Cuboid
Base of fourth metatarsal
Base of fifth metatarsal
Peroneus longus t

Soleus m
Flexor hallucis longus t
Talar dome
Kager triangle
Achilles t
Talus, posterior process
Talar body
Posterior subtalar joint
Calcaneal tuberosity
Calcaneus

Plantar calcaneocuboid lig — Abductor digiti minimi m — Long plantar lig — Plantar fascia, lateral cord

Figure 23.3.8

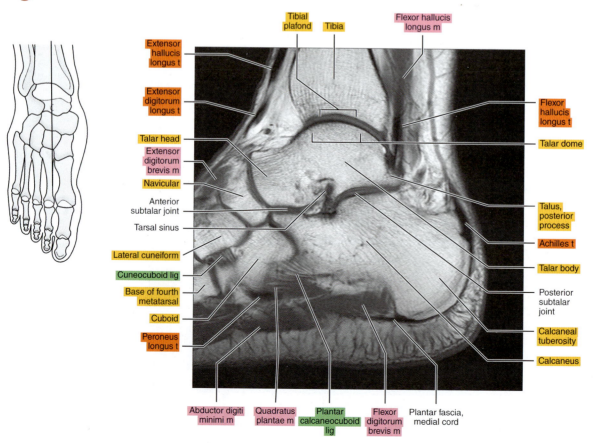

Tibial plafond — Tibia — Flexor hallucis longus m

Extensor hallucis longus t
Extensor digitorum longus t
Talar head
Extensor digitorum brevis m
Navicular
Anterior subtalar joint
Tarsal sinus
Lateral cuneiform
Cuneocuboid lig
Base of fourth metatarsal
Cuboid
Peroneus longus t

Flexor hallucis longus t
Talar dome
Talus, posterior process
Achilles t
Talar body
Posterior subtalar joint
Calcaneal tuberosity
Calcaneus

Abductor digiti minimi m — Quadratus plantae m — Plantar calcaneocuboid lig — Flexor digitorum brevis m — Plantar fascia, medial cord

Figure 23.3.9

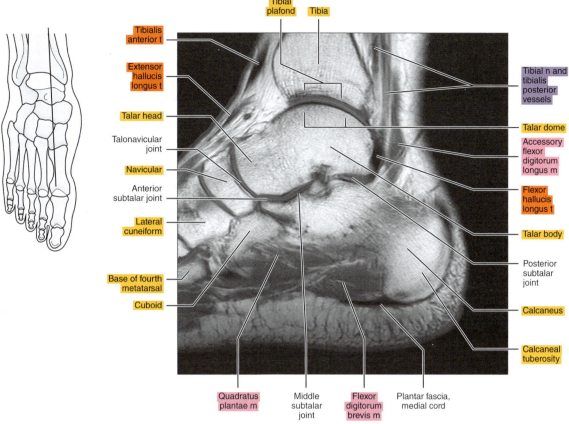

Tibial plafond

Tibia

Tibialis anterior t

Extensor hallucis longus t

Talar head

Talonavicular joint

Navicular

Anterior subtalar joint

Lateral cuneiform

Base of fourth metatarsal

Cuboid

Tibial n and tibialis posterior vessels

Talar dome

Accessory flexor digitorum longus m

Flexor hallucis longus t

Talar body

Posterior subtalar joint

Calcaneus

Calcaneal tuberosity

Quadratus plantae m

Middle subtalar joint

Flexor digitorum brevis m

Plantar fascia, medial cord

Figure 23.3.10

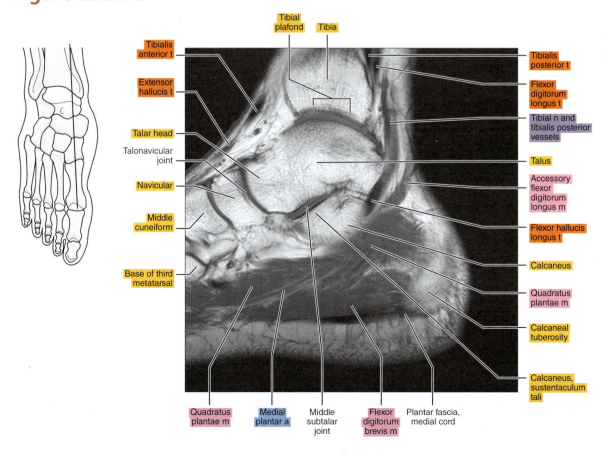

Tibial plafond

Tibia

Tibialis anterior t

Extensor hallucis t

Talar head

Talonavicular joint

Navicular

Middle cuneiform

Base of third metatarsal

Tibialis posterior t

Flexor digitorum longus t

Tibial n and tibialis posterior vessels

Talus

Accessory flexor digitorum longus m

Flexor hallucis longus t

Calcaneus

Quadratus plantae m

Calcaneal tuberosity

Calcaneus, sustentaculum tali

Quadratus plantae m

Medial plantar a

Middle subtalar joint

Flexor digitorum brevis m

Plantar fascia, medial cord

Figure 23.3.11

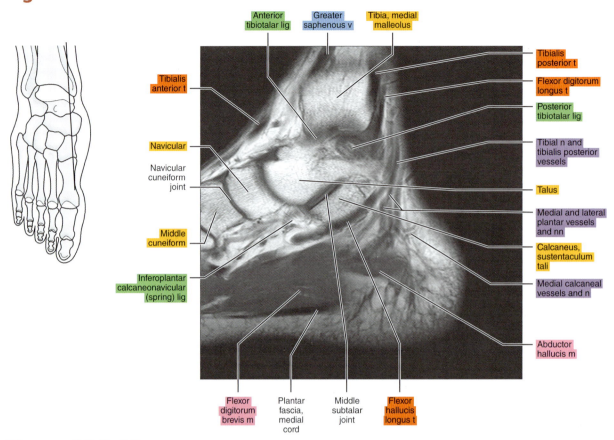

Anterior tibiotalar lig

Greater saphenous v

Tibia, medial malleolus

Tibialis anterior t

Navicular

Navicular cuneiform joint

Middle cuneiform

Inferoplantar calcaneonavicular (spring) lig

Tibialis posterior t

Flexor digitorum longus t

Posterior tibiotalar lig

Tibial n and tibialis posterior vessels

Talus

Medial and lateral plantar vessels and nn

Calcaneus, sustentaculum tali

Medial calcaneal vessels and n

Abductor hallucis m

Flexor digitorum brevis m

Plantar fascia, medial cord

Middle subtalar joint

Flexor hallucis longus t

Figure 23.3.12

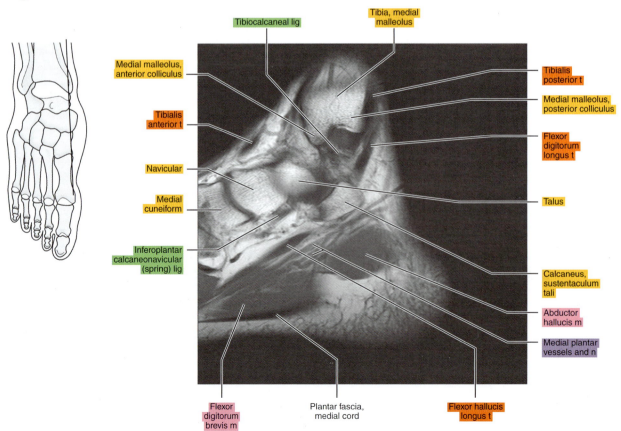

Tibiocalcaneal lig

Tibia, medial malleolus

Medial malleolus, anterior colliculus

Tibialis anterior t

Navicular

Medial cuneiform

Inferoplantar calcaneonavicular (spring) lig

Tibialis posterior t

Medial malleolus, posterior colliculus

Flexor digitorum longus t

Talus

Calcaneus, sustentaculum tali

Abductor hallucis m

Medial plantar vessels and n

Flexor digitorum brevis m

Plantar fascia, medial cord

Flexor hallucis longus t

Figure 23.3.13

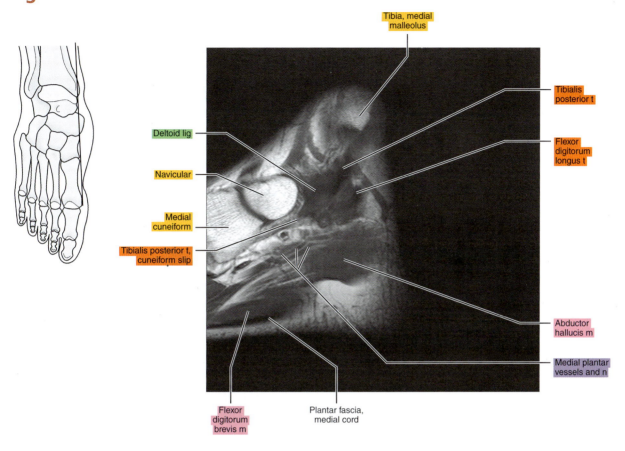

Tibia, medial malleolus

Tibialis posterior t

Deltoid lig

Flexor digitorum longus t

Navicular

Medial cuneiform

Tibialis posterior t, cuneiform slip

Abductor hallucis m

Medial plantar vessels and n

Flexor digitorum brevis m

Plantar fascia, medial cord

CORONAL
Figure 23.4.1

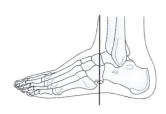

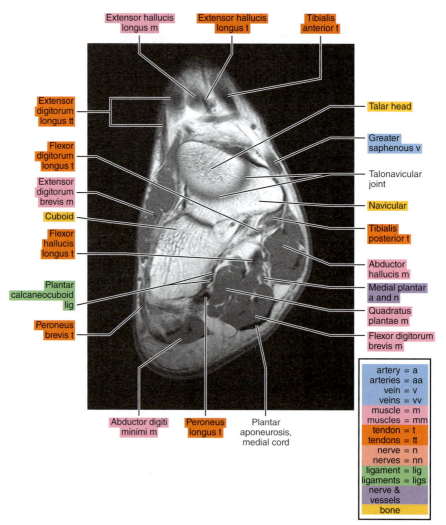

Extensor hallucis longus m

Extensor hallucis longus t

Tibialis anterior t

Extensor digitorum longus tt

Flexor digitorum longus t

Extensor digitorum brevis m

Cuboid

Flexor hallucis longus t

Plantar calcaneocuboid lig

Peroneus brevis t

Talar head

Greater saphenous v

Talonavicular joint

Navicular

Tibialis posterior t

Abductor hallucis m

Medial plantar a and n

Quadratus plantae m

Flexor digitorum brevis m

Abductor digiti minimi m

Peroneus longus t

Plantar aponeurosis, medial cord

artery = a
arteries = aa
vein = v
veins = vv
muscle = m
muscles = mm
tendon = t
tendons = tt
nerve = n
nerves = nn
ligament = lig
ligaments = ligs
nerve & vessels
bone

Figure 23.4.2

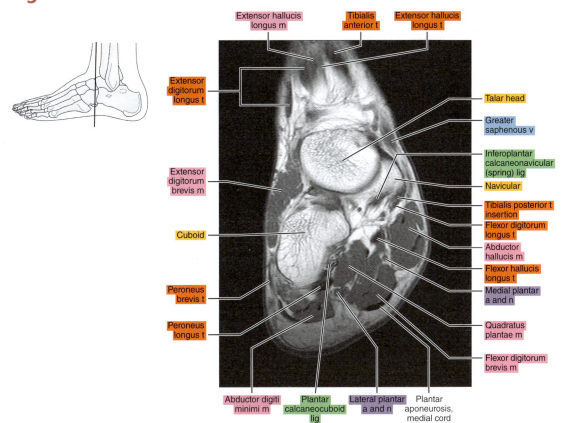

Extensor hallucis longus m

Tibialis anterior t

Extensor hallucis longus t

Extensor digitorum longus t

Extensor digitorum brevis m

Cuboid

Peroneus brevis t

Peroneus longus t

Talar head

Greater saphenous v

Inferoplantar calcaneonavicular (spring) lig

Navicular

Tibialis posterior t insertion

Flexor digitorum longus t

Abductor hallucis m

Flexor hallucis longus t

Medial plantar a and n

Quadratus plantae m

Flexor digitorum brevis m

Abductor digiti minimi m

Plantar calcaneocuboid lig

Lateral plantar a and n

Plantar aponeurosis, medial cord

Figure 23.4.3

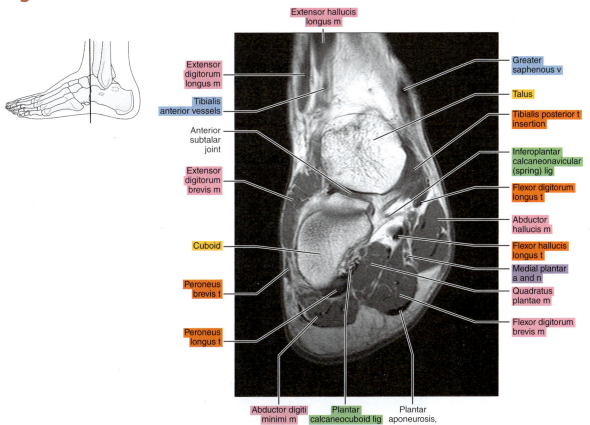

Extensor hallucis longus m

Extensor digitorum longus m

Tibialis anterior vessels

Anterior subtalar joint

Extensor digitorum brevis m

Cuboid

Peroneus brevis t

Peroneus longus t

Greater saphenous v

Talus

Tibialis posterior t insertion

Inferoplantar calcaneonavicular (spring) lig

Flexor digitorum longus t

Abductor hallucis m

Flexor hallucis longus t

Medial plantar a and n

Quadratus plantae m

Flexor digitorum brevis m

Abductor digiti minimi m

Plantar calcaneocuboid lig

Plantar aponeurosis, medial cord

Figure 23.4.4

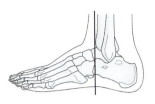

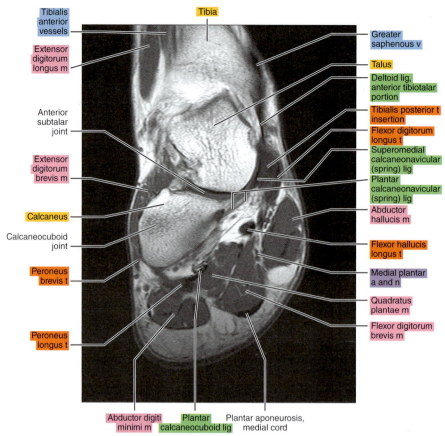

Tibialis anterior vessels

Extensor digitorum longus m

Anterior subtalar joint

Extensor digitorum brevis m

Calcaneus

Calcaneocuboid joint

Peroneus brevis t

Peroneus longus t

Tibia

Greater saphenous v

Talus

Deltoid lig, anterior tibiotalar portion

Tibialis posterior t insertion

Flexor digitorum longus t

Superomedial calcaneonavicular (spring) lig

Plantar calcaneonavicular (spring) lig

Abductor hallucis m

Flexor hallucis longus t

Medial plantar a and n

Quadratus plantae m

Flexor digitorum brevis m

Abductor digiti minimi m

Plantar calcaneocuboid lig

Plantar aponeurosis, medial cord

Figure 23.4.5

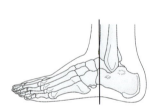

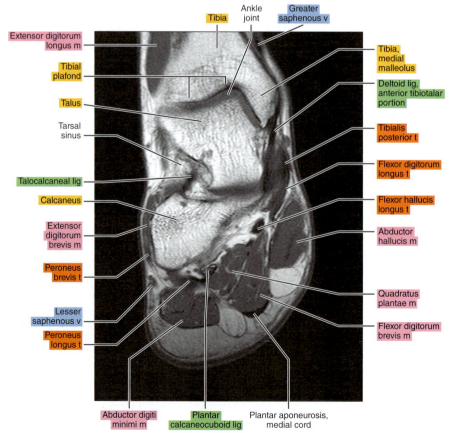

Extensor digitorum longus m

Tibial plafond

Talus

Tarsal sinus

Talocalcaneal lig

Calcaneus

Extensor digitorum brevis m

Peroneus brevis t

Lesser saphenous v

Peroneus longus t

Tibia

Ankle joint

Greater saphenous v

Tibia, medial malleolus

Deltoid lig, anterior tibiotalar portion

Tibialis posterior t

Flexor digitorum longus t

Flexor hallucis longus t

Abductor hallucis m

Quadratus plantae m

Flexor digitorum brevis m

Abductor digiti minimi m

Plantar calcaneocuboid lig

Plantar aponeurosis, medial cord

Figure 23.4.6

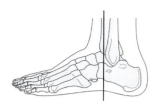

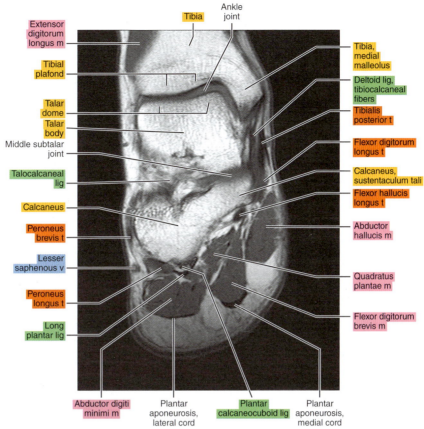

Ankle joint

Tibia

Extensor digitorum longus m

Tibial plafond

Talar dome

Talar body

Middle subtalar joint

Talocalcaneal lig

Calcaneus

Peroneus brevis t

Lesser saphenous v

Peroneus longus t

Long plantar lig

Tibia, medial malleolus

Deltoid lig, tibiocalcaneal fibers

Tibialis posterior t

Flexor digitorum longus t

Calcaneus, sustentaculum tali

Flexor hallucis longus t

Abductor hallucis m

Quadratus plantae m

Flexor digitorum brevis m

Abductor digiti minimi m

Plantar aponeurosis, lateral cord

Plantar calcaneocuboid lig

Plantar aponeurosis, medial cord

Figure 23.4.7

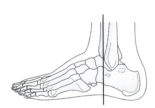

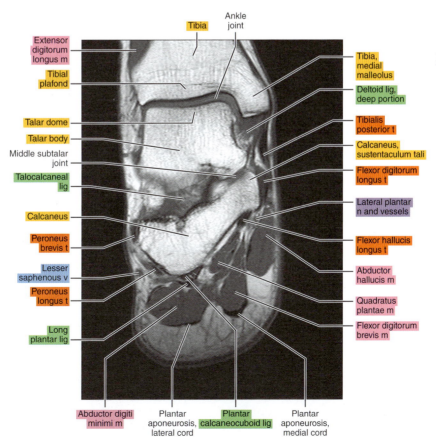

Ankle joint

Tibia

Extensor digitorum longus m

Tibial plafond

Talar dome

Talar body

Middle subtalar joint

Talocalcaneal lig

Calcaneus

Peroneus brevis t

Lesser saphenous v

Peroneus longus t

Long plantar lig

Tibia, medial malleolus

Deltoid lig, deep portion

Tibialis posterior t

Calcaneus, sustentaculum tali

Flexor digitorum longus t

Lateral plantar n and vessels

Flexor hallucis longus t

Abductor hallucis m

Quadratus plantae m

Flexor digitorum brevis m

Abductor digiti minimi m

Plantar aponeurosis, lateral cord

Plantar calcaneocuboid lig

Plantar aponeurosis, medial cord

Figure 23.4.8

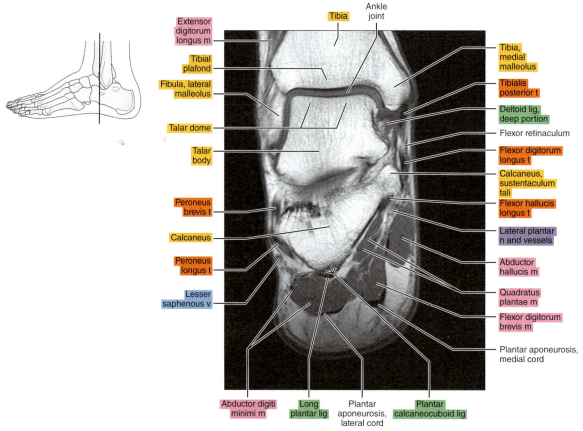

Extensor digitorum longus m
Tibial plafond
Fibula, lateral malleolus
Talar dome
Talar body
Peroneus brevis t
Calcaneus
Peroneus longus t
Lesser saphenous v

Ankle joint
Tibia

Tibia, medial malleolus
Tibialis posterior t
Deltoid lig, deep portion
Flexor retinaculum
Flexor digitorum longus t
Calcaneus, sustentaculum tali
Flexor hallucis longus t
Lateral plantar n and vessels
Abductor hallucis m
Quadratus plantae m
Flexor digitorum brevis m
Plantar aponeurosis, medial cord

Abductor digiti minimi m
Long plantar lig
Plantar aponeurosis, lateral cord
Plantar calcaneocuboid lig

Figure 23.4.9

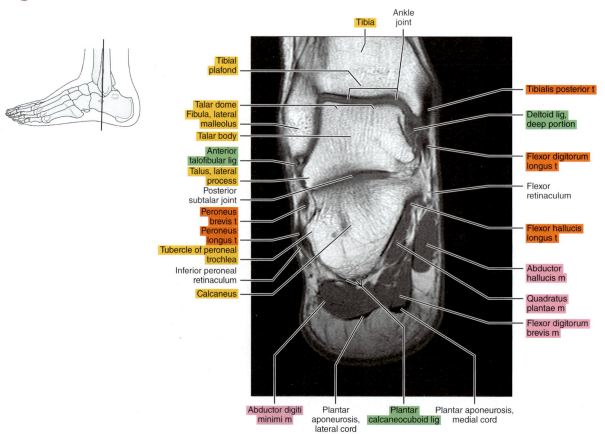

Ankle joint
Tibia

Tibial plafond
Talar dome
Fibula, lateral malleolus
Talar body
Anterior talofibular lig
Talus, lateral process
Posterior subtalar joint
Peroneus brevis t
Peroneus longus t
Tubercle of peroneal trochlea
Inferior peroneal retinaculum
Calcaneus

Tibialis posterior t
Deltoid lig, deep portion
Flexor digitorum longus t
Flexor retinaculum
Flexor hallucis longus t
Abductor hallucis m
Quadratus plantae m
Flexor digitorum brevis m

Abductor digiti minimi m
Plantar aponeurosis, lateral cord
Plantar calcaneocuboid lig
Plantar aponeurosis, medial cord

Figure 23.4.10

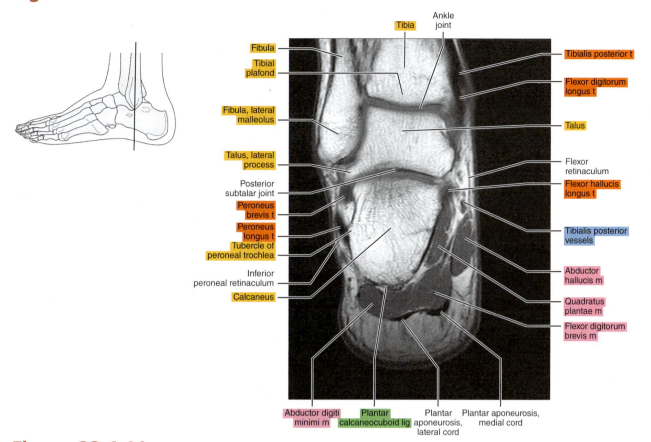

Ankle joint
Tibia
Fibula
Tibial plafond
Fibula, lateral malleolus
Talus, lateral process
Posterior subtalar joint
Peroneus brevis t
Peroneus longus t
Tubercle of peroneal trochlea
Inferior peroneal retinaculum
Calcaneus

Tibialis posterior t
Flexor digitorum longus t
Talus
Flexor retinaculum
Flexor hallucis longus t
Tibialis posterior vessels
Abductor hallucis m
Quadratus plantae m
Flexor digitorum brevis m

Abductor digiti minimi m
Plantar calcaneocuboid lig
Plantar aponeurosis, lateral cord
Plantar aponeurosis, medial cord

Figure 23.4.11

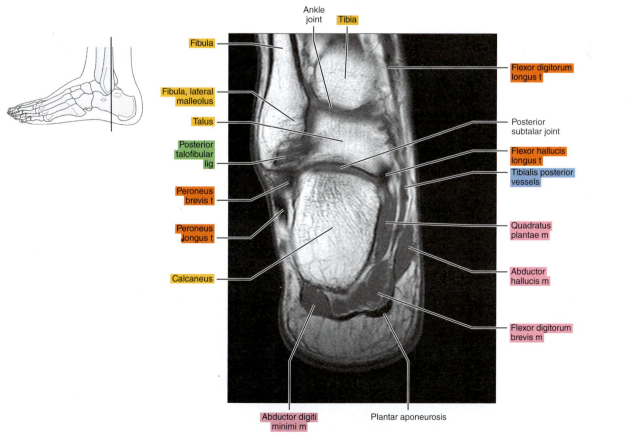

Ankle joint
Tibia
Fibula
Fibula, lateral malleolus
Talus
Posterior talofibular lig
Peroneus brevis t
Peroneus longus t
Calcaneus

Flexor digitorum longus t
Posterior subtalar joint
Flexor hallucis longus t
Tibialis posterior vessels
Quadratus plantae m
Abductor hallucis m
Flexor digitorum brevis m

Abductor digiti minimi m
Plantar aponeurosis

Figure 23.4.12

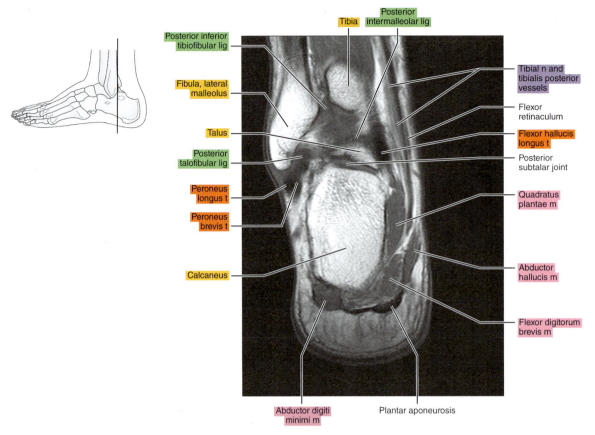

Posterior inferior tibiofibular lig

Fibula, lateral malleolus

Talus

Posterior talofibular lig

Peroneus longus t

Peroneus brevis t

Calcaneus

Tibia

Posterior intermalleolar lig

Tibial n and tibialis posterior vessels

Flexor retinaculum

Flexor hallucis longus t

Posterior subtalar joint

Quadratus plantae m

Abductor hallucis m

Flexor digitorum brevis m

Abductor digiti minimi m

Plantar aponeurosis

Figure 23.4.13

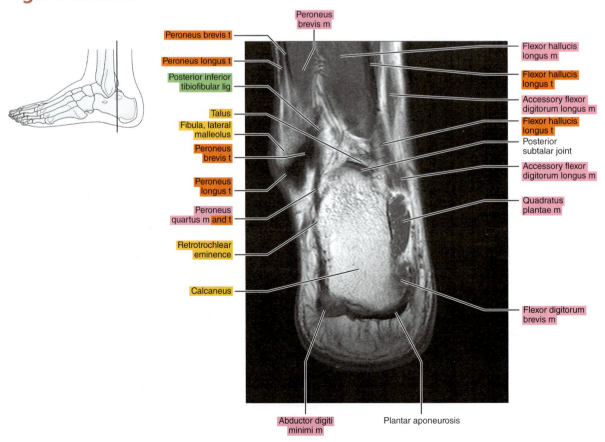

Peroneus brevis t

Peroneus longus t

Posterior inferior tibiofibular lig

Talus

Fibula, lateral malleolus

Peroneus brevis t

Peroneus longus t

Peroneus quartus m and t

Retrotrochlear eminence

Calcaneus

Peroneus brevis m

Flexor hallucis longus m

Flexor hallucis longus t

Accessory flexor digitorum longus m

Flexor hallucis longus t

Posterior subtalar joint

Accessory flexor digitorum longus m

Quadratus plantae m

Flexor digitorum brevis m

Abductor digiti minimi m

Plantar aponeurosis

Figure 23.4.14

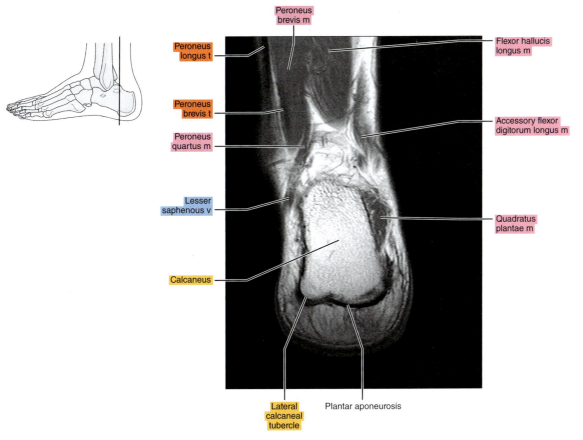

Peroneus brevis m

Peroneus longus t

Peroneus brevis t

Peroneus quartus m

Lesser saphenous v

Calcaneus

Flexor hallucis longus m

Accessory flexor digitorum longus m

Quadratus plantae m

Lateral calcaneal tubercle

Plantar aponeurosis

Figure 23.4.15

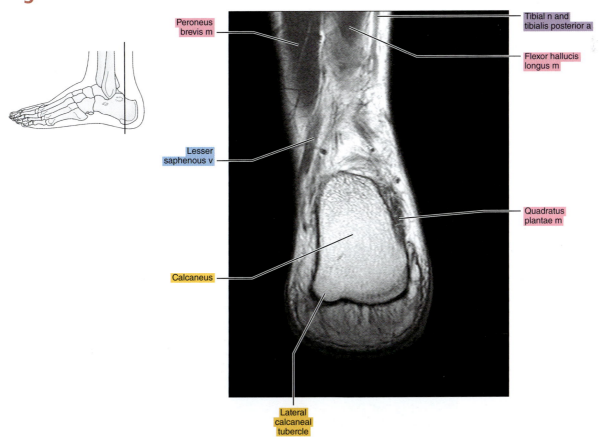

Peroneus brevis m

Lesser saphenous v

Calcaneus

Tibial n and tibialis posterior a

Flexor hallucis longus m

Quadratus plantae m

Lateral calcaneal tubercle

Figure 23.4.16

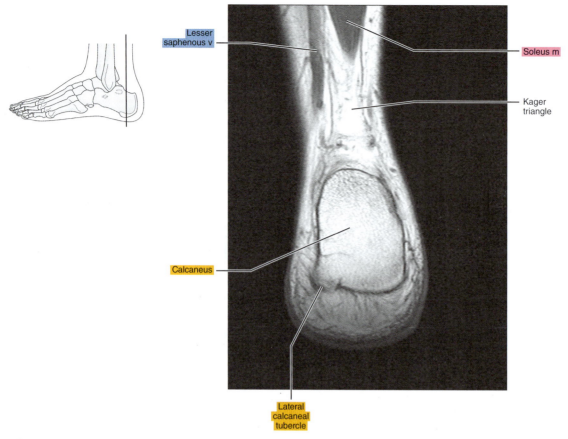

Lesser saphenous v

Soleus m

Kager triangle

Calcaneus

Lateral calcaneal tubercle

Figure 23.4.17

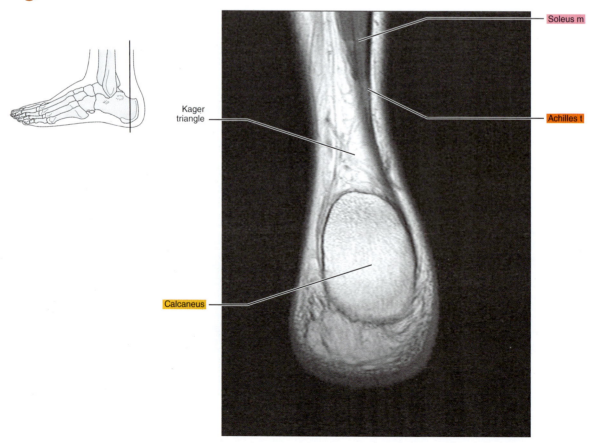

Soleus m

Kager triangle

Achilles t

Calcaneus

Figure 23.4.18

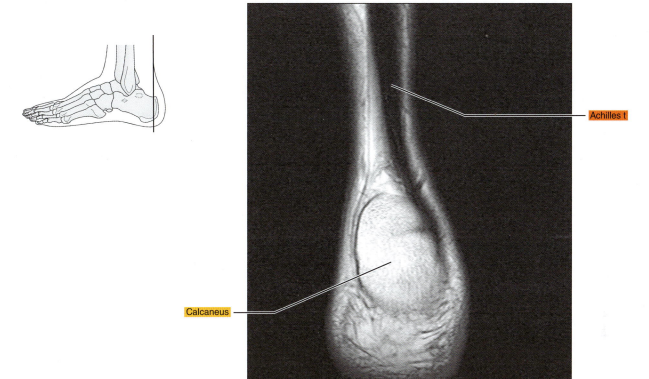

Chapter

24

MRI of the Foot

AXIAL
Figure 24.1.1

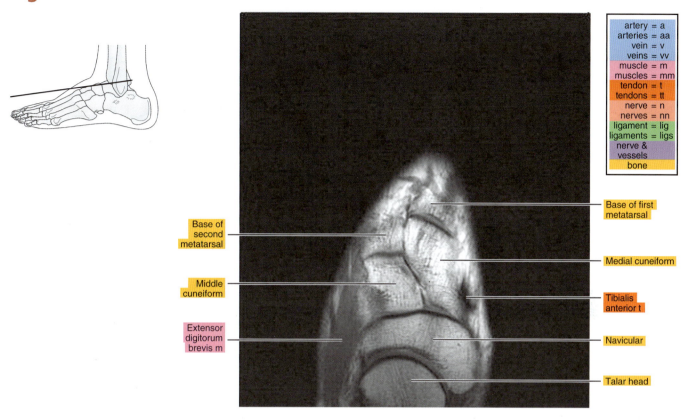

artery = a	
arteries = aa	
vein = v	
veins = vv	
muscle = m	
muscles = mm	
tendon = t	
tendons = tt	
nerve = n	
nerves = nn	
ligament = lig	
ligaments = ligs	
nerve & vessels	
bone	

Base of second metatarsal

Middle cuneiform

Extensor digitorum brevis m

Base of first metatarsal

Medial cuneiform

Tibialis anterior t

Navicular

Talar head

Figure 24.1.2

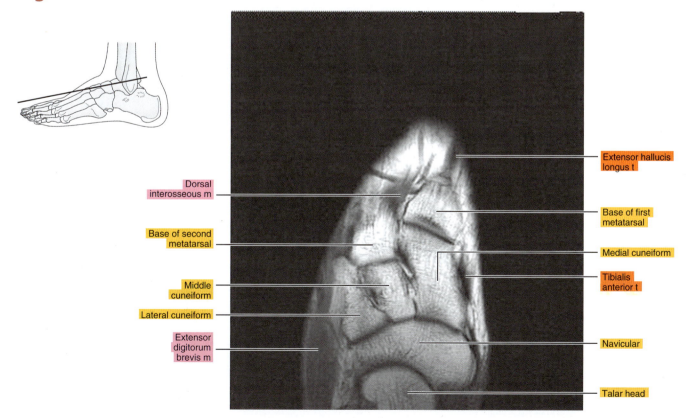

Dorsal interosseous m

Base of second metatarsal

Middle cuneiform

Lateral cuneiform

Extensor digitorum brevis m

Extensor hallucis longus t

Base of first metatarsal

Medial cuneiform

Tibialis anterior t

Navicular

Talar head

Figure 24.1.3

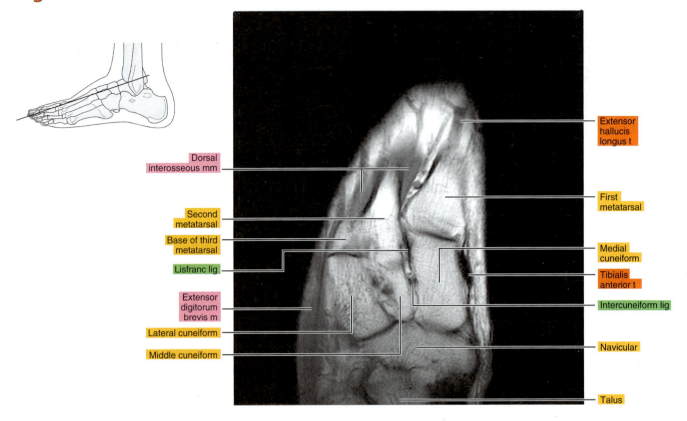

- Dorsal interosseous mm
- Second metatarsal
- Base of third metatarsal
- Lisfranc lig
- Extensor digitorum brevis m
- Lateral cuneiform
- Middle cuneiform
- Extensor hallucis longus t
- First metatarsal
- Medial cuneiform
- Tibialis anterior t
- Intercuneiform lig
- Navicular
- Talus

Figure 24.1.4

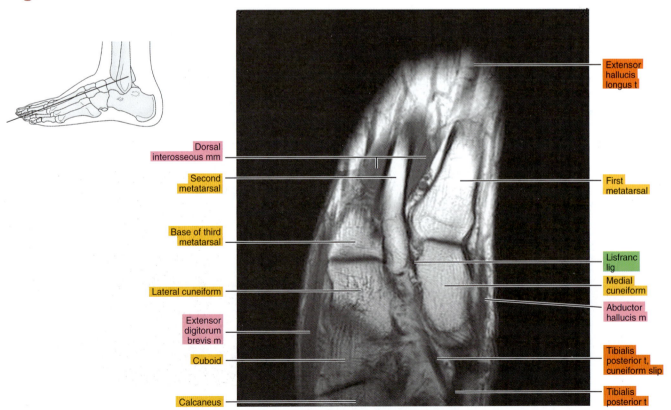

- Dorsal interosseous mm
- Second metatarsal
- Base of third metatarsal
- Lateral cuneiform
- Extensor digitorum brevis m
- Cuboid
- Calcaneus
- Extensor hallucis longus t
- First metatarsal
- Lisfranc lig
- Medial cuneiform
- Abductor hallucis m
- Tibialis posterior t, cuneiform slip
- Tibialis posterior t

Figure 24.1.5

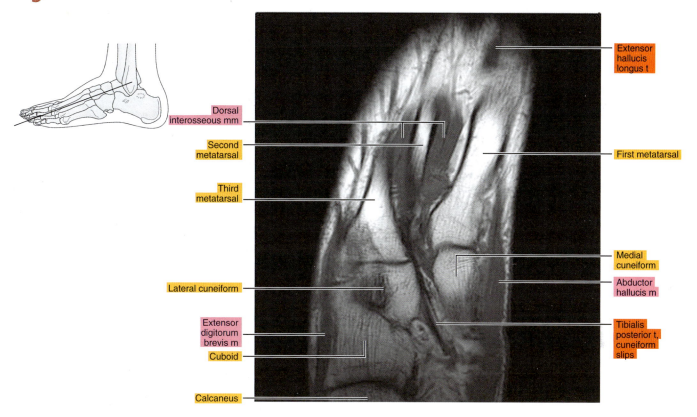

Extensor hallucis longus t

Dorsal interosseous mm

Second metatarsal

Third metatarsal

First metatarsal

Lateral cuneiform

Medial cuneiform

Abductor hallucis m

Extensor digitorum brevis m

Cuboid

Tibialis posterior t, cuneiform slips

Calcaneus

Figure 24.1.6

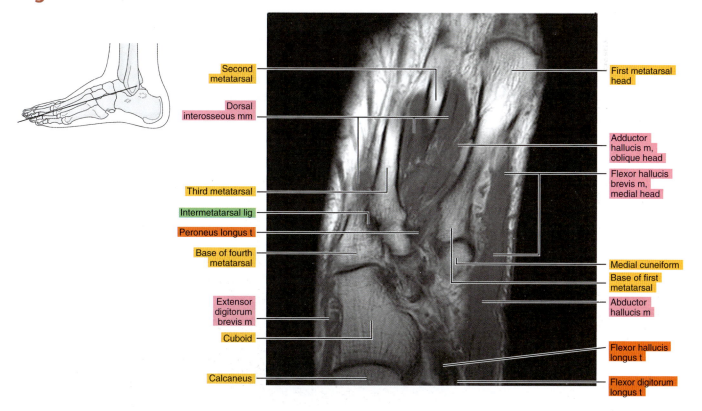

Second metatarsal

Dorsal interosseous mm

First metatarsal head

Adductor hallucis m, oblique head

Flexor hallucis brevis m, medial head

Third metatarsal

Intermetatarsal lig

Peroneus longus t

Base of fourth metatarsal

Medial cuneiform

Base of first metatarsal

Extensor digitorum brevis m

Cuboid

Abductor hallucis m

Flexor hallucis longus t

Calcaneus

Flexor digitorum longus t

Figure 24.1.7

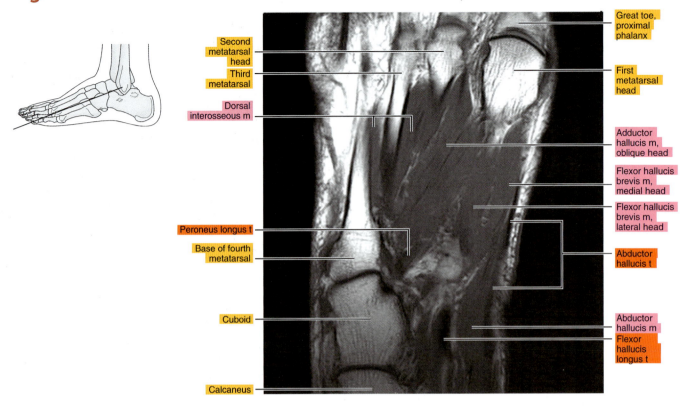

- Second metatarsal head
- Third metatarsal
- Dorsal interosseous m
- Peroneus longus t
- Base of fourth metatarsal
- Cuboid
- Calcaneus
- Great toe, proximal phalanx
- First metatarsal head
- Adductor hallucis m, oblique head
- Flexor hallucis brevis m, medial head
- Flexor hallucis brevis m, lateral head
- Abductor hallucis t
- Abductor hallucis m
- Flexor hallucis longus t

Figure 24.1.8

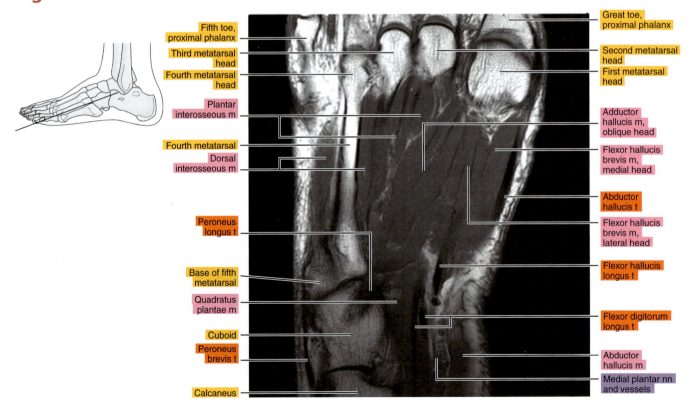

- Fifth toe, proximal phalanx
- Third metatarsal head
- Fourth metatarsal head
- Plantar interosseous m
- Fourth metatarsal
- Dorsal interosseous m
- Peroneus longus t
- Base of fifth metatarsal
- Quadratus plantae m
- Cuboid
- Peroneus brevis t
- Calcaneus
- Great toe, proximal phalanx
- Second metatarsal head
- First metatarsal head
- Adductor hallucis m, oblique head
- Flexor hallucis brevis m, medial head
- Abductor hallucis t
- Flexor hallucis brevis m, lateral head
- Flexor hallucis longus t
- Flexor digitorum longus t
- Abductor hallucis m
- Medial plantar nn and vessels

Figure 24.1.9

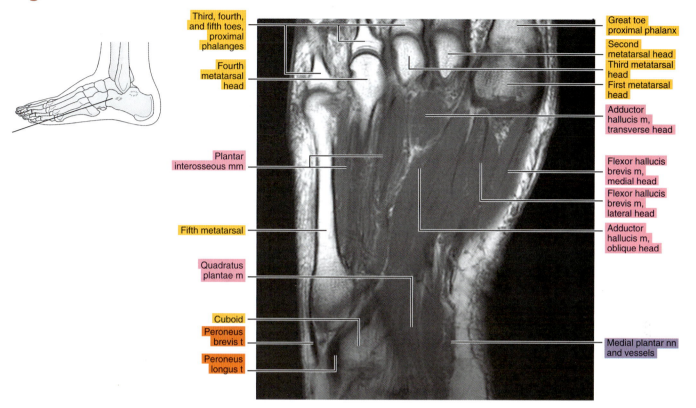

Third, fourth, and fifth toes, proximal phalanges

Fourth metatarsal head

Plantar interosseous mm

Fifth metatarsal

Quadratus plantae m

Cuboid

Peroneus brevis t

Peroneus longus t

Great toe proximal phalanx

Second metatarsal head

Third metatarsal head

First metatarsal head

Adductor hallucis m, transverse head

Flexor hallucis brevis m, medial head

Flexor hallucis brevis m, lateral head

Adductor hallucis m, oblique head

Medial plantar nn and vessels

Figure 24.1.10

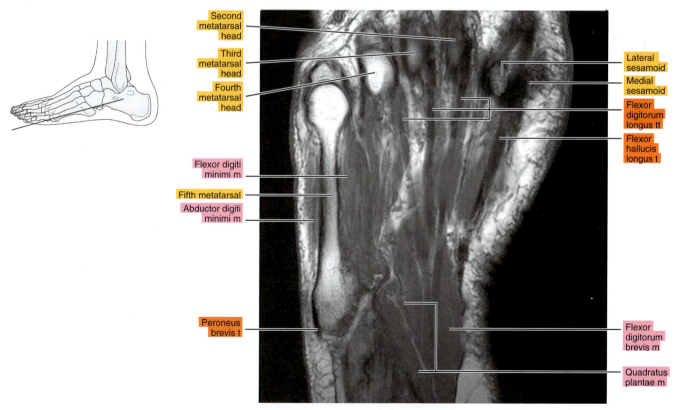

Second metatarsal head

Third metatarsal head

Fourth metatarsal head

Flexor digiti minimi m

Fifth metatarsal

Abductor digiti minimi m

Peroneus brevis t

Lateral sesamoid

Medial sesamoid

Flexor digitorum longus tt

Flexor hallucis longus t

Flexor digitorum brevis m

Quadratus plantae m

Figure 24.1.11

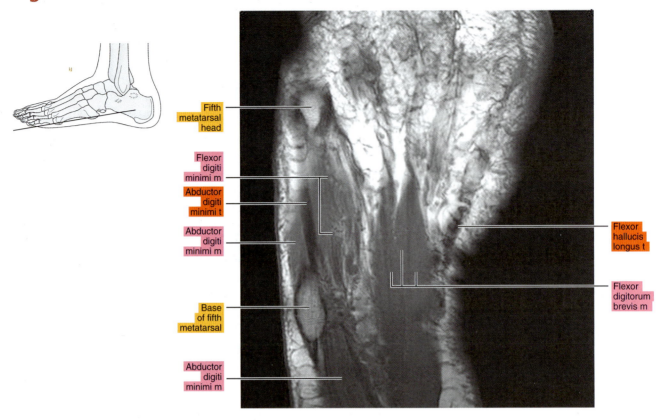

Fifth metatarsal head

Flexor digiti minimi m

Abductor digiti minimi t

Abductor digiti minimi m

Base of fifth metatarsal

Abductor digiti minimi m

Flexor hallucis longus t

Flexor digitorum brevis m

Figure 24.1.12

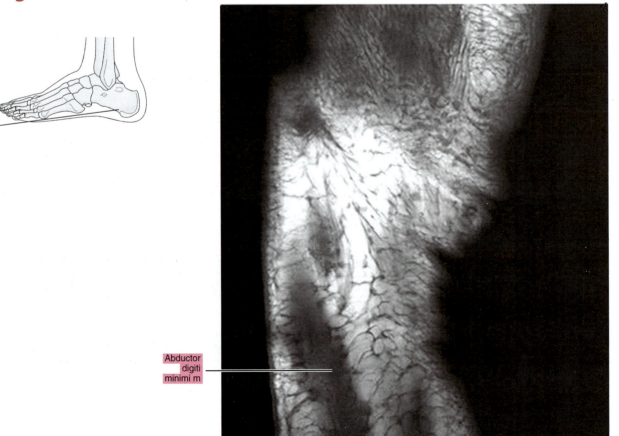

Abductor digiti minimi m

SAGITTAL
Figure 24.2.1

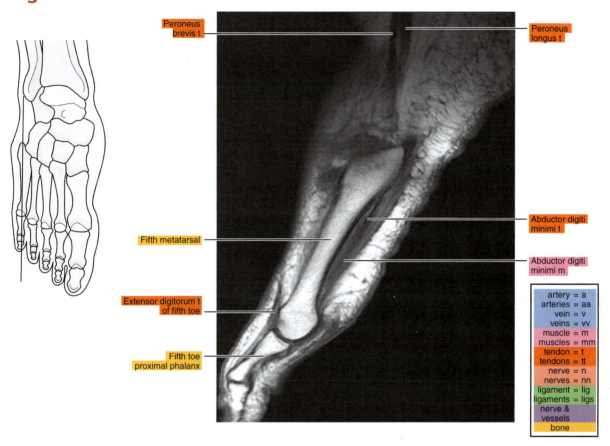

Peroneus brevis t

Peroneus longus t

Fifth metatarsal

Abductor digiti minimi t

Abductor digiti minimi m

Extensor digitorum t of fifth toe

Fifth toe proximal phalanx

artery = a	
arteries = aa	
vein = v	
veins = vv	
muscle = m	
muscles = mm	
tendon = t	
tendons = tt	
nerve = n	
nerves = nn	
ligament = lig	
ligaments = ligs	
nerve & vessels	
bone	

Figure 24.2.2

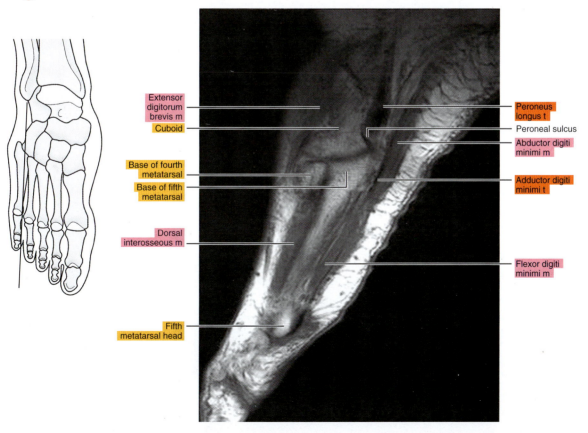

Extensor digitorum brevis m

Cuboid

Peroneus longus t

Peroneal sulcus

Abductor digiti minimi m

Base of fourth metatarsal

Base of fifth metatarsal

Adductor digiti minimi t

Dorsal interosseous m

Flexor digiti minimi m

Fifth metatarsal head

Figure 24.2.3

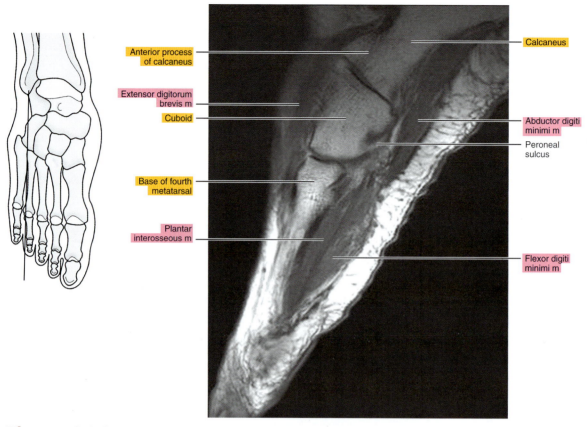

Anterior process of calcaneus

Calcaneus

Extensor digitorum brevis m

Cuboid

Abductor digiti minimi m

Peroneal sulcus

Base of fourth metatarsal

Plantar interosseous m

Flexor digiti minimi m

Figure 24.2.4

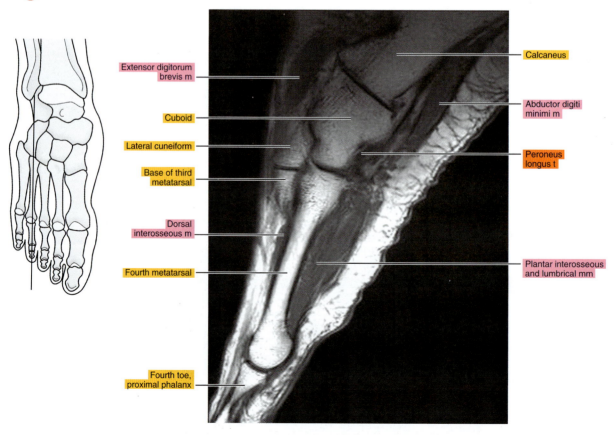

Extensor digitorum brevis m

Calcaneus

Cuboid

Abductor digiti minimi m

Lateral cuneiform

Peroneus longus t

Base of third metatarsal

Dorsal interosseous m

Fourth metatarsal

Plantar interosseous and lumbrical mm

Fourth toe, proximal phalanx

Figure 24.2.5

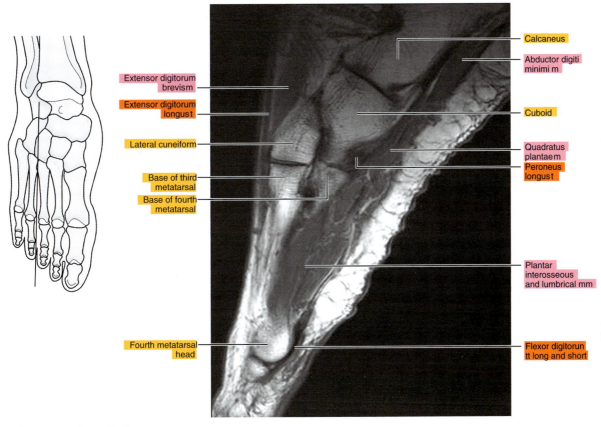

- Extensor digitorum brevis m
- Extensor digitorum longus t
- Lateral cuneiform
- Base of third metatarsal
- Base of fourth metatarsal
- Fourth metatarsal head
- Calcaneus
- Abductor digiti minimi m
- Cuboid
- Quadratus plantae m
- Peroneus longus t
- Plantar interosseous and lumbrical mm
- Flexor digitorun tt long and short

Figure 24.2.6

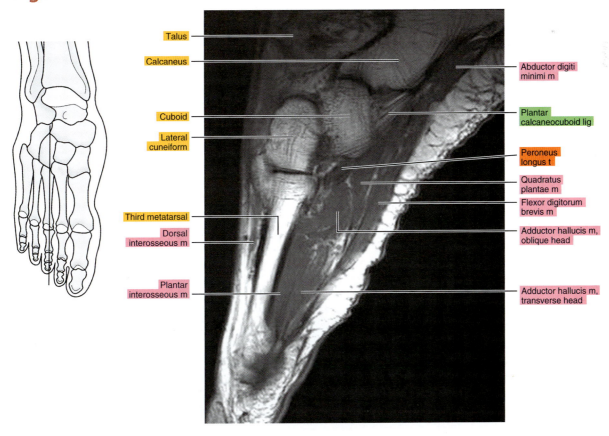

- Talus
- Calcaneus
- Cuboid
- Lateral cuneiform
- Third metatarsal
- Dorsal interosseous m
- Plantar interosseous m
- Abductor digiti minimi m
- Plantar calcaneocuboid lig
- Peroneus longus t
- Quadratus plantae m
- Flexor digitorum brevis m
- Adductor hallucis m, oblique head
- Adductor hallucis m, transverse head

Figure 24.2.7

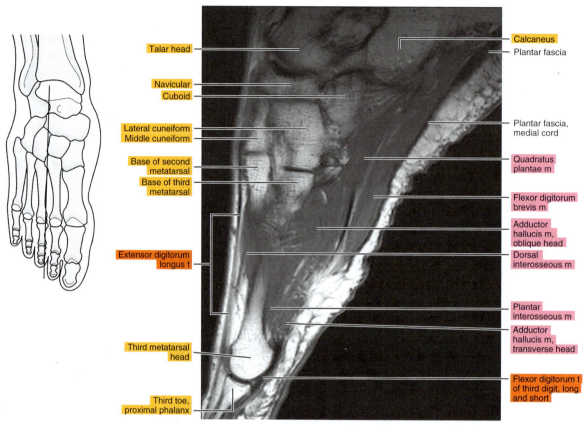

Talar head
Navicular
Cuboid
Lateral cuneiform
Middle cuneiform
Base of second metatarsal
Base of third metatarsal
Extensor digitorum longus t
Third metatarsal head
Third toe, proximal phalanx

Calcaneus
Plantar fascia
Plantar fascia, medial cord
Quadratus plantae m
Flexor digitorum brevis m
Adductor hallucis m, oblique head
Dorsal interosseous m
Plantar interosseous m
Adductor hallucis m, transverse head
Flexor digitorum t of third digit, long and short

Figure 24.2.8

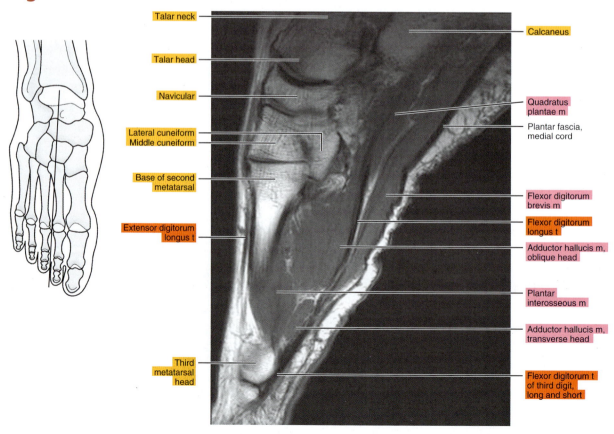

Talar neck
Talar head
Navicular
Lateral cuneiform
Middle cuneiform
Base of second metatarsal
Extensor digitorum longus t
Third metatarsal head

Calcaneus
Quadratus plantae m
Plantar fascia, medial cord
Flexor digitorum brevis m
Flexor digitorum longus t
Adductor hallucis m, oblique head
Plantar interosseous m
Adductor hallucis m, transverse head
Flexor digitorum t of third digit, long and short

Figure 24.2.9

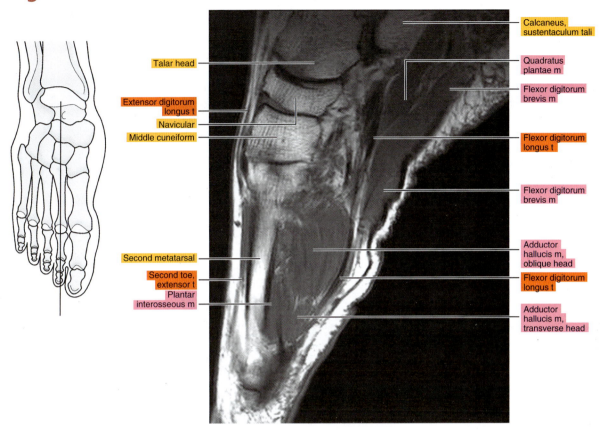

- Calcaneus, sustentaculum tali
- Talar head
- Quadratus plantae m
- Flexor digitorum brevis m
- Extensor digitorum longus t
- Navicular
- Middle cuneiform
- Flexor digitorum longus t
- Flexor digitorum brevis m
- Second metatarsal
- Adductor hallucis m, oblique head
- Second toe, extensor t
- Flexor digitorum longus t
- Plantar interosseous m
- Adductor hallucis m, transverse head

Figure 24.2.10

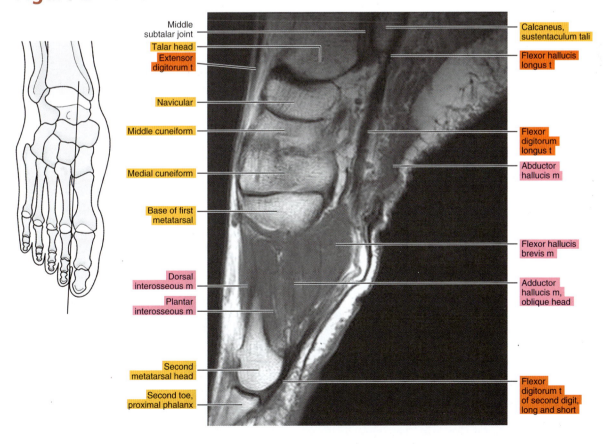

- Middle subtalar joint
- Calcaneus, sustentaculum tali
- Talar head
- Flexor hallucis longus t
- Extensor digitorum t
- Navicular
- Middle cuneiform
- Flexor digitorum longus t
- Medial cuneiform
- Abductor hallucis m
- Base of first metatarsal
- Flexor hallucis brevis m
- Dorsal interosseous m
- Adductor hallucis m, oblique head
- Plantar interosseous m
- Second metatarsal head
- Flexor digitorum t of second digit, long and short
- Second toe, proximal phalanx

Figure 24.2.11

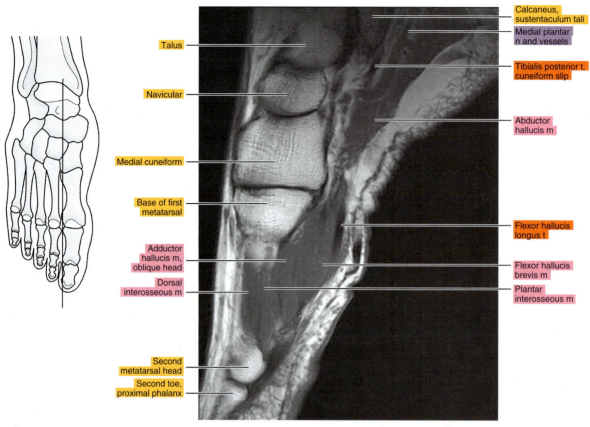

Calcaneus, sustentaculum tali

Medial plantar n and vessels

Talus

Tibialis posterior t, cuneiform slip

Navicular

Abductor hallucis m

Medial cuneiform

Base of first metatarsal

Flexor hallucis longus t

Adductor hallucis m, oblique head

Flexor hallucis brevis m

Dorsal interosseous m

Plantar interosseous m

Second metatarsal head

Second toe, proximal phalanx

Figure 24.2.12

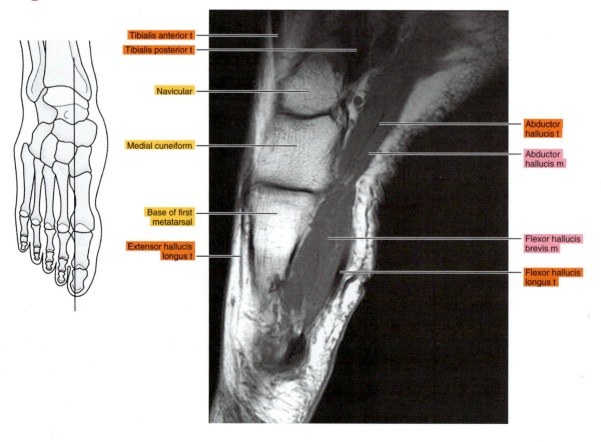

Tibialis anterior t

Tibialis posterior t

Navicular

Abductor hallucis t

Abductor hallucis m

Medial cuneiform

Base of first metatarsal

Flexor hallucis brevis m

Extensor hallucis longus t

Flexor hallucis longus t

Figure 24.2.13

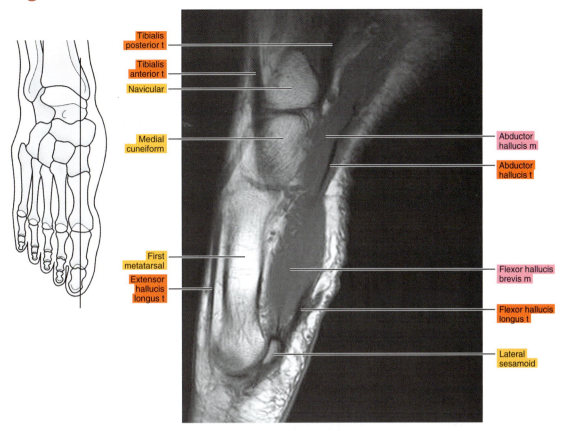

Tibialis posterior t
Tibialis anterior t
Navicular
Medial cuneiform
First metatarsal
Extensor hallucis longus t
Abductor hallucis m
Abductor hallucis t
Flexor hallucis brevis m
Flexor hallucis longus t
Lateral sesamoid

Figure 24.2.14

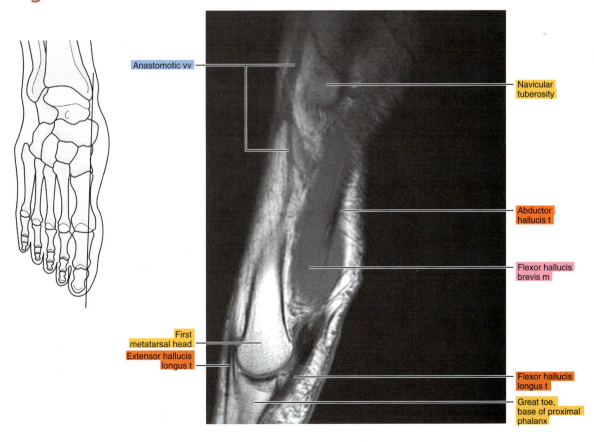

Anastomotic vv
Navicular tuberosity
Abductor hallucis t
Flexor hallucis brevis m
First metatarsal head
Extensor hallucis longus t
Flexor hallucis longus t
Great toe, base of proximal phalanx

Figure 24.2.15

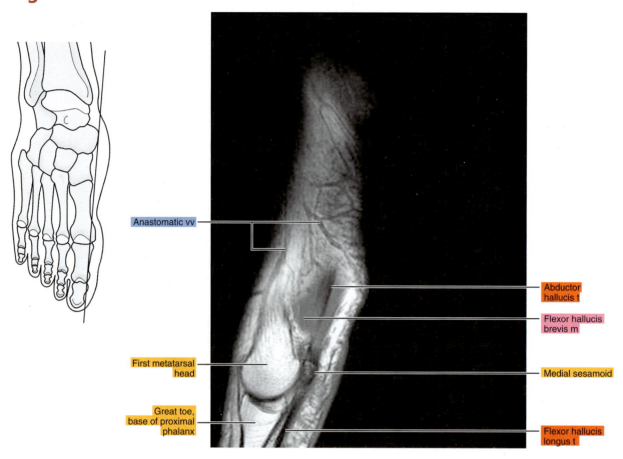

Anastomatic vv

Abductor hallucis t

Flexor hallucis brevis m

First metatarsal head

Medial sesamoid

Great toe, base of proximal phalanx

Flexor hallucis longus t

CORONAL
Figure 24.3.1

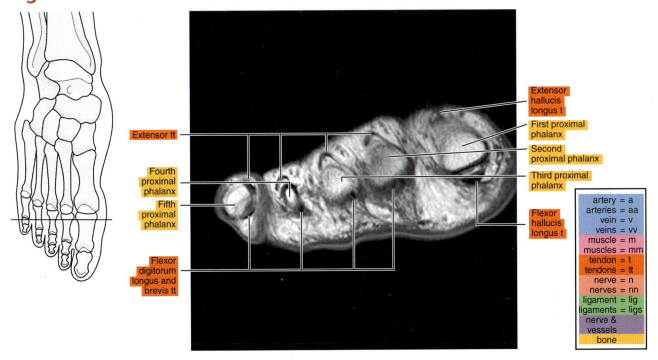

Extensor hallucis longus t

First proximal phalanx

Second proximal phalanx

Third proximal phalanx

Flexor hallucis longus t

Extensor tt

Fourth proximal phalanx

Fifth proximal phalanx

Flexor digitorum longus and brevis tt

artery = a	
arteries = aa	
vein = v	
veins = vv	
muscle = m	
muscles = mm	
tendon = t	
tendons = tt	
nerve = n	
nerves = nn	
ligament = lig	
ligaments = ligs	
nerve & vessels	
bone	

Figure 24.3.2

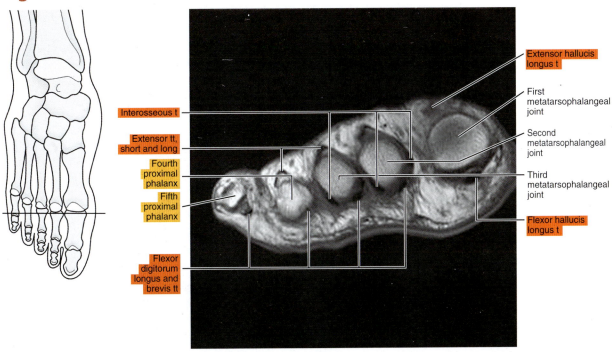

Extensor hallucis longus t

First metatarsophalangeal joint

Second metatarsophalangeal joint

Third metatarsophalangeal joint

Flexor hallucis longus t

Interosseous t

Extensor tt, short and long

Fourth proximal phalanx

Fifth proximal phalanx

Flexor digitorum longus and brevis tt

Figure 24.3.3

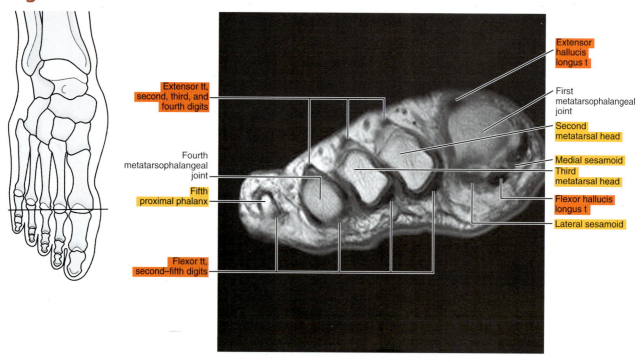

Extensor hallucis longus t

First metatarsophalangeal joint

Second metatarsal head

Medial sesamoid

Third metatarsal head

Flexor hallucis longus t

Lateral sesamoid

Extensor tt, second, third, and fourth digits

Fourth metatarsophalangeal joint

Fifth proximal phalanx

Flexor tt, second–fifth digits

Figure 24.3.4

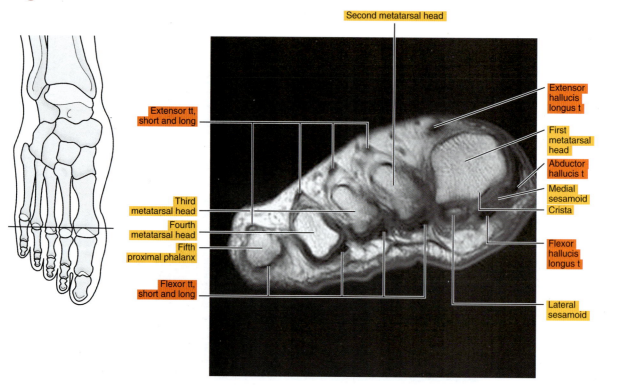

Second metatarsal head

Extensor hallucis longus t

First metatarsal head

Abductor hallucis t

Medial sesamoid

Crista

Flexor hallucis longus t

Lateral sesamoid

Extensor tt, short and long

Third metatarsal head

Fourth metatarsal head

Fifth proximal phalanx

Flexor tt, short and long

Figure 24.3.5

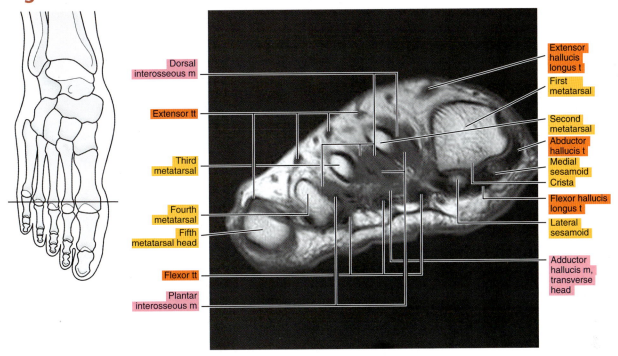

Dorsal interosseous m

Extensor tt

Third metatarsal

Fourth metatarsal

Fifth metatarsal head

Flexor tt

Plantar interosseous m

Extensor hallucis longus t

First metatarsal

Second metatarsal

Abductor hallucis t

Medial sesamoid

Crista

Flexor hallucis longus t

Lateral sesamoid

Adductor hallucis m, transverse head

Figure 24.3.6

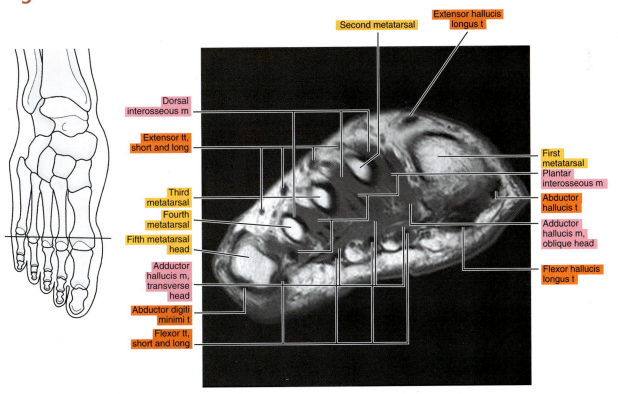

Second metatarsal

Extensor hallucis longus t

Dorsal interosseous m

Extensor tt, short and long

Third metatarsal

Fourth metatarsal

Fifth metatarsal head

Adductor hallucis m, transverse head

Abductor digiti minimi t

Flexor tt, short and long

First metatarsal

Plantar interosseous m

Abductor hallucis t

Adductor hallucis m, oblique head

Flexor hallucis longus t

Figure 24.3.7

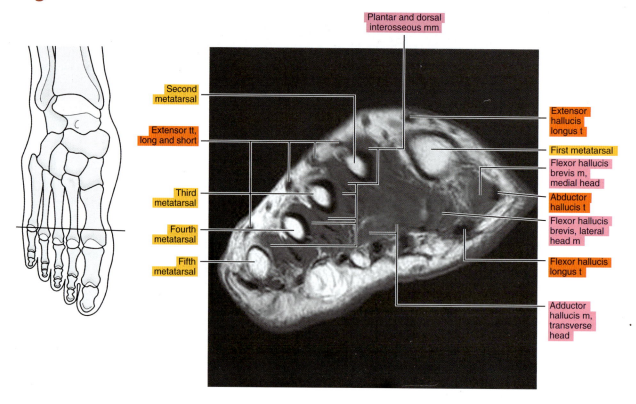

Plantar and dorsal interosseous mm

Second metatarsal

Extensor tt, long and short

Third metatarsal

Fourth metatarsal

Fifth metatarsal

Extensor hallucis longus t

First metatarsal

Flexor hallucis brevis m, medial head

Abductor hallucis t

Flexor hallucis brevis, lateral head m

Flexor hallucis longus t

Adductor hallucis m, transverse head

Figure 24.3.8

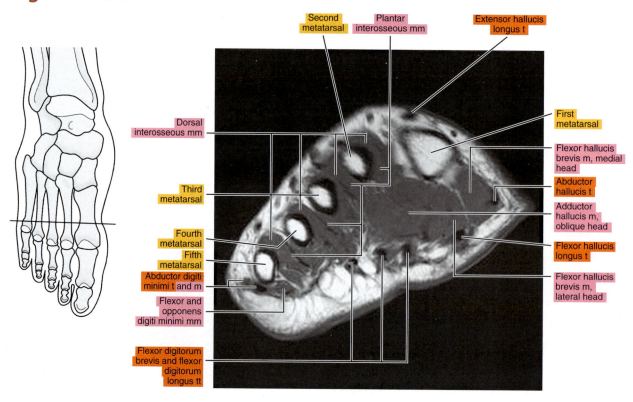

Second metatarsal

Plantar interosseous mm

Extensor hallucis longus t

Dorsal interosseous mm

Third metatarsal

Fourth metatarsal

Fifth metatarsal

Abductor digiti minimi t and m

Flexor and opponens digiti minimi mm

Flexor digitorum brevis and flexor digitorum longus tt

First metatarsal

Flexor hallucis brevis m, medial head

Abductor hallucis t

Adductor hallucis m, oblique head

Flexor hallucis longus t

Flexor hallucis brevis m, lateral head

Figure 24.3.9

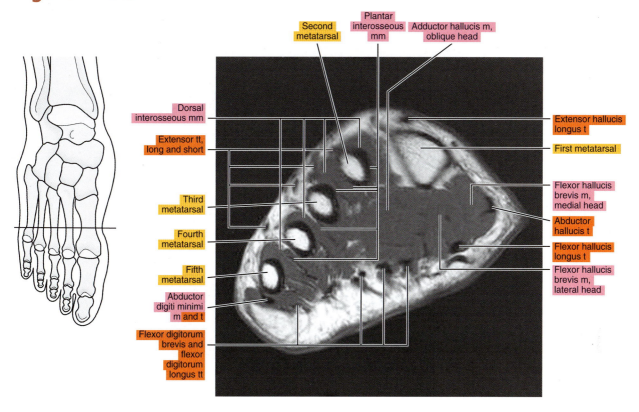

Second metatarsal

Plantar interosseous mm

Adductor hallucis m, oblique head

Dorsal interosseous mm

Extensor tt, long and short

Third metatarsal

Fourth metatarsal

Fifth metatarsal

Abductor digiti minimi m and t

Flexor digitorum brevis and flexor digitorum longus tt

Extensor hallucis longus t

First metatarsal

Flexor hallucis brevis m, medial head

Abductor hallucis t

Flexor hallucis longus t

Flexor hallucis brevis m, lateral head

Figure 24.3.10

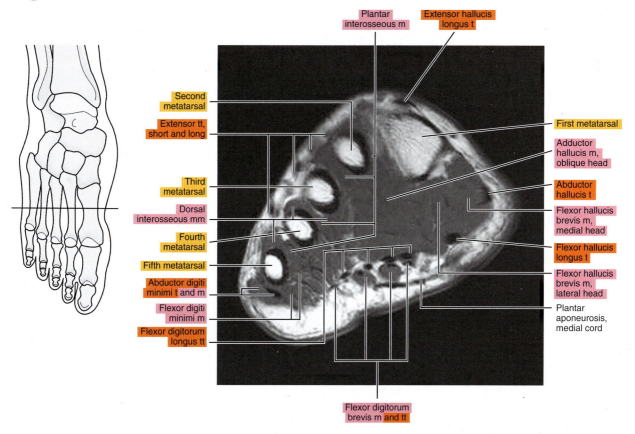

Plantar interosseous m

Extensor hallucis longus t

Second metatarsal

Extensor tt, short and long

Third metatarsal

Dorsal interosseous mm

Fourth metatarsal

Fifth metatarsal

Abductor digiti minimi t and m

Flexor digiti minimi m

Flexor digitorum longus tt

First metatarsal

Adductor hallucis m, oblique head

Abductor hallucis t

Flexor hallucis brevis m, medial head

Flexor hallucis longus t

Flexor hallucis brevis m, lateral head

Plantar aponeurosis, medial cord

Flexor digitorum brevis m and tt

Figure 24.3.11

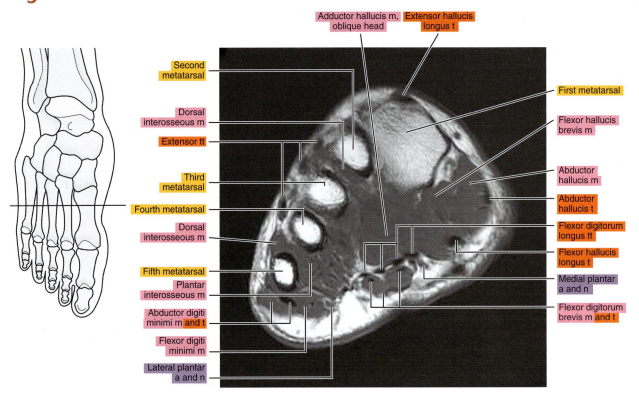

Adductor hallucis m, oblique head
Extensor hallucis longus t
Second metatarsal
Dorsal interosseous m
Extensor tt
Third metatarsal
Fourth metatarsal
Dorsal interosseous m
Fifth metatarsal
Plantar interosseous m
Abductor digiti minimi m and t
Flexor digiti minimi m
Lateral plantar a and n
First metatarsal
Flexor hallucis brevis m
Abductor hallucis m
Abductor hallucis t
Flexor digitorum longus tt
Flexor hallucis longus t
Medial plantar a and n
Flexor digitorum brevis m and t

Figure 24.3.12

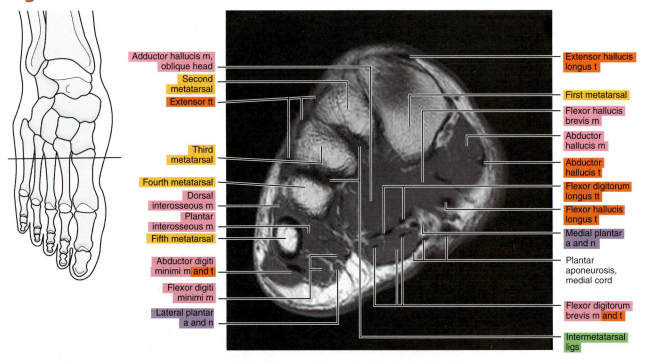

Adductor hallucis m, oblique head
Second metatarsal
Extensor tt
Third metatarsal
Fourth metatarsal
Dorsal interosseous m
Plantar interosseous m
Fifth metatarsal
Abductor digiti minimi m and t
Flexor digiti minimi m
Lateral plantar a and n
Extensor hallucis longus t
First metatarsal
Flexor hallucis brevis m
Abductor hallucis m
Abductor hallucis t
Flexor digitorum longus tt
Flexor hallucis longus t
Medial plantar a and n
Plantar aponeurosis, medial cord
Flexor digitorum brevis m and t
Intermetatarsal ligs

Figure 24.3.13

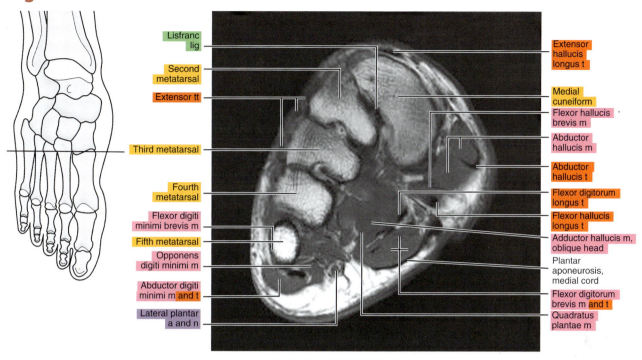

Lisfranc lig
Second metatarsal
Extensor tt
Third metatarsal
Fourth metatarsal
Flexor digiti minimi brevis m
Fifth metatarsal
Opponens digiti minimi m
Abductor digiti minimi m and t
Lateral plantar a and n

Extensor hallucis longus t
Medial cuneiform
Flexor hallucis brevis m
Abductor hallucis m
Abductor hallucis t
Flexor digitorum longus t
Flexor hallucis longus t
Adductor hallucis m, oblique head
Plantar aponeurosis, medial cord
Flexor digitorum brevis m and t
Quadratus plantae m

Figure 24.3.14

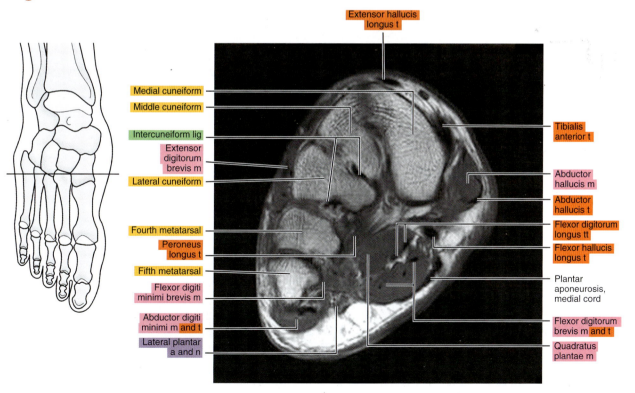

Extensor hallucis longus t

Medial cuneiform
Middle cuneiform
Intercuneiform lig
Extensor digitorum brevis m
Lateral cuneiform
Fourth metatarsal
Peroneus longus t
Fifth metatarsal
Flexor digiti minimi brevis m
Abductor digiti minimi m and t
Lateral plantar a and n

Tibialis anterior t
Abductor hallucis m
Abductor hallucis t
Flexor digitorum longus tt
Flexor hallucis longus t
Plantar aponeurosis, medial cord
Flexor digitorum brevis m and t
Quadratus plantae m

Figure 24.3.15

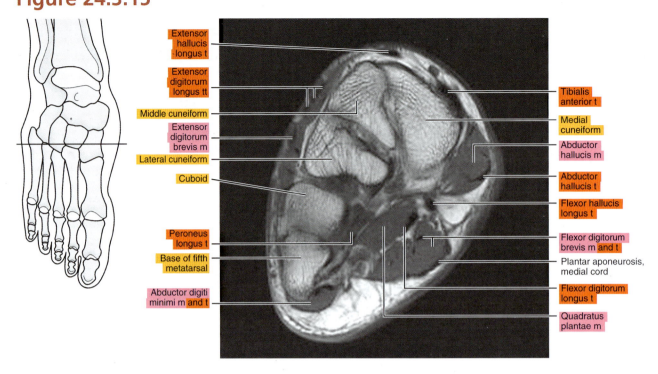

Extensor hallucis longus t
Extensor digitorum longus tt
Middle cuneiform
Extensor digitorum brevis m
Lateral cuneiform
Cuboid
Peroneus longus t
Base of fifth metatarsal
Abductor digiti minimi m and t

Tibialis anterior t
Medial cuneiform
Abductor hallucis m
Abductor hallucis t
Flexor hallucis longus t
Flexor digitorum brevis m and t
Plantar aponeurosis, medial cord
Flexor digitorum longus t
Quadratus plantae m

Figure 24.3.16

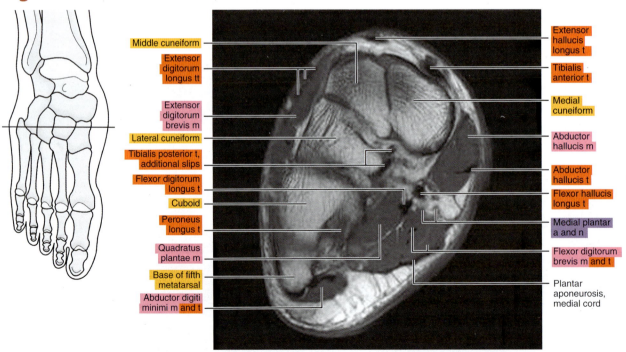

Middle cuneiform
Extensor digitorum longus tt
Extensor digitorum brevis m
Lateral cuneiform
Tibialis posterior t, additional slips
Flexor digitorum longus t
Cuboid
Peroneus longus t
Quadratus plantae m
Base of fifth metatarsal
Abductor digiti minimi m and t

Extensor hallucis longus t
Tibialis anterior t
Medial cuneiform
Abductor hallucis m
Abductor hallucis t
Flexor hallucis longus t
Medial plantar a and n
Flexor digitorum brevis m and t
Plantar aponeurosis, medial cord

Figure 24.3.17

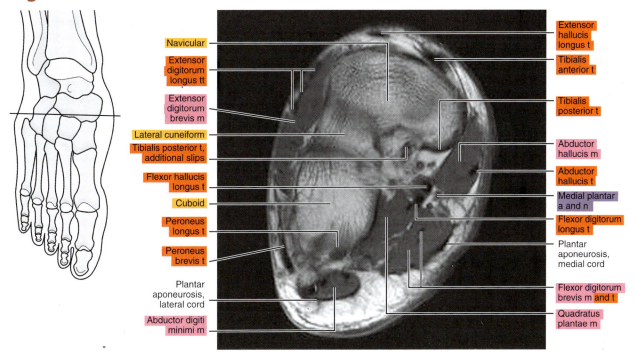

Navicular

Extensor digitorum longus tt

Extensor digitorum brevis m

Lateral cuneiform

Tibialis posterior t, additional slips

Flexor hallucis longus t

Cuboid

Peroneus longus t

Peroneus brevis t

Plantar aponeurosis, lateral cord

Abductor digiti minimi m

Extensor hallucis longus t

Tibialis anterior t

Tibialis posterior t

Abductor hallucis m

Abductor hallucis t

Medial plantar a and n

Flexor digitorum longus t

Plantar aponeurosis, medial cord

Flexor digitorum brevis m and t

Quadratus plantae m

Figure 24.3.18

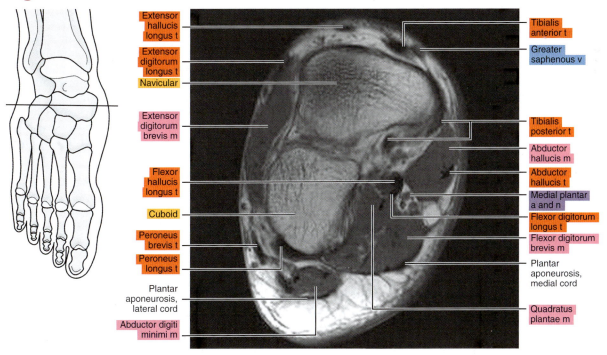

Extensor hallucis longus t

Extensor digitorum longus t

Navicular

Extensor digitorum brevis m

Flexor hallucis longus t

Cuboid

Peroneus brevis t

Peroneus longus t

Plantar aponeurosis, lateral cord

Abductor digiti minimi m

Tibialis anterior t

Greater saphenous v

Tibialis posterior t

Abductor hallucis m

Abductor hallucis t

Medial plantar a and n

Flexor digitorum longus t

Flexor digitorum brevis m

Plantar aponeurosis, medial cord

Quadratus plantae m

Table 24-1. Muscles of the Foot

MUSCLE	ORIGIN	INSERTION	NERVE SUPPLY
Extensor digitorum brevis	Distal part of the lateral and superior surfaces of the calcaneus and the apex of the inferior extensor retinaculum.	As the fiber bundles extend distally, they become grouped into four bellies. Those fibers of the most medial and largest belly are known as extensor hallucis brevis. The tendon of this muscle inserts onto the base of the first metatarsal. The remaining fiber bundles have more variable insertions. The second toe fibers usually insert onto the middle dorsal aspect of the base of the proximal phalanx and are often united with the long extensor tendon. The three more lateral tendons are usually fused with the lateral margins of the corresponding long extensor tendons near the bases of the respective middle phalanges and usually extend to the bases of the corresponding proximal phalanges.	Deep peroneal.
Flexor digitorum	Medial process of the tuber calcanei, posterior third of the plantar aponeurosis, and medial and lateral intermuscular septa.	Tendons of the short (brevis) flexors pass superficial to those of the long flexor into the osteofibrous canals on the flexor surface of the digits. On the proximal phalanx of each toe, the tendon of the short flexor divides and forms an opening through which the tendon of the long flexor passes. The tendons of the short flexor insert onto the base of the middle phalanx.	Surface near the medial edge of the muscle.
Quadratus plantae (flexor accessorius)	Two heads: a small lateral and a large medial one. (1) Lateral head arises from an elongated tendon from the lateral process of the tuberosity of the calcaneus and from the lateral margin of the long plantar ligament. (2) Medial head originates from the medial surface of the calcaneus in front of the tuberosity and from adjacent ligaments.	The two heads are separated at their origin by a short triangular space. The heads fuse to form a single belly, but the fiber bundles of each head are separately inserted. From the lateral head, the fibers insert into the lateral margin of the flexor tendon. The medial head inserts as an aponeurosis into the deep surface of the flexor tendon.	Lateral plantar nerve branch that passes obliquely across the superficial surface of the muscle, parallel with the tendon of the flexor digitorum longus.
Lumbricals	Three lateral lumbricals arise from the adjacent sides of the digital tendons of the flexor digitorum longus. The first lumbrical arises on the medial margin of the second toe.	Fiber bundles of each muscle converge on both sides of a tendon that becomes free near the metatarsophalangeal joint and is inserted onto the medial side of the proximal phalanx of the appropriate toe. A tendinous expansion is inserted into the aponeurosis of the extensor muscle.	Three lateral lumbricals are usually supplied by branches of the deep ramus of the lateral plantar nerve. Medial lumbrical is supplied by the first common plantar digital branch of the medial plantar nerve. This nerve may supply the two more medial muscles, or the medial muscles may receive a double nerve supply.

Table 24-1. Muscles of the Foot

MUSCLE	ORIGIN	INSERTION	NERVE SUPPLY
Abductor hallucis	Medial border of the medial process of the tuber calcanei, flexor retinaculum, and plantar aponeurosis.	Along with the tendon of the medial belly of flexor brevis onto the base of the proximal phalanx of the great toe.	Branch of the medial plantar.
Flexor hallucis brevis	From the plantar surface of the lateral cuneiform and cuboid bones.	The medial and lateral sides of the base of the proximal phalanx of the great toe.	Branch from the medial plantar or first plantar digital. Rarely, the lateral body may receive a branch from the lateral plantar.
Adductor hallucis, oblique head	Tuberosity of the cuboid and sheath of the tendon of the peroneus longus, the plantar calcaneocuboid ligament, the third cuneiform, and bases of the second and third metatarsals.	By a flat tendon that inserts in common with that of the flexor brevis onto the lateral part of the plantar surface of the base of the proximal phalanx and by a slip into the aponeurosis of the long extensor muscle on the back of the great toe.	Branch of the deep ramus of the lateral plantar.
Adductor hallucis, transverse head	Joint capsules of the third, fourth, and fifth metatarsophalangeal joints and the deep transverse metatarsal ligaments.	By a common tendon that splits and passes on each side of the tendon of the oblique head and is inserted into the sheath on the tendon of the long flexor of the great toe.	Branch from the deep ramus of the lateral plantar.
Abductor digiti minimi	Lateral and medial processes of the tuber calcanei and lateral and plantar surfaces of the body of the bone in front of these, lateral intermuscular septum, deep surface of the lateral plantar fascia, and fibrous band extending from the calcaneus to the lateral side of the base of the fifth metatarsal.	Onto the lateral surface of the proximal phalanx of the little toe and the metatarsophalangeal capsule.	Lateral plantar.
Flexor digiti minimi brevis	Sheath of the peroneus longus, tuberosity of the cuboid, and base of the fifth metatarsal.	By short tendinous bands onto the base of the proximal phalanx of the little toe, the capsule of the corresponding joint, and the aponeurosis on the dorsal surface of the toe.	Branch from the superficial ramus of the lateral plantar.
Opponens digiti minimi	An inconstant muscle, it may arise from the sheath of the peroneus longus and the tuberosity of the cuboid by a thin tendon that passes over the tuberosity of the fifth metatarsal.	Onto the lateral surface of the fifth metatarsal.	Branch from the nerve to the flexor brevis and the superficial ramus of the lateral plantar.

continued

Table 24-1. Muscles of the Foot–cont'd

MUSCLE	ORIGIN	INSERTION	NERVE SUPPLY
Interosseous, dorsal	Each of the three lateral dorsal interosseous muscles arises from the sides of the shaft and the plantar surface of the bases of the metatarsals, bounding the space in which each lies, from the fascia covering it dorsally, and from the fibrous prolongations from the long plantar ligament. The first (medial) has a similar origin, except that its medial origin is by a tendinous slip from the peroneus longus tendon and, occasionally, by fiber bundles from the medial side of the proximal end of the first metatarsal.	The first and second interosseous muscles onto each side of the base of the proximal phalanx of the second toe; the third and fourth onto the lateral side of the bases of the proximal phalanges of the third and fourth toes. Each tendon adheres to the capsule of the adjacent joint.	Deep branch of the lateral plantar. The interosseous muscles of the fourth interspace are usually supplied by a branch from the superficial ramus of the lateral plantar.
Interosseous, plantar	The plantar interosseous muscle arises from the proximal third of the medial plantar surface of the shaft, from the base of the metatarsal on which it lies, and from the fascial expansions of the long plantar ligament.	Onto a tubercle on the medial side of the base of the proximal phalanx of the digit to which it goes.	Lateral plantar.

Section VII

Pelvis

CT of the Male Pelvis

AXIAL
Figure 25.1.1

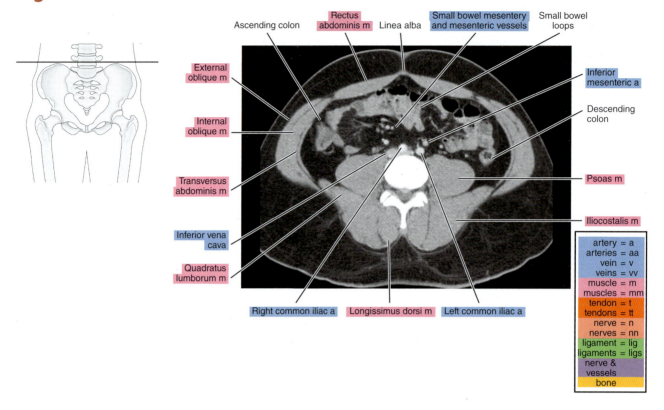

Ascending colon
Rectus abdominis m
Linea alba
Small bowel mesentery and mesenteric vessels
Small bowel loops
External oblique m
Inferior mesenteric a
Internal oblique m
Descending colon
Transversus abdominis m
Psoas m
Iliocostalis m
Inferior vena cava
Quadratus lumborum m
Right common iliac a
Longissimus dorsi m
Left common iliac a

artery = a
arteries = aa
vein = v
veins = vv
muscle = m
muscles = mm
tendon = t
tendons = tt
nerve = n
nerves = nn
ligament = lig
ligaments = ligs
nerve & vessels
bone

Figure 25.1.2

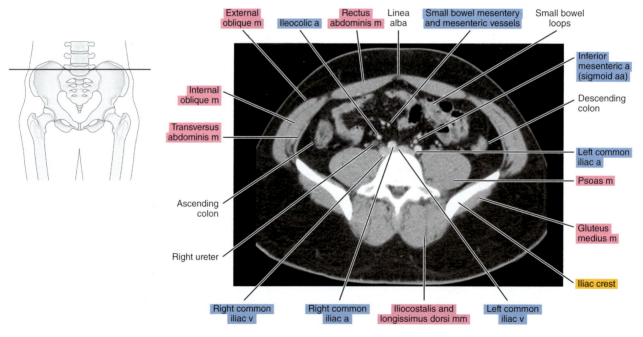

External oblique m
Ileocolic a
Rectus abdominis m
Linea alba
Small bowel mesentery and mesenteric vessels
Small bowel loops
Inferior mesenteric a (sigmoid aa)
Internal oblique m
Descending colon
Transversus abdominis m
Left common iliac a
Psoas m
Ascending colon
Gluteus medius m
Right ureter
Iliac crest
Right common iliac v
Right common iliac a
Iliocostalis and longissimus dorsi mm
Left common iliac v

Figure 25.1.3

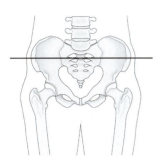

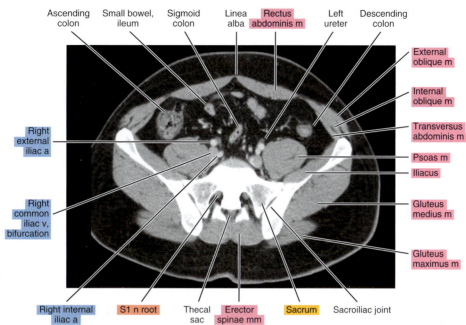

Ascending colon · Small bowel, ileum · Sigmoid colon · Linea alba · Rectus abdominis m · Left ureter · Descending colon · External oblique m · Internal oblique m · Transversus abdominis m · Psoas m · Iliacus · Gluteus medius m · Gluteus maximus m · Right external iliac a · Right common iliac v, bifurcation · Right internal iliac a · S1 n root · Thecal sac · Erector spinae mm · Sacrum · Sacroiliac joint

Figure 25.1.4

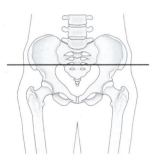

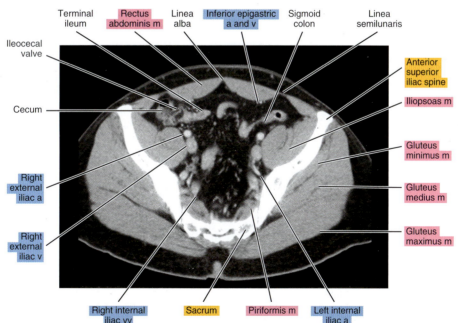

Terminal ileum · Rectus abdominis m · Linea alba · Inferior epigastric a and v · Sigmoid colon · Linea semilunaris · Ileocecal valve · Anterior superior iliac spine · Iliopsoas m · Cecum · Gluteus minimus m · Gluteus medius m · Gluteus maximus m · Right external iliac a · Right external iliac v · Right internal iliac vv · Sacrum · Piriformis m · Left internal iliac a

Figure 25.1.5

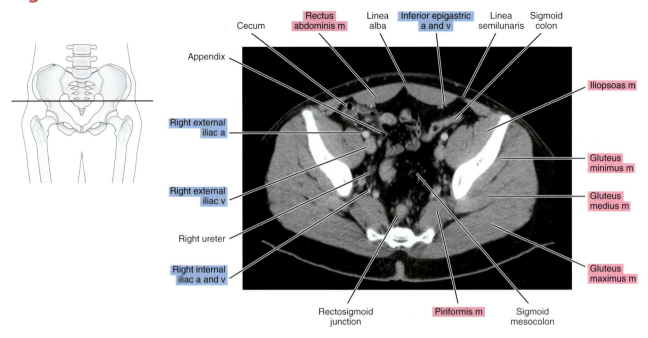

Cecum — Rectus abdominis m — Linea alba — Inferior epigastric a and v — Linea semilunaris — Sigmoid colon

Appendix

Iliopsoas m

Right external iliac a

Right external iliac v

Right ureter

Right internal iliac a and v

Gluteus minimus m

Gluteus medius m

Gluteus maximus m

Rectosigmoid junction — Piriformis m — Sigmoid mesocolon

Figure 25.1.6

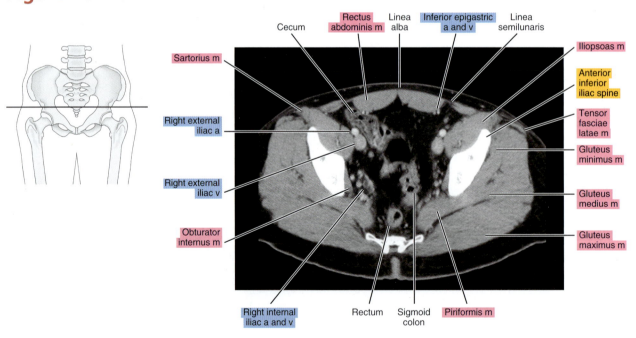

Cecum — Rectus abdominis m — Linea alba — Inferior epigastric a and v — Linea semilunaris

Sartorius m

Iliopsoas m

Anterior inferior iliac spine

Right external iliac a

Tensor fasciae latae m

Gluteus minimus m

Right external iliac v

Gluteus medius m

Obturator internus m

Gluteus maximus m

Right internal iliac a and v — Rectum — Sigmoid colon — Piriformis m

Figure 25.1.7

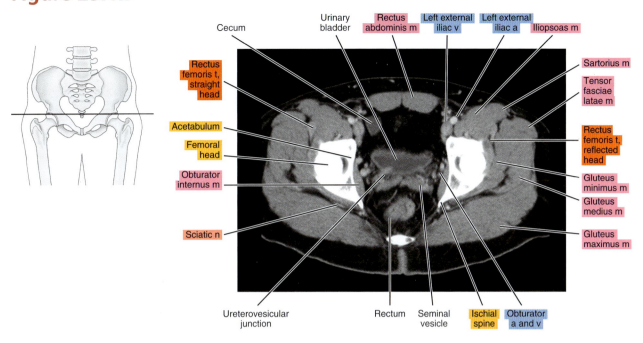

Cecum

Urinary bladder

Rectus abdominis m

Left external iliac v

Left external iliac a

Iliopsoas m

Rectus femoris t, straight head

Sartorius m

Tensor fasciae latae m

Acetabulum

Femoral head

Rectus femoris t, reflected head

Obturator internus m

Gluteus minimus m

Gluteus medius m

Sciatic n

Gluteus maximus m

Ureterovesicular junction

Rectum

Seminal vesicle

Ischial spine

Obturator a and v

Figure 25.1.8

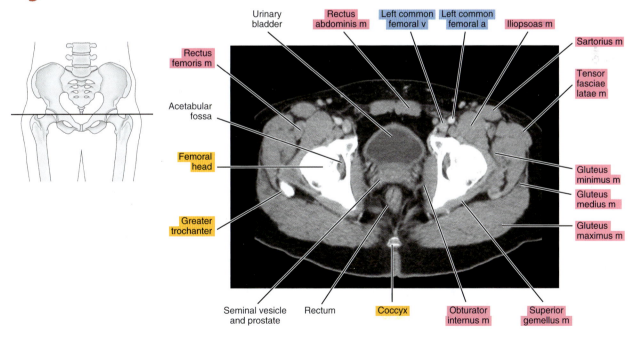

Urinary bladder

Rectus abdominis m

Left common femoral v

Left common femoral a

Iliopsoas m

Rectus femoris m

Sartorius m

Tensor fasciae latae m

Acetabular fossa

Femoral head

Gluteus minimus m

Gluteus medius m

Greater trochanter

Gluteus maximus m

Seminal vesicle and prostate

Rectum

Coccyx

Obturator internus m

Superior gemellus m

Figure 25.1.9

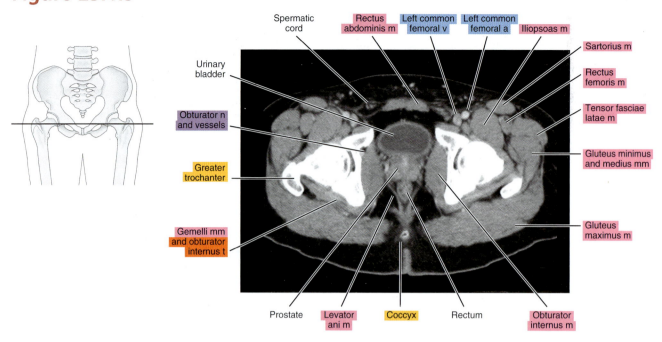

Spermatic cord
Rectus abdominis m
Left common femoral v
Left common femoral a
Iliopsoas m
Sartorius m
Rectus femoris m
Tensor fasciae latae m
Gluteus minimus and medius mm
Urinary bladder
Obturator n and vessels
Greater trochanter
Gemelli mm and obturator internus t
Gluteus maximus m
Prostate
Levator ani m
Coccyx
Rectum
Obturator internus m

Figure 25.1.10

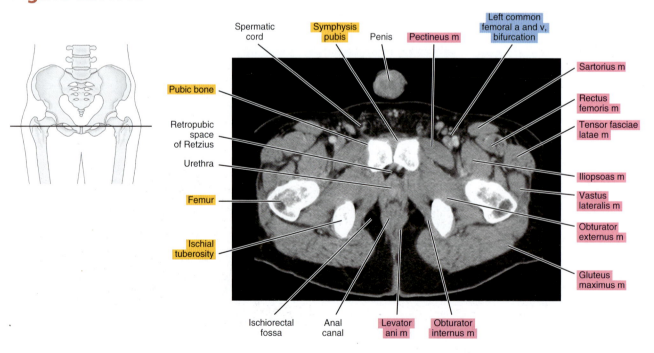

Spermatic cord
Symphysis pubis
Penis
Pectineus m
Left common femoral a and v, bifurcation
Sartorius m
Pubic bone
Rectus femoris m
Tensor fasciae latae m
Retropubic space of Retzius
Urethra
Iliopsoas m
Femur
Vastus lateralis m
Obturator externus m
Ischial tuberosity
Gluteus maximus m
Ischiorectal fossa
Anal canal
Levator ani m
Obturator internus m

Figure 25.1.11

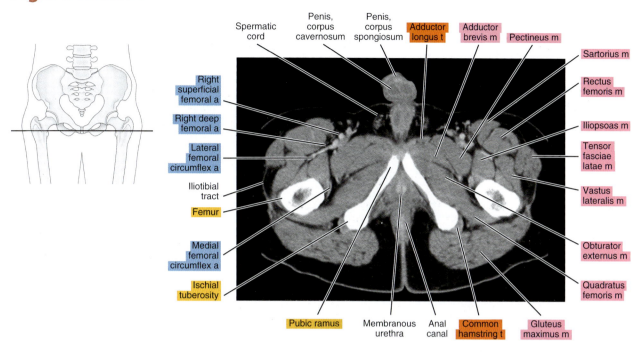

Figure 25.1.12

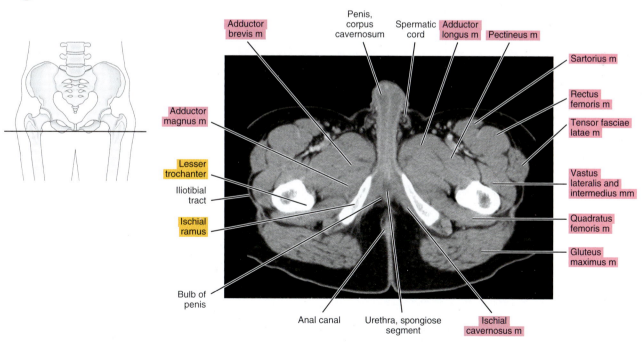

SAGITTAL
Figure 25.2.1

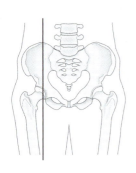

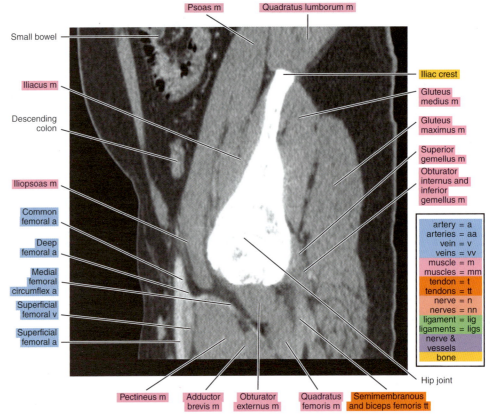

Psoas m

Quadratus lumborum m

Small bowel

Iliacus m

Descending colon

Iliopsoas m

Common femoral a

Deep femoral a

Medial femoral circumflex a

Superficial femoral v

Superficial femoral a

Iliac crest

Gluteus medius m

Gluteus maximus m

Superior gemellus m

Obturator internus and inferior gemellus m

artery = a	
arteries = aa	
vein = v	
veins = vv	
muscle = m	
muscles = mm	
tendon = t	
tendons = tt	
nerve = n	
nerves = nn	
ligament = lig	
ligaments = ligs	
nerve & vessels	
bone	

Hip joint

Pectineus m

Adductor brevis m

Obturator externus m

Quadratus femoris m

Semimembranous and biceps femoris tt

Figure 25.2.2

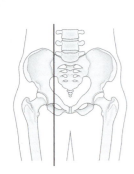

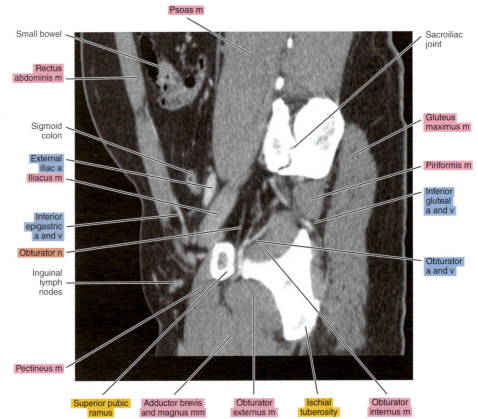

Psoas m

Small bowel

Rectus abdominis m

Sigmoid colon

External iliac a

Iliacus m

Inferior epigastric a and v

Obturator n

Inguinal lymph nodes

Pectineus m

Sacroiliac joint

Gluteus maximus m

Piriformis m

Inferior gluteal a and v

Obturator a and v

Superior pubic ramus

Adductor brevis and magnus mm

Obturator externus m

Ischial tuberosity

Obturator internus m

Figure 25.2.3

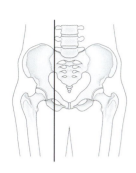

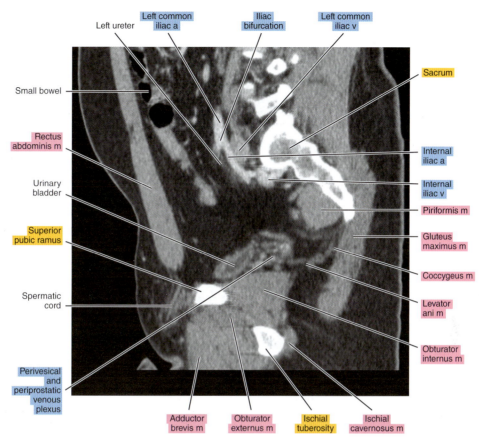

Left ureter

Left common iliac a

Iliac bifurcation

Left common iliac v

Small bowel

Sacrum

Rectus abdominis m

Internal iliac a

Urinary bladder

Internal iliac v

Superior pubic ramus

Piriformis m

Gluteus maximus m

Spermatic cord

Coccygeus m

Levator ani m

Obturator internus m

Perivesical and periprostatic venous plexus

Adductor brevis m

Obturator externus m

Ischial tuberosity

Ischial cavernosus m

Figure 25.2.4

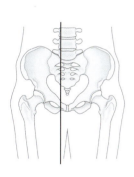

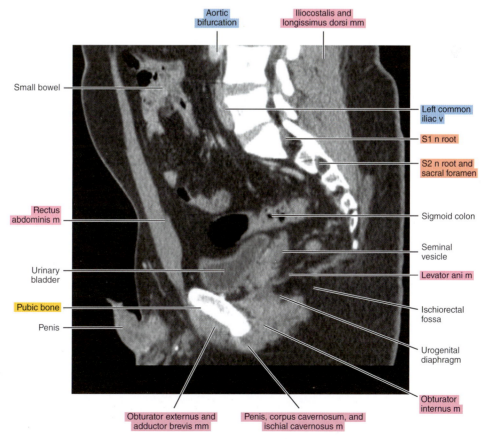

Aortic bifurcation

Iliocostalis and longissimus dorsi mm

Small bowel

Left common iliac v

S1 n root

S2 n root and sacral foramen

Rectus abdominis m

Sigmoid colon

Seminal vesicle

Urinary bladder

Levator ani m

Pubic bone

Ischiorectal fossa

Penis

Urogenital diaphragm

Obturator internus m

Obturator externus and adductor brevis mm

Penis, corpus cavernosum, and ischial cavernosus m

Figure 25.2.5

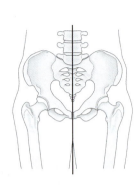

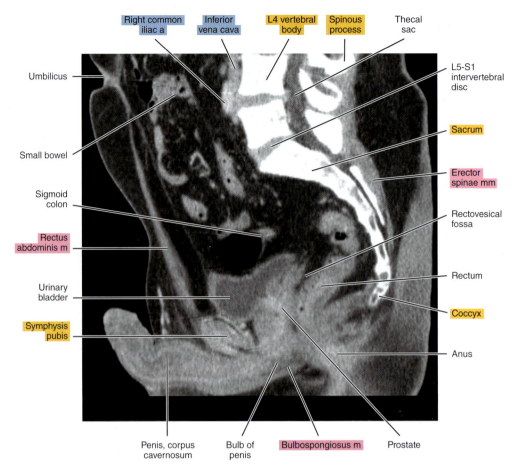

Right common iliac a

Inferior vena cava

L4 vertebral body

Spinous process

Thecal sac

Umbilicus

Small bowel

Sigmoid colon

Rectus abdominis m

Urinary bladder

Symphysis pubis

L5-S1 intervertebral disc

Sacrum

Erector spinae mm

Rectovesical fossa

Rectum

Coccyx

Anus

Penis, corpus cavernosum

Bulb of penis

Bulbospongiosus m

Prostate

CORONAL
Figure 25.3.1

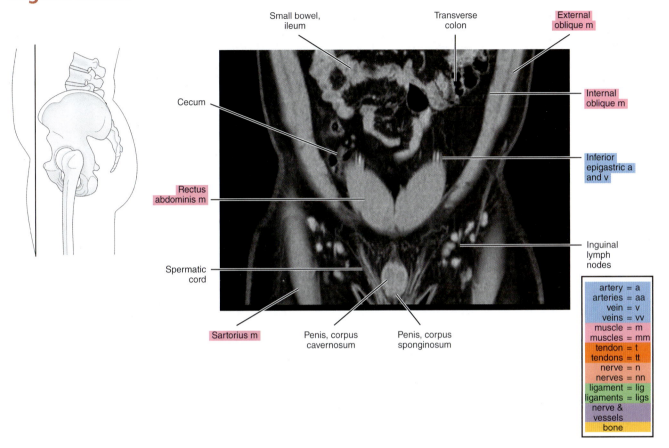

Small bowel, ileum

Transverse colon

External oblique m

Cecum

Internal oblique m

Inferior epigastric a and v

Rectus abdominis m

Inguinal lymph nodes

Spermatic cord

Sartorius m

Penis, corpus cavernosum

Penis, corpus sponginosum

artery = a	
arteries = aa	
vein = v	
veins = vv	
muscle = m	
muscles = mm	
tendon = t	
tendons = tt	
nerve = n	
nerves = nn	
ligament = lig	
ligaments = ligs	
nerve & vessels	
bone	

Figure 25.3.2

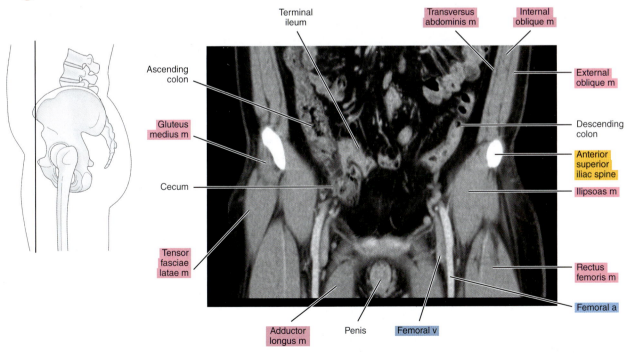

Terminal ileum

Transversus abdominis m

Internal oblique m

Ascending colon

External oblique m

Gluteus medius m

Descending colon

Anterior superior iliac spine

Cecum

Ilipsoas m

Tensor fasciae latae m

Rectus femoris m

Femoral a

Adductor longus m

Penis

Femoral v

Figure 25.3.3

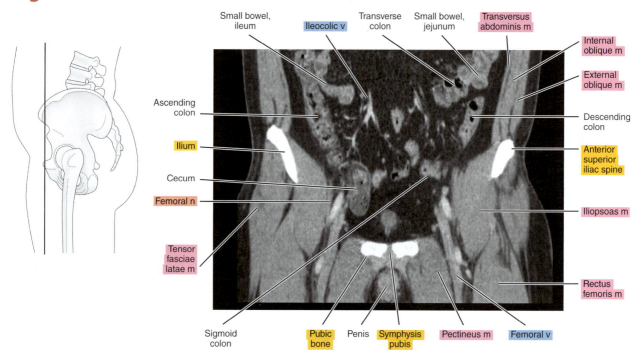

Small bowel, ileum
Ileocolic v
Transverse colon
Small bowel, jejunum
Transversus abdominis m
Internal oblique m
External oblique m
Ascending colon
Descending colon
Ilium
Anterior superior iliac spine
Cecum
Femoral n
Iliopsoas m
Tensor fasciae latae m
Rectus femoris m
Sigmoid colon
Pubic bone
Penis
Symphysis pubis
Pectineus m
Femoral v

Figure 25.3.4

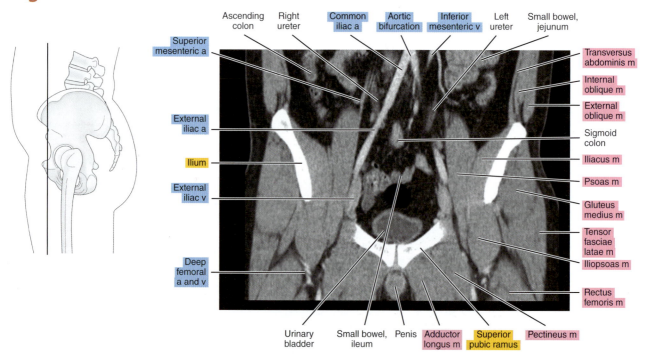

Superior mesenteric a
Ascending colon
Right ureter
Common iliac a
Aortic bifurcation
Inferior mesenteric v
Left ureter
Small bowel, jejunum
Transversus abdominis m
Internal oblique m
External oblique m
External iliac a
Sigmoid colon
Ilium
Iliacus m
External iliac v
Psoas m
Gluteus medius m
Tensor fasciae latae m
Iliopsoas m
Deep femoral a and v
Rectus femoris m
Urinary bladder
Small bowel, ileum
Penis
Adductor longus m
Superior pubic ramus
Pectineus m

Figure 25.3.5

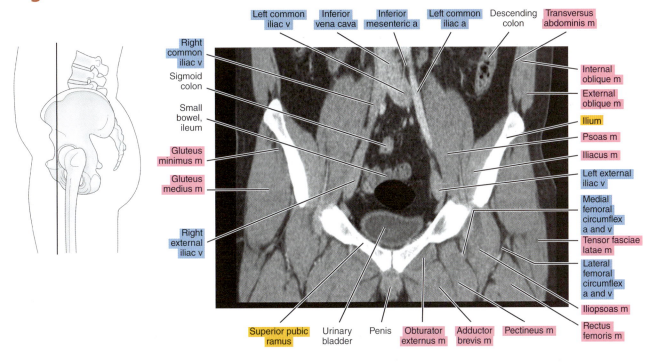

Left common iliac v | Inferior vena cava | Inferior mesenteric a | Left common iliac a | Descending colon | Transversus abdominis m

Right common iliac v
Sigmoid colon
Small bowel, ileum
Gluteus minimus m
Gluteus medius m
Right external iliac v

Internal oblique m
External oblique m
Ilium
Psoas m
Iliacus m
Left external iliac v
Medial femoral circumflex a and v
Tensor fasciae latae m
Lateral femoral circumflex a and v
Iliopsoas m
Rectus femoris m

Superior pubic ramus | Urinary bladder | Penis | Obturator externus m | Adductor brevis m | Pectineus m

Figure 25.3.6

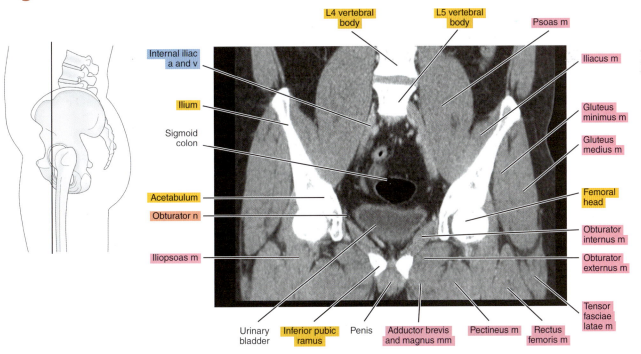

L4 vertebral body | L5 vertebral body | Psoas m

Internal iliac a and v
Ilium
Sigmoid colon
Acetabulum
Obturator n
Iliopsoas m

Iliacus m
Gluteus minimus m
Gluteus medius m
Femoral head
Obturator internus m
Obturator externus m
Tensor fasciae latae m

Urinary bladder | Inferior pubic ramus | Penis | Adductor brevis and magnus mm | Pectineus m | Rectus femoris m

Figure 25.3.7

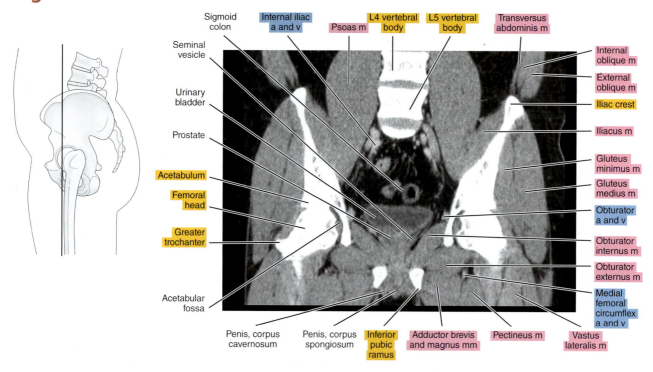

Figure 25.3.8

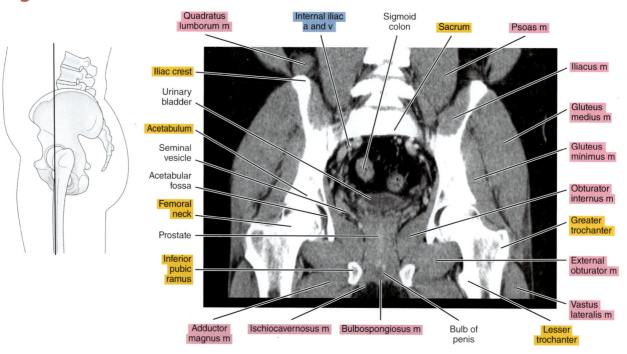

Figure 25.3.9

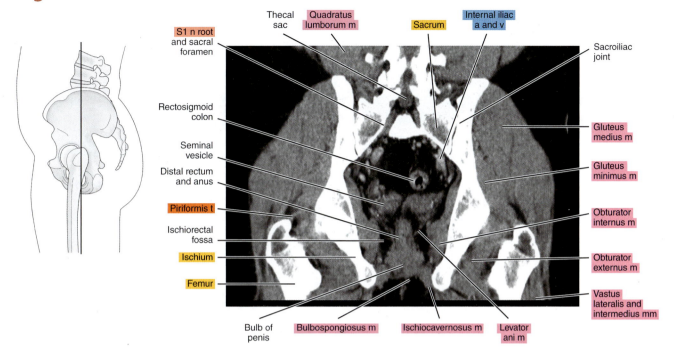

S1 n root and sacral foramen
Thecal sac
Quadratus lumborum m
Sacrum
Internal iliac a and v
Sacroiliac joint
Rectosigmoid colon
Gluteus medius m
Seminal vesicle
Gluteus minimus m
Distal rectum and anus
Piriformis t
Obturator internus m
Ischiorectal fossa
Ischium
Obturator externus m
Femur
Vastus lateralis and intermedius mm
Bulb of penis
Bulbospongiosus m
Ischiocavernosus m
Levator ani m

Figure 25.3.10

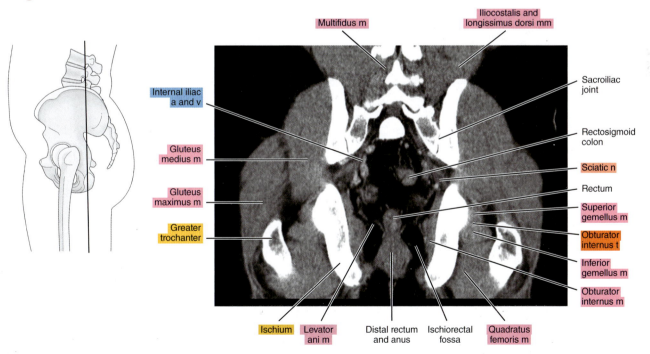

Multifidus m
Iliocostalis and longissimus dorsi mm
Internal iliac a and v
Sacroiliac joint
Gluteus medius m
Rectosigmoid colon
Sciatic n
Gluteus maximus m
Rectum
Superior gemellus m
Greater trochanter
Obturator internus t
Inferior gemellus m
Obturator internus m
Ischium
Levator ani m
Distal rectum and anus
Ischiorectal fossa
Quadratus femoris m

Figure 25.3.11

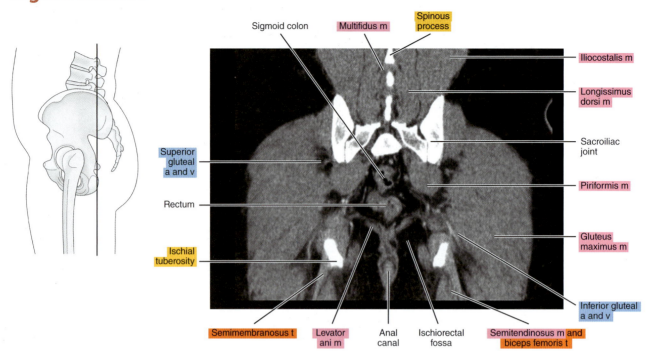

Sigmoid colon

Multifidus m

Spinous process

Iliocostalis m

Longissimus dorsi m

Sacroiliac joint

Piriformis m

Gluteus maximus m

Superior gluteal a and v

Rectum

Ischial tuberosity

Inferior gluteal a and v

Semimembranosus t

Levator ani m

Anal canal

Ischiorectal fossa

Semitendinosus m and biceps femoris t

Chapter

26

CT of the Female Pelvis

AXIAL
Figure 26.1.1

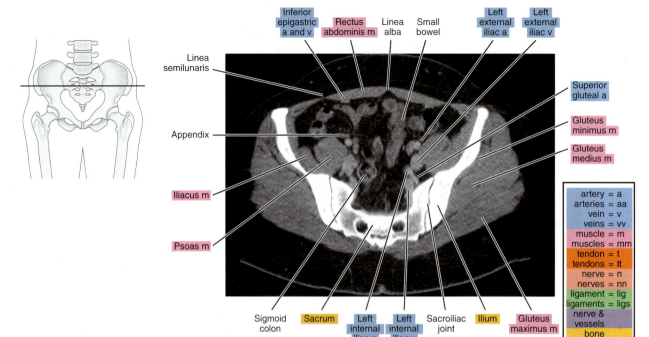

Inferior epigastric a and v · Rectus abdominis m · Linea alba · Small bowel · Left external iliac a · Left external iliac v

Linea semilunaris

Superior gluteal a

Gluteus minimus m

Gluteus medius m

Appendix

Iliacus m

Psoas m

artery = a
arteries = aa
vein = v
veins = vv
muscle = m
muscles = mm
tendon = t
tendons = tt
nerve = n
nerves = nn
ligament = lig
ligaments = ligs
nerve & vessels
bone

Sigmoid colon · Sacrum · Left internal iliac a · Left internal iliac v · Sacroiliac joint · Ilium · Gluteus maximus m

Figure 26.1.2

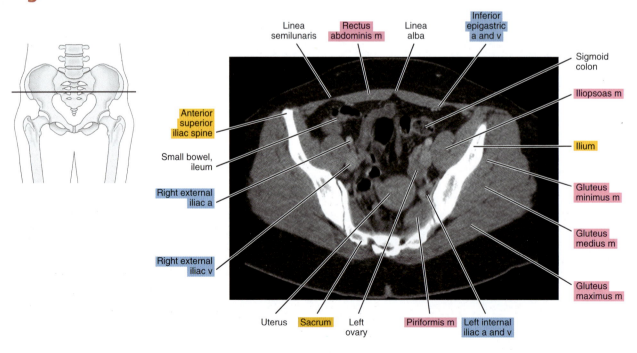

Linea semilunaris · Rectus abdominis m · Linea alba · Inferior epigastric a and v

Sigmoid colon

Iliopsoas m

Anterior superior iliac spine

Ilium

Small bowel, ileum

Gluteus minimus m

Right external iliac a

Gluteus medius m

Right external iliac v

Gluteus maximus m

Uterus · Sacrum · Left ovary · Piriformis m · Left internal iliac a and v

Figure 26.1.3

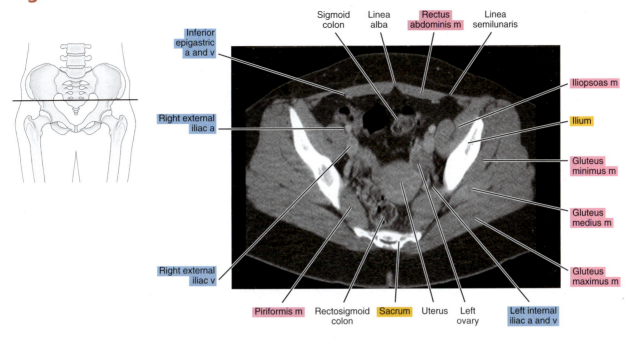

Sigmoid colon
Linea alba
Rectus abdominis m
Linea semilunaris
Inferior epigastric a and v
Iliopsoas m
Right external iliac a
Ilium
Gluteus minimus m
Gluteus medius m
Right external iliac v
Gluteus maximus m
Piriformis m
Rectosigmoid colon
Sacrum
Uterus
Left ovary
Left internal iliac a and v

Figure 26.1.4

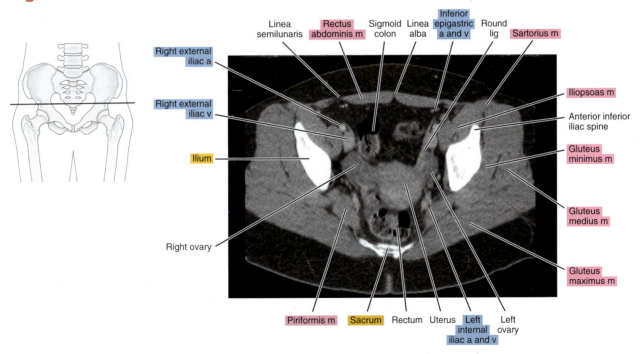

Linea semilunaris
Rectus abdominis m
Sigmoid colon
Linea alba
Inferior epigastric a and v
Round lig
Sartorius m
Right external iliac a
Iliopsoas m
Right external iliac v
Anterior inferior iliac spine
Ilium
Gluteus minimus m
Gluteus medius m
Right ovary
Gluteus maximus m
Piriformis m
Sacrum
Rectum
Uterus
Left internal iliac a and v
Left ovary

Figure 26.1.5

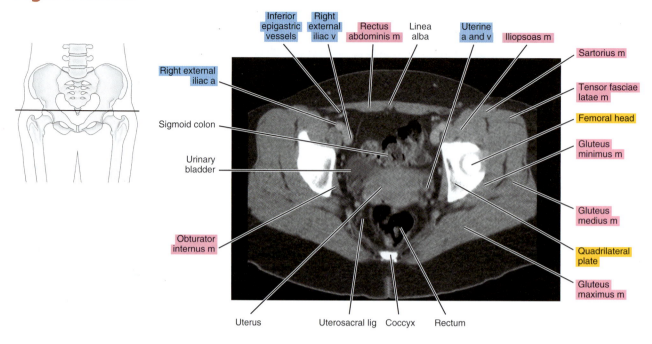

Inferior epigastric vessels · Right external iliac v · Rectus abdominis m · Linea alba · Uterine a and v · Iliopsoas m · Sartorius m · Tensor fasciae latae m · Femoral head · Gluteus minimus m · Gluteus medius m · Quadrilateral plate · Gluteus maximus m · Right external iliac a · Sigmoid colon · Urinary bladder · Obturator internus m · Uterus · Uterosacral lig · Coccyx · Rectum

Figure 26.1.6

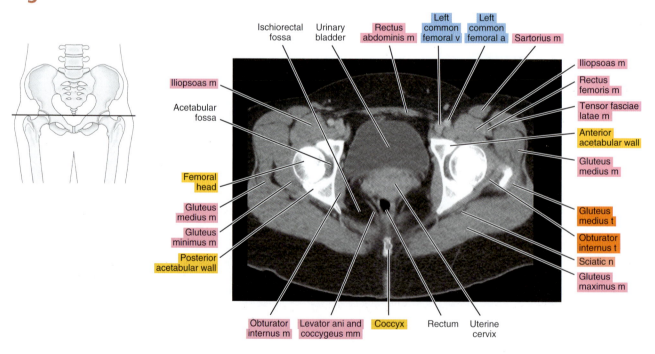

Ischiorectal fossa · Urinary bladder · Rectus abdominis m · Left common femoral v · Left common femoral a · Sartorius m · Iliopsoas m · Rectus femoris m · Tensor fasciae latae m · Anterior acetabular wall · Gluteus medius m · Gluteus medius t · Obturator internus t · Sciatic n · Gluteus maximus m · Iliopsoas m · Acetabular fossa · Femoral head · Gluteus medius m · Gluteus minimus m · Posterior acetabular wall · Obturator internus m · Levator ani and coccygeus mm · Coccyx · Rectum · Uterine cervix

Figure 26.1.7

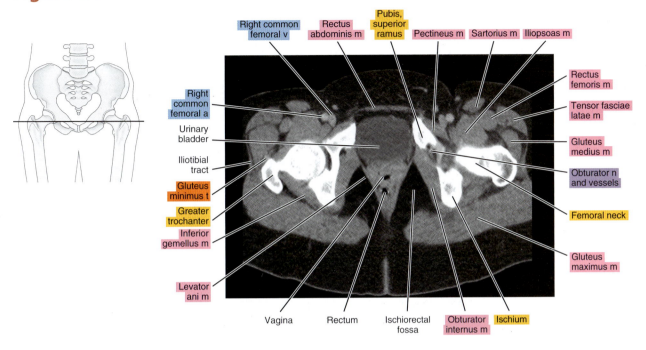

Right common femoral v
Rectus abdominis m
Pubis, superior ramus
Pectineus m
Sartorius m
Iliopsoas m
Rectus femoris m
Tensor fasciae latae m
Gluteus medius m
Obturator n and vessels
Femoral neck
Gluteus maximus m

Right common femoral a
Urinary bladder
Iliotibial tract
Gluteus minimus t
Greater trochanter
Inferior gemellus m
Levator ani m

Vagina
Rectum
Ischiorectal fossa
Obturator internus m
Ischium

Figure 26.1.8

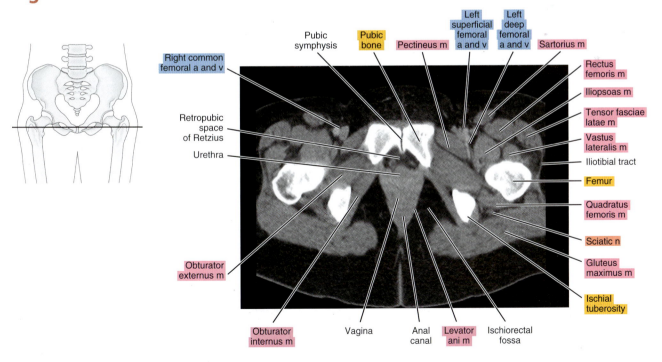

Pubic symphysis
Pubic bone
Pectineus m
Left superficial femoral a and v
Left deep femoral a and v
Sartorius m
Rectus femoris m
Iliopsoas m
Tensor fasciae latae m
Vastus lateralis m
Iliotibial tract
Femur
Quadratus femoris m
Sciatic n
Gluteus maximus m
Ischial tuberosity

Right common femoral a and v
Retropubic space of Retzius
Urethra
Obturator externus m

Obturator internus m
Vagina
Anal canal
Levator ani m
Ischiorectal fossa

Figure 26.1.9

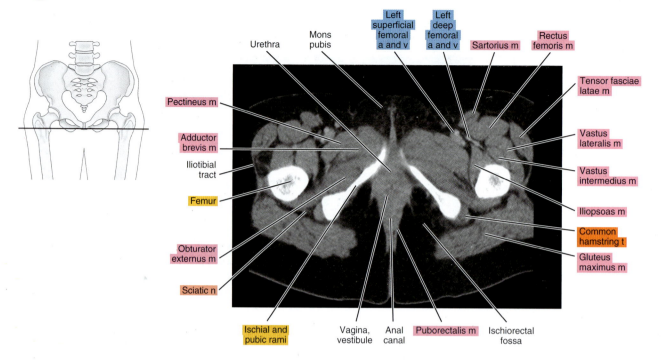

Urethra

Mons pubis

Left superficial femoral a and v

Left deep femoral a and v

Sartorius m

Rectus femoris m

Pectineus m

Adductor brevis m

Iliotibial tract

Femur

Obturator externus m

Sciatic n

Tensor fasciae latae m

Vastus lateralis m

Vastus intermedius m

Iliopsoas m

Common hamstring t

Gluteus maximus m

Ischial and pubic rami

Vagina, vestibule

Anal canal

Puborectalis m

Ischiorectal fossa

SAGITTAL
Figure 26.2.1

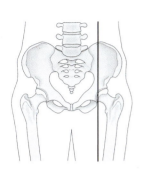

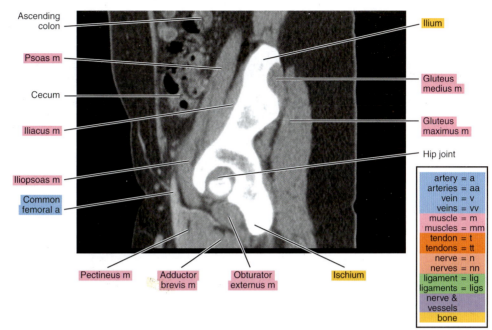

Ascending colon

Psoas m

Cecum

Iliacus m

Iliopsoas m

Common femoral a

Ilium

Gluteus medius m

Gluteus maximus m

Hip joint

| artery = a |
| arteries = aa |
| vein = v |
| veins = vv |
| muscle = m |
| muscles = mm |
| tendon = t |
| tendons = tt |
| nerve = n |
| nerves = nn |
| ligament = lig |
| ligaments = ligs |
| nerve & vessels |
| bone |

Pectineus m

Adductor brevis m

Obturator externus m

Ischium

Figure 26.2.2

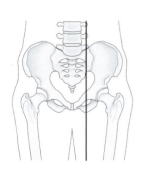

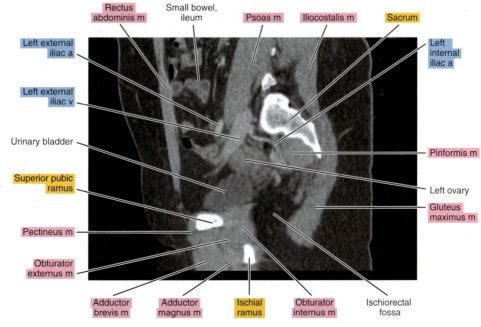

Rectus abdominis m

Small bowel, ileum

Psoas m

Iliocostalis m

Sacrum

Left external iliac a

Left internal iliac a

Left external iliac v

Urinary bladder

Superior pubic ramus

Piriformis m

Left ovary

Gluteus maximus m

Pectineus m

Obturator externus m

Adductor brevis m

Adductor magnus m

Ischial ramus

Obturator internus m

Ischiorectal fossa

Figure 26.2.3

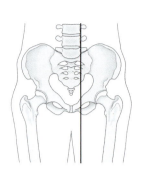

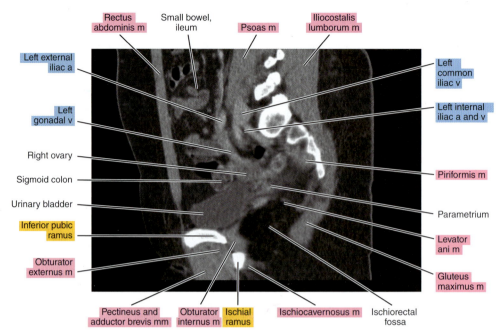

Rectus abdominis m — Small bowel, ileum — Psoas m — Iliocostalis lumborum m

Left external iliac a

Left gonadal v

Right ovary

Sigmoid colon

Urinary bladder

Inferior pubic ramus

Obturator externus m

Left common iliac v

Left internal iliac a and v

Piriformis m

Parametrium

Levator ani m

Gluteus maximus m

Pectineus and adductor brevis mm — Obturator internus m — Ischial ramus — Ischiocavernosus m — Ischiorectal fossa

Figure 26.2.4

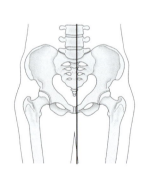

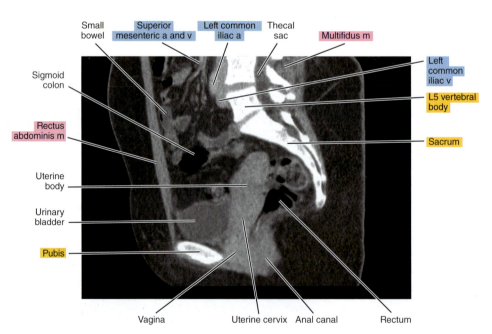

Small bowel — Superior mesenteric a and v — Left common iliac a — Thecal sac — Multifidus m

Sigmoid colon

Rectus abdominis m

Uterine body

Urinary bladder

Pubis

Left common iliac v

L5 vertebral body

Sacrum

Vagina — Uterine cervix — Anal canal — Rectum

Figure 26.2.5

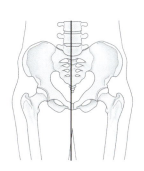

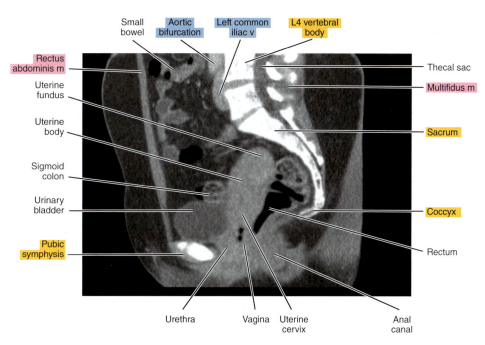

Small bowel

Aortic bifurcation

Left common iliac v

L4 vertebral body

Rectus abdominis m

Uterine fundus

Uterine body

Sigmoid colon

Urinary bladder

Pubic symphysis

Thecal sac

Multifidus m

Sacrum

Coccyx

Rectum

Urethra

Vagina

Uterine cervix

Anal canal

CORONAL
Figure 26.3.1

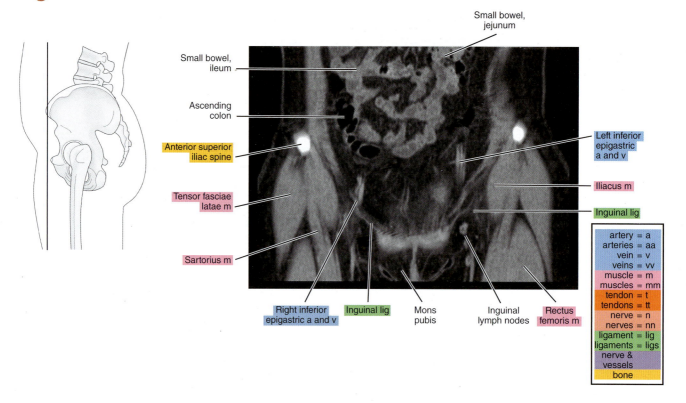

Small bowel, jejunum

Small bowel, ileum

Ascending colon

Anterior superior iliac spine

Tensor fasciae latae m

Sartorius m

Left inferior epigastric a and v

Iliacus m

Inguinal lig

Right inferior epigastric a and v

Inguinal lig

Mons pubis

Inguinal lymph nodes

Rectus femoris m

artery = a	
arteries = aa	
vein = v	
veins = vv	
muscle = m	
muscles = mm	
tendon = t	
tendons = tt	
nerve = n	
nerves = nn	
ligament = lig	
ligaments = ligs	
nerve & vessels	
bone	

Figure 26.3.2

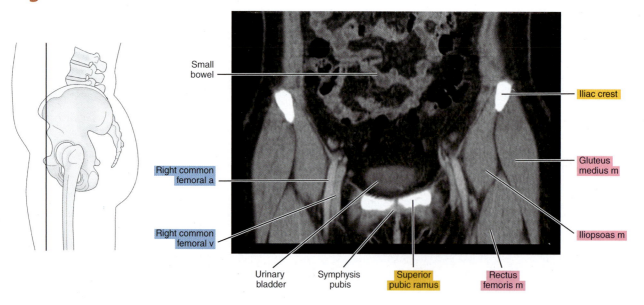

Small bowel

Iliac crest

Right common femoral a

Gluteus medius m

Right common femoral v

Iliopsoas m

Urinary bladder

Symphysis pubis

Superior pubic ramus

Rectus femoris m

Figure 26.3.3

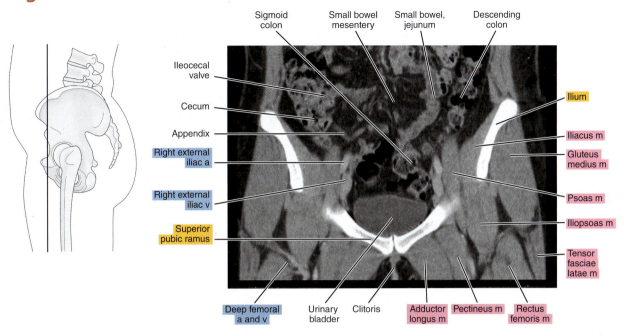

Sigmoid colon
Small bowel mesentery
Small bowel, jejunum
Descending colon
Ileocecal valve
Cecum
Appendix
Right external iliac a
Right external iliac v
Superior pubic ramus
Ilium
Iliacus m
Gluteus medius m
Psoas m
Iliopsoas m
Tensor fasciae latae m
Deep femoral a and v
Urinary bladder
Clitoris
Adductor longus m
Pectineus m
Rectus femoris m

Figure 26.3.4

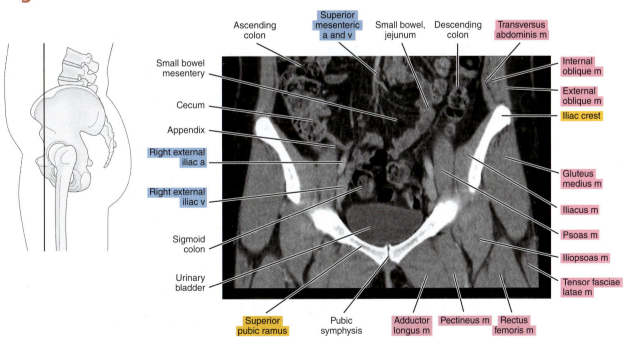

Ascending colon
Superior mesenteric a and v
Small bowel, jejunum
Descending colon
Transversus abdominis m
Small bowel mesentery
Cecum
Appendix
Right external iliac a
Right external iliac v
Sigmoid colon
Urinary bladder
Internal oblique m
External oblique m
Iliac crest
Gluteus medius m
Iliacus m
Psoas m
Iliopsoas m
Tensor fasciae latae m
Superior pubic ramus
Pubic symphysis
Adductor longus m
Pectineus m
Rectus femoris m

Figure 26.3.5

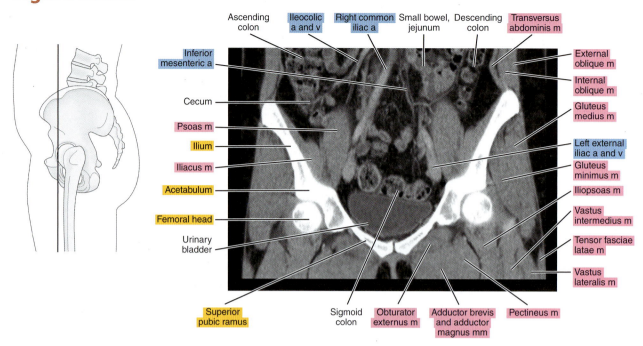

Ascending colon
Ileocolic a and v
Right common iliac a
Small bowel, jejunum
Descending colon
Transversus abdominis m
Inferior mesenteric a
External oblique m
Internal oblique m
Cecum
Gluteus medius m
Psoas m
Ilium
Left external iliac a and v
Iliacus m
Gluteus minimus m
Acetabulum
Iliopsoas m
Femoral head
Vastus intermedius m
Urinary bladder
Tensor fasciae latae m
Vastus lateralis m
Superior pubic ramus
Sigmoid colon
Obturator externus m
Adductor brevis and adductor magnus mm
Pectineus m

Figure 26.3.6

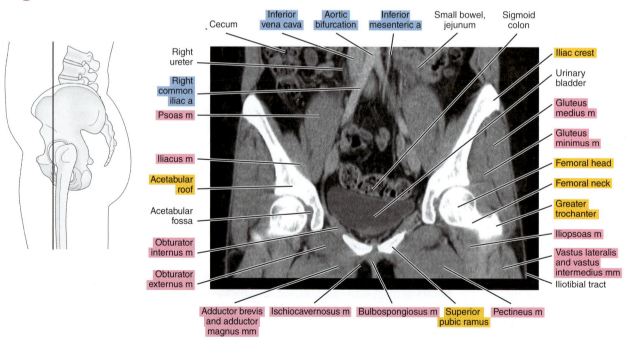

Cecum
Inferior vena cava
Aortic bifurcation
Inferior mesenteric a
Small bowel, jejunum
Sigmoid colon
Right ureter
Iliac crest
Right common iliac a
Urinary bladder
Psoas m
Gluteus medius m
Gluteus minimus m
Iliacus m
Femoral head
Acetabular roof
Femoral neck
Acetabular fossa
Greater trochanter
Obturator internus m
Iliopsoas m
Obturator externus m
Vastus lateralis and vastus intermedius mm
Iliotibial tract
Adductor brevis and adductor magnus mm
Ischiocavernosus m
Bulbospongiosus m
Superior pubic ramus
Pectineus m

Figure 26.3.7

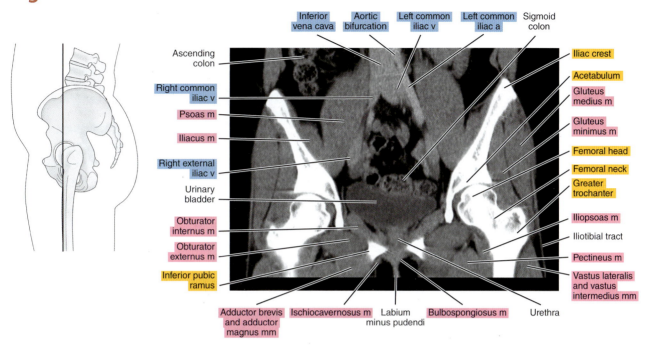

Figure 26.3.8

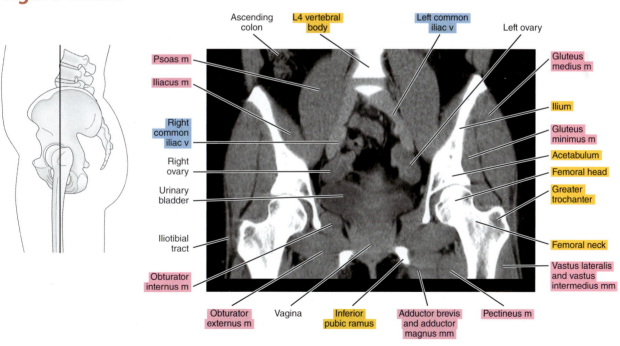

Figure 26.3.9

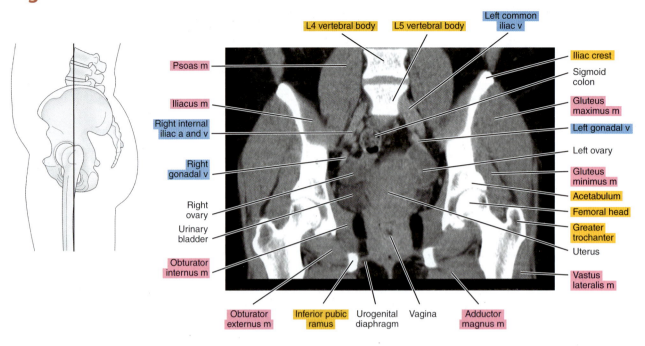

L4 vertebral body — L5 vertebral body — Left common iliac v — Iliac crest — Psoas m — Sigmoid colon — Iliacus m — Gluteus maximus m — Right internal iliac a and v — Left gonadal v — Right gonadal v — Left ovary — Right ovary — Gluteus minimus m — Urinary bladder — Acetabulum — Femoral head — Obturator internus m — Greater trochanter — Uterus — Vastus lateralis m — Obturator externus m — Inferior pubic ramus — Urogenital diaphragm — Vagina — Adductor magnus m

Figure 26.3.10

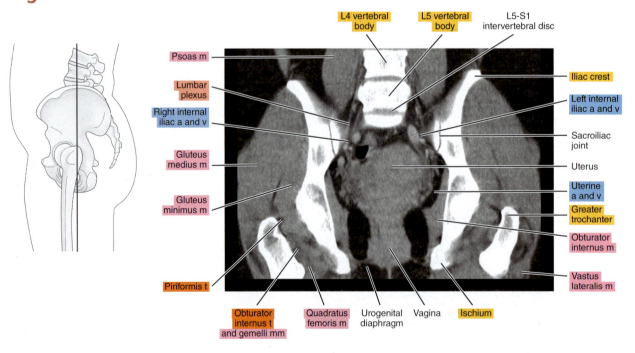

L4 vertebral body — L5 vertebral body — L5-S1 intervertebral disc — Psoas m — Iliac crest — Lumbar plexus — Left internal iliac a and v — Right internal iliac a and v — Sacroiliac joint — Gluteus medius m — Uterus — Gluteus minimus m — Uterine a and v — Greater trochanter — Obturator internus m — Piriformis t — Vastus lateralis m — Obturator internus t and gemelli mm — Quadratus femoris m — Urogenital diaphragm — Vagina — Ischium

Figure 26.3.11

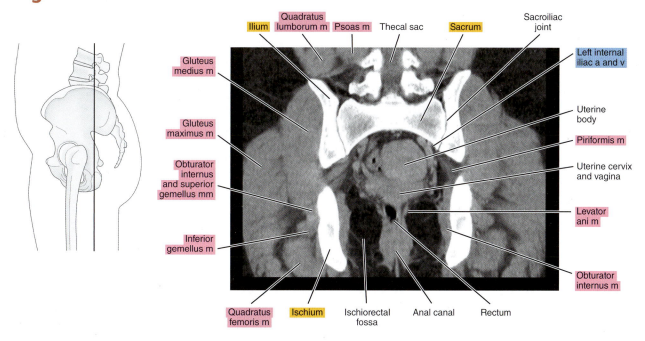

Figure 26.3.12

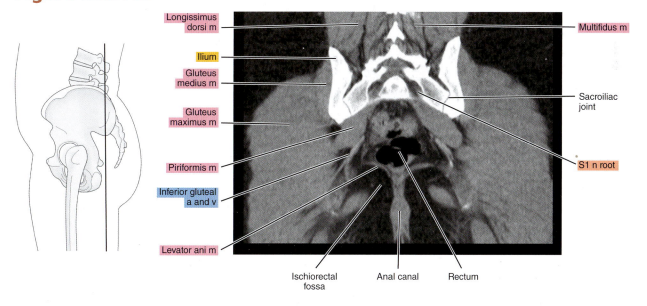

Chapter 27

MRI of the Male Pelvis

AXIAL
Figure 27.1.1

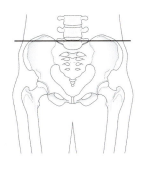

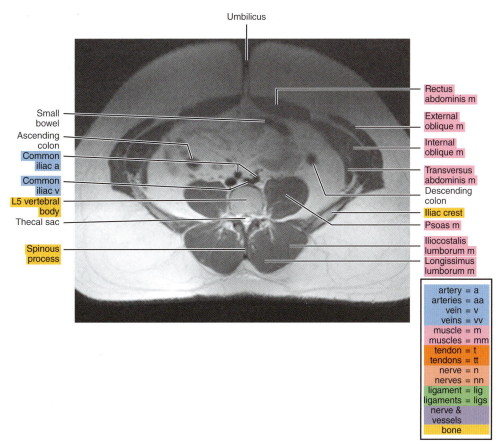

Umbilicus

Small bowel

Ascending colon

Common iliac a

Common iliac v

L5 vertebral body

Thecal sac

Spinous process

Rectus abdominis m

External oblique m

Internal oblique m

Transversus abdominis m

Descending colon

Iliac crest

Psoas m

Iliocostalis lumborum m

Longissimus lumborum m

artery	= a
arteries	= aa
vein	= v
veins	= vv
muscle	= m
muscles	= mm
tendon	= t
tendons	= tt
nerve	= n
nerves	= nn
ligament	= lig
ligaments	= ligs
nerve & vessels	
bone	

Figure 27.1.2

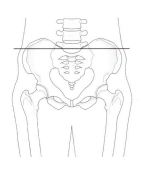

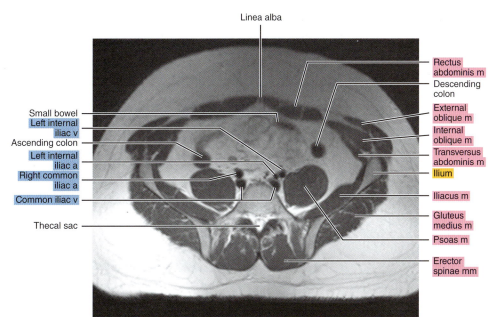

Linea alba

Small bowel

Left internal iliac v

Ascending colon

Left internal iliac a

Right common iliac a

Common iliac v

Thecal sac

Rectus abdominis m

Descending colon

External oblique m

Internal oblique m

Transversus abdominis m

Ilium

Iliacus m

Gluteus medius m

Psoas m

Erector spinae mm

Figure 27.1.3

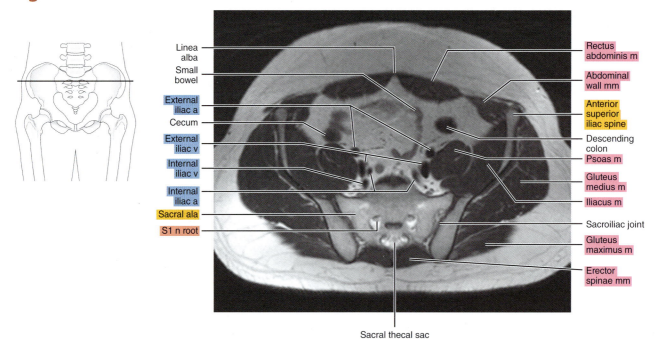

Linea alba
Small bowel
External iliac a
Cecum
External iliac v
Internal iliac v
Internal iliac a
Sacral ala
S1 n root

Rectus abdominis m
Abdominal wall mm
Anterior superior iliac spine
Descending colon
Psoas m
Gluteus medius m
Iliacus m
Sacroiliac joint
Gluteus maximus m
Erector spinae mm

Sacral thecal sac

Figure 27.1.4

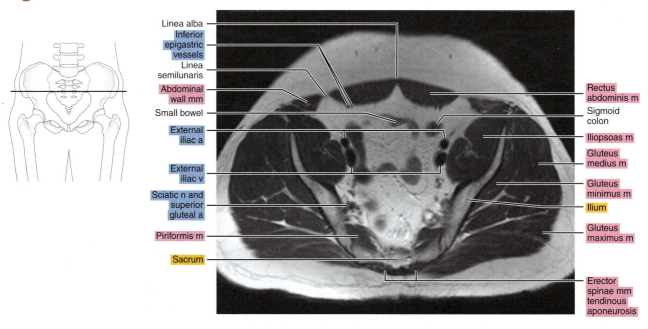

Linea alba
Inferior epigastric vessels
Linea semilunaris
Abdominal wall mm
Small bowel
External iliac a
External iliac v
Sciatic n and superior gluteal a
Piriformis m
Sacrum

Rectus abdominis m
Sigmoid colon
Iliopsoas m
Gluteus medius m
Gluteus minimus m
Ilium
Gluteus maximus m
Erector spinae mm tendinous aponeurosis

Figure 27.1.5

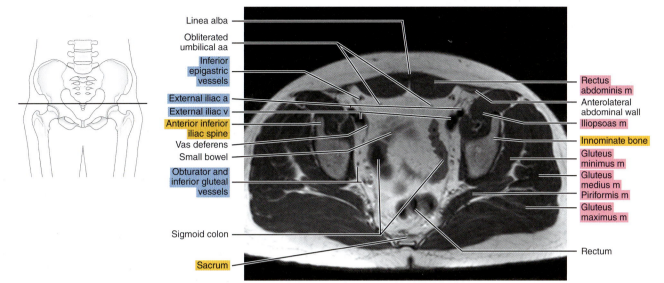

Linea alba
Obliterated umbilical aa
Inferior epigastric vessels
External iliac a
External iliac v
Anterior inferior iliac spine
Vas deferens
Small bowel
Obturator and inferior gluteal vessels
Sigmoid colon
Sacrum

Rectus abdominis m
Anterolateral abdominal wall
Iliopsoas m
Innominate bone
Gluteus minimus m
Gluteus medius m
Piriformis m
Gluteus maximus m
Rectum

Figure 27.1.6

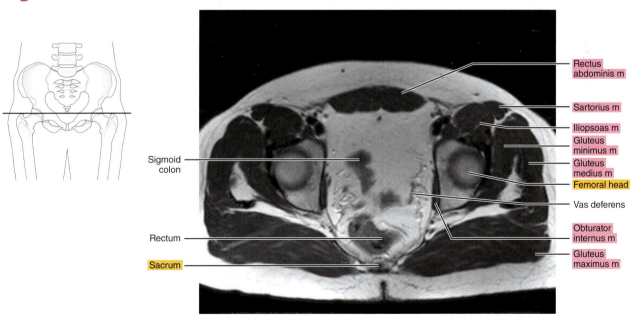

Sigmoid colon
Rectum
Sacrum

Rectus abdominis m
Sartorius m
Iliopsoas m
Gluteus minimus m
Gluteus medius m
Femoral head
Vas deferens
Obturator internus m
Gluteus maximus m

Figure 27.1.7

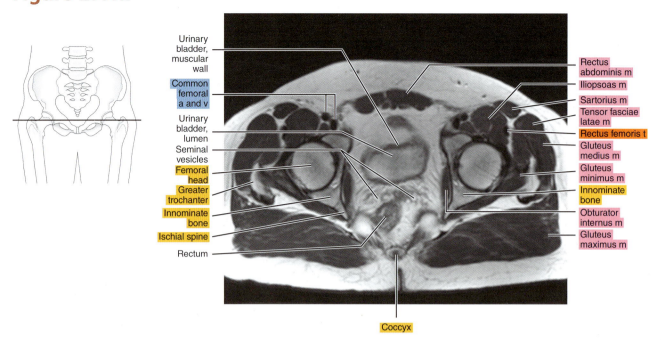

Urinary bladder, muscular wall

Common femoral a and v

Urinary bladder, lumen

Seminal vesicles

Femoral head

Greater trochanter

Innominate bone

Ischial spine

Rectum

Rectus abdominis m

Iliopsoas m

Sartorius m

Tensor fasciae latae m

Rectus femoris t

Gluteus medius m

Gluteus minimus m

Innominate bone

Obturator internus m

Gluteus maximus m

Coccyx

Figure 27.1.8

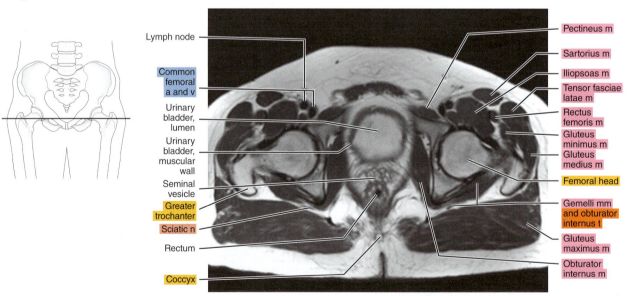

Lymph node

Common femoral a and v

Urinary bladder, lumen

Urinary bladder, muscular wall

Seminal vesicle

Greater trochanter

Sciatic n

Rectum

Coccyx

Pectineus m

Sartorius m

Iliopsoas m

Tensor fasciae latae m

Rectus femoris m

Gluteus minimus m

Gluteus medius m

Femoral head

Gemelli mm and obturator internus t

Gluteus maximus m

Obturator internus m

Figure 27.1.9

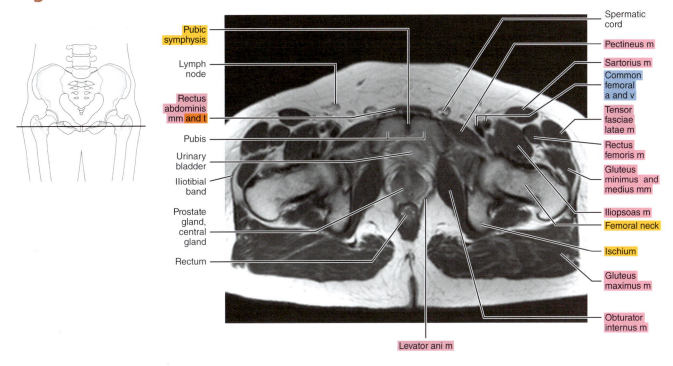

Pubic symphysis

Lymph node

Rectus abdominis mm and t

Pubis

Urinary bladder

Iliotibial band

Prostate gland, central gland

Rectum

Spermatic cord

Pectineus m

Sartorius m

Common femoral a and v

Tensor fasciae latae m

Rectus femoris m

Gluteus minimus and medius mm

Iliopsoas m

Femoral neck

Ischium

Gluteus maximus m

Obturator internus m

Levator ani m

Figure 27.1.10

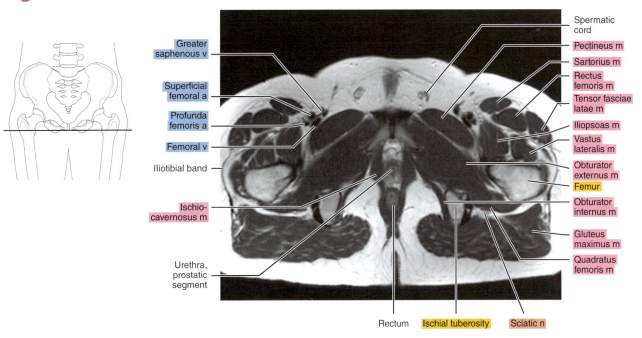

Greater saphenous v

Superficial femoral a

Profunda femoris a

Femoral v

Iliotibial band

Ischio-cavernosus m

Urethra, prostatic segment

Spermatic cord

Pectineus m

Sartorius m

Rectus femoris m

Tensor fasciae latae m

Iliopsoas m

Vastus lateralis m

Obturator externus m

Femur

Obturator internus m

Gluteus maximus m

Quadratus femoris m

Rectum   Ischial tuberosity   Sciatic n

Figure 27.1.11

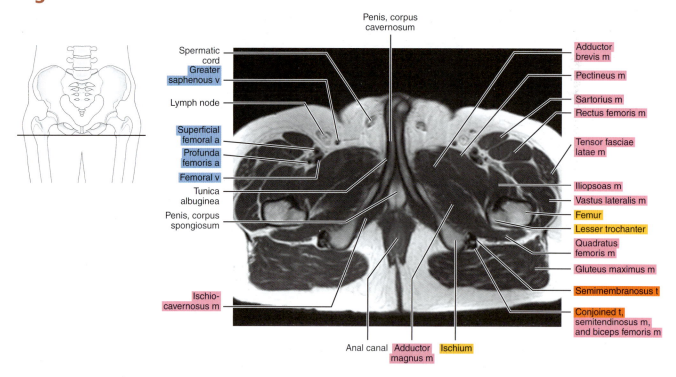

Penis, corpus cavernosum

Spermatic cord
Greater saphenous v
Lymph node
Superficial femoral a
Profunda femoris a
Femoral v
Tunica albuginea
Penis, corpus spongiosum
Ischio-cavernosus m

Adductor brevis m
Pectineus m
Sartorius m
Rectus femoris m
Tensor fasciae latae m
Iliopsoas m
Vastus lateralis m
Femur
Lesser trochanter
Quadratus femoris m
Gluteus maximus m
Semimembranosus t
Conjoined t, semitendinosus m, and biceps femoris m

Anal canal   Adductor magnus m   Ischium

Figure 27.1.12

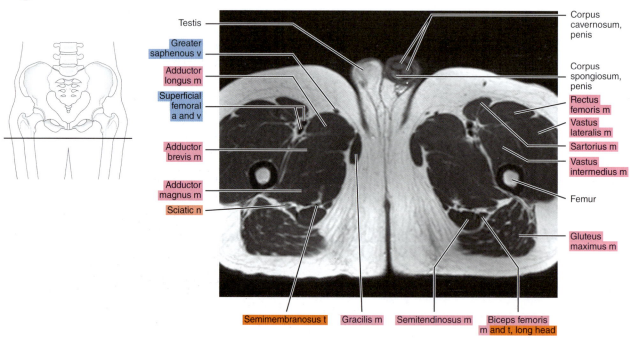

Testis
Greater saphenous v
Adductor longus m
Superficial femoral a and v
Adductor brevis m
Adductor magnus m
Sciatic n

Corpus cavernosum, penis
Corpus spongiosum, penis
Rectus femoris m
Vastus lateralis m
Sartorius m
Vastus intermedius m
Femur
Gluteus maximus m

Semimembranosus t   Gracilis m   Semitendinosus m   Biceps femoris m and t, long head

SAGITTAL
Figure 27.2.1

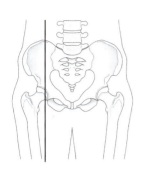

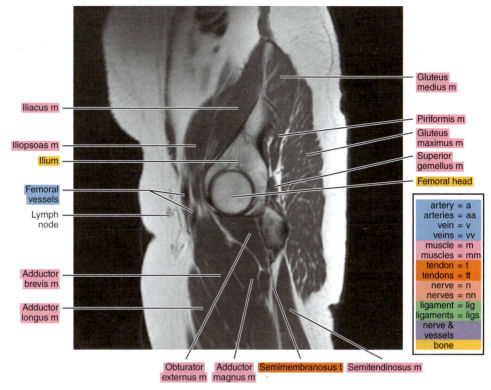

Iliacus m

Iliopsoas m

Ilium

Femoral vessels

Lymph node

Adductor brevis m

Adductor longus m

Gluteus medius m

Piriformis m

Gluteus maximus m

Superior gemellus m

Femoral head

artery = a	
arteries = aa	
vein = v	
veins = vv	
muscle = m	
muscles = mm	
tendon = t	
tendons = tt	
nerve = n	
nerves = nn	
ligament = lig	
ligaments = ligs	
nerve & vessels	
bone	

Obturator externus m

Adductor magnus m

Semimembranosus t

Semitendinosus m

Figure 27.2.2

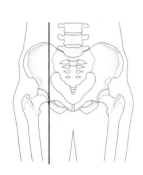

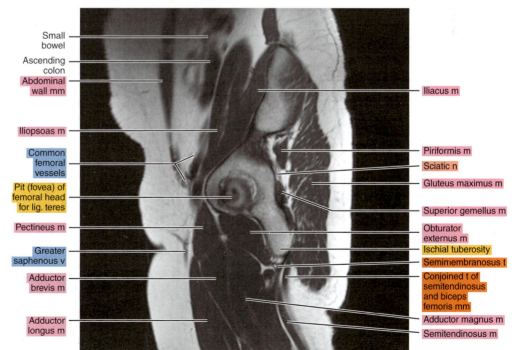

Small bowel

Ascending colon

Abdominal wall mm

Iliopsoas m

Common femoral vessels

Pit (fovea) of femoral head for lig. teres

Pectineus m

Greater saphenous v

Adductor brevis m

Adductor longus m

Iliacus m

Piriformis m

Sciatic n

Gluteus maximus m

Superior gemellus m

Obturator externus m

Ischial tuberosity

Semimembranosus t

Conjoined t of semitendinosus and biceps femoris mm

Adductor magnus m

Semitendinosus m

Figure 27.2.3

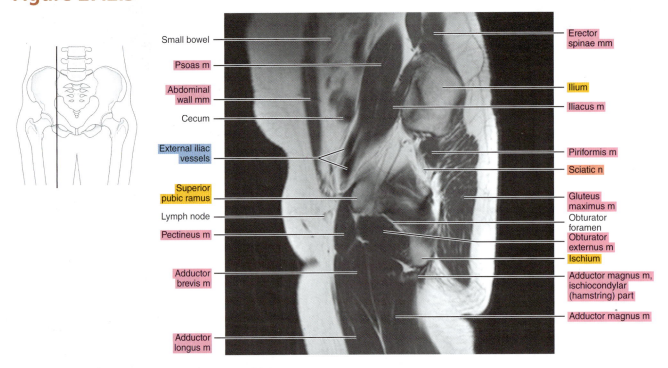

Small bowel
Psoas m
Abdominal wall mm
Cecum
External iliac vessels
Superior pubic ramus
Lymph node
Pectineus m
Adductor brevis m
Adductor longus m

Erector spinae mm
Ilium
Iliacus m
Piriformis m
Sciatic n
Gluteus maximus m
Obturator foramen
Obturator externus m
Ischium
Adductor magnus m, ischiocondylar (hamstring) part
Adductor magnus m

Figure 27.2.4

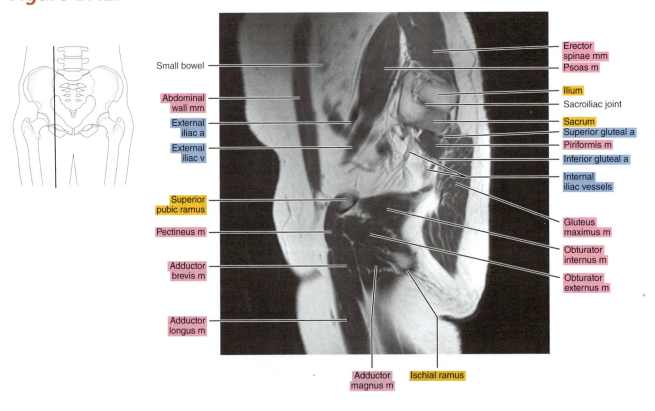

Small bowel
Abdominal wall mm
External iliac a
External iliac v
Superior pubic ramus
Pectineus m
Adductor brevis m
Adductor longus m

Erector spinae mm
Psoas m
Ilium
Sacroiliac joint
Sacrum
Superior gluteal a
Piriformis m
Inferior gluteal a
Internal iliac vessels
Gluteus maximus m
Obturator internus m
Obturator externus m

Adductor magnus m
Ischial ramus

Figure 27.2.5

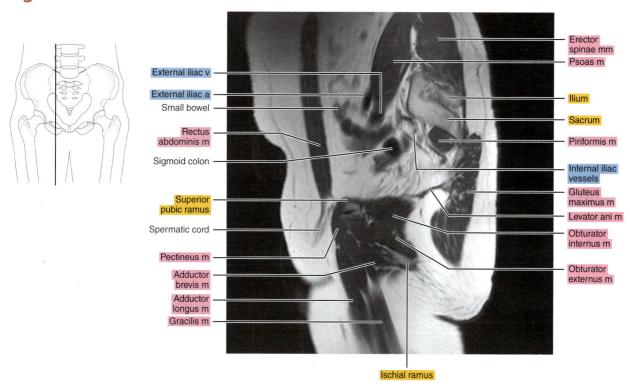

External iliac v
External iliac a
Small bowel
Rectus abdominis m
Sigmoid colon
Superior pubic ramus
Spermatic cord
Pectineus m
Adductor brevis m
Adductor longus m
Gracilis m

Erector spinae mm
Psoas m
Ilium
Sacrum
Piriformis m
Internal iliac vessels
Gluteus maximus m
Levator ani m
Obturator internus m
Obturator externus m

Ischial ramus

Figure 27.2.6

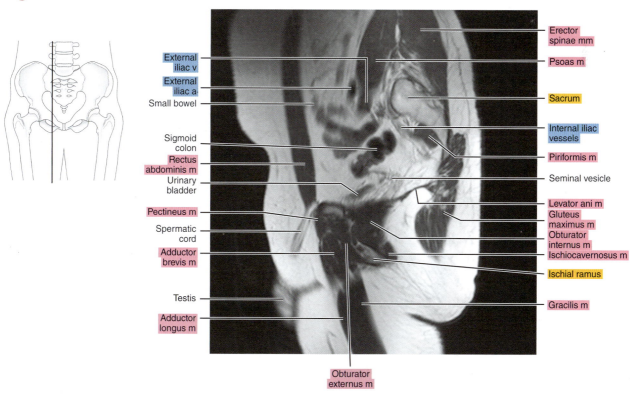

External iliac v
External iliac a
Small bowel
Sigmoid colon
Rectus abdominis m
Urinary bladder
Pectineus m
Spermatic cord
Adductor brevis m
Testis
Adductor longus m

Erector spinae mm
Psoas m
Sacrum
Internal iliac vessels
Piriformis m
Seminal vesicle
Levator ani m
Gluteus maximus m
Obturator internus m
Ischiocavernosus m
Ischial ramus
Gracilis m

Obturator externus m

Figure 27.2.7

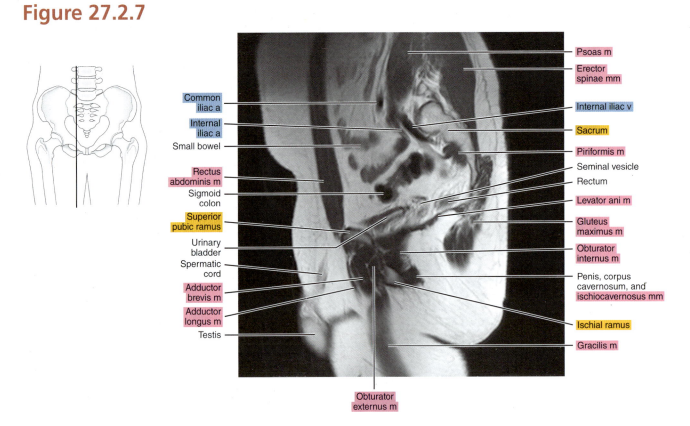

Common iliac a
Internal iliac a
Small bowel
Rectus abdominis m
Sigmoid colon
Superior pubic ramus
Urinary bladder
Spermatic cord
Adductor brevis m
Adductor longus m
Testis

Psoas m
Erector spinae mm
Internal iliac v
Sacrum
Piriformis m
Seminal vesicle
Rectum
Levator ani m
Gluteus maximus m
Obturator internus m
Penis, corpus cavernosum, and ischiocavernosus mm
Ischial ramus
Gracilis m

Obturator externus m

Figure 27.2.8

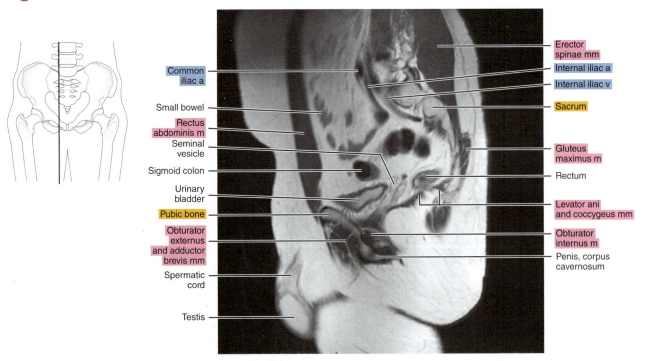

Common iliac a
Small bowel
Rectus abdominis m
Seminal vesicle
Sigmoid colon
Urinary bladder
Pubic bone
Obturator externus and adductor brevis mm
Spermatic cord
Testis

Erector spinae mm
Internal iliac a
Internal iliac v
Sacrum
Gluteus maximus m
Rectum
Levator ani and coccygeus mm
Obturator internus m
Penis, corpus cavernosum

Figure 27.2.9

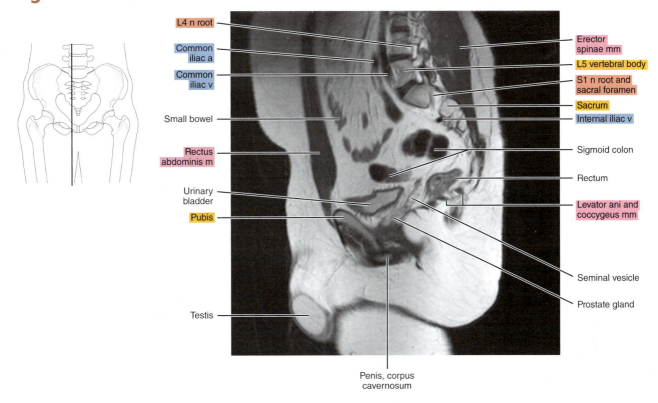

L4 n root

Common iliac a

Common iliac v

Small bowel

Rectus abdominis m

Urinary bladder

Pubis

Testis

Erector spinae mm

L5 vertebral body

S1 n root and sacral foramen

Sacrum

Internal iliac v

Sigmoid colon

Rectum

Levator ani and coccygeus mm

Seminal vesicle

Prostate gland

Penis, corpus cavernosum

Figure 27.2.10

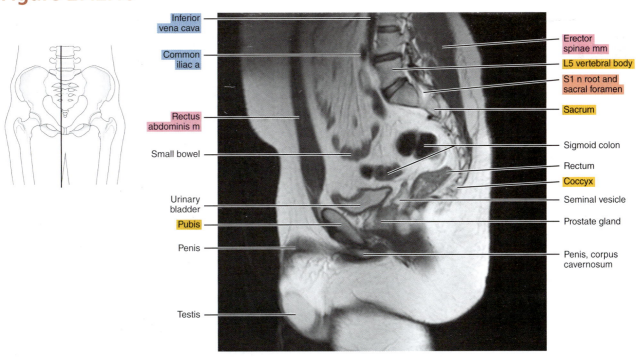

Inferior vena cava

Common iliac a

Rectus abdominis m

Small bowel

Urinary bladder

Pubis

Penis

Testis

Erector spinae mm

L5 vertebral body

S1 n root and sacral foramen

Sacrum

Sigmoid colon

Rectum

Coccyx

Seminal vesicle

Prostate gland

Penis, corpus cavernosum

Figure 27.2.11

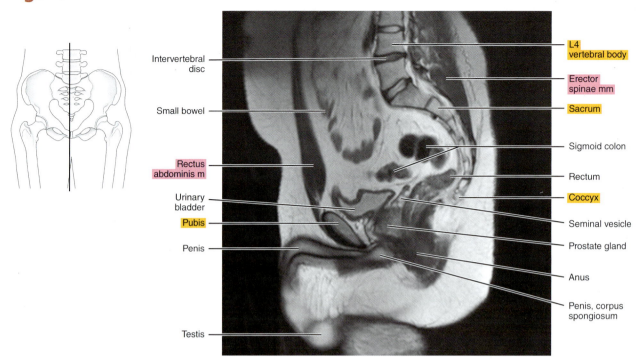

Intervertebral disc

Small bowel

Rectus abdominis m

Urinary bladder

Pubis

Penis

Testis

L4 vertebral body

Erector spinae mm

Sacrum

Sigmoid colon

Rectum

Coccyx

Seminal vesicle

Prostate gland

Anus

Penis, corpus spongiosum

Figure 27.2.12

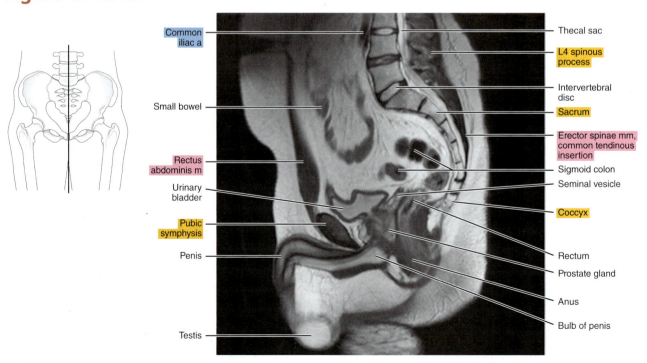

Common iliac a

Small bowel

Rectus abdominis m

Urinary bladder

Pubic symphysis

Penis

Testis

Thecal sac

L4 spinous process

Intervertebral disc

Sacrum

Erector spinae mm, common tendinous insertion

Sigmoid colon

Seminal vesicle

Coccyx

Rectum

Prostate gland

Anus

Bulb of penis

CORONAL
Figure 27.3.1

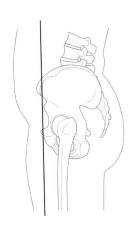

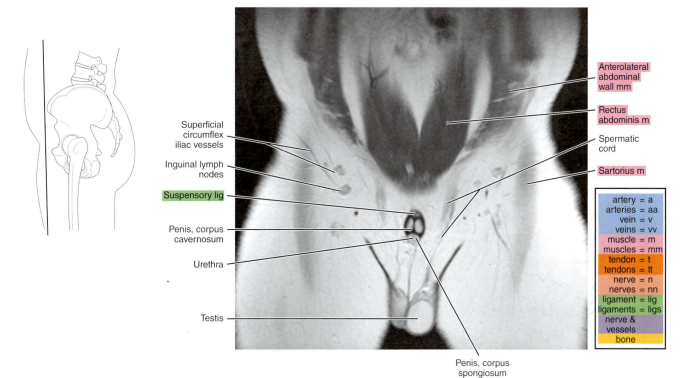

Anterolateral abdominal wall mm

Rectus abdominis m

Spermatic cord

Sartorius m

Superficial circumflex iliac vessels

Inguinal lymph nodes

Suspensory lig

Penis, corpus cavernosum

Urethra

Testis

Penis, corpus spongiosum

artery = a	
arteries = aa	
vein = v	
veins = vv	
muscle = m	
muscles = mm	
tendon = t	
tendons = tt	
nerve = n	
nerves = nn	
ligament = lig	
ligaments = ligs	
nerve & vessels	
bone	

Figure 27.3.2

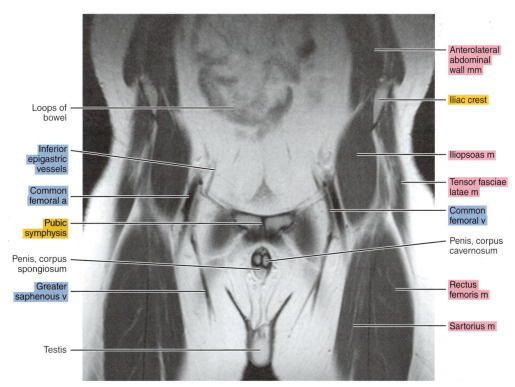

Anterolateral abdominal wall mm

Iliac crest

Iliopsoas m

Tensor fasciae latae m

Common femoral v

Penis, corpus cavernosum

Rectus femoris m

Sartorius m

Loops of bowel

Inferior epigastric vessels

Common femoral a

Pubic symphysis

Penis, corpus spongiosum

Greater saphenous v

Testis

Figure 27.3.3

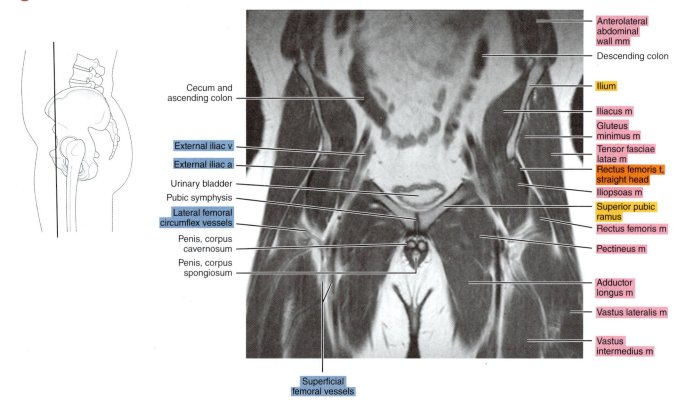

Cecum and ascending colon

External iliac v
External iliac a
Urinary bladder
Pubic symphysis
Lateral femoral circumflex vessels
Penis, corpus cavernosum
Penis, corpus spongiosum

Superficial femoral vessels

Anterolateral abdominal wall mm
Descending colon
Ilium
Iliacus m
Gluteus minimus m
Tensor fasciae latae m
Rectus femoris t, straight head
Iliopsoas m
Superior pubic ramus
Rectus femoris m
Pectineus m
Adductor longus m
Vastus lateralis m
Vastus intermedius m

Figure 27.3.4

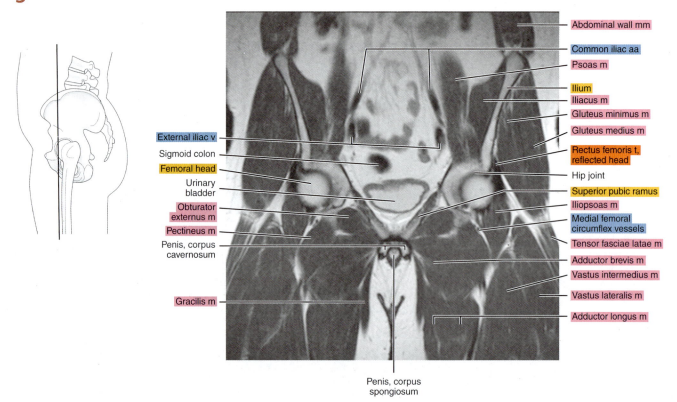

External iliac v
Sigmoid colon
Femoral head
Urinary bladder
Obturator externus m
Pectineus m
Penis, corpus cavernosum
Gracilis m

Abdominal wall mm
Common iliac aa
Psoas m
Ilium
Iliacus m
Gluteus minimus m
Gluteus medius m
Rectus femoris t, reflected head
Hip joint
Superior pubic ramus
Iliopsoas m
Medial femoral circumflex vessels
Tensor fasciae latae m
Adductor brevis m
Vastus intermedius m
Vastus lateralis m
Adductor longus m

Penis, corpus spongiosum

Figure 27.3.5

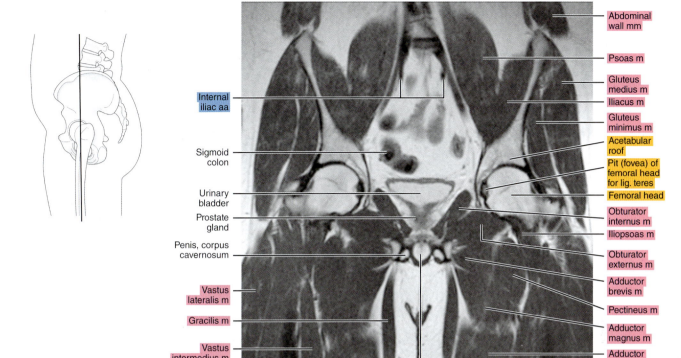

Internal iliac aa

Sigmoid colon

Urinary bladder

Prostate gland

Penis, corpus cavernosum

Vastus lateralis m

Gracilis m

Vastus intermedius m

Abdominal wall mm

Psoas m

Gluteus medius m

Iliacus m

Gluteus minimus m

Acetabular roof

Pit (fovea) of femoral head for lig. teres

Femoral head

Obturator internus m

Iliopsoas m

Obturator externus m

Adductor brevis m

Pectineus m

Adductor magnus m

Adductor longus m

Penis, corpus spongiosum

Figure 27.3.6

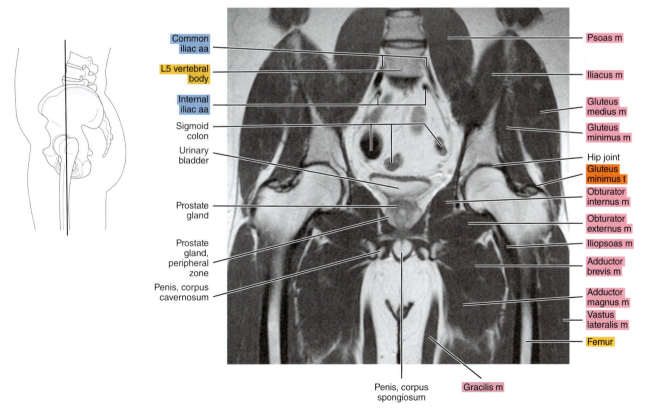

Common iliac aa

L5 vertebral body

Internal iliac aa

Sigmoid colon

Urinary bladder

Prostate gland

Prostate gland, peripheral zone

Penis, corpus cavernosum

Psoas m

Iliacus m

Gluteus medius m

Gluteus minimus m

Hip joint

Gluteus minimus t

Obturator internus m

Obturator externus m

Iliopsoas m

Adductor brevis m

Adductor magnus m

Vastus lateralis m

Femur

Penis, corpus spongiosum

Gracilis m

Figure 27.3.7

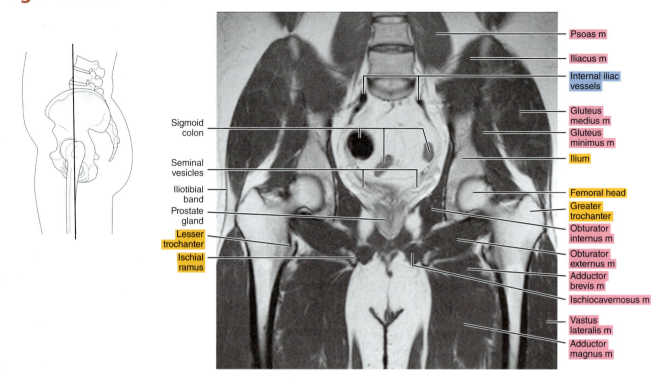

Sigmoid colon
Seminal vesicles
Iliotibial band
Prostate gland
Lesser trochanter
Ischial ramus

Psoas m
Iliacus m
Internal iliac vessels
Gluteus medius m
Gluteus minimus m
Ilium
Femoral head
Greater trochanter
Obturator internus m
Obturator externus m
Adductor brevis m
Ischiocavernosus m
Vastus lateralis m
Adductor magnus m

Figure 27.3.8

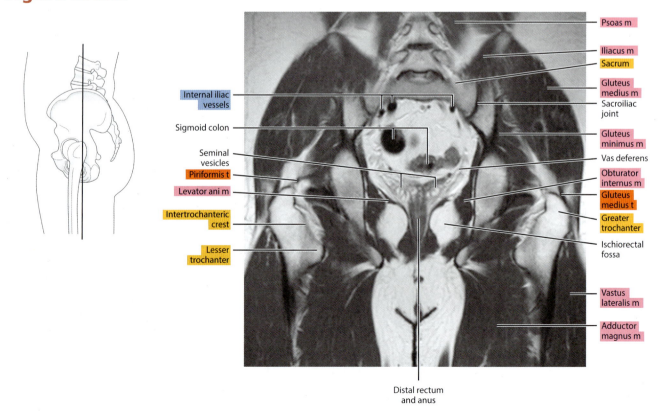

Internal iliac vessels
Sigmoid colon
Seminal vesicles
Piriformis t
Levator ani m
Intertrochanteric crest
Lesser trochanter

Psoas m
Iliacus m
Sacrum
Gluteus medius m
Sacroiliac joint
Gluteus minimus m
Vas deferens
Obturator internus m
Gluteus medius t
Greater trochanter
Ischiorectal fossa
Vastus lateralis m
Adductor magnus m

Distal rectum and anus

Figure 27.3.9

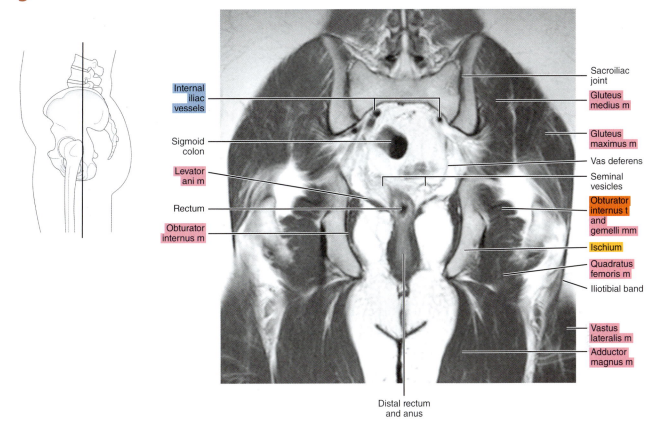

Internal iliac vessels

Sigmoid colon

Levator ani m

Rectum

Obturator internus m

Sacroiliac joint

Gluteus medius m

Gluteus maximus m

Vas deferens

Seminal vesicles

Obturator internus t and gemelli mm

Ischium

Quadratus femoris m

Iliotibial band

Vastus lateralis m

Adductor magnus m

Distal rectum and anus

Figure 27.3.10

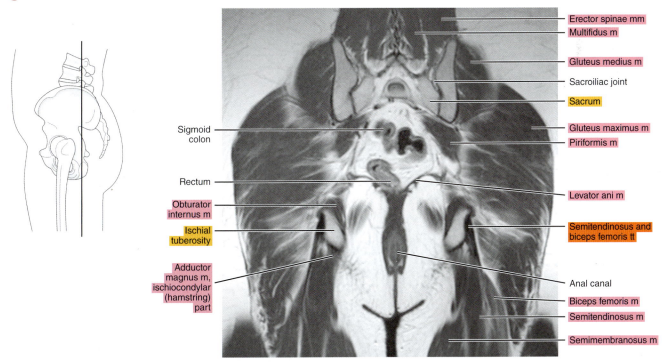

Sigmoid colon

Rectum

Obturator internus m

Ischial tuberosity

Adductor magnus m, ischiocondylar (hamstring) part

Erector spinae mm

Multifidus m

Gluteus medius m

Sacroiliac joint

Sacrum

Gluteus maximus m

Piriformis m

Levator ani m

Semitendinosus and biceps femoris tt

Anal canal

Biceps femoris m

Semitendinosus m

Semimembranosus m

Figure 27.3.11

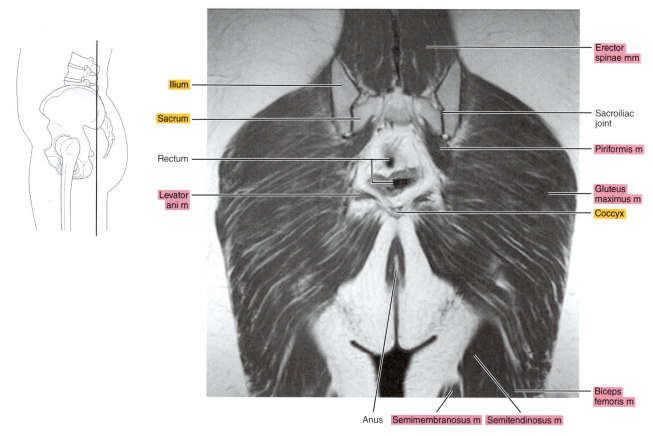

Erector spinae mm

Ilium

Sacrum

Sacroiliac joint

Rectum

Piriformis m

Levator ani m

Gluteus maximus m

Coccyx

Biceps femoris m

Anus   Semimembranosus m   Semitendinosus m

Figure 27.3.12

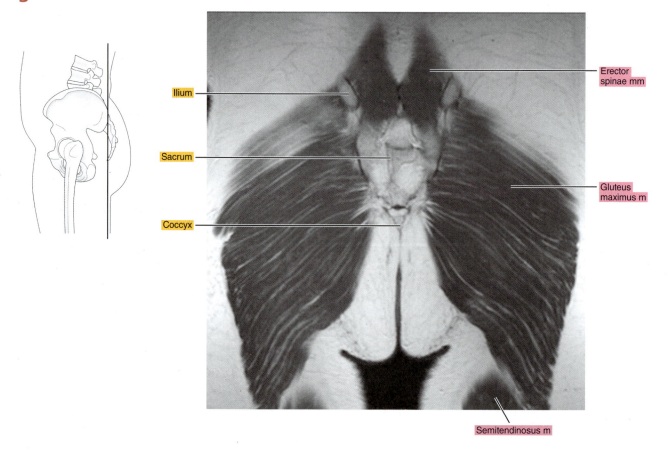

Ilium

Erector spinae mm

Sacrum

Gluteus maximus m

Coccyx

Semitendinosus m

Chapter

28

MRI of the Female Pelvis

AXIAL
Figure 28.1.1

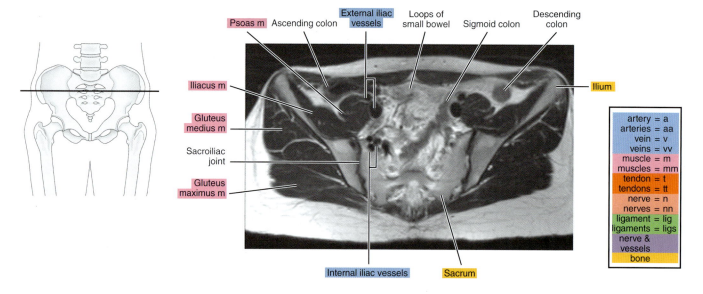

Psoas m Ascending colon External iliac vessels Loops of small bowel Sigmoid colon Descending colon

Iliacus m

Gluteus medius m

Sacroiliac joint

Gluteus maximus m

Ilium

Internal iliac vessels Sacrum

artery	= a
arteries	= aa
vein	= v
veins	= vv
muscle	= m
muscles	= mm
tendon	= t
tendons	= tt
nerve	= n
nerves	= nn
ligament	= lig
ligaments	= ligs
nerve & vessels	
bone	

Figure 28.1.2

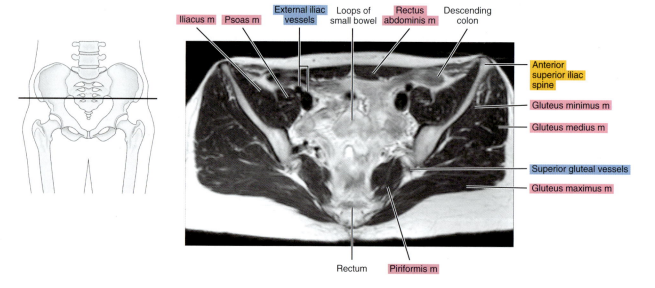

Iliacus m Psoas m External iliac vessels Loops of small bowel Rectus abdominis m Descending colon

Anterior superior iliac spine

Gluteus minimus m

Gluteus medius m

Superior gluteal vessels

Gluteus maximus m

Rectum Piriformis m

Figure 28.1.3

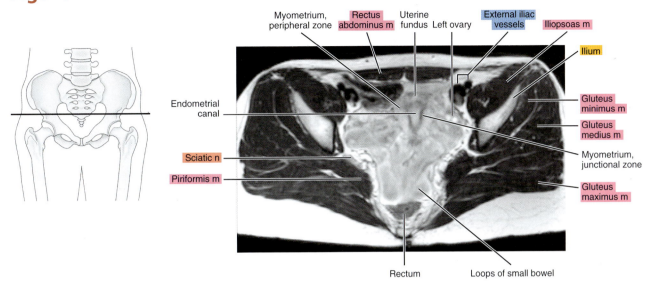

Myometrium, peripheral zone
Rectus abdominus m
Uterine fundus
Left ovary
External iliac vessels
Iliopsoas m
Ilium
Endometrial canal
Gluteus minimus m
Gluteus medius m
Sciatic n
Myometrium, junctional zone
Piriformis m
Gluteus maximus m
Rectum
Loops of small bowel

Figure 28.1.4

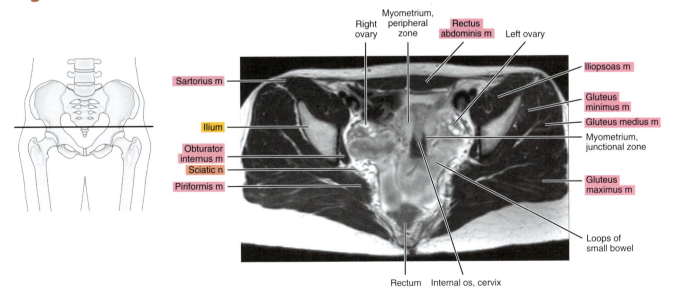

Right ovary
Myometrium, peripheral zone
Rectus abdominis m
Left ovary
Sartorius m
Iliopsoas m
Gluteus minimus m
Ilium
Gluteus medius m
Obturator internus m
Myometrium, junctional zone
Sciatic n
Piriformis m
Gluteus maximus m
Loops of small bowel
Rectum
Internal os, cervix

Figure 28.1.5

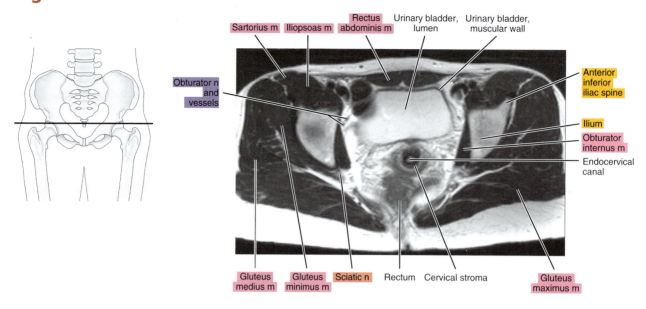

Sartorius m · Iliopsoas m · Rectus abdominis m · Urinary bladder, lumen · Urinary bladder, muscular wall · Anterior inferior iliac spine · Obturator n and vessels · Ilium · Obturator internus m · Endocervical canal · Gluteus medius m · Gluteus minimus m · Sciatic n · Rectum · Cervical stroma · Gluteus maximus m

Figure 28.1.6

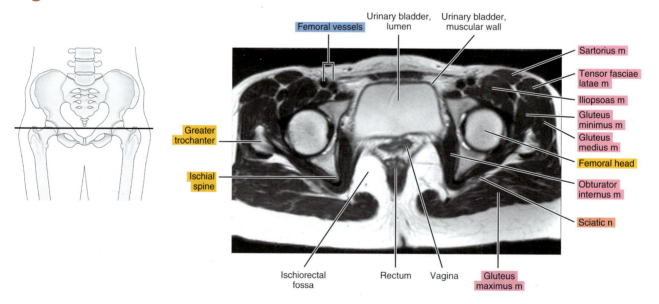

Femoral vessels · Urinary bladder, lumen · Urinary bladder, muscular wall · Sartorius m · Tensor fasciae latae m · Iliopsoas m · Gluteus minimus m · Gluteus medius m · Femoral head · Obturator internus m · Sciatic n · Greater trochanter · Ischial spine · Ischiorectal fossa · Rectum · Vagina · Gluteus maximus m

Figure 28.1.7

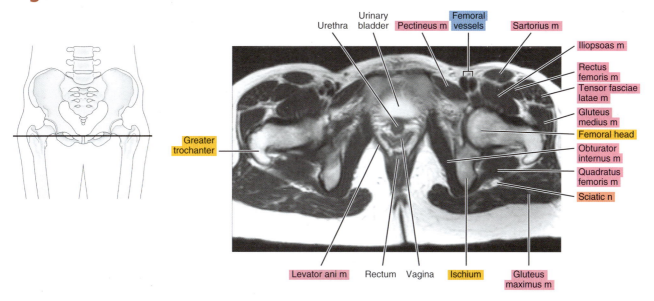

Urethra
Urinary bladder
Pectineus m
Femoral vessels
Sartorius m
Iliopsoas m
Rectus femoris m
Tensor fasciae latae m
Gluteus medius m
Femoral head
Obturator internus m
Quadratus femoris m
Sciatic n
Greater trochanter
Levator ani m
Rectum
Vagina
Ischium
Gluteus maximus m

Figure 28.1.8

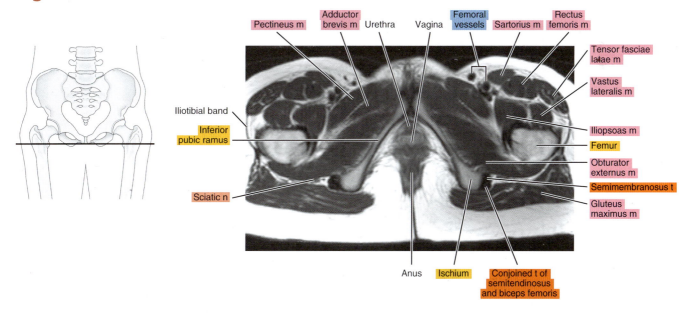

Pectineus m
Adductor brevis m
Urethra
Vagina
Femoral vessels
Sartorius m
Rectus femoris m
Tensor fasciae latae m
Vastus lateralis m
Iliopsoas m
Femur
Obturator externus m
Semimembranosus t
Gluteus maximus m
Iliotibial band
Inferior pubic ramus
Sciatic n
Anus
Ischium
Conjoined t of semitendinosus and biceps femoris

SAGITTAL
Figure 28.2.1

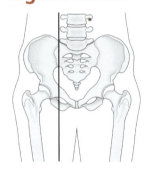

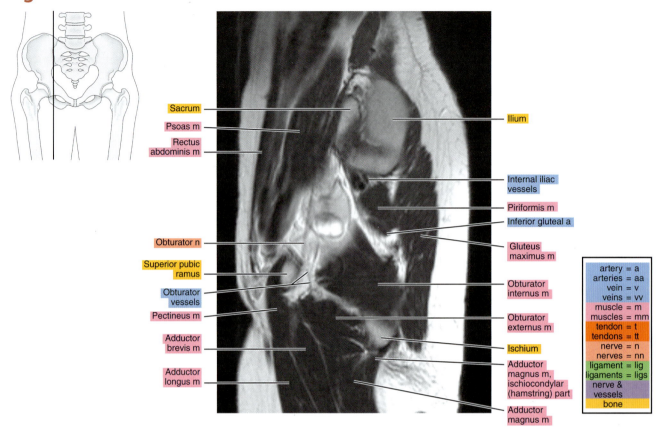

Sacrum

Psoas m

Rectus abdominis m

Obturator n

Superior pubic ramus

Obturator vessels

Pectineus m

Adductor brevis m

Adductor longus m

Ilium

Internal iliac vessels

Piriformis m

Inferior gluteal a

Gluteus maximus m

Obturator internus m

Obturator externus m

Ischium

Adductor magnus m, ischiocondylar (hamstring) part

Adductor magnus m

artery = a
arteries = aa
vein = v
veins = vv
muscle = m
muscles = mm
tendon = t
tendons = tt
nerve = n
nerves = nn
ligament = lig
ligaments = ligs
nerve & vessels
bone

Figure 28.2.2

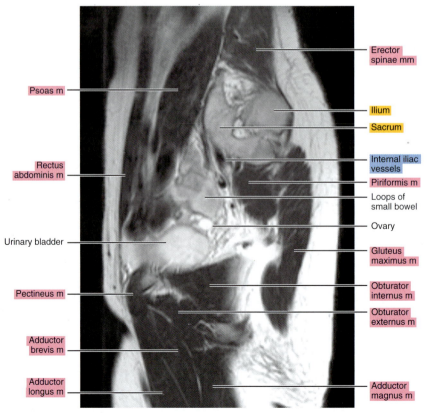

Psoas m

Rectus abdominis m

Urinary bladder

Pectineus m

Adductor brevis m

Adductor longus m

Erector spinae mm

Ilium

Sacrum

Internal iliac vessels

Piriformis m

Loops of small bowel

Ovary

Gluteus maximus m

Obturator internus m

Obturator externus m

Adductor magnus m

Figure 28.2.3

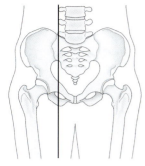

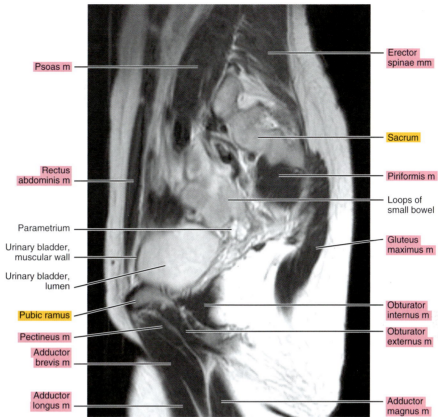

Psoas m

Rectus abdominis m

Parametrium

Urinary bladder, muscular wall

Urinary bladder, lumen

Pubic ramus

Pectineus m

Adductor brevis m

Adductor longus m

Erector spinae mm

Sacrum

Piriformis m

Loops of small bowel

Gluteus maximus m

Obturator internus m

Obturator externus m

Adductor magnus m

Figure 28.2.4

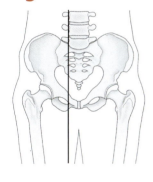

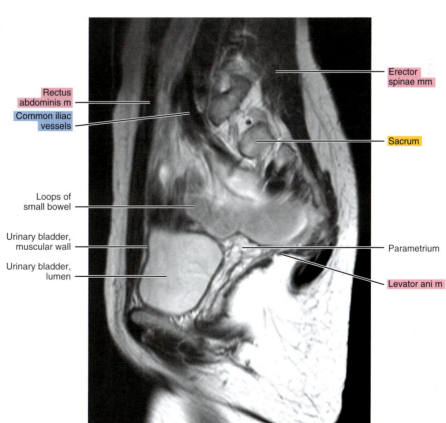

Rectus abdominis m

Common iliac vessels

Loops of small bowel

Urinary bladder, muscular wall

Urinary bladder, lumen

Erector spinae mm

Sacrum

Parametrium

Levator ani m

Figure 28.2.5

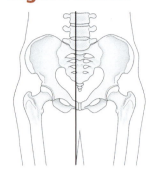

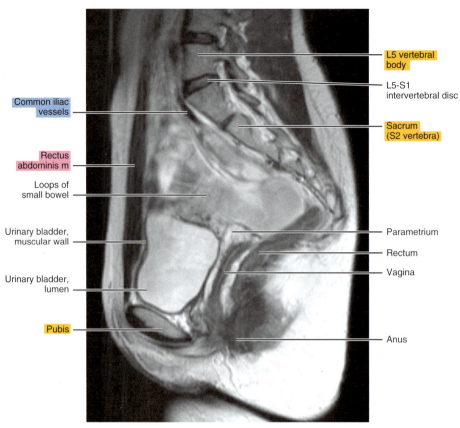

- L5 vertebral body
- L5-S1 intervertebral disc
- Common iliac vessels
- Sacrum (S2 vertebra)
- Rectus abdominis m
- Loops of small bowel
- Urinary bladder, muscular wall
- Parametrium
- Rectum
- Vagina
- Urinary bladder, lumen
- Pubis
- Anus

Figure 28.2.6

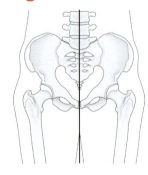

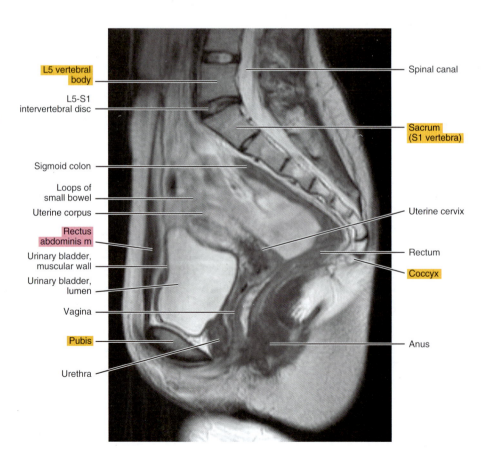

- L5 vertebral body
- L5-S1 intervertebral disc
- Spinal canal
- Sacrum (S1 vertebra)
- Sigmoid colon
- Loops of small bowel
- Uterine corpus
- Uterine cervix
- Rectus abdominis m
- Urinary bladder, muscular wall
- Rectum
- Coccyx
- Urinary bladder, lumen
- Vagina
- Pubis
- Anus
- Urethra

Figure 28.2.7

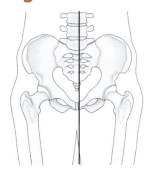

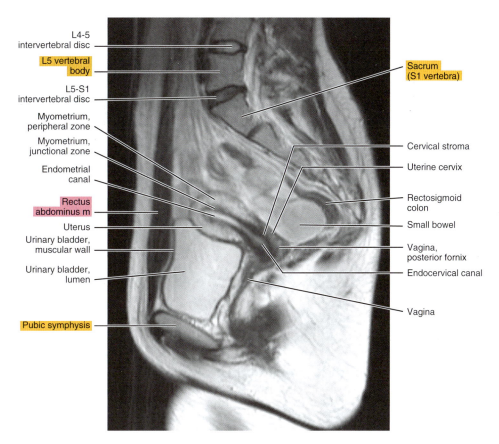

L4-5 intervertebral disc

L5 vertebral body

L5-S1 intervertebral disc

Myometrium, peripheral zone

Myometrium, junctional zone

Endometrial canal

Rectus abdominus m

Uterus

Urinary bladder, muscular wall

Urinary bladder, lumen

Pubic symphysis

Sacrum (S1 vertebra)

Cervical stroma

Uterine cervix

Rectosigmoid colon

Small bowel

Vagina, posterior fornix

Endocervical canal

Vagina

CORONAL
Figure 28.3.1

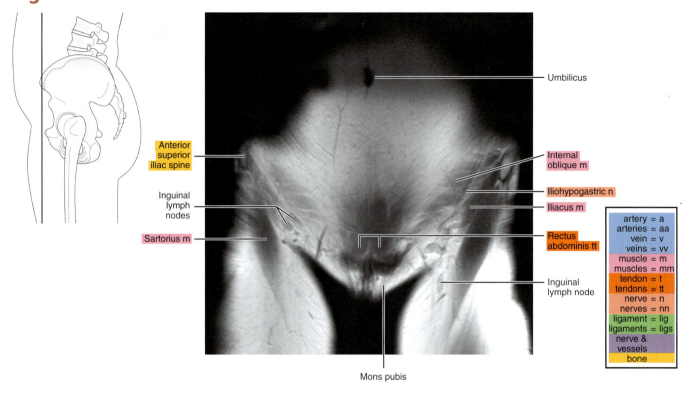

Umbilicus

Anterior superior iliac spine

Inguinal lymph nodes

Sartorius m

Internal oblique m

Iliohypogastric n

Iliacus m

Rectus abdominis tt

Inguinal lymph node

Mons pubis

artery = a	
arteries = aa	
vein = v	
veins = vv	
muscle = m	
muscles = mm	
tendon = t	
tendons = tt	
nerve = n	
nerves = nn	
ligament = lig	
ligaments = ligs	
nerve & vessels	
bone	

Figure 28.3.2

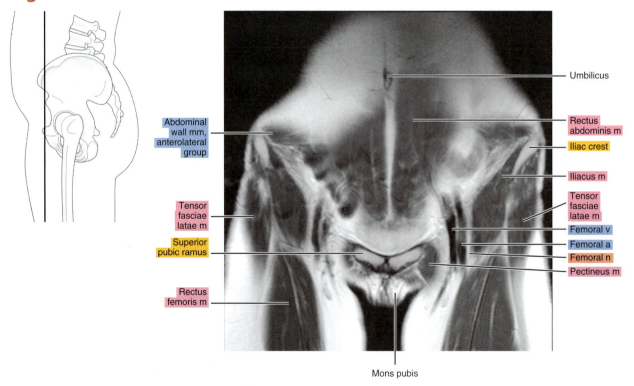

Umbilicus

Abdominal wall mm, anterolateral group

Rectus abdominis m

Iliac crest

Iliacus m

Tensor fasciae latae m

Tensor fasciae latae m

Femoral v

Superior pubic ramus

Femoral a

Femoral n

Pectineus m

Rectus femoris m

Mons pubis

Figure 28.3.3

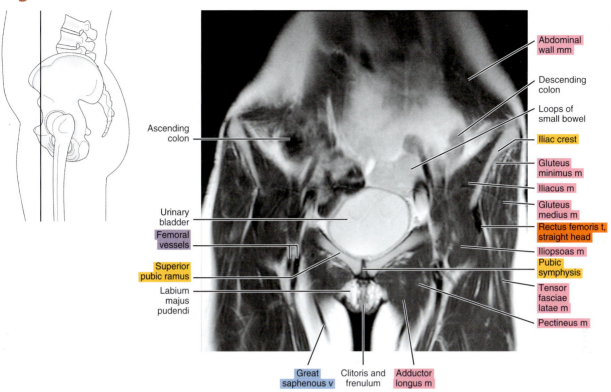

Ascending colon

Urinary bladder

Femoral vessels

Superior pubic ramus

Labium majus pudendi

Abdominal wall mm

Descending colon

Loops of small bowel

Iliac crest

Gluteus minimus m

Iliacus m

Gluteus medius m

Rectus femoris t, straight head

Iliopsoas m

Pubic symphysis

Tensor fasciae latae m

Pectineus m

Great saphenous v   Clitoris and frenulum   Adductor longus m

Figure 28.3.4

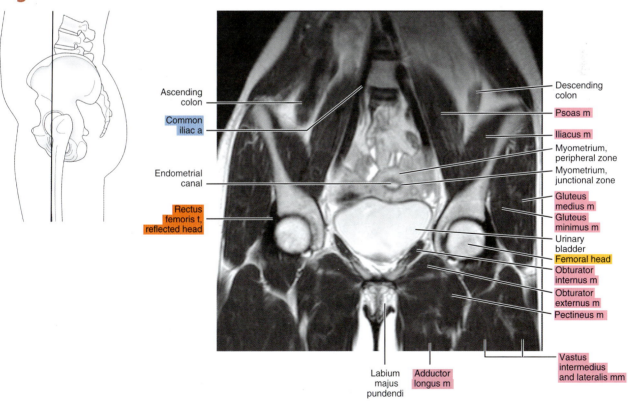

Ascending colon

Common iliac a

Endometrial canal

Rectus femoris t, reflected head

Descending colon

Psoas m

Iliacus m

Myometrium, peripheral zone

Myometrium, junctional zone

Gluteus medius m

Gluteus minimus m

Urinary bladder

Femoral head

Obturator internus m

Obturator externus m

Pectineus m

Vastus intermedius and lateralis mm

Labium majus pundendi   Adductor longus m

Figure 28.3.5

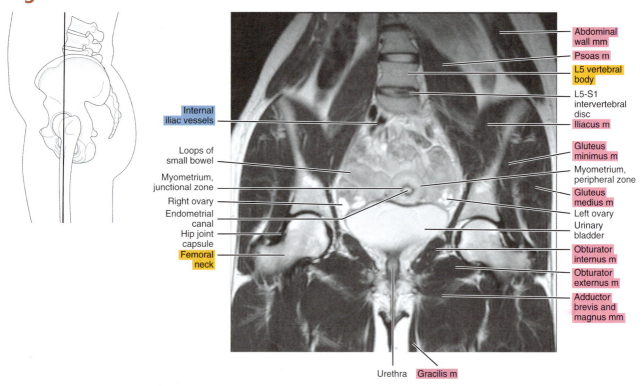

Abdominal wall mm
Psoas m
L5 vertebral body
L5-S1 intervertebral disc
Iliacus m
Gluteus minimus m
Myometrium, peripheral zone
Gluteus medius m
Left ovary
Urinary bladder
Obturator internus m
Obturator externus m
Adductor brevis and magnus mm

Internal iliac vessels
Loops of small bowel
Myometrium, junctional zone
Right ovary
Endometrial canal
Hip joint capsule
Femoral neck

Urethra   Gracilis m

Figure 28.3.6

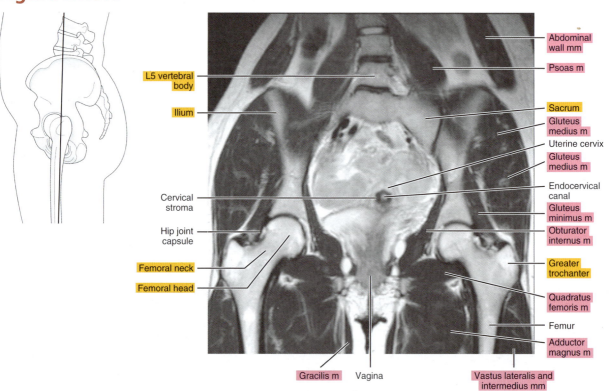

L5 vertebral body
Ilium
Cervical stroma
Hip joint capsule
Femoral neck
Femoral head

Abdominal wall mm
Psoas m
Sacrum
Gluteus medius m
Uterine cervix
Gluteus medius m
Endocervical canal
Gluteus minimus m
Obturator internus m
Greater trochanter
Quadratus femoris m
Femur
Adductor magnus m

Gracilis m   Vagina   Vastus lateralis and intermedius mm

Figure 28.3.7

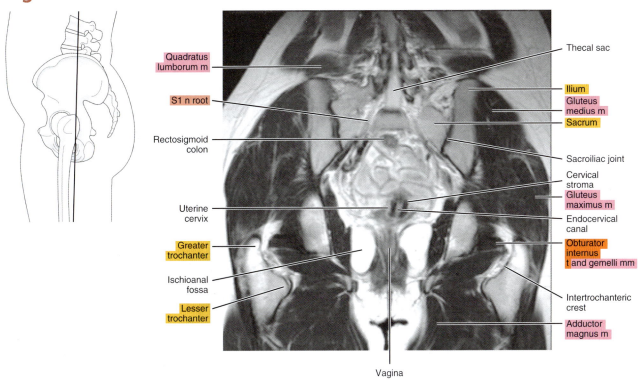

Quadratus lumborum m

S1 n root

Rectosigmoid colon

Uterine cervix

Greater trochanter

Ischioanal fossa

Lesser trochanter

Thecal sac

Ilium

Gluteus medius m

Sacrum

Sacroiliac joint

Cervical stroma

Gluteus maximus m

Endocervical canal

Obturator internus t and gemelli mm

Intertrochanteric crest

Adductor magnus m

Vagina

Figure 28.3.8

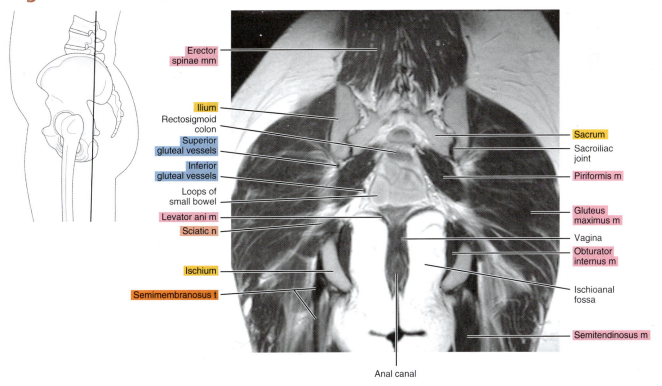

Erector spinae mm

Ilium

Rectosigmoid colon

Superior gluteal vessels

Inferior gluteal vessels

Loops of small bowel

Levator ani m

Sciatic n

Ischium

Semimembranosus t

Sacrum

Sacroiliac joint

Piriformis m

Gluteus maximus m

Vagina

Obturator internus m

Ischioanal fossa

Semitendinosus m

Anal canal

Figure 28.3.9

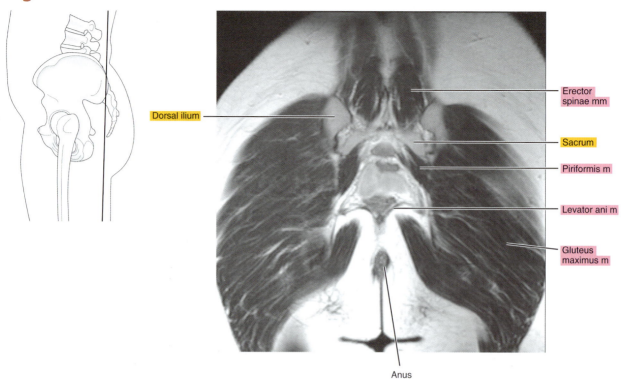

Dorsal ilium

Erector spinae mm

Sacrum

Piriformis m

Levator ani m

Gluteus maximus m

Anus

Index

Note: Page numbers followed by *f* indicate figures; *t*, tables. *a.* = artery; *ABER* = abduction external rotation; *lig.* = ligament; *ligs.* = ligaments; *m.* = muscle; *n.* = nerve; *t.* = tendon; *v.* = vein

A

A1 pulley
  axial view, of hand, 266*f*, 268*f*
  sagittal view, of hand, 274*f*
A2 pulley
  axial view, of hand, 268*f*
  sagittal view, of hand, 274*f*
A3 pulley, sagittal view, of hand, 274*f*
A4 pulley, sagittal view, of hand, 274*f*
A5 pulley, sagittal view, of hand, 274*f*
Abdominal aorta
  coronal view, of thorax CT, 48*f*, 49*f*
  sagittal view
    of heart MRI, 59*f*
    of thorax CT, 45*f*
Abdominal wall m.
  axial view, of male pelvis MRI, 596*f*, 597*f*
  coronal view
    of female pelvis MRI, 622*f*, 623*f*, 624*f*
    of lumbar spine, 320*f*, 321*f*
    of male pelvis MRI, 607*f*, 608*f*, 609*f*
  sagittal view, of male pelvis MRI, 601*f*, 602*f*
Abductor digiti minimi m.
  axial view of ankle, 509*f*, 510*f*
  coronal view
    of ankle, 524*f*, 525*f*, 526*f*, 527*f*, 528*f*, 529*f*, 530*f*
    of hand, 280*f*, 281*f*
  oblique axial view, of ankle, 514*f*, 515*f*, 516*f*
  origin, insertion, and nerve supply of, 284*t*
  sagittal view
    of ankle, 518*f*, 519*f*, 520*f*
    of hand, 276*f*, 277*f*, 278*f*
Abductor digiti minimi t.
  axial view
    of foot, 540*f*
    of hand, 262*f*, 263*f*, 264*f*, 266*f*, 267*f*
  coronal view, of foot, 551*f*, 552*f*, 553*f*, 554*f*, 555*f*, 556*f*
  oblique axial view, of ankle, 516*f*
  sagittal view, of foot, 541*f*
Abductor hallucis m.
  axial view, of ankle, 507*f*, 508*f*, 509*f*
  coronal view, of ankle, 524*f*, 525*f*, 526*f*, 527*f*, 528*f*, 529*f*, 530*f*
  oblique axial view, of ankle, 514*f*, 515*f*, 516*f*
  sagittal view, of ankle, 522*f*, 523*f*
Abductor hallucis t.
  oblique axial view, of ankle, 515*f*, 516*f*
Abductor pollicis brevis m.
  axial view, of hand, 262*f*, 263*f*, 264*f*, 265*f*
  coronal view, of hand, 279*f*
  origin, insertion, and nerve supply of, 284*t*
  sagittal view, of hand, 280*f*, 281*f*, 282*f*
Abductor pollicis brevis t., sagittal view, of hand, 270*f*, 271*f*

Abductor pollicis longus m.
  axial view, of forearm, 210*f*, 211*f*, 212*f*, 213*f*, 214*f*, 215*f*, 216*f*, 217*f*, 218*f*
  coronal view, of forearm, 230*f*, 231*f*
  oblique sagittal view, of elbow, 193*f*
  origin, insertion, and nerve supply of, 233*t*–234*t*
  sagittal view, of forearm, 221*f*, 222*f*, 223*f*
Abductor pollicis longus t.
  axial view, of forearm, 214*f*, 215*f*, 216*f*
  coronal view, of hand, 279*f*, 280*f*
  sagittal view, of forearm, 221*f*
Accessory cephalic v.
  axial view
    of elbow, 179*f*, 180*f*, 181*f*, 182*f*, 183*f*, 184*f*, 185*f*, 186*f*, 187*f*, 188*f*, 189*f*
    of forearm, 209*f*
  oblique coronal, of elbow, 199*f*, 200*f*
  oblique sagittal view, of elbow, 190*f*, 191*f*, 192*f*
  sagittal view, of forearm, 219*f*
Accessory collateral ligs.
  axial view, of hand, 268*f*
  coronal view, of hand, 281*f*
Accessory flexor digitorum longus m.
  axial view, of ankle, 503*f*, 504*f*, 505*f*, 506*f*, 507*f*
  coronal view, of ankle, 530*f*, 531*f*
  sagittal view, of ankle, 521*f*
Accessory hemiazygos v.
  axial view, of thoracic spine, 297*f*
  sagittal view
    of abdomen CT, 333*f*
    of thoracic spine, 300*f*
Acetabular fossa
  axial view
    of female pelvis CT, 582*f*
    of hip, 377*f*
    of hip arthrogram, 405*f*, 406*f*, 407*f*
    of male pelvis CT, 567*f*
  coronal view
    of female pelvis CT, 590*f*
    of hip, 395*f*, 396*f*
    of hip arthrogram, 417*f*
    of male pelvis CT, 576*f*
  sagittal view
    of hip, 390*f*
    of hip arthrogram, 413*f*
Acetabular lig., transverse
  axial view, of hip arthrogram, 406*f*, 407*f*
  coronal view, of hip arthrogram, 414*f*, 415*f*, 416*f*, 417*f*
  sagittal view, of hip arthrogram, 412*f*, 413*f*
Acetabular roof
  coronal view
    of female pelvis CT, 590*f*
    of hip, 395*f*, 396*f*
    of male pelvis MRI, 609*f*
  sagittal view
    of hip, 388*f*, 389*f*

Acetabular roof (Continued)
  of hip arthrogram, 409*f*, 410*f*, 411*f*, 412*f*
Acetabular wall, anterior
  axial view
    of female pelvis CT, 582*f*
    of hip, 376*f*, 377*f*
  sagittal view
    of hip, 389*f*, 390*f*
    of hip arthrogram, 411*f*, 412*f*
Acetabular wall, posterior
  axial view
    of female pelvis CT, 582*f*
    of hip, 376*f*, 377*f*
  sagittal view
    of hip, 389*f*
    of hip arthrogram, 411*f*
Acetabulum
  axial view, of male pelvis CT, 567*f*
  coronal view
    of female pelvis CT, 590*f*, 591*f*, 592*f*
    of hip, 395*f*
    of male pelvis CT, 575*f*, 576*f*
Achilles t.
  axial view
    of ankle, 501*f*, 502*f*, 503*f*, 504*f*, 505*f*, 506*f*, 507*f*, 508*f*, 509*f*
    of leg, 479*f*, 480*f*, 481*f*, 482*f*, 483*f*
  coronal view
    of ankle, 532*f*, 533*f*
    of leg, 494*f*, 495*f*
  gastrocnemius part, coronal view, of leg, 495*f*
  oblique axial view, of ankle, 511*f*, 512*f*
  sagittal view
    of ankle, 518*f*, 519*f*, 520*f*
    of leg, 488*f*, 489*f*
Acromioclavicular joint
  axial view
    of pectoral girdle and chest wall, 69*f*
    of shoulder, 99*f*, 100*f*
  coronal view
    of arm, 171*f*, 172*f*
    of pectoral girdle and chest wall, 90*f*, 91*f*
  oblique coronal view
    of shoulder, 121*f*, 122*f*
    of shoulder arthrogram, 143*f*
  oblique sagittal view
    of shoulder, 114*f*, 115*f*
    of shoulder arthrogram, 138*f*
Acromioclavicular lig.
  oblique sagittal view, of shoulder, 115*f*
Acromion
  ABER view, of shoulder arthrogram, 148*f*, 150*f*, 151*f*
  angle of, oblique coronal view of shoulder, 125*f*, 126*f*
  axial view
    of pectoral girdle and chest wall, 69*f*

Acromion (Continued)
of shoulder, 99f, 100f
coronal view
of arm, 171f, 172f, 173f
of pectoral girdle and chest wall, 90f, 91f, 92f, 93f
oblique coronal view
of shoulder, 122f, 123f, 124f, 125f
of shoulder arthrogram, 142f, 143f, 144f, 145f, 146f, 147f
oblique sagittal view
of shoulder, 112f, 113f, 114f, 115f
of shoulder arthrogram, 136f, 137f, 138f, 139f, 140f, 141f
sagittal view
of arm, 165f, 166f, 167f
of pectoral girdle and chest wall, 79f, 80f
Adductor aponeurosis, sagittal view, of hand, 274f, 275f
Adductor brevis m.
axial view
of female pelvis CT, 584f
of female pelvis MRI, 617f
of hip, 379f, 380f, 381f, 382f
of male pelvis CT, 569f
of male pelvis MRI, 600f
of thigh, 420f, 421f, 422f
coronal view
of female pelvis CT, 590f, 591f
of female pelvis MRI, 624f
of hip, 394f, 395f, 396f
of male pelvis CT, 575f, 576f
of male pelvis MRI, 608f, 609f, 610f
of thigh, 440f, 441f
origin, insertion, and nerve supply of, 445t
sagittal view
of female pelvis CT, 585f, 586f
of female pelvis MRI, 618f, 619f
of hip, 388f, 389f, 390f, 391f, 392f
of male pelvis CT, 570f, 571f
of male pelvis MRI, 601f, 602f, 603f, 604f
of thigh, 434f, 435f, 436f
Adductor canal, axial view, of thigh, 426f
Adductor longus m.
axial view
of hip, 379f, 380f, 381f, 382f
of male pelvis CT, 569f
of male pelvis MRI, 600f
of thigh, 420f, 421f, 422f, 423f, 424f, 425f
coronal view
of female pelvis CT, 589f
of female pelvis MRI, 623f
of hip, 393f, 394f, 395f
of male pelvis CT, 573f, 574f
of male pelvis MRI, 608f, 609f
of thigh, 439f, 440f, 441f
origin, insertion, and nerve supply of, 445t
sagittal view
of female pelvis MRI, 618f, 619f
of hip, 389f, 390f, 391f, 392f
of male pelvis MRI, 601f, 602f, 603f, 604f
of thigh, 433f, 434f, 436f
Adductor longus t., axial view, of male pelvis CT, 569f
Adductor magnus m.
axial view
of hip, 380f, 381f, 382f
of male pelvis CT, 569f
of male pelvis MRI, 600f
of thigh, 420f, 421f, 422f, 423f, 424f, 425f, 426f
coronal view
of female pelvis CT, 590f, 591f, 592f
of female pelvis MRI, 624f, 625f
of hip, 396f, 397f
of male pelvis CT, 575f, 576f
of male pelvis MRI, 609f, 610f, 611f
of thigh, 441f, 442f
origin, insertion, and nerve supply of, 445t
sagittal view
of female pelvis CT, 585f
of female pelvis MRI, 618f, 619f
of hip, 386f, 387f, 388f, 389f, 390f, 391f, 392f
of male pelvis CT, 570f
of male pelvis MRI, 601f, 602f

Adductor magnus m. (Continued)
of thigh, 430f, 431f, 432f, 433f, 434f, 435f, 436f
Adductor magnus m., ischiocondylar (hamstring) part
coronal view, of male pelvis MRI, 611f
sagittal view
of female pelvis MRI, 618f
of male pelvis MRI, 602f
Adductor magnus t.
axial view, of knee, 447f, 448f, 449f
coronal view
of knee, 468f
of thigh, 443f
sagittal view
of knee, 461f
of thigh, 433f
Adductor pollicis brevis m., origin, insertion, and nerve supply of, 284t
Adductor pollicis m.
axial view of hand, 263f, 264f, 265f, 266f
sagittal view of hand, 270f, 271f, 272f
Adductor pollicis m., oblique head
coronal view, of hand, 280f, 281f
sagittal view
of hand, 272f, 273f, 274f
Adductor pollicis m., transverse head
coronal view, of hand, 280f, 281f
sagittal view
of hand, 272f, 273f, 274f
Adductor pollicis t., axial view, of hand, 266f
Adductor tubercle, sagittal view, of knee, 461f
Adenoid tonsils, axial view, of brain CT, 8f
Adrenal gland
axial view
of abdomen CT, 327f, 328f
of abdomen MRI, 346f, 347f, 348f, 349f, 350f
coronal view
of abdomen CT, 342f, 343f
of abdomen MRI, 367f, 368f
sagittal view
of abdomen CT, 333f, 336f
of abdomen MRI, 355f, 356f, 360f
Adrenal v., axial view, of abdomen CT, 327f
Anal canal
axial view
of female pelvis CT, 583f, 584f
of male pelvis CT, 568f, 569f
of male pelvis MRI, 600f
coronal view
of female pelvis CT, 593f
of female pelvis MRI, 625f
of male pelvis CT, 578f
of male pelvis MRI, 611f
sagittal view, of female pelvis CT, 586f, 587f
Anconeus m.
axial view
of elbow, 180f, 181f, 182f, 183f, 184f, 185f, 186f, 187f, 188f, 189f
of forearm, 209f, 210f
coronal view, of forearm, 231f
oblique coronal view, of elbow, 205f, 206f, 207f
oblique sagittal view, of elbow, 192f, 193f, 194f
origin, insertion, and nerve supply of, 233t–234t
sagittal view, of forearm, 223f, 224f
Ankle joint
axial view, of ankle, 504f
coronal view, of ankle, 526f, 527f, 528f, 529f
sagittal view, of ankle, 518f, 519f, 520f
Annular lig.
axial view, of elbow, 184f
oblique coronal, of elbow, 203f, 204f
oblique sagittal view, of elbow, 192f, 193f
Anterior bands
ABER view, of shoulder arthrogram, 150f, 151f
axial view
of elbow, 182f
of shoulder arthrogram, 135f
coronal view, of arm, 170f
oblique coronal view, of shoulder arthrogram, 144f
oblique sagittal view
of elbow, 197f
of shoulder arthrogram, 139f

Anterior scalene m., coronal view of cervical spine MRI, 294f
Anus
axial view, of female pelvis MRI, 617f
coronal view
of female pelvis MRI, 626f
of male pelvis CT, 577f
of male pelvis MRI, 610f, 611f, 612f
sagittal view
of female pelvis MRI, 620f
of male pelvis CT, 572f
of male pelvis MRI, 606f
Aorta
axial view
of abdomen CT, 326f, 327f, 328f, 329f, 330f
of abdomen MRI, 346f, 347f, 348f, 349f, 350f, 351f, 352f, 353f
of heart MRI, 56f, 57f
of lumbar spine, 310f
of thoracic spine, 297f, 298f
of thorax CT, 39f, 42f
coronal view
of abdomen CT, 339f, 340f, 341f, 342f, 343f
of abdomen MRI, 364f, 365f, 366f, 367f, 368f
of lumbar spine, 317f, 318f
sagittal view
of abdomen CT, 334f
of abdomen MRI, 356f, 357f
of thoracic spine, 300f
Aorta, abdominal
coronal view, of thorax CT, 48f, 49f
sagittal view
of heart MRI, 59f
of thorax CT, 45f
Aorta, ascending
axial view
of heart MRI, 54f, 55f
of pectoral girdle and chest wall, 73f, 74f, 75f
of thorax CT, 38f, 39f
coronal view
of heart MRI, 61f, 62f
of pectoral girdle and chest wall, 90f
sagittal view
of heart MRI, 59f
of thorax CT, 45f
Aorta, descending
axial view
of heart MRI, 54f, 55f
of thorax CT, 38f, 39f, 40f, 41f
coronal view, of heart MRI, 63f
sagittal view
of abdomen CT, 333f
of heart MRI, 58f
of thorax CT, 44f
Aortic arch
axial view
of heart MRI, 54f
of thorax CT, 37f, 38f
coronal view
of heart MRI, 62f
of thorax CT, 47f, 48f, 49f
sagittal view
of heart MRI, 58f, 59f
of thorax CT, 44f, 45f
Aortic bifurcation
axial view, of abdomen CT, 331f
coronal view
of abdomen CT, 339f
of female pelvis CT, 590f, 591f
of male pelvis CT, 574f
sagittal view
of female pelvis CT, 587f
of male pelvis CT, 571f
Aortic outflow tract, axial view, of heart MRI, 56f
Aortic root
axial view, of heart MRI, 56f
coronal view, of heart MRI, 61f
sagittal view
of heart MRI, 59f
of thorax CT, 44f, 45f
Aortic valve leaflets
axial view, of thorax CT, 40f
coronal view, of thorax CT, 49f
Aortic valve plane, coronal view, of thorax CT, 48f

Aorticopulmonary window, sagittal view, of heart MRI, 59f
Appendix
  axial view
    of female pelvis CT, 580f
    of male pelvis CT, 566f
  coronal view, of female pelvis CT, 589f
Arcuate lig., median, sagittal view, of abdomen CT, 334f
Articular cartilage
  axial view
    of knee, 449f
    of shoulder, 131f, 132f, 133f
  coronal view, of knee, 466f, 467f, 468f
  oblique coronal view, of shoulder, 123f, 145f
  sagittal view, of knee, 455f, 456f, 457f, 460f, 461f
Articular recess, superior, coronal view, of hip arthrogram, 414f, 415f, 416f, 417f, 418f
Articulating process (facet)
  inferior, sagittal view, of thoracic spine, 300f, 301f
  superior, sagittal view, of thoracic spine, 300f, 301f
Atrial appendage
  axial view
    of heart MRI, 56f
    of thorax CT, 39f
  coronal view, of thorax CT, 47f
  sagittal view
    of heart MRI, 59f
    of thorax CT, 44f
Atrium
  left
    axial view
      of heart MRI, 56f
      of thorax CT, 39f, 40f
    coronal view
      of abdomen MRI, 366f
      of heart MRI, 62f
      of thorax CT, 49f, 50f
    sagittal view
      of abdomen CT, 334f
      of heart MRI, 59f
      of thorax CT, 44f, 45f
  right
    axial view
      of heart MRI, 56f, 57f
      of thorax CT, 39f, 40f
    coronal view
      of abdomen CT, 341f
      of heart MRI, 61f, 62f
      of thorax CT, 47f, 48f, 49f
    sagittal view
      of abdomen CT, 335f
      of heart MRI, 59f, 60f
      of thorax CT, 46f
Axillary a.
  axial view
    of pectoral girdle and chest wall, 71f, 72f, 73f
    of shoulder, 104f, 105f, 106f, 107f, 108f
  coronal view
    of heart MRI, 62f
    of pectoral girdle and chest wall, 91f, 92f
  oblique coronal view, of shoulder, 112f, 119f, 120f, 121f
  oblique sagittal view, of shoulder, 115f, 116f, 117f, 118f
  sagittal view, of pectoral girdle and chest wall, 81f, 82f, 83f, 84f
Axillary lymph node, oblique sagittal view, of shoulder, 116f
Axillary n.
  axial view
    of pectoral girdle and chest wall, 73f, 74f
    of shoulder, 108f
  coronal view
    of arm, 173f
    of pectoral girdle and chest wall, 93f
  oblique coronal view
    of shoulder, 122f, 125f, 126f, 127f
    of shoulder arthrogram, 147f
  oblique sagittal view
    of shoulder, 112f, 113f
    of shoulder arthrogram, 139f

Axillary n. (Continued)
  sagittal view
    of arm, 163f, 164f, 166f, 167f
    of pectoral girdle and chest wall, 80f
Axillary neurovascular bundle
  axial view, of pectoral girdle and chest wall, 74f
  coronal view, of arm, 171f
  sagittal view, of arm, 166f, 167f
Axillary pouch
  axial view, of shoulder arthrogram, 135f
  oblique sagittal view, of shoulder arthrogram, 139f, 140f
Axillary recess, oblique coronal view, of shoulder arthrogram, 144f, 145f, 146f, 147f
Axillary v.
  axial view
    of pectoral girdle and chest wall, 71f, 72f, 73f
    of shoulder, 104f, 105f, 106f, 107f, 108f
  coronal view
    of heart MRI, 62f
    of pectoral girdle and chest wall, 91f, 92f
  oblique coronal view, of shoulder, 119f, 120f, 121f
  oblique sagittal view, of shoulder, 116f, 117f, 118f
  sagittal view, of pectoral girdle and chest wall, 82f, 83f, 84f
Azygos v.
  axial view
    of abdomen MRI, 346f, 347f
    of heart MRI, 55f, 56f, 57f
    of lumbar spine, 310f
    of thoracic spine, 297f, 298f
    of thorax CT, 38f, 39f, 41f, 42f
  coronal view
    of abdomen MRI, 368f
    of lumbar spine, 317f
  sagittal view, of lumbar spine, 316f
Azygos v., arch
  axial view, of thorax CT, 38f
  coronal view, of heart MRI, 62f
  sagittal view, of thorax CT, 45f

B
Basilar a.
  axial view
    of brain CT, 7f, 8f
    of brain MRI, 23f
  coronal view, of brain CT, 15f
  sagittal view, of brain MRI, 30f
Basilic v.
  axial view
    of arm, 155f, 156f, 157f, 158f, 159f, 160f
    of elbow, 180f, 181f, 182f, 183f, 184f, 185f, 186f, 187f, 188f, 189f
  coronal view
    of arm, 169f, 170f, 171f, 172f
    of elbow, 203f, 204f, 205f
  oblique coronal view
    of elbow, 203f, 204f, 205f
    of shoulder, 123f
  oblique sagittal view, of elbow, 197f, 198f
  sagittal view
    of arm, 165f, 166f
    of forearm, 219f
Basilic v., median
  axial view
    of elbow, 183f, 184f, 185f, 186f, 187f, 188f, 189f
    of forearm, 209f, 210f, 211f, 212f, 213f, 214f, 215f, 216f
  coronal view
    of elbow, 199f, 200f
    of forearm, 225f
  oblique coronal, of elbow, 199f, 200f
  oblique sagittal view, of elbow, 196f
Basivertebral v.
  axial view, of lumbar spine, 312f
  coronal view, of lumbar spine, 319f
Basivertebral venous plexus
  axial view
    of lumbar spine, 310f
    of thoracic spine, 298f
  coronal view, of thoracic spine, 302f

Basivertebral venous plexus (Continued)
  sagittal view
    of lumbar spine, 316f
    of thoracic spine, 301f
Biceps anchor
  ABER view, of shoulder arthrogram, 148f
  oblique coronal view, of shoulder, 122f
  oblique sagittal view, of shoulder, 115f, 139f, 140f
Biceps brachii m.
  ABER view, of shoulder arthrogram, 149f, 150f
  axial view
    of arm, 157f, 158f, 159f, 160f
    of elbow, 179f, 180f, 181f
  coronal view.
    of arm, 168f, 170f
    of elbow, 199f, 200f, 201f, 202f
    of pectoral girdle and chest wall, 91f, 92f, 93f
  oblique coronal view, of elbow, 199f, 200f, 201f, 202f
  oblique sagittal view, of elbow, 190f, 191f, 192f, 193f, 194f, 195f, 196f
  origin, insertion, and nerve supply of, 177t
  sagittal view
    of arm, 162f, 163f, 164f, 165f, 166f, 167f
    of elbow, 190f, 191f, 192f, 193f, 194f, 195f, 196f
Biceps brachii m., long head.
  axial view
    of arm, 155f, 156f
    of pectoral girdle and chest wall, 74f, 75f, 76f, 77f
  coronal view
    of arm, 169f, 170f
    of pectoral girdle and chest wall, 89f, 91f, 92f
    of shoulder, 123f
  oblique coronal view, of shoulder, 123f
  sagittal view
    of arm, 163f, 164f
    of pectoral girdle and chest wall, 79f
Biceps brachii m., short head
  axial view
    of arm, 155f, 156f
    of pectoral girdle and chest wall, 73f, 74f, 75f, 76f, 77f
    of shoulder, 104f, 105f, 106f, 107f, 108f
  coronal view
    of arm, 169f, 170f
    of pectoral girdle and chest wall, 91f, 92f
    of shoulder, 120f, 121f, 122f, 123f, 124f
  oblique coronal view, of shoulder, 120f, 121f, 122f, 123f, 124f
  oblique sagittal view, of shoulder, 112f, 113f, 114f
  sagittal view
    of arm, 165f, 166f
    of pectoral girdle and chest wall, 79f, 80f, 81f
    of shoulder, 112f, 113f, 114f
Biceps brachii t.
  ABER view, of shoulder arthrogram, 148f
  axial view
    of arm, 159f, 160f
    of elbow, 179f, 180f, 181f, 182f, 183f, 184f, 185f, 186f, 187f
    of forearm, 209f
  coronal view
    of arm, 168f
    of elbow, 201f, 202f, 203f
    of forearm, 227f, 228f
  oblique coronal, of elbow, 201f, 202f, 203f
  oblique sagittal view, of elbow, 194f
  sagittal view
    of arm, 164f
    of elbow, 194f
    of forearm, 220f, 221f
    of pectoral girdle and chest wall, 79f
Biceps brachii t., long head
  ABER view, of shoulder arthrogram, 148f, 149f
  axial view
    of pectoral girdle and chest wall, 71f, 72f, 73f
    of shoulder, 102f, 103f, 104f, 105f, 106f, 107f, 108f
    of shoulder arthrogram, 131f, 132f, 133f, 134f
  coronal view
    of arm, 169f

Biceps brachii t., long head (Continued)
  of pectoral girdle and chest wall, 90f, 91f
  oblique coronal view
    of shoulder, 122f, 123f, 124f
    of shoulder arthrogram, 142f, 143f, 144f, 145f
  oblique sagittal view
    of shoulder, 110f, 111f, 112f, 113f, 114f
    of shoulder arthrogram, 136f, 137f, 138f, 139f
Biceps brachii t., short head
  ABER view, of shoulder arthrogram, 148f
  axial view
    of pectoral girdle and chest wall, 71f, 72f, 73f
    of shoulder, 105f, 106f, 107f
    of shoulder arthrogram, 134f, 135f
  oblique coronal view
    of shoulder, 121f, 122f
    of shoulder arthrogram, 142f, 143f
  oblique sagittal view
    of shoulder, 113f
    of shoulder arthrogram, 138f
Biceps femoris m.
  axial view, of thigh, 423f
  coronal view
    of knee, 469f, 470f, 471f, 472f
    of leg, 494f
    of male pelvis MRI, 611f, 612f
  origin, insertion, and nerve supply of, 445t
  sagittal view, of knee, 454f
Biceps femoris m., long head
  axial view
    of hip, 380f, 382f
    of knee, 447f
    of male pelvis MRI, 600f
    of thigh, 422f, 423f, 424f, 425f, 426f, 427f
  coronal view
    of thigh, 442f, 443f, 444f
  origin, insertion, and nerve supply of,
    400t–401t
  sagittal view
    of knee, 455f
    of thigh, 428f, 429f, 430f
Biceps femoris m., short head
  axial view
    of knee, 447f, 448f, 449f, 450f
    of thigh, 424f, 425f, 426f, 427f
  coronal view
    of knee, 471f
    of thigh, 441f
  sagittal view
    of knee, 454f, 455f
    of thigh, 428f, 429f
Biceps femoris t.
  axial view
    of knee, 447f, 448f, 449f, 450f, 451f
    of thigh, 420f, 421f
  coronal view
    of knee, 469f, 470f, 471f
    of leg, 494f, 495f
    of male pelvis CT, 578f
    of male pelvis MRI, 611f
  sagittal view
    of knee, 454f
    of leg, 484f
    of male pelvis CT, 570f
Biceps femoris t., long head, axial view
  of hip, 382f
  of male pelvis MRI, 600f
Biceps m., short head, and coracobrachialis m.,
  conjoined tendon of, 71f, 104f
Bicipital aponeurosis, axial view, of elbow, 183f,
  184f
Bicipital (intertubercular) groove, axial view
  of shoulder, 104f
  of shoulder arthrogram, 134f, 135f
Bile duct, common
  axial view
    of abdomen CT, 328f
    of abdomen MRI, 350f, 351f, 352f
  coronal view
    of abdomen CT, 339f
    of abdomen MRI, 365f, 366f
  sagittal view
    of abdomen CT, 335f
    of abdomen MRI, 360f
Blumensaat's line, sagittal view, of knee, 458f

Brachial a.
  axial view
    of arm, 155f, 156f, 157f, 158f, 159f, 160f
    of elbow, 179f, 180f, 181f, 182f, 183f
  coronal view
    of arm, 168f, 171f
    of pectoral girdle and chest wall, 92f
  oblique coronal view
    of elbow, 201f
    of shoulder, 122f, 123f
  oblique sagittal view, of elbow, 195f, 196f
  sagittal view
    of arm, 165f
    of elbow, 195f, 196f
Brachial a., deep
  axial view, of pectoral girdle and chest wall,
    75f, 77f
  coronal view, of pectoral girdle and chest wall,
    93f
  oblique coronal view, of shoulder, 123f, 125f
  sagittal view, of pectoral girdle and chest wall,
    80f
Brachial neurovascular bundle
  axial view, of pectoral girdle and chest wall,
    75f, 76f, 77f
  coronal view
    of arm, 170f, 171f
    of pectoral girdle and chest wall, 93f
  sagittal view, of pectoral girdle and chest wall,
    80f
Brachial plexus
  coronal view, of pectoral girdle and chest wall,
    91f, 92f
  oblique sagittal view, of shoulder, 116f, 118f
  sagittal view
    of cervical spine MRI, 291f
    of pectoral girdle and chest wall, 83f, 84f, 85f
    of thoracic spine, 299f
Brachial v.
  axial view, of arm, 157f, 158f, 159f
  coronal view
    of arm, 168f, 170f, 171f
    of pectoral girdle and chest wall, 92f
  sagittal view, of arm, 165f
Brachialis m.
  axial view
    of arm, 155f, 156f, 157f, 158f, 159f, 160f
    of elbow, 179f, 180f, 181f, 182f, 183f, 184f,
      185f
  coronal view
    of arm, 168f, 169f, 170f, 171f
    of elbow, 201f, 202f, 203f, 204f
  oblique coronal, of elbow, 201f, 202f, 203f, 204f
  oblique sagittal view, of elbow, 191f, 192f,
    193f, 194f, 195f, 196f, 197f
  origin, insertion, and nerve supply of, 177t
  sagittal view
    of arm, 161f, 162f, 163f, 164f, 165f
    of elbow, 191f, 192f, 193f, 194f, 195f, 196f,
      197f
    of forearm, 223f
Brachialis t.
  axial view, of elbow, 179f, 180f, 181f, 182f,
    183f, 184f, 185f, 186f
  oblique coronal, of elbow, 201f
  sagittal view, of arm, 164f
Brachiocephalic a.
  axial view
    of pectoral girdle and chest wall, 71f, 72f
    of thorax CT, 37f
  coronal view, of thorax CT, 47f, 48f, 49f
  sagittal view, of thorax CT, 46f
Brachiocephalic trunk
  coronal view, of pectoral girdle and chest wall,
    90f
  sagittal view, of heart MRI, 59f
Brachiocephalic v.
  axial view
    of pectoral girdle and chest wall, 71f, 72f, 73f
    of thorax CT, 37f
  coronal view
    of heart MRI, 62f
    of pectoral girdle and chest wall, 90f, 91f
    of thorax CT, 47f, 48f, 49f
  sagittal view

Brachiocephalic v. (Continued)
    of heart MRI, 59f
    of pectoral girdle and chest wall, 87f
    of thorax CT, 44f, 45f, 46f
Brachioradialis m.
  axial view
    of arm, 158f, 159f, 160f
    of elbow, 179f, 180f, 181f, 182f, 183f, 184f,
      185f, 186f, 187f, 188f, 189f
    of forearm, 209f, 220f, 221f, 222f, 223f
  coronal view
    of arm, 168f, 169f, 170f, 171f, 172f
    of elbow, 199f, 200f, 201f, 202f, 203f, 204f,
      205f, 206f
    of forearm, 227f, 228f, 229f, 230f
  oblique coronal, of elbow, 199f, 200f, 201f,
    202f, 203f, 204f, 205f, 206f
  oblique sagittal view, of elbow, 190f, 191f,
    192f, 193f, 194f
  origin, insertion, and nerve supply of, 233t–234t
  sagittal view
    of arm, 161f, 162f
    of elbow, 190f, 191f, 192f, 193f, 194f
    of forearm, 219f
Brachioradialis t., axial view, of forearm, 213f,
  214f, 216f, 217f, 218f
Breast
  coronal view, of abdomen MRI, 362f, 363f, 364f
  sagittal view, of abdomen MRI, 354f
Bronchus
  axial view
    of heart MRI, 55f
    of pectoral girdle and chest wall, 74f
    of thorax CT, 38f
  coronal view, of thorax CT, 50f
  sagittal view
    of heart MRI, 58f, 59f
    of thorax CT, 43f, 44f
Bulbospongiosus m.
  coronal view
    of female pelvis CT, 590f, 591f
    of male pelvis CT, 576f, 577f
  sagittal view, of male pelvis CT, 572f

C

C1 lateral mass, axial view, of cervical spine MRI,
  288f
C1 posterior arch
  axial view, of cervical spine MRI, 288f
  coronal view, of cervical spine MRI, 295f
C1 pulley, sagittal view, of hand, 274f
C1 transverse process, sagittal view, of cervical
  spine MRI, 291f
C5-6 disc level, axial view, of pectoral girdle and
  chest wall, 68f
C6 spinous process, axial view, of cervical spine
  MRI, 290f
C7 transverse process, coronal view, of cervical
  spine MRI, 294f
C7 vertebral body, axial view, of pectoral girdle
  and chest wall, 69f
Calcaneal tubercle
  axial view, of ankle, 507f, 508f
  lateral, coronal view, of ankle, 531f, 532f
Calcaneal tuberosity
  axial view, of ankle, 507f, 508f, 509f, 510f
  sagittal view, of ankle, 518f, 519f, 520f, 521f
Calcaneal vessels, medial, sagittal view, of ankle,
  522f
Calcaneocuboid joint
  axial view, of ankle, 508f
  coronal view, of ankle, 526f
  oblique axial view, of ankle, 515f
Calcaneocuboid lig., plantar
  axial view, of ankle, 508f, 509f
  coronal view, of ankle, 524f, 525f, 526f, 527f,
    528f, 529f
  sagittal view, of ankle, 519f, 520f
Calcaneofibular lig., axial view, of ankle, 506f,
  507f
Calcaneonavicular (spring) lig.
  inferoplantar
    axial view, of ankle, 507f
    coronal view, of ankle, 525f

Calcaneonavicular (spring) lig. (Continued)
  oblique axial view, of ankle, 514f
    sagittal view, of ankle, 522f
  medioplantar, axial view, of ankle, 507f
  plantar, oblique axial view, of ankle, 514f
  superomedial, coronal view, of ankle, 526f
Calcaneus
  axial view, of ankle, 507f, 508f, 509f
  coronal view
    of ankle, 526f, 527f, 528f, 529f, 530f, 531f,
      532f, 533f
    of leg, 492f, 493f, 494f
  oblique axial view, of ankle, 512f, 513f, 514f
  sagittal view, of ankle, 518f, 519f, 520f, 521f
Calcar femorale
  axial view, of hip, 379f, 380f, 381f
  coronal view, of hip, 396f
Calvarium
  axial view
    of brain CT, 4f, 5f, 6f
    of brain MRI, 19f, 20f, 21f
  coronal view, of brain CT, 13f, 14f, 15f, 16f, 17f
  coronal view, of cervical spine MRI, 295f
  sagittal view, of brain MRI, 28f, 29f, 30f, 31f,
    32f
Capitate
  coronal view, of hand, 280f, 281f, 282f
  sagittal view, of hand, 273f, 274f
Capitellum
  axial view, of elbow, 181f, 182f, 183f
  oblique coronal, of elbow, 203f, 204f
  oblique sagittal view, of elbow, 192f, 193f, 194f
  sagittal view
    of arm, 162f, 163f
    of elbow, 192f, 193f, 194f
Capsular insertion, axial view, of shoulder
    arthrogram, 133f, 134f
Capsular lig.
  lateral, coronal view, of knee, 469f
  oblique coronal view, of shoulder, 123f, 124f,
    125f
Cardiac septum, coronal view, of heart MRI, 61f
Carina, axial view, of heart MRI, 54f
Carotid a., axial view
  of pectoral girdle and chest wall, 68f
  of thorax CT, 36f, 37f
Carotid a., common
  axial view
    of pectoral girdle and chest wall, 70f, 71f
    of thorax CT, 36f
  coronal view
    of pectoral girdle and chest wall, 90f
    of thorax CT, 48f, 49f
  sagittal view, of thorax CT, 44f, 45f
Carpal lig., palmar, axial view, of wrist, 238f, 239f,
    240f
Carpometacarpal joint
  2nd, sagittal view, of hand, 272f
  3rd, sagittal view, of hand, 274f
Cauda equina
  coronal view
    of lumbar spine, 320f
    of thoracic spine, 302f
  sagittal view, of thoracic spine, 301f
Caudate lobe of liver
  axial view
    of abdomen CT, 327f
    of abdomen MRI, 346f, 347f
  coronal view
    of abdomen CT, 341f
    of abdomen MRI, 366f, 367f
  sagittal view
    of abdomen CT, 334f, 335f, 336f
    of abdomen MRI, 359f, 360f
Caudate nucleus body
  axial view
    of brain CT, 5f
    of brain MRI, 20f
  coronal view, of brain CT, 15f
Caudate nucleus head
  axial view
    of brain CT, 6f
    of brain MRI, 21f
  coronal view, of brain CT, 14f
  sagittal view, of brain MRI, 29f

C5-C6 facet joint, coronal view, of cervical spine
    MRI, 294f
Cecum
  axial view
    of male pelvis CT, 565f, 566f, 567f
    of male pelvis MRI, 596f
  coronal view
    of abdomen CT, 339f
    of female pelvis CT, 589f, 590f
    of male pelvis CT, 573f, 574f
    of male pelvis MRI, 608f
  sagittal view
    of abdomen MRI, 361f
    of female pelvis CT, 585f
    of male pelvis MRI, 602f
Celiac a.
  axial view, of heart MRI, 59f
  coronal view
    of abdomen MRI, 365f, 366f
    of thorax CT, 49f
  sagittal view
    of abdomen MRI, 357f
    of thorax CT, 44f
Celiac trunk
  axial view
    of abdomen CT, 327f, 328f
    of abdomen MRI, 349f
  coronal view, of abdomen CT, 340f, 341f
  sagittal view, of abdomen CT, 334f
Central sulcus, axial view
  of brain CT, 4f
  of brain MRI, 19f, 20f
Centrum semiovale
  axial view
    of brain CT, 4f, 5f
    of brain MRI, 19f, 20f
  coronal view, of brain CT, 14f, 15f, 16f
  sagittal view
    of brain CT, 11f
    of brain MRI, 26f, 29f, 30f, 31f
Cephalic v.
  axial view
    of arm, 155f, 156f
    of elbow, 179f, 180f, 181f, 182f, 183f, 184f,
      185f, 186f, 187f, 188f, 189f
    of forearm, 209f, 210f, 211f, 212f, 213f, 214f,
      215f, 216f, 217f, 218f
    of pectoral girdle and chest wall, 71f, 74f,
      75f, 76f, 77f
    of shoulder, 103f, 104f, 105f, 106f, 107f, 108f
  coronal view
    of arm, 168f
    of elbow, 199f, 200f
    of forearm, 227f, 228f, 229f
    of pectoral girdle and chest wall, 88f, 89f,
      90f, 91f
  oblique coronal view
    of elbow, 199f, 200f
    of shoulder, 119f, 120f, 121f
  oblique sagittal view
    of elbow, 192f, 193f, 194f
    of shoulder, 111f, 112f, 113f, 114f, 115f, 116f,
      117f, 118f
  sagittal view
    of forearm, 219f, 220f
    of pectoral girdle and chest wall, 79f, 82f, 83f
Cerebellar hemisphere
  axial view
    of brain CT, 7f, 8f
    of brain MRI, 23f, 24f
  coronal view, of brain CT, 16f, 17f
  sagittal view
    of brain CT, 10f, 11f, 12f
    of brain MRI, 25f, 26f, 27f, 31f, 32f
Cerebellar tonsils
  axial view
    of brain CT, 8f
    of brain MRI, 24f
  sagittal view, of cervical spine MRI, 293f
Cerebellar vermis
  axial view
    of brain CT, 6f, 7f, 8f
    of brain MRI, 22f, 23f, 24f
  coronal view, of brain CT, 16f, 17f
  sagittal view

Cerebellar vermis (Continued)
  of brain CT, 10f
  of brain MRI, 25f, 31f, 32f
Cerebellopontine angle cistern, axial view, of
    brain CT, 7f
Cerebellopontine angle, sagittal view, of brain
    CT, 10f
Cerebellum, sagittal view, of cervical spine MRI,
    291f, 292f
Cerebral aqueduct
  axial view
    of brain CT, 7f
    of brain MRI, 22f
  sagittal view, of brain MRI, 25f
Cerebral peduncle
  axial view
    of brain CT, 7f
    of brain MRI, 22f
  coronal view, of brain CT, 15f
  sagittal view, of brain MRI, 30f
Cerebrospinal fluid
  axial view, of cervical spine MRI, 290f
  coronal view, of cervical spine MRI, 294f, 295f
Cervical a. and v., superficial, coronal view, of
    thoracic spine, 304f
Cervical lymph node, coronal view, of cervical
    spine MRI, 294f
Cervical spinal cord
  axial view
    of brain CT, 9f
    of cervical spine MRI, 290f
  coronal view, of cervical spine MRI, 294f
  sagittal view, of cervical spine MRI, 293f
Cervical stroma
  axial view, of female pelvis MRI, 616f
  coronal view, of female pelvis MRI, 624f, 625f
  sagittal view, of female pelvis MRI, 621f
Cervical vessels, transverse
  axial view, of pectoral girdle and chest
    wall, 69f
  coronal view, of pectoral girdle and chest
    wall, 92f, 93f
Cervicomedullary junction, axial view, of brain
    MRI, 24f
Cervix, axial view, of female pelvis MRI, 615f
Choroid plexus
  axial view
    of brain CT, 5f
    of brain MRI, 21f
  coronal view, of brain CT, 16f
  sagittal view
    of brain CT, 11f
    of brain MRI, 31f
Cingulate gyrus, sagittal view, of brain MRI, 25f
Circumflex a.
  axial view
    of heart MRI, 56f
    of thorax CT, 41f
  coronal view, of thorax CT, 48f, 49f
  posterior, sagittal view, of pectoral girdle and
    chest wall, 80f
Circumflex femoral a.
  lateral
    axial view, of male pelvis CT, 569f
    coronal view, of male pelvis CT, 575f
  medial
    axial view, of male pelvis CT, 569f
    coronal view, of male pelvis CT, 575f, 576f
  sagittal view, of male pelvis CT, 570f
Circumflex femoral v.
  lateral, coronal view, of male pelvis CT, 575f
  medial, coronal view, of male pelvis CT, 575f,
    576f
Circumflex femoral vessels
  lateral
    axial view, of hip, 379f
    coronal view, of male pelvis MRI, 608f
    sagittal view, of hip, 384f, 385f, 386f
  medial
    axial view, of hip, 379f
    coronal view, of male pelvis MRI, 608f
    sagittal view, of hip, 387f, 389f, 390f
Circumflex humeral a.
  anterior
    oblique coronal view, of shoulder, 122f, 123f

Circumflex humeral a. *(Continued)*
oblique sagittal view, of shoulder, 111f, 112f, 113f, 115f
sagittal view, of pectoral girdle and chest wall, 79f
posterior
axial view
of pectoral girdle and chest wall, 72f, 73f
of shoulder, 107f, 108f
coronal view
of arm, 173f
of pectoral girdle and chest wall, 93f
oblique coronal view, of shoulder, 122f, 123f, 124f, 125f, 126f, 127f
oblique sagittal view, of shoulder, 112f, 113f, 114f, 115f
sagittal view
of arm, 163f, 164f, 166f, 167f
of pectoral girdle and chest wall, 79f
Circumflex humeral vessels
oblique coronal view, of shoulder arthrogram, 147f
oblique sagittal view, of shoulder arthrogram, 139f, 140f
Circumflex iliac v., superficial, coronal view, of hip, 393f
Circumflex iliac vessels, superficial, coronal view, of male pelvis MRI, 607f
Circumflex scapular a.
axial view, of pectoral girdle and chest wall, 73f
coronal view
of arm, 172f
of pectoral girdle and chest wall, 92f, 93f, 94f
oblique coronal view, of shoulder, 122f, 123f, 124f, 125f, 126f, 127f
oblique sagittal view, of shoulder, 116f, 117f
sagittal view, of arm, 167f
Circumflex vessels, oblique coronal view, of shoulder, 125f
Clavicle
axial view
of pectoral girdle and chest wall, 70f, 71f, 72f
of shoulder, 101f, 102f
of shoulder arthrogram, 131f
of thorax CT, 36f
coronal view
of arm, 171f, 172f
of pectoral girdle and chest wall, 88f, 89f, 90f
distal
axial view
of pectoral girdle and chest wall, 69f
of shoulder, 99f, 100f
coronal view, of pectoral girdle and chest wall, 91f
sagittal view, of pectoral girdle and chest wall, 81f
medial, sagittal view, of pectoral girdle and chest wall, 87f
oblique coronal view
of shoulder, 119f, 120f, 121f, 122f
of shoulder arthrogram, 142f, 143f
oblique sagittal view
of shoulder, 115f, 116f, 117f, 118f
of shoulder arthrogram, 139f, 140f, 141f
sagittal view
of heart MRI, 58f, 60f
of pectoral girdle and chest wall, 81f
of thorax CT, 43f
Clavicular head
coronal view
of heart MRI, 61f
of thorax CT, 47f
sagittal view, of thorax CT, 44f, 46f
Clitoris, coronal view
of female pelvis CT, 589f
of female pelvis MRI, 623f
Clivus, sagittal view, of cervical spine MRI, 293f
Coccygeus m.
axial view
of female pelvis CT, 582f
of hip, 377f
sagittal view
of male pelvis CT, 571f
of male pelvis MRI, 604f, 605f

Coccyx
axial view
of female pelvis CT, 582f
of male pelvis CT, 567f, 568f
of male pelvis MRI, 598f
coronal view, of male pelvis MRI, 612f
sagittal view
of female pelvis CT, 587f
of female pelvis MRI, 620f
of male pelvis CT, 572f
of male pelvis MRI, 605f, 606f
Collateral ligs
accessory
axial view, of hand, 268f
coronal view, of hand, 281f
sagittal view, of hand, 270f
Colon
axial view, of abdomen CT, 329f, 330f, 331f
coronal view, of abdomen MRI, 362f, 363f, 364f, 365f, 366f, 367f
sagittal view
of abdomen CT, 332f, 337f
of abdomen MRI, 354f, 355f, 361f
Colon, ascending
axial view
of abdomen CT, 330f, 331f
of abdomen MRI, 353f
of female pelvis MRI, 614f
of male pelvis CT, 564f, 565f
of male pelvis MRI, 595f
coronal view
of abdomen CT, 340f, 341f
of abdomen MRI, 363f, 364f, 365f, 366f, 367f
of female pelvis CT, 588f, 590f, 591f
of female pelvis MRI, 623f
of male pelvis CT, 573f, 574f
of male pelvis MRI, 608f
sagittal view
of abdomen CT, 337f
of abdomen MRI, 361f
of female pelvis CT, 585f
of male pelvis MRI, 601f
Colon, descending
axial view
of abdomen CT, 330f, 331f
of abdomen MRI, 351f, 352f, 353f
of female pelvis MRI, 614f
of male pelvis CT, 564f, 565f
of male pelvis MRI, 595f, 596f
coronal view
of abdomen CT, 340f, 342f, 343f
of abdomen MRI, 364f, 365f, 366f, 367f
of female pelvis CT, 589f, 590f
of female pelvis MRI, 623f
of male pelvis CT, 573f, 574f, 575f
of male pelvis MRI, 608f
sagittal view
of abdomen CT, 332f
of abdomen MRI, 354f, 355f
of male pelvis CT, 570f
Colon, hepatic flexure
axial view
of abdomen CT, 329f, 330f
of abdomen MRI, 351f, 352f
coronal view
of abdomen CT, 339f, 340f, 341f
of abdomen MRI, 362f, 363f
of thorax CT, 47f
sagittal view
of abdomen CT, 337f
of abdomen MRI, 361f
of thorax CT, 46f
Colon, rectosigmoid
axial view, of female pelvis CT, 581f
coronal view
of female pelvis MRI, 625f
of male pelvis CT, 577f
sagittal view, of female pelvis MRI, 621f
Colon, sigmoid
axial view
of female pelvis CT, 580f, 581f, 582f
of female pelvis MRI, 614f
of male pelvis CT, 565f, 566f
of male pelvis MRI, 596f, 597f
coronal view

Colon, sigmoid *(Continued)*
of abdomen CT, 338f
of abdomen MRI, 364f
of female pelvis CT, 589f, 590f, 591f, 592f
of male pelvis CT, 574f, 575f, 576f, 578f
of male pelvis MRI, 608f, 609f, 610f, 611f
sagittal view
of abdomen CT, 333f, 334f
of female pelvis CT, 586f, 587f
of female pelvis MRI, 620f
of male pelvis CT, 570f, 571f
of male pelvis MRI, 603f, 604f, 605f, 606f
Colon, splenic flexure
axial view
of abdomen CT, 329f, 330f
of abdomen MRI, 348f, 349f, 350f
coronal view
of abdomen CT, 339f, 340f, 341f, 342f
of abdomen MRI, 363f, 364f
sagittal view, of abdomen MRI, 354f
Colon, transverse
axial view
of abdomen CT, 330f, 331f
of abdomen MRI, 350f, 351f, 352f, 353f
coronal view
of abdomen CT, 338f, 339f
of abdomen MRI, 362f, 363f
of male pelvis CT, 573f, 574f
sagittal view
of abdomen CT, 332f, 333f, 334f, 335f, 336f
of abdomen MRI, 355f, 356f, 357f, 358f, 359f, 360f, 361f
Confluence of sinuses, sagittal view, of brain CT, 10f
Confluence of sinuses, sagittal view, of brain MRI, 25f
Conjoined t.
of coracobrachialis m. and biceps m., short head, 71f, 104f
of semitendinosus m. and biceps femoris m., long head
axial view
of female pelvis MRI, 617f
of hip, 380f, 381f, 382f
of male pelvis MRI, 600f
coronal view, of thigh, 442f, 443f
sagittal view, of male pelvis MRI, 601f
Conus medullaris
coronal view, of thoracic spine, 302f
sagittal view
of lumbar spine, 316f
of thoracic spine, 301f
Coracoacromial lig.
axial view
of shoulder, 101f, 102f, 103f
of shoulder arthrogram, 132f, 133f
oblique sagittal view
of shoulder, 113f, 114f
of shoulder arthrogram, 137f, 138f, 139f
sagittal view, of pectoral girdle and chest wall, 80f, 81f
Coracobrachialis m.
axial view
of arm, 155f
of pectoral girdle and chest wall, 72f, 73f, 74f, 75f, 76f, 77f
of shoulder, 104f, 105f, 106f, 107f, 108f
and biceps m., short head, conjoined tendon of, 71f, 104f
coronal view
of arm, 169f, 170f
of pectoral girdle and chest wall, 89f, 90f, 91f, 92f, 93f
oblique coronal view, of shoulder, 120f, 121f, 122f, 123f, 124f, 125f
oblique sagittal view
of shoulder, 113f, 114f, 115f
of shoulder arthrogram, 139f
origin, insertion, and nerve supply of, 177t
sagittal view
of arm, 165f, 166f, 167f
of pectoral girdle and chest wall, 80f, 81f
Coracobrachialis t.
ABER view, of shoulder arthrogram, 148f
axial view

Coracobrachialis t. *(Continued)*
　of pectoral girdle and chest wall, 71*f*
　of shoulder, 105*f*, 106*f*, 107*f*
　of shoulder arthrogram, 134*f*, 135*f*
　oblique coronal view
　　of shoulder, 120*f*
　　of shoulder arthrogram, 142*f*, 143*f*
　oblique sagittal view, of shoulder arthrogram,
　　138*f*
Coracoclavicular lig.
　axial view, of shoulder, 102*f*
　conoid portion
　　axial view, of shoulder, 101*f*, 102*f*
　　oblique coronal view, of shoulder, 119*f*, 120*f*
　　oblique sagittal view, of shoulder, 117*f*, 118*f*
　trapezoid portion
　　axial view, of shoulder, 101*f*, 102*f*
　　oblique coronal view, of shoulder, 120*f*
　　oblique sagittal view
　　　of shoulder, 116*f*, 117*f*
　　　of shoulder arthrogram, 140*f*, 141*f*
Coracohumeral lig.
　axial view
　　of shoulder, 102*f*
　　of shoulder arthrogram, 132*f*
　oblique coronal view
　　of shoulder, 120*f*, 121*f*, 122*f*
　　of shoulder arthrogram, 142*f*
　oblique sagittal view
　　of shoulder, 111*f*, 112*f*, 113*f*, 114*f*, 115*f*
　　of shoulder arthrogram, 138*f*
　sagittal view, of pectoral girdle and chest wall,
　　81*f*
Coracoid process
　ABER view, of shoulder arthrogram, 148*f*
　axial view
　　of pectoral girdle and chest wall, 71*f*
　　of shoulder, 102*f*, 103*f*, 104*f*
　　of shoulder arthrogram, 131*f*, 132*f*, 133*f*, 134*f*
　base
　　oblique coronal view, of shoulder
　　　arthrogram, 142*f*
　　oblique sagittal view, of shoulder, 116*f*
　coronal view, of pectoral girdle and chest wall,
　　89*f*, 90*f*, 91*f*
　oblique coronal view
　　of shoulder, 120*f*, 121*f*
　　of shoulder arthrogram, 142*f*
　oblique sagittal view
　　of shoulder, 113*f*, 114*f*, 115*f*
　　of shoulder arthrogram, 139*f*, 140*f*, 141*f*
　sagittal view, of pectoral girdle and chest wall,
　　81*f*
　tip, oblique sagittal view, of shoulder
　　arthrogram, 138*f*
Corona radiata
　axial view
　　of brain CT, 5*f*
　　of brain MRI, 20*f*
　coronal view, of brain CT, 14*f*, 15*f*, 16*f*
　sagittal view
　　of brain CT, 11*f*
　　of brain MRI, 26*f*, 29*f*, 30*f*, 31*f*
Coronary a., axial view
　of heart MRI, 56*f*, 57*f*
　of thorax CT, 39*f*, 42*f*
Coronary sinus, axial view, of heart MRI, 57*f*
Coronoid fossa
　axial view, of elbow, 180*f*, 181*f*
　oblique coronal, of elbow, 204*f*
　oblique sagittal view, of elbow, 195*f*
　sagittal view
　　of arm, 164*f*, 165*f*
　　of elbow, 195*f*
Coronoid process
　axial view, of elbow, 184*f*
　oblique coronal, of elbow, 203*f*, 204*f*
　oblique sagittal view, of elbow, 195*f*, 196*f*
　sagittal view
　　of arm, 163*f*, 164*f*
　　of elbow, 195*f*, 196*f*
Corpus cavernosum
　axial view
　　of male pelvis CT, 569*f*
　　of male pelvis MRI, 600*f*

Corpus cavernosum *(Continued)*
　coronal view
　　of male pelvis CT, 573*f*, 576*f*
　　of male pelvis MRI, 607*f*, 608*f*
　sagittal view
　　of male pelvis CT, 571*f*, 572*f*
　　of male pelvis MRI, 604*f*, 605*f*
Corpus spongiosum
　axial view
　　of male pelvis CT, 569*f*
　　of male pelvis MRI, 600*f*
　coronal view
　　of male pelvis CT, 573*f*, 576*f*
　　of male pelvis MRI, 607*f*, 608*f*, 609*f*
　sagittal view, of male pelvis MRI, 606*f*
Costal cartilage
　axial view
　　of abdomen CT, 326*f*
　　of abdomen MRI, 346*f*
　coronal view
　　of abdomen CT, 338*f*
　　of abdomen MRI, 362*f*
　　of pectoral girdle and chest wall, 88*f*
　sagittal view
　　of abdomen CT, 332*f*
　　of pectoral girdle and chest wall, 85*f*, 86*f*, 87*f*
Costochondral cartilage
　axial view, of pectoral girdle and chest wall, 73*f*
　coronal view, of heart MRI, 61*f*
Costoclavicular lig., coronal view, of pectoral
　　girdle and chest wall, 89*f*
Costotransverse foramen, axial view, of thoracic
　　spine, 297*f*, 298*f*
Costotransverse joint
　axial view
　　of pectoral girdle and chest wall, 70*f*
　　of thoracic spine, 297*f*, 298*f*
　coronal view
　　of pectoral girdle and chest wall, 95*f*, 96*f*
　　of thoracic spine, 303*f*
　sagittal view, of thoracic spine, 299*f*, 300*f*
Costovertebral joint
　axial view
　　of pectoral girdle and chest wall, 70*f*, 72*f*, 77*f*
　　of thoracic spine, 297*f*
　coronal view
　　of pectoral girdle and chest wall, 96*f*
　　of thoracic spine, 302*f*
　sagittal view, of thoracic spine, 300*f*
Cotyloid notch, 413*f*
Cruciate lig., anterior
　axial view, of knee, 450*f*
　coronal view
　　of knee, 468*f*
　　of leg, 493*f*
　sagittal view, of knee, 457*f*, 458*f*
Cruciate lig., posterior
　axial view, of knee, 450*f*, 451*f*
　coronal view
　　of knee, 467*f*, 468*f*, 469*f*
　　of leg, 493*f*, 494*f*
　sagittal view
　　of knee, 458*f*, 459*f*
　　of leg, 488*f*
Crural fascia, axial view, of leg, 474*f*, 475*f*, 476*f*,
　　477*f*, 478*f*, 479*f*, 480*f*, 482*f*
Crural septum
　anterior, axial view, of leg, 476*f*, 477*f*
　posterior, axial view, of leg, 479*f*, 480*f*, 481*f*
Cubital tunnel retinaculum, axial view, of elbow,
　　180*f*, 181*f*
Cubital v., median
　axial view, of elbow, 179*f*, 180*f*, 181*f*, 182*f*
　oblique coronal, of elbow, 199*f*, 200*f*, 201*f*, 202*f*
　oblique sagittal view, of elbow, 195*f*, 196*f*
　sagittal view
　　of elbow, 195*f*, 196*f*
　　of forearm, 219*f*
Cuboid
　axial view, of ankle, 507*f*, 508*f*, 509*f*
　coronal view, of ankle, 524*f*, 525*f*
　oblique axial view, of ankle, 515*f*, 516*f*
　sagittal view, of ankle, 518*f*, 519*f*, 520*f*, 521*f*
Cuboid sulcus, sagittal view, of ankle, 519*f*
Cuneiform joint, sagittal view, of ankle, 522*f*

Cuneiform, lateral
　axial view, of ankle, 506*f*, 507*f*
　oblique axial view, of ankle, 515*f*, 516*f*
　sagittal view, of ankle, 520*f*, 521*f*
Cuneiform, medial
　axial view, of ankle, 506*f*, 507*f*
　oblique axial view, of ankle, 515*f*, 516*f*
　sagittal view, of ankle, 522*f*, 523*f*
Cuneiform, middle
　axial view, of ankle, 506*f*, 507*f*
　oblique axial view, of ankle, 515*f*, 516*f*
　sagittal view, of ankle, 521*f*, 522*f*
Cuneocuboid lig.
　plantar, axial view, of ankle, 508*f*
　sagittal view, of ankle, 520*f*
Cystic duct, axial view, of abdomen MRI, 349*f*

D
Deltoid lig.
　axial view, of ankle, 504*f*, 505*f*, 506*f*
　coronal view, of ankle, 526*f*, 527*f*, 528*f*
　oblique axial view, of ankle, 513*f*
　sagittal view, of ankle, 523*f*
Deltoid m.
　anterior
　　axial view, of pectoral girdle and chest wall,
　　　70*f*, 71*f*, 72*f*
　　coronal view, of pectoral girdle and chest
　　　wall, 88*f*
　axial view
　　of arm, 155*f*
　　of pectoral girdle and chest wall, 70*f*, 71*f*,
　　　72*f*, 73*f*, 74*f*, 75*f*, 76*f*, 77*f*
　　of shoulder, 100*f*, 101*f*, 102*f*, 103*f*, 104*f*, 105*f*,
　　　106*f*, 107*f*, 108*f*
　　of shoulder arthrogram, 131*f*, 132*f*, 133*f*, 134*f*
　coronal view
　　of arm, 168*f*, 169*f*, 171*f*, 172*f*, 173*f*, 174*f*,
　　　175*f*, 176*f*
　　of pectoral girdle and chest wall, 89*f*, 90*f*,
　　　91*f*, 92*f*, 93*f*, 94*f*, 95*f*, 96*f*, 97*f*
　　of thoracic spine, 304*f*
　middle, axial view, of pectoral girdle and chest
　　wall, 70*f*
　oblique coronal view
　　of shoulder, 119*f*, 120*f*, 121*f*, 122*f*, 123*f*, 124*f*,
　　　125*f*, 126*f*, 127*f*, 128*f*
　　of shoulder arthrogram, 143*f*, 144*f*, 145*f*, 146*f*
　oblique sagittal view
　　of shoulder, 109*f*, 110*f*, 111*f*, 112*f*, 113*f*, 114*f*,
　　　115*f*, 116*f*, 117*f*, 118*f*
　　of shoulder arthrogram, 136*f*, 137*f*, 138*f*, 139*f*
　origin, insertion, and nerve supply of, 129*t*,
　　306*t*–308*t*
　posterior, axial view, of pectoral girdle and
　　chest wall, 70*f*, 71*f*
　sagittal view
　　of arm, 161*f*, 162*f*, 163*f*, 164*f*, 165*f*, 166*f*, 167*f*
　　of pectoral girdle and chest wall, 78*f*, 79*f*,
　　　80*f*, 81*f*, 82*f*
Deltoid t.
　coronal view, of arm, 173*f*, 174*f*
　oblique coronal view, of shoulder, 125*f*
Deltoid tuberosity
　axial view, of arm, 155*f*
　coronal view, of arm, 172*f*
　sagittal view, of pectoral girdle and chest wall,
　　78*f*, 79*f*
Deltopectoral triangle
　axial view, of shoulder, 105*f*, 106*f*, 107*f*, 108*f*
　oblique sagittal view, of shoulder, 113*f*
Diaphragm
　axial view
　　of abdomen MRI, 346*f*, 348*f*, 349*f*, 350*f*, 351*f*,
　　　352*f*
　　of thorax CT, 42*f*
　coronal view
　　of abdomen CT, 338*f*, 340*f*
　　of abdomen MRI, 365*f*, 366*f*, 367*f*
　sagittal view
　　of abdomen CT, 332*f*, 334*f*, 335*f*, 336*f*
　　of thorax CT, 43*f*, 46*f*
　urogenital
　　coronal view, of female pelvis CT, 592*f*

Diaphragm *(Continued)*
  sagittal view, of male pelvis CT, 571*f*
Diaphragm, crus
  axial view
    of abdomen CT, 327*f*, 328*f*, 329*f*
    of abdomen MRI, 346*f*, 347*f*
  coronal view
    of abdomen CT, 341*f*, 342*f*, 343*f*
    of abdomen MRI, 368*f*
    of lumbar spine, 318*f*, 319*f*, 320*f*
    of thoracic spine, 302*f*
  sagittal view, of abdomen CT, 334*f*, 335*f*, 336*f*
Digital a., palmar
  axial view, of hand, 265*f*, 268*f*
  coronal view, of hand, 280*f*, 281*f*
  sagittal view
    of hand, 275*f*
    of wrist, 246*f*, 247*f*
Digital n., palmar, axial view, of hand, 268*f*
Digital neurovascular structures, axial view, of
    hand, 268*f*
Digital v.
  dorsal, axial view, of hand, 268*f*
  palmar, axial view, of hand, 268*f*
Distal phalanx
  index finger, sagittal view, 269*f*, 272*f*, 273*f*
  long finger, sagittal view, 273*f*, 274*f*
  ring finger, sagittal view, 275*f*, 276*f*
  small finger, sagittal view, 278*f*
  thumb
    coronal view, 281*f*
    sagittal view, 269*f*
Dorsal nerve root ganglion, sagittal view, of
    thoracic spine, 300*f*, 301*f*
Dorsal ramus n. and vessels, coronal view, of
    lumbar spine, 319*f*, 321*f*
Dorsum sellae, axial view, of brain CT, 7*f*
Duodenal bulb
  axial view
    of abdomen CT, 329*f*
    of abdomen MRI, 350*f*
  coronal view
    of abdomen CT, 338*f*
    of abdomen MRI, 364*f*, 365*f*
  sagittal view, of abdomen MRI, 360*f*
Duodenojejunal junction, axial view, of abdomen
    MRI, 353*f*
Duodenum
  axial view, of abdomen CT, 328*f*
  sagittal view, of thorax CT, 45*f*
Duodenum, second portion
  axial view
    of abdomen CT, 329*f*, 330*f*
    of abdomen MRI, 350*f*, 351*f*, 352*f*, 353*f*
  coronal view
    of abdomen CT, 340*f*, 341*f*
    of abdomen MRI, 365*f*, 366*f*
    of thorax CT, 47*f*
  sagittal view
    of abdomen CT, 336*f*
    of abdomen MRI, 361*f*
Duodenum, third portion
  axial view
    of abdomen CT, 330*f*
    of abdomen MRI, 352*f*, 353*f*, 357*f*, 358*f*, 359*f*,
      360*f*
  coronal view, of abdomen CT, 340*f*
  sagittal view
    of abdomen CT, 333*f*, 334*f*, 335*f*
Dura mater, coronal view, of thoracic spine, 302*f*

E

Endocervical canal
  axial view, of female pelvis MRI, 616*f*
  coronal view, of female pelvis MRI, 624*f*, 625*f*
  sagittal view, of female pelvis MRI, 621*f*
Endometrial canal
  axial view, of female pelvis MRI, 615*f*
  coronal view, of female pelvis MRI, 623*f*, 624*f*
  sagittal view, of female pelvis MRI, 621*f*
Epicondyle, lateral
  axial view, of elbow, 180*f*, 181*f*, 182*f*
  coronal view
    of arm, 170*f*, 171*f*

Epicondyle, lateral *(Continued)*
  of elbow, 204*f*, 205*f*, 206*f*
  oblique coronal, of elbow, 204*f*, 205*f*, 206*f*
  oblique sagittal view, of elbow, 191*f*
Epicondyle, medial
  axial view, of elbow, 180*f*, 181*f*, 182*f*
  coronal view
    of arm, 169*f*, 170*f*
    of elbow, 204*f*, 205*f*
  oblique coronal, of elbow, 204*f*, 205*f*
  oblique sagittal view, of elbow, 197*f*, 198*f*
  sagittal view
    of arm, 166*f*, 167*f*
    of elbow, 197*f*, 198*f*
Epidural fat
  axial view, of cervical spine MRI, 290*f*
  coronal view
    of lumbar spine, 320*f*, 321*f*
    of thoracic spine, 302*f*
  sagittal view
    of cervical spine MRI, 293*f*
    of thoracic spine, 300*f*, 301*f*
Epidural space, posterior, sagittal view, of thoracic
    spine, 301*f*
Epidural v., axial view, of lumbar spine, 310*f*, 311*f*
Epidural vessels
  coronal view, of lumbar spine, 319*f*
  sagittal view, of thoracic spine, 301*f*
Epigastric a., inferior
  axial view
    of female pelvis CT, 580*f*, 581*f*
    of male pelvis CT, 566*f*
  coronal view
    of abdomen CT, 338*f*
    of female pelvis CT, 588*f*
    of male pelvis CT, 573*f*
  sagittal view, of male pelvis CT, 570*f*
Epigastric v., inferior
  axial view
    of female pelvis CT, 580*f*, 581*f*
    of male pelvis CT, 566*f*
  coronal view
    of abdomen CT, 338*f*
    of female pelvis CT, 588*f*
    of male pelvis CT, 573*f*
  sagittal view, of male pelvis CT, 570*f*
Epigastric vessels, inferior
  axial view
    of female pelvis CT, 582*f*
    of male pelvis MRI, 596*f*, 597*f*
  coronal view, of male pelvis MRI, 607*f*
  sagittal view, of abdomen CT, 336*f*
Epitrochlear lymph node, oblique coronal, of
    elbow, 203*f*
Erector spinae m.
  axial view
    of abdomen MRI, 347*f*, 349*f*, 350*f*, 351*f*, 352*f*,
      353*f*
    of male pelvis CT, 565*f*
    of male pelvis MRI, 595*f*, 596*f*
    of pectoral girdle and chest wall, 72*f*, 74*f*,
      75*f*, 76*f*, 77*f*
    of thoracic spine, 297*f*, 298*f*
  coronal view
    of female pelvis MRI, 625*f*, 626*f*
    of male pelvis MRI, 611*f*, 612*f*
    of pectoral girdle and chest wall, 96*f*, 97*f*
    of thoracic spine, 304*f*
  sagittal view
    of abdomen MRI, 355*f*, 357*f*, 359*f*, 360*f*
    of female pelvis MRI, 618*f*, 619*f*
    of male pelvis CT, 572*f*
    of male pelvis MRI, 602*f*, 603*f*, 604*f*, 605*f*,
      606*f*
    of pectoral girdle and chest wall, 87*f*
    of thoracic spine, 299*f*, 300*f*
Esophagus
  axial view
    of abdomen CT, 326*f*
    of abdomen MRI, 346*f*
    of cervical spine MRI, 290*f*
    of heart MRI, 54*f*, 55*f*, 56*f*, 57*f*
    of pectoral girdle and chest wall, 69*f*
    of thoracic spine, 298*f*
    of thorax CT, 36*f*, 37*f*, 39*f*, 40*f*, 41*f*, 42*f*

Esophagus *(Continued)*
  coronal view
    of abdomen MRI, 367*f*
    of thorax CT, 49*f*, 50*f*
  sagittal view
    of abdomen CT, 334*f*
    of abdomen MRI, 357*f*
    of thoracic spine, 300*f*, 301*f*
    of thorax CT, 44*f*, 45*f*
Ethmoid air cells
  axial view
    of brain CT, 8*f*
    of brain MRI, 22*f*, 23*f*
  coronal view, of brain CT, 13*f*
  sagittal view
    of brain CT, 10*f*
    of brain MRI, 25*f*
Extensor carpi radialis brevis m.
  axial view
    of elbow, 180*f*, 181*f*, 182*f*, 183*f*, 184*f*, 185*f*,
      186*f*, 187*f*, 188*f*, 189*f*
    of forearm, 209*f*, 210*f*, 211*f*, 212*f*, 213*f*, 214*f*
  coronal view
    of elbow, 201*f*, 202*f*, 203*f*, 204*f*
    of forearm, 229*f*, 230*f*, 231*f*, 232*f*
  oblique coronal, of elbow, 201*f*, 202*f*, 203*f*, 204*f*
  oblique sagittal view, of elbow, 190*f*, 191*f*,
    192*f*, 193*f*
  origin, insertion, and nerve supply of, 233*t*–234*t*
  sagittal view
    of elbow, 190*f*, 191*f*, 192*f*, 193*f*
    of forearm, 219*f*, 220*f*, 221*f*
Extensor carpi radialis brevis t.
  axial view
    of forearm, 214*f*, 215*f*, 216*f*, 217*f*
    of hand, 262*f*
  coronal view, of hand, 282*f*
Extensor carpi radialis longus m.
  axial view
    of arm, 158*f*, 159*f*, 160*f*
    of elbow, 179*f*, 180*f*, 181*f*, 182*f*, 183*f*, 184*f*,
      185*f*, 186*f*, 187*f*, 188*f*, 189*f*
    of forearm, 209*f*, 210*f*, 211*f*, 212*f*, 213*f*
  coronal view
    of arm, 171*f*
    of elbow, 199*f*, 200*f*, 201*f*, 202*f*, 203*f*, 204*f*,
      205*f*, 206*f*
    of forearm, 230*f*, 231*f*, 232*f*
  oblique coronal, of elbow, 199*f*, 200*f*, 201*f*,
    202*f*, 203*f*, 204*f*, 205*f*, 206*f*
  oblique sagittal view, of elbow, 190*f*, 191*f*,
    192*f*, 193*f*
  origin, insertion, and nerve supply of, 233*t*–234*t*
  sagittal view
    of arm, 161*f*
    of elbow, 190*f*, 191*f*, 192*f*, 193*f*
    of forearm, 219*f*, 220*f*
Extensor carpi radialis longus t
  axial view
    of forearm, 213*f*, 214*f*, 215*f*, 216*f*, 217*f*
    of hand, 262*f*
  coronal view
    of forearm, 230*f*
    of hand, 282*f*
  sagittal view, of forearm, 220*f*
Extensor carpi ulnaris m.
  axial view
    of elbow, 185*f*, 186*f*, 187*f*, 188*f*, 189*f*
    of forearm, 209*f*, 210*f*, 211*f*, 212*f*, 214*f*, 215*f*,
      216*f*, 217*f*, 218*f*, 219*f*
  coronal view
    of elbow, 204*f*, 205*f*, 206*f*
    of forearm, 229*f*, 230*f*, 231*f*, 232*f*
  oblique coronal view, of elbow, 204*f*, 205*f*, 206*f*
  oblique sagittal view, of elbow, 192*f*, 193*f*
  origin, insertion, and nerve supply of, 233*t*–234*t*
  sagittal view
    of elbow, 192*f*, 193*f*
    of forearm, 223*f*, 224*f*
Extensor carpi ulnaris t.
  axial view
    of elbow, 183*f*
    of forearm, 217*f*, 218*f*
  coronal view
    of elbow, 204*f*

Extensor carpi ulnaris t. *(Continued)*
  of forearm, 227*f*, 228*f*, 229*f*
  of hand, 281*f*, 282*f*
  oblique coronal, of elbow, 204*f*
  sagittal view, of hand, 276*f*
Extensor digiti minimi m.
  axial view
    of elbow, 187*f*, 188*f*, 189*f*
    of forearm, 209*f*, 210*f*, 211*f*, 212*f*, 213*f*, 214*f*
  coronal view, of forearm, 231*f*
  oblique sagittal view, of elbow, 192*f*
  origin, insertion, and nerve supply of, 233*t*–234*t*
Extensor digiti minimi t.
  axial view
    of elbow, 185*f*, 186*f*
    of forearm, 214*f*, 215*f*, 216*f*, 217*f*, 218*f*
    of hand, 262*f*, 263*f*, 264*f*, 265*f*, 266*f*, 267*f*
  coronal view
    of elbow, 204*f*
    of hand, 282*f*
  oblique coronal, of elbow, 204*f*
  oblique sagittal view, of elbow, 191*f*
  sagittal view
    of elbow, 191*f*
    of forearm, 222*f*, 223*f*
    of hand, 276*f*, 277*f*
Extensor digitorum brevis m.
  axial view, of ankle, 505*f*, 506*f*, 507*f*, 508*f*
  coronal view, of ankle, 524*f*, 525*f*, 526*f*
  oblique axial view, of ankle, 514*f*, 515*f*, 516*f*
  sagittal view, of ankle, 518*f*, 519*f*, 520*f*
Extensor digitorum longus m.
  axial view
    of ankle, 501*f*, 502*f*, 503*f*
    of knee, 452*f*, 453*f*
    of leg, 474*f*, 475*f*, 476*f*, 477*f*, 478*f*, 479*f*, 480*f*,
      481*f*, 482*f*, 483*f*
  coronal view
    of ankle, 525*f*, 526*f*, 527*f*, 528*f*
    of knee, 467*f*, 468*f*, 469*f*, 470*f*
    of leg, 492*f*, 493*f*
  oblique axial view, of ankle, 511*f*, 512*f*
  origin, insertion, and nerve supply of, 498*t*–499*t*
  sagittal view
    of ankle, 518*f*, 519*f*
    of knee, 455*f*
    of leg, 484*f*, 485*f*, 486*f*
Extensor digitorum longus t.
  axial view
    of ankle, 501*f*, 502*f*, 503*f*, 504*f*, 505*f*
    of leg, 476*f*, 477*f*, 478*f*, 479*f*, 480*f*, 481*f*, 482*f*,
      483*f*
  coronal view
    of ankle, 524*f*, 525*f*
    of leg, 492*f*
  oblique axial view, of ankle, 511*f*, 512*f*, 513*f*,
    514*f*, 515*f*, 516*f*
  sagittal view
    of ankle, 519*f*, 520*f*
    of leg, 484*f*, 485*f*, 486*f*
Extensor digitorum m.
  axial view
    of elbow, 184*f*, 185*f*, 186*f*, 187*f*, 188*f*, 189*f*
    of forearm, 209*f*, 210*f*, 211*f*, 212*f*, 213*f*, 214*f*,
      215*f*, 216*f*
  coronal view
    of elbow, 202*f*, 203*f*, 204*f*
    of forearm, 230*f*, 231*f*, 232*f*
  oblique coronal, of elbow, 202*f*, 203*f*, 204*f*
  oblique sagittal view, of elbow, 190*f*, 191*f*, 192*f*
  origin, insertion, and nerve supply of, 233*t*–234*t*
  sagittal view
    of elbow, 190*f*, 191*f*, 192*f*
    of forearm, 221*f*, 222*f*, 223*f*, 224*f*
Extensor digitorum t.
  axial view
    of elbow, 183*f*, 184*f*
    of forearm, 214*f*, 215*f*, 216*f*, 217*f*, 218*f*
    of hand, 262*f*, 263*f*, 264*f*, 265*f*, 266*f*, 267*f*,
      268*f*
  coronal view, of hand, 282*f*, 283*f*
  sagittal view
    of hand, 272*f*, 273*f*, 274*f*, 275*f*, 276*f*, 277*f*
Extensor expansion (hood)
  axial view, of hand, 267*f*, 268*f*

Extensor expansion (hood) *(Continued)*
  coronal view, of hand, 281*f*, 282*f*, 283*f*
  sagittal view, of hand, 269*f*, 270*f*, 277*f*
Extensor hallucis brevis m., oblique axial view, of
  ankle, 516*f*
Extensor hallucis longus m.
  axial view
    of ankle, 501*f*, 502*f*, 503*f*
    of leg, 481*f*, 482*f*, 483*f*
  coronal view
    of ankle, 524*f*, 525*f*
    of leg, 492*f*, 493*f*
  oblique axial view, of ankle, 511*f*, 512*f*, 513*f*,
    514*f*
  origin, insertion, and nerve supply of, 498*t*–499*t*
  sagittal view, of ankle, 519*f*
Extensor hallucis longus t.
  axial view
    of ankle, 501*f*, 502*f*, 503*f*, 504*f*
    of leg, 481*f*, 482*f*, 483*f*
  coronal view
    of ankle, 524*f*, 525*f*
    of leg, 492*f*, 493*f*
  oblique axial view, of ankle, 511*f*, 512*f*, 513*f*,
    514*f*, 515*f*, 516*f*
  sagittal view, of ankle, 520*f*, 521*f*
Extensor indicis m.
  axial view, of forearm, 216*f*, 217*f*, 218*f*
  coronal view, of forearm, 228*f*, 229*f*
  origin, insertion, and nerve supply of, 233*t*–234*t*
  sagittal view, of forearm, 223*f*
Extensor indicis t.
  axial view
    of forearm, 218*f*
    of hand, 262*f*, 263*f*, 264*f*, 265*f*, 266*f*, 267*f*,
      268*f*
  sagittal view, of forearm, 223*f*
Extensor pollicis brevis m.
  axial view of forearm, 214*f*, 215*f*, 216*f*, 217*f*,
    218*f*
  coronal view, of forearm, 229*f*
  origin, insertion, and nerve supply of, 233*t*–234*t*
  sagittal view, of forearm, 221*f*, 222*f*
Extensor pollicis brevis t.
  axial view
    of forearm, 217*f*, 218*f*
    of hand, 262*f*, 263*f*, 264*f*
  coronal view, of hand, 279*f*, 280*f*, 281*f*
  sagittal view, of forearm, 221*f*
Extensor pollicis longus m.
  axial view, of forearm, 210*f*, 211*f*, 212*f*, 213*f*,
    214*f*, 215*f*, 216*f*, 217*f*
  coronal view, of forearm, 229*f*, 230*f*
  origin, insertion, and nerve supply of, 233*t*–234*t*
  sagittal view, of forearm, 222*f*, 223*f*
Extensor pollicis longus t.
  axial view
    of forearm, 218*f*
    of hand, 262*f*, 263*f*, 264*f*, 265*f*, 266*f*
  coronal view
    of forearm, 229*f*
    of hand, 281*f*, 282*f*
Extensor retinaculum
  axial view, of ankle, 501*f*, 502*f*
  oblique axial view, of ankle, 511*f*, 514*f*, 515*f*
Extensor t., common
  axial view, of elbow, 182*f*
  oblique coronal, of elbow, 204*f*, 205*f*
External capsule
  axial view, of brain MRI, 21*f*
  sagittal view, of brain MRI, 29*f*
External capsule, coronal view, of brain CT, 15*f*

F

Facet joint
  axial view, of lumbar spine, 310*f*
  sagittal view, of thoracic spine, 300*f*, 301*f*
Falciform lig.
  axial view, of abdomen CT, 328*f*
  coronal view, of abdomen CT, 338*f*
  sagittal view, of abdomen CT, 336*f*
Falx cerebri
  axial view, of brain CT, 4*f*, 5*f*, 6*f*
  coronal view, of brain CT, 13*f*, 14*f*

Fat pad, anterior
  axial view, of elbow, 180*f*
  oblique sagittal view, of elbow, 194*f*, 195*f*
  sagittal view
    of arm, 164*f*, 165*f*
    of elbow, 194*f*, 195*f*
Fat pad, infrapatellar
  axial view, of knee, 450*f*, 451*f*, 452*f*
  coronal view
    of knee, 463*f*, 464*f*
    of leg, 492*f*
  sagittal view
    of knee, 456*f*, 457*f*, 458*f*, 459*f*
    of leg, 486*f*, 487*f*, 488*f*
Fat pad, posterior
  axial view, of elbow, 194*f*, 195*f*
  oblique sagittal view, of elbow, 193*f*, 194*f*, 195*f*
  sagittal view
    of arm, 164*f*, 165*f*
    of elbow, 193*f*, 194*f*, 195*f*
Femoral a.
  axial view
    of hip, 379*f*, 380*f*
    of hip arthrogram, 403*f*, 404*f*, 406*f*, 408*f*
  coronal view
    of female pelvis MRI, 622*f*
    of male pelvis CT, 573*f*
    of thigh, 438*f*, 441*f*
  sagittal view, of thigh, 434*f*
Femoral a., common
  axial view
    of female pelvis CT, 582*f*, 583*f*
    of hip, 376*f*, 377*f*
    of male pelvis CT, 567*f*, 568*f*
    of male pelvis MRI, 598*f*, 599*f*
  coronal view
    of female pelvis CT, 588*f*
    of hip, 393*f*, 394*f*
    of male pelvis MRI, 607*f*
  sagittal view
    of female pelvis CT, 585*f*
    of hip, 390*f*
    of male pelvis CT, 570*f*
Femoral a., deep
  axial view
    of female pelvis CT, 583*f*, 584*f*
    of hip, 378*f*
    of male pelvis CT, 569*f*
    of thigh, 420*f*, 421*f*, 422*f*, 423*f*
  coronal view
    of female pelvis CT, 589*f*
    of hip, 394*f*
    of male pelvis CT, 574*f*
  sagittal view
    of hip, 385*f*
    of male pelvis CT, 570*f*
    of thigh, 430*f*
Femoral a., superficial
  axial view
    of female pelvis CT, 583*f*, 584*f*
    of hip, 378*f*
    of male pelvis CT, 569*f*
    of male pelvis MRI, 599*f*, 600*f*
    of thigh, 420*f*, 421*f*, 422*f*, 423*f*, 424*f*, 425*f*,
      426*f*
  coronal view, of thigh, 440*f*
  sagittal view, of male pelvis CT, 570*f*
Femoral circumflex a.
  lateral
    axial view, of male pelvis CT, 569*f*
    coronal view, of male pelvis CT, 575*f*
  medial
    axial view, of male pelvis CT, 569*f*
    coronal view, of male pelvis CT, 575*f*
    sagittal view, of male pelvis CT, 570*f*
Femoral circumflex v.
  lateral, coronal view, of male pelvis CT, 575*f*
  medial, coronal view, of male pelvis CT, 575*f*,
    576*f*
Femoral circumflex vessels
  lateral
    axial view, of hip, 378*f*, 380*f*
    coronal view, of male pelvis MRI, 608*f*
    sagittal view, of hip, 384*f*, 385*f*, 386*f*
  medial

Femoral circumflex vessels *(Continued)*
  axial view, of hip, 378*f*, 380*f*
  coronal view, of male pelvis MRI, 608*f*
  sagittal view, of hip, 387*f*, 389*f*, 390*f*
Femoral condyle
  lateral
    axial view, of knee, 449*f*, 450*f*
    coronal view, of knee, 463*f*, 464*f*, 465*f*, 466*f*,
      467*f*, 468*f*, 469*f*, 470*f*
    sagittal view, of knee, 454*f*, 455*f*, 456*f*
  medial
    axial view, of knee, 449*f*, 450*f*
    coronal view, of knee, 464*f*, 465*f*, 466*f*, 467*f*,
      468*f*, 469*f*, 470*f*
    sagittal view, of knee, 460*f*, 461*f*, 462*f*
Femoral cortex
  anterior, coronal view, of thigh, 438*f*
  medial, sagittal view, of thigh, 431*f*
  posterior, coronal view, of thigh, 440*f*
Femoral diaphysis
  axial view, of thigh, 420*f*
  coronal view, of hip, 395*f*
  sagittal view, of hip, 385*f*, 386*f*
Femoral head
  axial view
    of female pelvis CT, 582*f*
    of female pelvis MRI, 616*f*, 617*f*
    of hip, 376*f*, 377*f*, 378*f*
    of hip arthrogram, 403*f*
    of male pelvis CT, 567*f*
    of male pelvis MRI, 597*f*, 598*f*
  coronal view
    of female pelvis CT, 590*f*, 591*f*, 592*f*
    of female pelvis MRI, 623*f*, 624*f*
    of hip, 395*f*, 396*f*
    of hip arthrogram, 414*f*, 417*f*
    of male pelvis CT, 575*f*, 576*f*
    of male pelvis MRI, 608*f*, 609*f*, 610*f*
  sagittal view
    of hip, 387*f*, 389*f*, 390*f*
    of hip arthrogram, 409*f*, 410*f*, 411*f*, 412*f*,
      413*f*
    of male pelvis MRI, 601*f*
Femoral lig., head
  coronal view, of male pelvis MRI, 609*f*
  sagittal view, of male pelvis MRI, 601*f*
Femoral n.
  axial view, of hip, 377*f*
  coronal view
    of female pelvis MRI, 622*f*
    of male pelvis CT, 574*f*
Femoral neck
  axial view
    of female pelvis CT, 583*f*
    of hip, 378*f*, 379*f*
    of hip arthrogram, 406*f*, 407*f*
    of male pelvis MRI, 599*f*
  coronal view
    of female pelvis CT, 590*f*, 591*f*
    of female pelvis MRI, 624*f*
    of hip, 396*f*
    of hip arthrogram, 415*f*, 416*f*, 417*f*
    of male pelvis CT, 576*f*
  sagittal view
    of hip, 387*f*
    of hip arthrogram, 409*f*
    of thigh, 431*f*
Femoral shaft, axial view, of thigh, 421*f*
Femoral trochlea
  axial view, of knee, 449*f*, 450*f*
  coronal view, of knee, 463*f*
Femoral v.
  axial view
    of hip, 378*f*, 379*f*, 380*f*
    of hip arthrogram, 403*f*, 404*f*, 406*f*, 408*f*
    of male pelvis MRI, 599*f*, 600*f*
  coronal view
    of female pelvis MRI, 622*f*
    of male pelvis CT, 573*f*, 574*f*
    of thigh, 438*f*, 441*f*
  sagittal view, of thigh, 435*f*
Femoral v., common
  axial view
    of female pelvis CT, 582*f*, 583*f*
    of hip, 376*f*, 377*f*, 378*f*

Femoral v., common *(Continued)*
    of male pelvis CT, 567*f*, 568*f*
    of male pelvis MRI, 598*f*, 599*f*
  coronal view
    of female pelvis CT, 588*f*
    of hip, 393*f*, 394*f*
    of male pelvis MRI, 607*f*
Femoral v., deep
  axial view
    of female pelvis CT, 583*f*, 584*f*
    of thigh, 420*f*, 421*f*, 422*f*, 423*f*
  coronal view
    of female pelvis CT, 589*f*
    of male pelvis CT, 574*f*
  sagittal view, of hip, 385*f*
Femoral v., superficial
  axial view
    of female pelvis CT, 583*f*, 584*f*
    of hip, 380*f*
    of male pelvis MRI, 600*f*
    of thigh, 421*f*, 422*f*, 423*f*, 424*f*, 425*f*, 426*f*
  coronal view, of thigh, 439*f*
  sagittal view, of male pelvis CT, 570*f*
Femoral vessels
  axial view, of female pelvis MRI, 616*f*, 617*f*
  common, sagittal view, of male pelvis MRI, 601*f*
  coronal view
    of female pelvis MRI, 623*f*
    of thigh, 438*f*
  sagittal view
    of hip, 390*f*
    of hip arthrogram, 413*f*
    of male pelvis MRI, 601*f*
Femoral vessels, deep
  axial view, of hip, 382*f*
  coronal view
    of hip, 394*f*
    of thigh, 439*f*, 440*f*
  sagittal view
    of hip, 388*f*
    of thigh, 432*f*, 433*f*
Femoral vessels, superficial
  axial view, of hip, 381*f*, 382*f*
  coronal view
    of male pelvis MRI, 608*f*
    of thigh, 439*f*, 440*f*
  sagittal view
    of hip, 388*f*
    of thigh, 432*f*, 433*f*, 434*f*
Femur
  axial view
    of female pelvis CT, 583*f*, 584*f*
    of female pelvis MRI, 617*f*
    of hip, 379*f*, 381*f*, 382*f*
    of knee, 447*f*, 448*f*, 449*f*
    of male pelvis CT, 568*f*, 569*f*
    of male pelvis MRI, 599*f*, 600*f*
    of thigh, 420*f*, 422*f*, 423*f*, 424*f*, 425*f*, 426*f*,
      427*f*
  coronal view
    of female pelvis MRI, 624*f*
    of knee, 464*f*, 466*f*, 467*f*
    of leg, 492*f*, 493*f*
    of male pelvis CT, 577*f*
    of male pelvis MRI, 609*f*
    of thigh, 439*f*, 440*f*
  sagittal view
    of knee, 455*f*, 456*f*, 457*f*, 458*f*, 459*f*
    of thigh, 429*f*, 430*f*, 431*f*, 432*f*
Fibula
  axial view
    of ankle, 501*f*, 502*f*, 503*f*
    of knee, 453*f*
    of leg, 474*f*, 475*f*, 476*f*, 477*f*, 478*f*, 479*f*, 480*f*,
      481*f*, 482*f*, 483*f*
  coronal view
    of ankle, 528*f*, 529*f*, 530*f*
    of leg, 492*f*, 493*f*, 494*f*, 495*f*
  oblique axial view, of ankle, 511*f*, 512*f*, 513*f*
  sagittal view
    of ankle, 517*f*, 518*f*
    of knee, 456*f*
    of leg, 486*f*
Fibular (lateral) collateral lig.
  axial view, of knee, 450*f*, 451*f*, 452*f*

Fibular (lateral) collateral lig. *(Continued)*
  coronal view
    of knee, 469*f*, 470*f*
    of leg, 494*f*
  sagittal view, of knee, 454*f*
Fibular head
  axial view, of knee, 452*f*
  coronal view
    of knee, 470*f*, 471*f*, 472*f*
    of leg, 494*f*, 495*f*
  sagittal view
    of knee, 454*f*, 455*f*
    of leg, 484*f*, 485*f*, 486*f*
Fibular notch, axial view, of ankle, 502*f*, 503*f*
Fibular shaft, sagittal view, of leg, 485*f*
Finger, index
  distal phalanx, sagittal view, 272*f*
  middle phalanx, sagittal view, 271*f*
  proximal phalanx
    coronal view, 281*f*, 282*f*
    sagittal view, 271*f*, 272*f*, 273*f*
  sagittal view, 270*f*, 273*f*
Finger, long
  distal phalanx, sagittal view, 273*f*, 274*f*
  middle phalanx
    coronal view, 280*f*
    sagittal view, 273*f*, 274*f*, 275*f*
  proximal phalanx
    coronal view, 281*f*, 282*f*
    sagittal view, 273*f*, 274*f*, 275*f*
Finger, ring
  distal phalanx, sagittal view, 276*f*
  middle phalanx
    coronal view, 280*f*
    sagittal view, 276*f*
  proximal phalanx
    coronal view, 281*f*, 282*f*
    sagittal view, 275*f*, 276*f*
Finger, small
  distal phalanx, sagittal view, 278*f*
  middle phalanx
    coronal view, 280*f*, 281*f*
    sagittal view, 277*f*, 278*f*
  proximal phalanx
    coronal view, 280*f*, 281*f*
    sagittal view, 277*f*, 278*f*
First rib
  coronal view, of cervical spine MRI, 294*f*
  sagittal view, of cervical spine MRI, 292*f*
Flexor carpi radialis m.
  axial view
    of elbow, 183*f*, 184*f*, 185*f*, 186*f*, 187*f*, 188*f*,
      189*f*
    of forearm, 209*f*, 210*f*, 211*f*, 212*f*, 213*f*, 214*f*
  coronal view
    of elbow, 199*f*, 200*f*, 201*f*, 202*f*
    of forearm, 225*f*, 226*f*, 227*f*, 228*f*
  oblique coronal, of elbow, 199*f*, 200*f*, 201*f*, 202*f*
  oblique sagittal view, of elbow, 194*f*, 195*f*,
    196*f*, 197*f*
  origin, insertion, and nerve supply of, 233*t*–234*t*
  sagittal view
    of arm, 166*f*, 167*f*
    of elbow, 194*f*, 195*f*, 196*f*, 197*f*
    of forearm, 219*f*, 220*f*, 221*f*
Flexor carpi radialis t.
  axial view
    of forearm, 213*f*, 214*f*, 215*f*, 216*f*, 217*f*, 218*f*
  coronal view
    of forearm, 228*f*
    of hand, 279*f*
  sagittal view, of hand, 272*f*, 273*f*
Flexor carpi ulnaris m.
  axial view
    of elbow, 182*f*, 183*f*, 184*f*, 185*f*, 186*f*, 187*f*,
      188*f*, 189*f*
    of forearm, 209*f*, 210*f*, 211*f*, 212*f*, 213*f*, 214*f*,
      215*f*, 216*f*, 217*f*, 218*f*
  coronal view
    of elbow, 203*f*, 204*f*, 205*f*, 206*f*
    of forearm, 225*f*, 226*f*, 227*f*
    of hand, 279*f*
  oblique coronal, of elbow, 203*f*, 204*f*, 205*f*, 206*f*
  oblique sagittal view, of elbow, 196*f*, 197*f*, 198*f*
  origin, insertion, and nerve supply of, 233*t*–234*t*

Flexor carpi ulnaris m. *(Continued)*
  sagittal view
    of elbow, 196f, 197f, 198f
    of forearm, 223f, 224f
Flexor carpi ulnaris t.
  axial view, of forearm, 213f, 216f, 217f, 218f
  sagittal view
    of forearm, 221f, 222f
    of hand, 275f
Flexor digiti minimi brevis m.
  axial view
    of hand, 262f, 263f, 264f, 265f, 266f
    origin, insertion, and nerve supply of, 284t
  sagittal view, of hand, 275f, 276f
Flexor digiti minimi m.
  coronal view, of hand, 280f
  sagittal view, of hand, 275f, 276f, 277f
Flexor digitorum brevis m.
  axial view, of ankle, 510f
  coronal view, of ankle, 524f, 525f, 526f, 527f,
    528f, 529f, 530f
  oblique axial view, of ankle, 514f, 515f, 516f
  sagittal view, of ankle, 520f, 521f, 522f, 523f
Flexor digitorum longus m.
  axial view
    of ankle, 501f
    of leg, 476f, 477f, 479f, 480f, 481f, 482f, 483f
  coronal view, of leg, 493f, 494f
  origin, insertion, and nerve supply of, 498t–499t
  sagittal view, of leg, 488f
Flexor digitorum longus t.
  axial view
    of ankle, 501f, 502f, 503f, 504f, 505f, 506f,
      507f, 508f
    of leg, 476f, 477f, 479f, 480f, 481f, 482f, 483f
  coronal view
    of ankle, 524f, 525f, 526f, 527f, 528f, 529f
    of leg, 493f
  oblique axial view, of ankle, 512f, 513f, 514f,
    515f, 516f
  sagittal view
    of ankle, 522f, 523f
    of leg, 488f
Flexor digitorum profundus m.
  axial view
    of elbow, 183f, 184f, 185f, 186f, 187f, 188f,
      189f
    of forearm, 209f, 210f, 211f, 212f, 213f, 214f,
      215f, 216f, 217f, 218f
  coronal view
    of elbow, 202f, 203f, 204f, 205f, 206f, 207f
    of forearm, 225f, 226f, 227f, 228f, 229f
  oblique coronal, of elbow, 202f, 203f, 204f,
    205f, 206f, 207f
  oblique sagittal view, of elbow, 194f, 195f,
    196f, 197f
  origin, insertion, and nerve supply of, 233t–234t
  sagittal view
    of elbow, 194f, 195f, 196f, 197f
    of forearm, 220f, 221f, 222f, 223f, 224f
Flexor digitorum profundus t.
  axial view
    of forearm, 218f
    of hand, 262f, 263f, 264f, 265f, 266f, 267f,
      268f, 272f
  coronal view
    of forearm, 225f, 226f, 227f, 228f
    of hand, 280f
  sagittal view
    of forearm, 220f
    of hand, 272f, 273f, 274f, 275f, 276f, 277f
Flexor digitorum superficialis m.
  axial view
    of elbow, 182f, 183f, 184f, 185f, 186f, 187f,
      188f, 189f
    of forearm, 209f, 210f, 211f, 212f, 213f, 214f,
      215f, 216f, 217f, 218f
  coronal view
    of elbow, 200f, 201f, 202f, 203f, 204f, 205f
    of forearm, 225f, 226f, 227f, 228f, 229f
  oblique coronal, of elbow, 200f, 201f, 202f,
    203f, 204f, 205f
  oblique sagittal view, of elbow, 196f, 197f, 198f
  origin, insertion, and nerve supply of, 233t–234t
  sagittal view

Flexor digitorum superficialis m. *(Continued)*
    of elbow, 196f, 197f, 198f
    of forearm, 219f, 220f, 221f, 222f, 223f
Flexor digitorum superficialis t.
  axial view
    of forearm, 211f, 218f
    of hand, 262f, 263f, 264f, 265f, 266f, 267f,
      268f
  coronal view
    of forearm, 226f
    of hand, 279f, 280f
  sagittal view, of hand, 265f, 272f, 273f, 274f,
    275f, 276f, 277f, 278f
Flexor hallucis longus fascia
  axial view, of ankle, 505f
  oblique axial view, of ankle, 512f
Flexor hallucis longus m.
  axial view
    of ankle, 501f, 502f, 503f, 504f, 505f
    of leg, 475f, 476f, 477f, 478f, 479f, 480f, 481f,
      482f, 483f
  coronal view
    of ankle, 530f, 531f
    of leg, 494f, 495f
  oblique axial view, of ankle, 511f
  origin, insertion, and nerve supply of, 498t–499t
  sagittal view
    of ankle, 518f, 519f, 520f
    of leg, 486f, 487f, 488f
Flexor hallucis longus t.
  axial view
    of ankle, 501f, 502f, 503f, 504f, 505f, 506f,
      507f
    of leg, 477f, 481f, 482f, 483f
  coronal view
    of ankle, 524f, 525f, 526f, 527f, 528f, 529f,
      530f
    of leg, 494f
  oblique axial view, of ankle, 511f, 512f, 513f,
    514f, 515f
  sagittal view
    of ankle, 520f, 521f, 522f
    of leg, 488f
Flexor hallucis t., oblique axial view, of ankle, 514f
Flexor pollicis brevis m.
  axial view, of hand, 262f, 263f, 264f, 265f
  coronal view, of hand, 279f, 280f
  deep, sagittal view, of hand, 271f, 272f
  origin, insertion, and nerve supply of, 284t
  sagittal view, of hand, 271f
  superficial, sagittal view, of hand, 271f, 272f,
    273f
Flexor pollicis longus m.
  axial view, of forearm, 211f, 212f, 213f, 214f,
    215f, 216f, 218f
  coronal view, of forearm, 228f, 229f, 230f
  origin, insertion, and nerve supply of, 233t–234t
  sagittal view, of forearm, 220f, 221f
Flexor pollicis longus t.
  axial view
    of forearm, 218f
    of hand, 262f, 263f, 264f, 265f, 266f, 267f
  coronal view, of hand, 279f, 280f, 281f
  sagittal view
    of forearm, 220f
    of hand, 270f, 271f, 272f, 273f
Flexor retinaculum
  axial view, of ankle, 501f, 502f, 503f, 504f, 505f,
    506f, 507f
  coronal view
    of ankle, 528f, 529f
    of hand, 279f
  oblique axial view, of ankle, 512f, 513f, 514f
  sagittal view, of hand, 273f, 274f
Flexor t.
  common
    axial view, of elbow, 181f, 182f
    coronal view, of arm, 170f
Foramen magnum
  axial view, of brain CT, 8f
  coronal view, of brain CT, 16f
Foramen of Luschka
  axial view
    of brain CT, 8f
    of brain MRI, 24f

Foramen of Magendie
  axial view, of brain CT, 8f
  sagittal view, of brain MRI, 25f
Forearm v.
  deep, oblique sagittal view, of elbow, 194f
  superficial
    oblique sagittal view, of elbow, 190f
    sagittal view, of forearm, 219f
Fornix, sagittal view, of brain MRI, 25f, 30f
Fovea
  axial view
    of hip, 377f
    of hip arthrogram, 405f
  coronal view, of hip arthrogram, 416f
Frenulum, coronal view, of female pelvis MRI,
    623f
Frontal lobe
  axial view
    of brain CT, 4f, 5f, 6f, 7f
    of brain MRI, 19f, 20f, 21f
  coronal view, of brain CT, 13f, 14f, 15f
  sagittal view
    of brain CT, 10f, 11f, 12f
    of brain MRI, 25f, 26f, 27f, 28f, 29f, 30f

G

Gallbladder
  axial view
    of abdomen CT, 328f, 329f
    of abdomen MRI, 350f, 351f
  body
    coronal view, of abdomen CT, 338f, 339f
    sagittal view, of abdomen CT, 337f
  coronal view, of abdomen MRI, 363f, 364f,
    365f
  fundus
    axial view, of abdomen CT, 330f
    coronal view, of abdomen CT, 338f
    sagittal view, of abdomen CT, 337f
  neck
    axial view, of abdomen MRI, 349f
    coronal view
      of abdomen CT, 339f, 340f
      of thorax CT, 47f
  sagittal view, of abdomen MRI, 361f
Gastric a.
  axial view, of abdomen MRI, 348f, 349f
  coronal view
    of abdomen CT, 339f, 340f, 341f, 342f
    of abdomen MRI, 365f
  sagittal view
    of abdomen CT, 333f, 334f
    of abdomen MRI, 357f
Gastric v.
  axial view, of abdomen CT, 327f
  coronal view, of abdomen CT, 340f, 341f, 342f,
    343f
  sagittal view, of abdomen CT, 333f
Gastrocnemius aponeurosis
  axial view, of leg, 474f, 476f
  sagittal view, of leg, 487f, 488f, 489f
Gastrocnemius m., lateral head
  axial view
    of knee, 449f, 450f, 451f, 452f, 453f
    of leg, 474f, 475f, 476f, 477f, 478f
  coronal view
    of knee, 469f, 470f, 471f, 472f
    of leg, 495f, 496f, 497f
  sagittal view
    of knee, 454f, 455f, 456f, 457f
    of leg, 484f, 485f, 486f, 487f
Gastrocnemius m., medial head
  axial view
    of knee, 448f, 449f, 450f, 451f, 452f
    of leg, 474f, 475f, 476f, 477f, 478f, 479f
  coronal view
    of knee, 468f, 469f, 470f, 471f, 472f
    of leg, 493f, 494f, 495f, 496f, 497f
  sagittal view
    of knee, 459f, 460f, 461f, 462f
    of leg, 487f, 488f, 489f, 490f, 491f
Gastrocnemius m., origin, insertion, and nerve
    supply of, 498t–499t

Gastrocnemius t., medial head, axial view, of knee, 450f
Gastrocolic lig.
   coronal view, of abdomen CT, 338f
   sagittal view, of abdomen CT, 334f
Gastrocolic trunk
   axial view, of abdomen CT, 330f
   coronal view, of abdomen CT, 339f
Gastroduodenal a.
   coronal view, of abdomen CT, 339f
   sagittal view, of abdomen CT, 335f
Gastroepiploic a.
   coronal view, of abdomen CT, 338f
   sagittal view, of abdomen CT, 334f
Gastroepiploic v.
   coronal view, of abdomen CT, 338f
   sagittal view, of abdomen CT, 334f
Gastroesophageal junction
   axial view, of abdomen MRI, 346f
   coronal view
      of abdomen CT, 341f, 342f
      of abdomen MRI, 366f
   sagittal view
      of abdomen CT, 333f
      of abdomen MRI, 356f, 357f
Gastrohepatic lig.
   axial view, of abdomen CT, 327f
   coronal view, of abdomen CT, 340f
   sagittal view, of abdomen CT, 333f
Gemellus m.
   axial view
      of male pelvis CT, 567f
      of male pelvis MRI, 598f
   coronal view
      of female pelvis CT, 592f
      of female pelvis MRI, 625f
      of male pelvis MRI, 611f
   sagittal view, of male pelvis CT, 570f
Gemellus m., inferior
   axial view, of female pelvis CT, 583f
   coronal view
      of female pelvis CT, 593f
      of hip, 397f
      of male pelvis CT, 577f
   origin, insertion, and nerve supply of, 400t–401t
Gemellus m., superior
   axial view, of male pelvis CT, 567f
   coronal view
      of female pelvis CT, 593f
      of hip, 397f
      of male pelvis CT, 577f
   origin, insertion, and nerve supply of, 400t–401t
   sagittal view
      of hip, 391f
      of male pelvis CT, 570f
      of male pelvis MRI, 601f
Genu of corpus callosum
   axial view
      of brain CT, 5f, 6f
      of brain MRI, 20f, 21f
   sagittal view
      of brain CT, 10f
      of brain MRI, 25f
Gerdy's tubercle
   axial view, of knee, 452f
   coronal view
      of knee, 465f
      of leg, 492f, 493f
   sagittal view, of knee, 455f
Gissane's angle, sagittal view, of ankle, 519f
Glenohumeral joint
   axial view, of pectoral girdle and chest wall, 71f
   coronal view, of arm, 171f, 172f
Glenohumeral lig., axial view, of shoulder, 107f
Glenohumeral lig., inferior
   ABER view, of shoulder arthrogram, 150f, 151f
   axial view
      of shoulder, 107f
      of shoulder arthrogram, 135f
   oblique coronal view, of shoulder arthrogram, 143f, 144f
   oblique sagittal view, of shoulder arthrogram, 139f, 140f
Glenohumeral lig., middle
   ABER view, of shoulder arthrogram, 148f, 149f

Glenohumeral lig., middle (Continued)
   axial view
      of shoulder, 103f
      of shoulder arthrogram, 132f, 133f, 134f
   oblique coronal view, of shoulder arthrogram, 142f, 143f
   oblique sagittal view, of shoulder arthrogram, 139f, 140f
Glenohumeral lig., superior
   ABER view, of shoulder arthrogram, 148f
   axial view
      of shoulder, 103f
      of shoulder arthrogram, 131f, 132f
   oblique sagittal view
      of shoulder, 112f, 113f, 114f
      of shoulder arthrogram, 139f, 140f
Glenoid
   ABER view, of shoulder arthrogram, 148f, 149f, 150f, 151f, 152f, 153f
   axial view
      of pectoral girdle and chest wall, 70f, 71f, 72f
      of shoulder, 102f, 103f, 104f, 105f
      of shoulder arthrogram, 132f, 134f
      of thorax CT, 36f
   coronal view
      of arm, 172f, 173f
      of pectoral girdle and chest wall, 92f
   oblique coronal view
      of shoulder, 122f, 123f, 124f, 125f
      of shoulder arthrogram, 143f, 144f, 145f, 146f
   oblique sagittal view
      of shoulder, 115f
      of shoulder arthrogram, 140f, 141f
   sagittal view
      of arm, 166f, 167f
      of pectoral girdle and chest wall, 80f
Glenoid fossa, oblique sagittal view, of shoulder arthrogram, 140f
Glenoid, inferior
   ABER view, of shoulder arthrogram, 152f
   axial view, of shoulder arthrogram, 135f
Glenoid labrum
   axial view, of shoulder, 103f, 104f, 105f, 106f
   coronal view
      of arm, 171f, 172f
      of pectoral girdle and chest wall, 91f
Glenoid neck, axial view, of shoulder, 105f
Glenoid, posterior
   coronal view, of pectoral girdle and chest wall, 93f
   oblique coronal view, of shoulder arthrogram, 146f
Glenoid, superior
   axial view, of shoulder arthrogram, 131f
   coronal view, of pectoral girdle and chest wall, 92f
Globe
   axial view, of brain MRI, 22f, 23f
   coronal view, of brain CT, 13f
   sagittal view, of brain MRI, 26f, 27f, 28f
Globus pallidus
   axial view
      of brain CT, 6f
      of brain MRI, 21f
   sagittal view
      of brain CT, 11f
      of brain MRI, 26f, 30f
Gluteal a., inferior
   axial view, of hip, 376f, 377f
   coronal view
      of female pelvis CT, 593f
      of hip, 397f, 398f
      of lumbar spine, 318f
      of male pelvis CT, 578f
   sagittal view
      of female pelvis MRI, 618f
      of lumbar spine, 315f
      of male pelvis CT, 570f
      of male pelvis MRI, 602f
Gluteal a., superior
   axial view
      of female pelvis CT, 580f
      of hip, 374f
      of male pelvis MRI, 596f
   coronal view

Gluteal a., superior (Continued)
      of hip, 397f, 398f
      of lumbar spine, 318f
      of male pelvis CT, 578f
   sagittal view
      of hip, 392f
      of lumbar spine, 315f
      of male pelvis MRI, 602f
Gluteal a., trunk, coronal view, of lumbar spine, 318f
Gluteal tuberosity, axial view, of hip, 381f
Gluteal v., inferior
   axial view, of hip, 376f
   coronal view
      of female pelvis CT, 593f
      of lumbar spine, 318f
      of male pelvis CT, 578f
   sagittal view, of male pelvis CT, 570f
Gluteal v., superior
   axial view, of hip, 374f
   coronal view
      of lumbar spine, 318f
      of male pelvis CT, 578f
   sagittal view, of hip, 392f
Gluteal vessels, inferior
   axial view, of male pelvis MRI, 597f
   coronal view
      of female pelvis MRI, 625f
      of lumbar spine, 319f, 320f, 321f
   sagittal view, of hip, 391f
Gluteal vessels, superior
   axial view, of female pelvis MRI, 614f
   coronal view
      of female pelvis MRI, 625f
      of lumbar spine, 319f, 320f
   sagittal view, of hip, 390f, 391f
Gluteus maximus m.
   axial view
      of female pelvis CT, 580f, 581f, 582f, 583f, 584f
      of female pelvis MRI, 614f, 615f, 616f, 617f
      of hip, 374f, 375f, 376f, 377f, 378f, 379f, 380f, 381f, 382f
      of lumbar spine, 313f
      of male pelvis CT, 565f, 566f, 567f, 568f, 569f
      of male pelvis MRI, 596f, 597f, 599f, 600f
      of thigh, 420f, 421f, 422f
   coronal view
      of female pelvis CT, 592f, 593f
      of female pelvis MRI, 625f, 626f
      of hip, 397f, 398f, 399f
      of lumbar spine, 314f, 320f, 321f
      of male pelvis CT, 577f, 578f
      of male pelvis MRI, 611f, 612f
      of thigh, 441f, 442f, 443f
   origin, insertion, and nerve supply of, 400t–401t
   sagittal view
      of abdomen MRI, 354f, 361f
      of female pelvis CT, 585f, 586f
      of female pelvis MRI, 618f, 619f
      of hip, 383f, 384f, 385f, 386f, 387f, 388f, 389f, 390f, 391f, 392f
      of lumbar spine, 315f
      of male pelvis CT, 570f, 571f
      of male pelvis MRI, 601f, 602f, 603f, 604f
      of thigh, 428f, 429f, 430f, 431f, 432f, 433f, 434f, 435f, 436f
Gluteus medius m.
   axial view
      of female pelvis CT, 580f, 581f, 582f, 583f
      of female pelvis MRI, 614f, 615f, 616f, 617f
      of hip, 374f, 375f, 376f, 377f, 378f, 379f
      of lumbar spine, 311f, 312f, 314f
      of male pelvis CT, 564f, 565f, 566f, 567f
      of male pelvis MRI, 595f, 596f, 597f, 598f, 599f
   coronal view
      of abdomen CT, 343f
      of abdomen MRI, 366f, 367f, 368f
      of female pelvis CT, 588f, 589f, 590f, 591f, 592f, 593f
      of female pelvis MRI, 623f, 624f, 625f
      of hip, 394f, 395f, 396f, 397f
      of lumbar spine, 319f, 320f, 321f
      of male pelvis CT, 573f, 574f, 575f, 576f, 577f

Gluteus medius m. (Continued)
  origin, insertion, and nerve supply of, 400t–401t
  sagittal view
    of abdomen CT, 332f
    of abdomen MRI, 354f, 355f, 361f
    of female pelvis CT, 585f
    of hip, 383f, 384f, 385f, 386f, 387f, 388f, 389f
    of lumbar spine, 314f
    of male pelvis CT, 570f
    of male pelvis MRI, 601f
Gluteus medius t.
  axial view
    of female pelvis CT, 582f
    of hip, 376f, 377f
    of hip arthrogram, 403f, 404f, 405f
  coronal view, of male pelvis MRI, 610f
  sagittal view, of hip, 386f
Gluteus minimus m.
  axial view
    of female pelvis CT, 580f, 581f, 582f
    of female pelvis MRI, 614f, 615f, 616f
    of hip, 374f, 375f, 376f
    of male pelvis CT, 565f, 566f, 567f, 568f
    of male pelvis MRI, 597f, 598f, 599f
  coronal view
    of female pelvis CT, 590f, 591f, 592f
    of female pelvis MRI, 623f, 624f
    of hip, 394f, 395f, 396f, 397f
    of lumbar spine, 318f
    of male pelvis CT, 575f, 576f, 577f
    of male pelvis MRI, 608f, 609f, 610f
  origin, insertion, and nerve supply of, 400t–401t
  sagittal view, of hip, 383f, 384f, 385f, 386f, 387f, 388f, 389f
Gluteus minimus t.
  axial view
    of hip, 377f, 378f
    of hip arthrogram, 405f
  sagittal view, of hip, 384f, 385f
Gonadal v.
  axial view, of abdomen CT, 330f, 331f
  coronal view
    of abdomen CT, 341f
    of female pelvis CT, 592f
  sagittal view
    of abdomen CT, 333f, 336f
    of female pelvis CT, 586f
Gracilis m.
  axial view
    of hip, 381f, 382f
    of knee, 447f
    of male pelvis MRI, 600f
    of thigh, 420f, 421f, 422f, 423f, 424f, 425f, 426f, 427f
  coronal view
    of female pelvis MRI, 624f
    of hip, 394f, 395f, 396f
    of knee, 472f
    of male pelvis MRI, 608f, 609f
    of thigh, 441f, 442f, 443f, 444f
  origin, insertion, and nerve supply of, 445t
  sagittal view
    of male pelvis MRI, 603f, 604f
    of thigh, 433f, 434f, 435f, 436f
Gracilis t.
  axial view, of knee, 447f, 448f, 449f, 450f, 451f, 452f
  coronal view
    of knee, 469f, 470f, 471f, 472f
    of leg, 495f
  sagittal view, of knee, 461f, 462f
Greater saphenous v.
  axial view
    of ankle, 501f, 502f, 503f, 504f, 505f
    of hip, 379f, 380f, 381f, 382f
    of knee, 447f, 448f, 449f, 450f, 451f, 452f, 453f
    of leg, 474f, 475f, 476f, 477f, 478f, 479f, 480f, 481f, 482f, 483f
    of male pelvis MRI, 599f, 600f
    of thigh, 420f, 423f, 426f, 427f
  coronal view
    of ankle, 524f, 525f, 526f
    of female pelvis MRI, 623f
    of hip, 393f

Greater saphenous v. (Continued)
    of knee, 468f, 469f
    of leg, 493f, 494f
    of male pelvis MRI, 607f
    of thigh, 437f, 438f, 439f, 440f, 441f, 442f
  oblique axial view, of ankle, 511f, 512f, 513f, 514f
  sagittal view
    of ankle, 522f
    of hip, 389f, 390f
    of leg, 490f, 491f
    of male pelvis MRI, 601f
    of thigh, 435f, 436f
Greater sciatic foramen, coronal view, of hip, 397f
Greater sciatic notch, sagittal view, of hip, 391f
Greater trochanter
  axial view
    of female pelvis CT, 583f
    of female pelvis MRI, 616f, 617f
    of hip, 377f, 378f
    of hip arthrogram, 406f
    of male pelvis CT, 567f
    of male pelvis MRI, 598f
  coronal view
    of female pelvis CT, 590f, 591f, 592f
    of female pelvis MRI, 624f, 625f
    of hip, 396f, 397f
    of hip arthrogram, 417f, 418f
    of male pelvis CT, 576f, 577f
    of male pelvis MRI, 610f
    of thigh, 439f, 440f
  sagittal view
    of hip, 384f, 385f, 386f, 387f
    of thigh, 428f, 429f
Greater tuberosity of humerus
  ABER view, of shoulder arthrogram, 149f, 150f, 151f, 152f
  axial view
    of pectoral girdle and chest wall, 70f, 72f
    of shoulder, 102f, 103f, 104f
    of shoulder arthrogram, 132f, 133f, 134f
  coronal view
    of arm, 170f, 171f, 172f
    of pectoral girdle and chest wall, 90f, 91f, 92f
  oblique coronal view
    of shoulder, 123f, 124f, 125f
    of shoulder arthrogram, 143f, 144f, 145f, 146f
  oblique sagittal view
    of shoulder, 109f, 110f
    of shoulder arthrogram, 136f
  sagittal view
    of arm, 163f
    of pectoral girdle and chest wall, 78f
Gyrus rectus
  axial view
    of brain CT, 7f
    of brain MRI, 22f
  coronal view, of brain CT, 13f, 14f
  sagittal view, of brain MRI, 28f, 29f

H
Hamate
  coronal view, of hand, 281f, 282f
  sagittal view, of hand, 274f, 275f
Hamate, hook
  coronal view, of hand, 279f, 280f
  sagittal view, of hand, 275f
Hamstring fascia, axial view, of thigh, 423f, 424f
Hamstring t., common, axial view
    of female pelvis CT, 584f
    of hip, 379f
    of male pelvis CT, 569f
Head of caudate nucleus, sagittal view, of brain MRI, 25f
Heart
  axial view
    of abdomen CT, 326f
    of abdomen MRI, 346f, 347f
  coronal view, of abdomen MRI, 363f, 364f, 365f, 366f, 367f
  sagittal view, of abdomen MRI, 354f, 355f, 356f, 357f, 358f, 359f
Hemiazygos v.
  axial view

Hemiazygos v. (Continued)
    of abdomen MRI, 348f
    of thoracic spine, 298f
    of thorax CT, 41f, 42f
  coronal view, of thoracic spine, 302f
  sagittal view, of thoracic spine, 300f
Hemidiaphragm
  coronal view, of thorax CT, 51f, 52f
  sagittal view, of abdomen MRI, 357f
Hepatic a
  axial view
    of abdomen CT, 327f, 328f
    of abdomen MRI, 348f, 349f
  coronal view, of abdomen CT, 339f
  sagittal view
    of abdomen CT, 335f, 336f
    of abdomen MRI, 360f
Hepatic a., common
  axial view
    of abdomen CT, 328f
    of abdomen MRI, 349f
  coronal view
    of abdomen CT, 340f, 341f
    of abdomen MRI, 365f
  sagittal view
    of abdomen CT, 335f
    of abdomen MRI, 358f
Hepatic a., proper
  coronal view, of abdomen CT, 340f
  sagittal view
    of abdomen CT, 335f, 336f
    of abdomen MRI, 359f
Hepatic duct, common, sagittal view, of abdomen CT, 336f
Hepatic v.
  axial view
    of abdomen CT, 326f, 327f, 328f
    of abdomen MRI, 346f
  coronal view
    of abdomen CT, 339f, 342f
    of abdomen MRI, 365f, 367f
Hepatic v., middle
  axial view
    of abdomen CT, 326f, 327f
    of abdomen MRI, 346f
  coronal view
    of abdomen CT, 339f, 341f
    of abdomen MRI, 365f
Hepatoduodenal lig., coronal view, of abdomen CT, 339f
Hilum, posterior, coronal view, of heart MRI, 63f
Hip
  coronal view, of male pelvis MRI, 608f, 609f
  sagittal view
    of female pelvis CT, 585f
    of male pelvis CT, 570f
Hip capsule
  axial view, 376f
  coronal view, 624f
Hippocampus
  axial view, of brain MRI, 22f
  sagittal view, of brain MRI, 26f
Humeral circumflex a., anterior.
  oblique coronal view, of shoulder, 122f, 123f
  oblique sagittal view, of shoulder, 111f, 112f, 113f, 115f
  sagittal view, of pectoral girdle and chest wall, 79f
Humeral circumflex a., posterior
  axial view
    of pectoral girdle and chest wall, 72f, 73f
    of shoulder, 107f, 108f
  coronal view
    of arm, 173f
    of pectoral girdle and chest wall, 79f
  oblique coronal view, of shoulder, 122f, 123f, 124f, 125f, 126f, 127f
  oblique sagittal view, of shoulder, 112f, 113f, 114f, 115f
  sagittal view, of pectoral girdle and chest wall, 93f
Humeral circumflex vessels
  oblique sagittal view, of shoulder arthrogram, 139f, 140f
  posterior

Humeral circumflex vessels (Continued)
  oblique coronal view, of shoulder
    arthrogram, 147f
  oblique sagittal view, of shoulder
    arthrogram, 140f
Humeral diaphysis
  ABER view, of shoulder arthrogram, 150f, 151f
  axial view
    of pectoral girdle and chest wall, 74f, 76f
    of shoulder, 108f
  coronal view
    of arm, 170f, 171f
    of pectoral girdle and chest wall, 92f, 93f,
      94f, 95f
  oblique coronal view
    of shoulder, 125f
    of shoulder arthrogram, 147f
  oblique sagittal view
    of shoulder, 113f
    of shoulder arthrogram, 139f
  sagittal view, of pectoral girdle and chest wall,
    79f
Humeral epiphysis, oblique sagittal view, of
    shoulder, 109f, 110f, 112f, 113f, 114f
Humeral head
  ABER view, of shoulder arthrogram, 149f, 150f,
    151f, 152f
  articular cartilage, 102f
  axial view
    of elbow, 187f
    of pectoral girdle and chest wall, 70f, 71f
    of shoulder, 102f, 103f
    of shoulder arthrogram, 131f, 132f, 133f
    of thorax CT, 36f
  coronal view
    of arm, 170f, 171f, 172f, 173f
    of pectoral girdle and chest wall, 90f, 91f, 92f
    medial, sagittal view, of pectoral girdle and
      chest wall, 80f
  oblique coronal view
    of shoulder, 122f, 123f, 124f, 125f, 126f
    of shoulder arthrogram, 143f, 144f, 145f
  oblique sagittal view
    of elbow, 197f, 198f
    of shoulder, 111f, 112f, 113f
    of shoulder arthrogram, 136f, 137f, 138f, 139f
  posterior
    ABER view, of shoulder arthrogram, 152f,
      153f
    oblique coronal view, of shoulder
      arthrogram, 147f
  sagittal view
    of arm, 163f, 164f, 165f, 166f
    of pectoral girdle and chest wall, 78f, 79f, 80f
Humeral lig., transverse, axial view, of shoulder,
    103f
Humeral metaphysis, oblique sagittal view, of
    shoulder, 110f
Humeral physis, oblique sagittal view, of shoulder,
    109f, 110f, 111f
Humeral surgical neck
  ABER view, of shoulder arthrogram, 149f, 150f,
    151f
  axial view
    of pectoral girdle and chest wall, 72f
    of shoulder arthrogram, 135f
  oblique coronal view
    of shoulder, 124f, 125f
    of shoulder arthrogram, 145f, 146f
  oblique sagittal view, of shoulder arthrogram,
    137f, 138f
Humerus
  axial view
    of arm, 155f, 156f, 157f, 158f, 159f, 160f
    of pectoral girdle and chest wall, 73f
    of shoulder, 105f, 106f, 107f
  coronal view
    of arm, 172f
    of elbow, 204f, 205f
    of shoulder, 126f
    of shoulder arthrogram, 147f
  oblique coronal view
    of elbow, 204f, 205f
    of shoulder, 126f
    of shoulder arthrogram, 147f

Humerus (Continued)
  oblique sagittal view
    of elbow, 193f, 194f, 195f
    of shoulder, 111f, 112f
  sagittal view
    of arm, 163f, 164f
    of elbow, 193f, 194f, 195f
    of shoulder, 111f, 112f
  spiral groove, coronal view, of arm, 172f
Humphrey's lig., sagittal view, of knee, 459f

I

Ileocecal valve
  axial view, of male pelvis CT, 565f
  coronal view
    of abdomen CT, 339f
    of female pelvis CT, 589f
Ileocolic a.
  axial view, of male pelvis CT, 564f
  coronal view, of female pelvis CT, 590f
Ileocolic v., coronal view
  of female pelvis CT, 590f
  of male pelvis CT, 574f
Ileum
  axial view
    of abdomen CT, 330f, 331f
    of female pelvis CT, 580f
    of male pelvis CT, 565f
  coronal view
    of abdomen CT, 338f, 339f
    of female pelvis CT, 588f
    of male pelvis CT, 573f, 574f, 575f
  sagittal view, of female pelvis CT, 585f, 586f
Iliac a., common
  axial view
    of abdomen CT, 331f
    of lumbar spine, 311f
    of male pelvis CT, 564f
    of male pelvis MRI, 595f
  coronal view
    of abdomen CT, 339f
    of abdomen MRI, 364f
    of female pelvis CT, 590f, 591f
    of female pelvis MRI, 623f
    of lumbar spine, 317f
    of male pelvis CT, 574f, 575f
    of male pelvis MRI, 608f, 609f
  sagittal view
    of abdomen CT, 333f, 334f, 335f
    of abdomen MRI, 359f
    of female pelvis CT, 586f
    of lumbar spine, 316f
    of male pelvis CT, 571f, 572f
    of male pelvis MRI, 604f, 605f, 606f
Iliac a., external
  axial view
    of female pelvis CT, 580f, 581f, 582f
    of hip, 375f
    of lumbar spine, 312f, 313f
    of male pelvis CT, 565f, 566f, 567f
    of male pelvis MRI, 596f, 597f
  coronal view
    of female pelvis CT, 589f, 590f
    of hip, 395f
    of lumbar spine, 317f
    of male pelvis CT, 574f
    of male pelvis MRI, 608f
  sagittal view
    of abdomen CT, 335f
    of female pelvis CT, 585f, 586f
    of male pelvis CT, 570f
    of male pelvis MRI, 602f, 603f
Iliac a., internal
  axial view
    of female pelvis CT, 580f, 581f
    of lumbar spine, 312f, 313f
    of male pelvis CT, 565f, 566f
    of male pelvis MRI, 595f, 596f
  coronal view
    of female pelvis CT, 592f, 593f
    of male pelvis CT, 575f, 576f, 577f
    of male pelvis MRI, 609f
  sagittal view
    of female pelvis CT, 585f, 586f

Iliac a., internal (Continued)
    of lumbar spine, 315f
    of male pelvis CT, 571f
    of male pelvis MRI, 604f
Iliac bifurcation, sagittal view, of male pelvis CT,
    571f
Iliac circumflex v., superficial, coronal view, of
    hip, 393f
Iliac circumflex vessels, superficial, coronal view,
    of male pelvis MR, 607f
Iliac crest
  axial view
    of abdomen CT, 331f
    of lumbar spine, 311f
    of male pelvis CT, 564f
    of male pelvis MRI, 595f
  coronal view
    of female pelvis CT, 588f, 589f, 590f, 591f,
      592f
    of female pelvis MRI, 622f, 623f
    of lumbar spine, 321f
    of male pelvis CT, 576f
    of male pelvis MRI, 607f
  sagittal view
    of abdomen CT, 337f
    of hip, 386f
    of male pelvis CT, 570f
Iliac spine, anterior inferior
  axial view
    of female pelvis CT, 581f
    of female pelvis MRI, 616f
    of hip, 375f
    of male pelvis CT, 565f, 566f
    of male pelvis MRI, 597f
  coronal view, of hip, 394f
  sagittal view, of hip, 385f, 386f, 387f
Iliac spine, anterior superior
  axial view
    of female pelvis CT, 580f
    of female pelvis MRI, 614f
    of male pelvis CT, 565f
    of male pelvis MRI, 596f
  coronal view
    of female pelvis CT, 588f
    of female pelvis MRI, 622f
    of hip, 394f
    of male pelvis CT, 573f, 575f
  sagittal view, of hip, 385f, 386f
Iliac v., common
  axial view
    of abdomen CT, 331f
    of lumbar spine, 311f, 312f
    of male pelvis CT, 564f, 565f
    of male pelvis MRI, 595f
  coronal view
    of abdomen CT, 339f
    of female pelvis CT, 591f, 592f
    of lumbar spine, 317f
    of male pelvis CT, 575f
  sagittal view
    of abdomen CT, 334f, 335f
    of female pelvis CT, 586f, 587f
    of lumbar spine, 316f
    of male pelvis CT, 571f
    of male pelvis MRI, 604f
Iliac v., external
  axial view
    of female pelvis CT, 580f, 581f, 582f
    of hip, 375f
    of lumbar spine, 313f
    of male pelvis CT, 566f, 567f
    of male pelvis MRI, 596f, 597f
  coronal view
    of female pelvis CT, 589f, 590f, 591f
    of hip, 395f
    of male pelvis CT, 574f, 575f
    of male pelvis MRI, 608f
  sagittal view
    of female pelvis CT, 585f
    of male pelvis MRI, 602f, 603f
Iliac v., internal
  axial view
    of female pelvis CT, 580f, 581f
    of lumbar spine, 312f, 313f
    of male pelvis CT, 566f

Iliac v., internal *(Continued)*
  of male pelvis MRI, 595*f*, 596*f*
  coronal view
    of female pelvis CT, 592*f*, 593*f*
    of male pelvis CT, 575*f*, 576*f*, 577*f*
  sagittal view
    of female pelvis CT, 586*f*
    of male pelvis CT, 571*f*
    of male pelvis MRI, 604*f*, 605*f*
Iliac vessels, common, sagittal view
  of abdomen MRI, 356*f*, 359*f*
  of female pelvis MRI, 619*f*, 620*f*
Iliac vessels, coronal view, of lumbar spine, 318*f*
Iliac vessels, external
  axial view
    of female pelvis MRI, 614*f*, 615*f*
    of hip, 374*f*
  coronal view, of hip, 395*f*, 396*f*
  sagittal view
    of hip, 391*f*
    of male pelvis MRI, 602*f*
Iliac vessels, internal
  axial view
    of female pelvis MRI, 614*f*
    of hip, 374*f*
  coronal view
    of female pelvis MRI, 624*f*
    of male pelvis MRI, 610*f*, 611*f*
  sagittal view
    of female pelvis MRI, 618*f*
    of male pelvis MRI, 602*f*, 603*f*
Iliac wing, coronal view, of hip, 394*f*
Iliacus, axial view, of male pelvis CT, 565*f*
Iliacus m.
  axial view
    of female pelvis CT, 580*f*
    of female pelvis MRI, 614*f*
    of lumbar spine, 311*f*, 313*f*, 314*f*
    of male pelvis MRI, 595*f*, 596*f*
  coronal view
    of abdomen CT, 341*f*
    of abdomen MRI, 365*f*
    of female pelvis CT, 588*f*, 589*f*, 590*f*, 591*f*, 592*f*
    of female pelvis MRI, 622*f*, 623*f*, 624*f*
    of hip, 395*f*
    of lumbar spine, 317*f*, 318*f*, 319*f*
    of male pelvis CT, 574*f*, 575*f*, 576*f*
    of male pelvis MRI, 608*f*, 609*f*, 610*f*
  origin, insertion, and nerve supply of, 400*t*–401*t*
  sagittal view
    of abdomen CT, 332*f*
    of abdomen MRI, 354*f*, 355*f*, 361*f*
    of female pelvis CT, 585*f*
    of lumbar spine, 314*f*
    of male pelvis CT, 570*f*
    of male pelvis MRI, 601*f*, 602*f*
Iliocostalis cervicis m., origin, insertion, and nerve supply of, 306*t*–308*t*
Iliocostalis lumborum m.
  axial view
    of abdomen MRI, 347*f*, 348*f*, 350*f*, 351*f*, 352*f*, 353*f*
    of lumbar spine, 310*f*, 311*f*, 312*f*, 313*f*
  coronal view
    of abdomen MRI, 368*f*, 369*f*
    of lumbar spine, 314*f*, 321*f*, 322*f*
  origin, insertion, and nerve supply of, 306*t*–308*t*
  sagittal view
    of abdomen MRI, 355*f*, 361*f*
    of female pelvis CT, 586*f*
    of lumbar spine, 314*f*
Iliocostalis m.
  axial view
    of abdomen CT, 326*f*, 328*f*, 330*f*, 331*f*
    of male pelvis CT, 564*f*
    of male pelvis MRI, 595*f*
  coronal view
    of abdomen CT, 343*f*
    of male pelvis CT, 577*f*, 578*f*
  sagittal view
    of abdomen CT, 332*f*, 333*f*, 334*f*, 337*f*
    of female pelvis CT, 585*f*
    of male pelvis CT, 571*f*

Iliocostalis thoracis m.
  axial view, of thoracic spine, 297*f*
  origin, insertion, and nerve supply of, 306*t*–308*t*
Iliofemoral lig.
  axial view, of hip arthrogram, 403*f*, 404*f*, 405*f*, 406*f*, 407*f*, 408*f*
  coronal view, of hip arthrogram, 414*f*, 415*f*, 416*f*, 417*f*, 418*f*
  sagittal view, of hip arthrogram, 409*f*, 410*f*, 411*f*
Iliohypogastric n., coronal view, of female pelvis MRI, 622*f*
Iliolumbar a.
  axial view, of lumbar spine, 313*f*
  coronal view, of lumbar spine, 318*f*
  sagittal view, of lumbar spine, 315*f*
Iliolumbar lig.
  axial view, of lumbar spine, 311*f*
  coronal view, of lumbar spine, 320*f*
  transverse part, sagittal view, of lumbar spine, 314*f*
Iliolumbar v., axial view, of lumbar spine, 313*f*
Iliolumbar vessels
  axial view, of lumbar spine, 312*f*
  iliac branches, coronal view, of lumbar spine, 319*f*
Iliopsoas m.
  axial view
    of female pelvis CT, 580*f*, 581*f*, 582*f*, 583*f*, 584*f*
    of female pelvis MRI, 615*f*, 616*f*, 617*f*
    of hip, 374*f*, 375*f*, 376*f*, 377*f*, 378*f*, 379*f*, 380*f*
    of male pelvis CT, 565*f*, 566*f*, 567*f*, 568*f*, 569*f*
    of male pelvis MRI, 596*f*, 597*f*, 598*f*, 599*f*, 600*f*
  coronal view
    of female pelvis CT, 588*f*, 589*f*, 590*f*, 591*f*
    of female pelvis MRI, 623*f*
    of hip, 394*f*, 395*f*, 396*f*
    of lumbar spine, 317*f*
    of male pelvis CT, 574*f*, 575*f*
    of male pelvis MRI, 607*f*, 608*f*
    of thigh, 438*f*, 439*f*
  sagittal view
    of female pelvis CT, 585*f*
    of hip, 386*f*, 387*f*, 390*f*, 391*f*
    of lumbar spine, 314*f*
    of male pelvis CT, 570*f*
    of male pelvis MRI, 601*f*
    of thigh, 432*f*, 433*f*, 434*f*
Iliopsoas t.
  axial view
    of hip, 374*f*, 375*f*, 376*f*, 377*f*, 378*f*, 379*f*, 380*f*
    of hip arthrogram, 403*f*, 404*f*, 405*f*, 406*f*, 407*f*, 408*f*
  coronal view, of hip, 395*f*, 396*f*
  sagittal view
    of hip, 389*f*, 390*f*
    of hip arthrogram, 410*f*, 411*f*, 412*f*
Iliotibial band
  axial view
    of female pelvis MRI, 617*f*
    of hip, 374*f*, 375*f*, 376*f*, 377*f*, 378*f*, 379*f*, 380*f*, 381*f*, 382*f*
    of knee, 447*f*, 448*f*, 449*f*, 450*f*, 451*f*, 452*f*
    of male pelvis MRI, 599*f*
    of thigh, 420*f*, 421*f*, 422*f*, 423*f*, 424*f*, 425*f*, 426*f*, 427*f*
  coronal view
    of hip, 395*f*, 396*f*, 397*f*
    of knee, 464*f*, 465*f*, 466*f*, 467*f*, 468*f*, 469*f*
    of leg, 492*f*, 493*f*
    of male pelvis MRI, 610*f*, 611*f*
    of thigh, 441*f*
  sagittal view
    of hip, 383*f*, 384*f*
    of thigh, 428*f*
Iliotibial tract
  axial view
    of female pelvis CT, 583*f*, 584*f*
    of hip, 379*f*
    of male pelvis CT, 569*f*
  coronal view
    of female pelvis CT, 590*f*, 591*f*
    of thigh, 440*f*

Ilium
  axial view
    of female pelvis CT, 580*f*, 581*f*
    of female pelvis MRI, 614*f*, 615*f*, 616*f*
    of hip, 374*f*, 375*f*, 376*f*
    of lumbar spine, 311*f*, 312*f*, 313*f*, 314*f*
    of male pelvis MRI, 595*f*
  coronal view
    of abdomen CT, 343*f*
    of abdomen MRI, 367*f*, 368*f*
    of female pelvis CT, 589*f*, 590*f*, 591*f*, 593*f*
    of female pelvis MRI, 624*f*, 625*f*
    of hip, 395*f*, 397*f*, 398*f*
    of hip arthrogram, 414*f*, 415*f*, 416*f*, 417*f*, 418*f*
    of lumbar spine, 317*f*, 318*f*, 319*f*, 320*f*, 322*f*
    of male pelvis CT, 574*f*, 575*f*
    of male pelvis MRI, 608*f*, 610*f*, 612*f*
  sagittal view
    of abdomen CT, 332*f*
    of abdomen MRI, 354*f*, 355*f*, 361*f*
    of female pelvis CT, 585*f*
    of female pelvis MRI, 618*f*
    of hip, 385*f*, 386*f*, 387*f*, 390*f*, 391*f*, 392*f*
    of hip arthrogram, 409*f*, 410*f*, 411*f*, 412*f*, 413*f*
    of lumbar spine, 315*f*
    of male pelvis MRI, 601*f*, 602*f*, 603*f*
Inferior articular recess, 408*f*
Inferior nasal conchae, sagittal view, of brain MRI, 28*f*, 29*f*
Inferior oblique capitis m
  axial view, of brain CT, 9*f*
  coronal view, of cervical spine MRI, 295*f*
  sagittal view, of cervical spine MRI, 31*f*, 32*f*, 291*f*, 292*f*
Inferior rectus m
  axial view, of brain MRI, 23*f*
  coronal view, of brain CT, 13*f*, 14*f*
  sagittal view, of brain MRI, 28*f*
Inferior rectus m., sagittal view, of brain MRI, 29*f*
Inferior vena cava
  axial view
    of abdomen CT, 326*f*, 327*f*, 328*f*, 329*f*, 330*f*, 331*f*
    of abdomen MRI, 346*f*, 347*f*, 348*f*, 349*f*, 350*f*, 351*f*, 352*f*, 353*f*
    of heart MRI, 57*f*
    of lumbar spine, 310*f*
    of male pelvis CT, 564*f*
    of thorax CT, 41*f*
  coronal view
    of abdomen CT, 339*f*, 340*f*, 341*f*, 342*f*
    of abdomen MRI, 365*f*, 366*f*, 367*f*
    of female pelvis CT, 590*f*, 591*f*
    of lumbar spine, 317*f*, 318*f*
    of male pelvis CT, 575*f*
    of thorax CT, 38*f*, 50*f*
  sagittal view
    of abdomen CT, 335*f*
    of abdomen MRI, 359*f*, 360*f*
    of heart MRI, 60*f*
    of lumbar spine, 315*f*, 316*f*
    of male pelvis CT, 572*f*
    of male pelvis MRI, 605*f*
    of thorax CT, 45*f*, 46*f*
Infraglenoid tubercle
  ABER view, of shoulder arthrogram, 153*f*
  axial view, of shoulder arthrogram, 135*f*
  oblique sagittal view
    of shoulder, 115*f*
    of shoulder arthrogram, 141*f*
Infrahyoid m.
  axial view, of pectoral girdle and chest wall, 68*f*
  coronal view, of pectoral girdle and chest wall, 89*f*
Infrapatellar fat pad
  axial view, of knee, 450*f*, 451*f*, 452*f*
  coronal view
    of knee, 463*f*, 464*f*
    of leg, 492*f*
  sagittal view
    of knee, 456*f*, 457*f*, 458*f*, 459*f*
    of leg, 486*f*, 487*f*, 488*f*

Infraspinatus m.
  ABER view, of shoulder arthrogram, 151f, 152f
  axial view
    of heart MRI, 54f
    of pectoral girdle and chest wall, 70f, 71f,
      72f, 73f, 74f
    of shoulder, 101f, 102f, 103f, 104f, 105f, 106f
    of shoulder arthrogram, 131f, 132f, 133f
  coronal view
    of arm, 157f, 173f, 174f, 175f
    of pectoral girdle and chest wall, 93f, 94f,
      95f, 96f, 97f
    of thoracic spine, 302f, 303f, 304f, 305f
  oblique coronal view
    of shoulder, 124f, 125f, 126f, 127f
    of shoulder arthrogram, 145f, 146f, 147f
  oblique sagittal view
    of shoulder, 113f, 114f, 115f, 116f, 117f, 118f
    of shoulder arthrogram, 139f, 140f, 141f
  origin, insertion, and nerve supply of, 129t,
    306t–308t
  sagittal view
    of arm, 163f, 164f, 165f, 166f, 167f
    of pectoral girdle and chest wall, 78f, 80f,
      81f, 82f, 83f, 84f
Infraspinatus t.
  ABER view, of shoulder arthrogram, 150f, 151f
  axial view
    of shoulder, 102f, 103f, 104f
    of shoulder arthrogram, 131f, 132f
  oblique coronal view
    of shoulder, 125f, 126f, 127f
    of shoulder arthrogram, 145f, 146f, 147f
  oblique sagittal view
    of shoulder, 110f, 111f, 112f, 113f
    of shoulder arthrogram, 136f, 137f, 138f,
      139f, 140f, 141f
  sagittal view
    of arm, 165f
    of pectoral girdle and chest wall, 80f
Infundibulum, sagittal view, of brain MRI, 25f, 30f
Inguinal lig., coronal view
  of female pelvis CT, 588f
  of hip, 393f
Inguinal lymph nodes
  coronal view
    of female pelvis CT, 588f
    of female pelvis MRI, 622f
    of male pelvis CT, 573f
    of male pelvis MRI, 607f
  sagittal view, of male pelvis CT, 570f
Innominate bone, axial view, of male pelvis MRI,
    597f, 598f
Insular cortex
  axial view
    of brain CT, 6f
    of brain MRI, 21f
  coronal view, of brain CT, 14f, 15f
  sagittal view, of brain MRI, 27f, 29f, 30f
Intercarpal lig., coronal view, of hand, 281f
Interclavicular lig., coronal view, of pectoral girdle
    and chest wall, 89f
Intercondylar eminence, coronal view, of knee,
    467f, 468f
Intercondylar fossa, axial view, of knee, 449f, 450f
Intercondylar notch
  coronal view
    of knee, 467f, 468f
    of leg, 493f
Intercostal a.
  coronal view
    of pectoral girdle and chest wall, 94f, 95f
    of thoracic spine, 302f, 303f
  sagittal view
    of abdomen CT, 333f
    of thoracic spine, 299f
Intercostal m.
  axial view
    of abdomen CT, 328f
    of pectoral girdle and chest wall, 76f
  coronal view
    of pectoral girdle and chest wall, 96f, 97f
    of thoracic spine, 302f, 303f
  sagittal view
    of abdomen CT, 332f

Intercostal m. (Continued)
    of pectoral girdle and chest wall, 84f, 86f
Intercostal n.
  coronal view, of thoracic spine, 302f, 303f
  sagittal view, of thoracic spine, 299f
Intercostal neurovascular bundle, sagittal view
    of pectoral girdle and chest wall, 85f, 87f
    of thoracic spine, 300f
Intercostal v.
  axial view, of thorax CT, 41f
  coronal view
    of pectoral girdle and chest wall, 94f, 95f
    of thoracic spine, 302f
  sagittal view
    of abdomen CT, 333f
    of thoracic spine, 299f
Intercostal vessels
  axial view
    of abdomen CT, 332f
    of thoracic spine, 297f
  coronal view, of pectoral girdle and chest wall,
    95f, 96f
  sagittal view, of abdomen CT, 332f
Interhemispheric fissure, axial view, of brain MRI,
    19f, 20f
Interlobar a.
  axial view, of thorax CT, 39f
  coronal view, of thorax CT, 48f, 50f, 51f
Intermalleolar lig., posterior, coronal view, of
    ankle, 530f
Intermuscular septum, lateral
  axial view
    of elbow, 183f
    of thigh, 421f
  oblique coronal, of elbow, 204f
  sagittal view, of thigh, 428f, 429f
Internal capsule
  axial view
    of brain CT, 6f
    of brain MRI, 21f
  coronal view, of brain CT, 15f
  sagittal view, of brain MRI, 29f
Internal carotid a.
  axial view, of cervical spine MRI, 288f, 289f
  sagittal view
    of brain MRI, 26f
    of cervical spine MRI, 292f
Internal cerebral vv., sagittal view, of brain MRI,
    31f
Internal jugular v.
  axial view, of cervical spine MRI, 288f, 289f
  coronal view, of cervical spine MRI, 294f
  sagittal view
    of brain CT, 11f
    of cervical spine MRI, 291f
Interosseous a., anterior
  axial view
    of elbow, 187f, 188f, 189f
    of forearm, 211f
  coronal view
    of elbow, 203f, 204f
    of forearm, 228f, 229f
  oblique coronal, of elbow, 203f, 204f
  oblique sagittal view, of elbow, 194f, 195f
  sagittal view
    of elbow, 194f, 195f
    of forearm, 221f, 222f
Interosseous a., common
  axial view
    of elbow, 187f, 188f
    of forearm, 209f
  oblique coronal, of elbow, 202f, 203f
  sagittal view, of forearm, 222f
Interosseous a., oblique coronal, of elbow, 203f
Interosseous a., posterior
  axial view
    of elbow, 189f
    of forearm, 210f, 211f, 212f, 213f, 218f
  coronal view, of forearm, 231f, 232f
  oblique sagittal view, of elbow, 193f
  sagittal view
    of elbow, 193f
    of forearm, 221f, 222f, 223f
Interosseous m.
  axial view, of hand, 268f

Interosseous m. (Continued)
  origin, insertion, and nerve supply of, 284t
Interosseous m. dorsal
  1st
    axial view, of hand, 263f, 264f, 266f, 267f
    coronal view, of hand, 281f, 282f
    sagittal view, of hand, 270f, 271f, 272f
  2nd
    axial view, of hand, 263f, 264f, 265f, 266f,
      267f
    coronal view, of hand, 281f, 282f, 283f
    sagittal view, of hand, 273f, 274f
  3rd
    axial view, of hand, 264f, 265f, 266f, 267f
    coronal view, of hand, 281f, 282f
    sagittal view, of hand, 275f
  4th
    axial view, of hand, 263f, 264f, 265f, 266f,
      267f
    coronal view, of hand, 281f, 282f
    sagittal view, of hand, 276f
Interosseous m., palmar
  1st
    axial view, of hand, 264f, 265f, 266f, 267f
    coronal view, of hand, 281f
  2nd
    axial view, of hand, 265f, 266f
    coronal view, of hand, 281f
  3rd
    axial view, of hand, 263f, 264f, 265f, 266f
    coronal view, of hand, 281f
    sagittal view
      of hand, 275f, 276f
      of wrist, 250f
    axial view, of hand, 264f, 265f
Interosseous membrane
  axial view
    of ankle, 501f
    of forearm, 212f, 213f, 214f, 215f
    of leg, 475f, 476f, 477f, 480f, 481f, 482f, 483f
  oblique sagittal view, of elbow, 194f
Interosseous n., anterior
  axial view
    of elbow, 183f, 184f, 185f, 186f
    of forearm, 210f, 211f, 212f, 213f, 214f, 215f,
      216f, 217f
  coronal view
    of elbow, 203f, 204f
    of forearm, 228f, 229f
  oblique coronal, of elbow, 203f, 204f
  oblique sagittal view, of elbow, 194f, 195f
  sagittal view
    of elbow, 194f, 195f
    of forearm, 221f
Interosseous n., posterior
  axial view, of forearm, 210f, 211f, 212f, 213f,
    214f, 215f, 216f, 217f
  coronal view
    of elbow, 204f
    of forearm, 231f, 232f
  oblique coronal, of elbow, 204f
  oblique sagittal view, of elbow, 193f
  sagittal view
    of elbow, 193f
    of forearm, 222f, 223f
Interosseous sacroiliac lig.
  coronal view, of lumbar spine, 321f, 322f
  sagittal view, of lumbar spine, 315f
Interosseous t., coronal view, of hand, 281f
Interosseous v., posterior, sagittal view, of
    forearm, 222f
Interosseous vessels, posterior, oblique coronal, of
    elbow, 204f
Interphalangeal joint
  distal, sagittal view, of hand, 272f, 273f, 276f
  proximal, sagittal view, of hand, 272f, 274f,
    276f, 277f, 278f
  sagittal view, of hand, 269f
Interspinales cervicis m., origin, insertion, and
    nerve supply of, 306t–308t
Interspinales lumborum m., origin, insertion, and
    nerve supply of, 306t–308t
Interspinales thoracis m.
  axial view, of thoracic spine, 298f
  origin, insertion, and nerve supply of, 306t–308t

Interspinales thoracis m. *(Continued)*
  sagittal view, of thoracic spine, 301*f*
Interspinous lig.
  axial view, of cervical spine MRI, 288*f*
  coronal view, of thoracic spine, 304*f*
  sagittal view
    of cervical spine MRI, 293*f*
    of lumbar spine, 316*f*
    of thoracic spine, 301*f*
Intertransversarii anteriores cervicis m., origin,
    insertion, and nerve supply of,
    306*t*–308*t*
Intertransversarii laterales lumbar m., origin,
    insertion, and nerve supply of,
    306*t*–308*t*
Intertransversarii thoracis m., origin, insertion,
    and nerve supply of, 306*t*–308*t*
Intertransversarius m.
  coronal view, of lumbar spine, 320*f*
  sagittal view, of thoracic spine, 300*f*
Intertrochanteric crest, coronal view
  of female pelvis MRI, 625*f*
  of male pelvis MRI, 610*f*
Interventricular septum
  axial view, of thorax CT, 40*f*, 41*f*
  sagittal view, of thorax CT, 43*f*, 44*f*
Intervertebral disc
  coronal view, of pectoral girdle and chest wall,
    94*f*
  sagittal view
    of abdomen MRI, 358*f*, 359*f*
    of male pelvis MRI, 606*f*
    of thoracic spine, 301*f*
Intraventricular septum, axial view, of heart MRI,
    56*f*
Ischial ramus
  axial view
    of female pelvis CT, 587*f*
    of male pelvis CT, 569*f*
  coronal view
    of male pelvis CT, 576*f*
    of male pelvis MRI, 610*f*
  sagittal view
    of female pelvis CT, 585*f*, 586*f*
    of male pelvis MRI, 602*f*, 603*f*, 604*f*
Ischial spine, axial view
  of female pelvis MRI, 616*f*
  of hip, 377*f*
  of hip arthrogram, 405*f*
  of male pelvis CT, 567*f*
  of male pelvis MRI, 598*f*
Ischial tuberosity
  axial view
    of female pelvis CT, 583*f*
    of hip, 378*f*, 379*f*, 380*f*
    of male pelvis CT, 568*f*, 569*f*
    of male pelvis MRI, 599*f*
  coronal view
    of male pelvis CT, 578*f*
    of male pelvis MRI, 611*f*
  sagittal view
    of male pelvis CT, 570*f*, 571*f*
    of male pelvis MRI, 601*f*
Ischioanal fossa, coronal view, of female pelvis
    MRI, 625*f*
Ischiocavernosus m.
  axial view
    of male pelvis CT, 569*f*
    of male pelvis MRI, 599*f*, 600*f*
  coronal view
    of female pelvis CT, 590*f*, 591*f*
    of male pelvis CT, 576*f*, 577*f*
    of male pelvis MRI, 610*f*
  sagittal view
    of female pelvis CT, 586*f*
    of male pelvis CT, 571*f*
    of male pelvis MRI, 603*f*, 604*f*
Ischiofemoral lig.
  axial view, of hip arthrogram, 404*f*, 405*f*, 406*f*,
    407*f*
  coronal view, of hip arthrogram, 418*f*
  sagittal view, of hip arthrogram, 409*f*, 410*f*,
    411*f*
Ischiorectal fossa
  axial view

Ischiorectal fossa *(Continued)*
    of female pelvis CT, 582*f*, 583*f*, 584*f*
    of female pelvis MRI, 616*f*
    of male pelvis CT, 568*f*
  coronal view
    of female pelvis CT, 593*f*
    of male pelvis CT, 577*f*, 578*f*
    of male pelvis MRI, 610*f*
  sagittal view
    of female pelvis CT, 585*f*, 586*f*
    of male pelvis CT, 571*f*
Ischium
  axial view
    of female pelvis CT, 583*f*
    of female pelvis MRI, 617*f*
    of hip, 378*f*
    of hip arthrogram, 407*f*, 408*f*
    of male pelvis MRI, 599*f*, 600*f*
    of thigh, 420*f*
  coronal view
    of female pelvis CT, 592*f*, 593*f*
    of female pelvis MRI, 625*f*
    of hip, 396*f*, 397*f*
    of hip arthrogram, 415*f*, 416*f*, 417*f*
    of male pelvis CT, 577*f*
    of male pelvis MRI, 611*f*
    of thigh, 442*f*, 443*f*
  sagittal view
    of female pelvis CT, 585*f*
    of female pelvis MRI, 618*f*
    of hip, 390*f*, 391*f*, 392*f*
    of hip arthrogram, 412*f*, 413*f*
    of male pelvis MRI, 602*f*
    of thigh, 434*f*, 435*f*

J
Jejunum
  axial view
    of abdomen CT, 329*f*, 330*f*, 331*f*
    of abdomen MRI, 349*f*, 350*f*, 351*f*, 352*f*, 353*f*
  coronal view
    of abdomen CT, 338*f*, 340*f*, 341*f*, 342*f*
    of abdomen MRI, 363*f*, 364*f*, 365*f*, 366*f*, 367*f*
    of female pelvis CT, 588*f*, 589*f*, 590*f*
    of male pelvis CT, 574*f*
  sagittal view, of abdomen CT, 332*f*
Joint capsule
  axial view, of lumbar spine, 310*f*
  coronal view
    of hand, 281*f*
    of hip, 624*f*
  oblique sagittal view, of shoulder arthrogram,
    139*f*
Jugular v.
  axial view, of thorax CT, 36*f*
  coronal view, of thorax CT, 47*f*, 48*f*
Jugular v., anterior
  axial view, of pectoral girdle and chest wall,
    70*f*, 71*f*
  coronal view, of pectoral girdle and chest wall,
    89*f*
  sagittal view, of pectoral girdle and chest wall,
    86*f*, 87*f*
Jugular v., external
  axial view, of pectoral girdle and chest wall, 70*f*
  coronal view, of pectoral girdle and chest wall,
    90*f*, 91*f*
  sagittal view, of pectoral girdle and chest wall,
    84*f*, 85*f*
Jugular v., internal
  axial view, of pectoral girdle and chest wall, 70*f*
  coronal view, of pectoral girdle and chest wall,
    90*f*
  sagittal view, of pectoral girdle and chest wall,
    87*f*

K
Kager's triangle.
  axial view, of ankle, 504*f*, 505*f*, 506*f*, 507*f*
  coronal view, of ankle, 532*f*
  sagittal view, of ankle, 519*f*, 520*f*
Kidney
  left

Kidney *(Continued)*
  axial view
    of abdomen CT, 328*f*, 329*f*, 330*f*
    of abdomen MRI, 348*f*, 349*f*, 350*f*, 351*f*,
      352*f*, 353*f*
    of lumbar spine, 314*f*
  coronal view
    of abdomen CT, 342*f*, 343*f*
    of abdomen MRI, 367*f*, 368*f*, 369*f*
    of lumbar spine, 320*f*
    of thoracic spine, 302*f*
    of thorax CT, 51*f*
  sagittal view
    of abdomen MRI, 354*f*, 355*f*, 356*f*
    of heart MRI, 58*f*
    of thoracic spine, 299*f*
    of thorax CT, 43*f*
  sagittal view, of abdomen CT, 332*f*
  left inferior pole
    axial view, of abdomen CT, 330*f*
    coronal view, of abdomen CT, 342*f*
  left superior pole
    axial view, of abdomen CT, 327*f*, 328*f*
    sagittal view, of abdomen CT, 333*f*
  left upper pole, axial view, of abdomen MRI,
    348*f*
  right
    axial view
      of abdomen CT, 328*f*, 329*f*, 330*f*
      of abdomen MRI, 349*f*, 350*f*, 351*f*, 352*f*,
        353*f*
      of lumbar spine, 314*f*
    coronal view
      of abdomen CT, 342*f*, 343*f*
      of abdomen MRI, 367*f*, 368*f*, 369*f*
      of lumbar spine, 321*f*
      of thoracic spine, 302*f*
      of thorax CT, 51*f*
    sagittal view
      of abdomen CT, 336*f*, 337*f*
      of abdomen MRI, 360*f*, 361*f*
  right inferior pole
    axial view, of abdomen CT, 330*f*
    coronal view
      of abdomen CT, 341*f*
      of lumbar spine, 319*f*
  right superior pole
    axial view, of abdomen CT, 327*f*, 328*f*
    sagittal view, of abdomen CT, 336*f*
  right upper pole, axial view, of abdomen MRI,
    348*f*
  sagittal view, of lumbar spine, 315*f*

L
L1
  transverse process, 321*f*
  vertebra, 319*f*
L2
  nerve, 320*f*
  pedicle, 320*f*
  spinal ganglion, 320*f*
  spinous process, 322*f*
  vertebra, 310*f*
  vertebral body, 341*f*
L3
  nerve, 319*f*
  nerve root, 310*f*
  pedicle, 319*f*
  spinous process, 316*f*
  transverse process, 315*f*
  vertebral body, 342*f*
L3–4 disc, 310*f*
L4
  dorsal ramus of spinal n., 319*f*
  inferior facet, 311*f*, 312*f*
  nerve, 319*f*
  nerve root, sagittal view, 605*f*
  spinous process, 311*f*, 606*f*
  vertebral body
    coronal view, 575*f*, 576*f*, 591*f*
    sagittal view, 572*f*, 587*f*, 606*f*
L4–5
  annulus fibrosus, 316*f*
  facet joint, 312*f*

L4–5 *(Continued)*
 intervertebral disc, 621*f*
 nucleus pulposus, 316*f*, 318*f*
L4–5 disc, 311*f*
L5
 inferior facet, 316*f*
 lamina, 312*f*
 laminar arch, 320*f*
 lateral recess, 311*f*, 312*f*
 nerve, 312*f*, 319*f*, 320*f*
 nerve root, 316*f*
 pars interarticularis, 316*f*
 pedicle, 311*f*, 312*f*, 316*f*
 spinal ganglion, 312*f*
 spinous process, 312*f*, 313*f*, 321*f*, 322*f*
 superior facet, 311*f*, 312*f*, 316*f*
 transverse process, 320*f*
 vertebra, 311*f*, 312*f*, 318*f*
 vertebral body
  axial view, 595*f*
  coronal view, 575*f*, 576*f*, 592*f*, 609*f*, 624*f*
  sagittal view, 586*f*, 605*f*, 620*f*, 621*f*
L5–S1
 articular facet, 312*f*
 facet joint, 313*f*
 intervertebral disc
  axial view, 312*f*
  coronal view, 318*f*, 592*f*, 624*f*
  sagittal view, 316*f*, 572*f*, 620*f*, 621*f*
Labium majus pudendi, coronal view, of female
  pelvis MRI, 623*f*
Labium minus pudendi, coronal view, of female
  pelvis CT, 591*f*
Labrum, anterior
 ABER view, of shoulder arthrogram, 149*f*, 150*f*,
  151*f*, 152*f*
 axial view
  of hip arthrogram, 403*f*, 404*f*, 405*f*, 406*f*
  of shoulder, 104*f*
  of shoulder arthrogram, 131*f*, 132*f*, 133*f*, 134*f*
 oblique sagittal view, of shoulder arthrogram,
  139*f*, 140*f*
 sagittal view, of hip arthrogram, 409*f*, 410*f*,
  411*f*
Labrum, anterior superior, coronal view, of hip
  arthrogram, 414*f*, 415*f*
Labrum, inferior
 ABER view, of shoulder arthrogram, 151*f*, 152*f*
 axial view, of shoulder, 106*f*
 coronal view, of hip arthrogram, 418*f*
 oblique coronal view, of shoulder, 123*f*
 sagittal view, of hip arthrogram, 412*f*
Labrum, oblique coronal view, of shoulder
  arthrogram, 143*f*, 144*f*, 145*f*
Labrum, posterior
 ABER view, of shoulder arthrogram, 150*f*, 151*f*,
  152*f*
 axial view
  of hip arthrogram, 403*f*, 404*f*, 405*f*, 406*f*
  of shoulder, 104*f*, 105*f*
  of shoulder arthrogram, 131*f*, 132*f*, 133*f*,
   134*f*, 135*f*
 coronal view, of hip arthrogram, 417*f*, 418*f*
 oblique coronal view, of shoulder arthrogram,
  146*f*
 oblique sagittal view
  of shoulder, 115*f*
  of shoulder arthrogram, 140*f*
 sagittal view, of hip arthrogram, 409*f*, 410*f*,
  411*f*
Labrum, superior
 ABER view, of shoulder arthrogram, 149*f*
 axial view, of shoulder arthrogram, 131*f*
 coronal view, of hip arthrogram, 415*f*, 416*f*,
  417*f*
 oblique coronal view, of shoulder, 122*f*, 123*f*,
  124*f*
 oblique sagittal view
  of shoulder, 115*f*
  of shoulder arthrogram, 139*f*
 sagittal view, of hip arthrogram, 409*f*
Lacrimal gland
 axial view
  of brain CT, 7*f*
  of brain MRI, 22*f*

Lacrimal gland *(Continued)*
  coronal view, of brain CT, 13*f*
  sagittal view, of brain MRI, 28*f*
Lamina, axial view, of lumbar spine, 310*f*
Lamina papyracea
 axial view, of brain CT, 7*f*, 8*f*
 coronal view, of brain CT, 13*f*
Laryngeal n., recurrent, axial view, of thorax CT,
  36*f*
Lateral meniscus
 anterior horn, sagittal view, of knee, 455*f*, 456*f*,
  457*f*
 body
  coronal view, of knee, 467*f*, 469*f*
  sagittal view, of knee, 454*f*
 coronal view, of knee, 467*f*
 posterior horn
  coronal view, of knee, 469*f*
  sagittal view, of knee, 455*f*, 456*f*, 457*f*
 sagittal view, of knee, 455*f*
Lateral recess, sagittal view, of thoracic spine,
  301*f*
Lateral rectus m.
 axial view
  of brain CT, 8*f*
  of brain MRI, 22*f*
 coronal view, of brain CT, 13*f*, 14*f*
 sagittal view, of brain MRI, 28*f*, 29*f*
Lateral ventricle body, axial view
 of brain CT, 5*f*
 of brain MRI, 20*f*
Lateral ventricle, sagittal view, of brain MRI, 25*f*,
  26*f*
Latissimus dorsi m.
 axial view
  of abdomen CT, 326*f*, 330*f*, 331*f*
  of abdomen MRI, 346*f*, 347*f*, 348*f*, 349*f*, 350*f*,
   353*f*
  of pectoral girdle and chest wall, 73*f*, 74*f*,
   75*f*, 76*f*, 77*f*
  of shoulder, 108*f*
 coronal view
  of abdomen MRI, 368*f*, 369*f*
  of arm, 171*f*, 172*f*, 173*f*, 174*f*, 175*f*
  of pectoral girdle and chest wall, 92*f*, 93*f*,
   94*f*, 95*f*, 96*f*, 97*f*
  of thoracic spine, 302*f*, 303*f*, 304*f*
 oblique coronal view, of shoulder, 123*f*, 124*f*,
  125*f*, 126*f*, 127*f*, 128*f*
 oblique sagittal view, of shoulder, 114*f*, 115*f*,
  116*f*, 117*f*, 118*f*
 origin, insertion, and nerve supply of, 129*t*,
  306*t*–308*t*
 sagittal view
  of abdomen CT, 332*f*, 333*f*, 337*f*
  of arm, 165*f*, 166*f*, 167*f*
  of pectoral girdle and chest wall, 80*f*, 81*f*,
   82*f*, 83*f*, 84*f*, 85*f*, 86*f*
Latissimus dorsi t.
 axial view
  of pectoral girdle and chest wall, 74*f*
  of shoulder, 107*f*, 108*f*
 coronal view, of arm, 171*f*
 oblique sagittal view, of shoulder, 113*f*, 114*f*
 sagittal view, of arm, 165*f*, 166*f*
Left brachial plexus, coronal view, of cervical
  spine MRI, 294*f*
Left internal carotid a.
 brain CT, 8*f*
 brain MRI, 24*f*
Left vertebral a., axial view, of brain MRI, 24*f*
Lens
 axial view, of brain MRI, 22*f*
 sagittal view, of brain MRI, 26*f*
Lens, coronal view, of brain CT, 13*f*
Lesser saphenous v.
 axial view
  of ankle, 501*f*, 502*f*, 503*f*, 504*f*, 505*f*, 506*f*
  of knee, 447*f*, 448*f*, 449*f*, 450*f*, 452*f*, 453*f*
  of leg, 474*f*, 475*f*, 476*f*, 477*f*, 478*f*, 479*f*
 coronal view
  of ankle, 526*f*, 527*f*, 528*f*, 531*f*, 532*f*
  of leg, 495*f*
 oblique axial view, of ankle, 511*f*, 512*f*, 513*f*
 sagittal view

Lesser saphenous v. *(Continued)*
 of ankle, 517*f*, 518*f*
 of knee, 458*f*
Lesser trochanter
 axial view
  of hip, 381*f*
  of male pelvis CT, 569*f*
  of male pelvis MRI, 600*f*
  of thigh, 420*f*
 coronal view
  of female pelvis MRI, 625*f*
  of hip, 396*f*
  of hip arthrogram, 418*f*
  of male pelvis CT, 576*f*
  of male pelvis MRI, 610*f*
  of thigh, 441*f*
 sagittal view
  of hip, 387*f*, 388*f*
  of thigh, 431*f*, 432*f*
Lesser tuberosity of humerus
 ABER view, of shoulder arthrogram, 148*f*
 axial view
  of pectoral girdle and chest wall, 72*f*
  of shoulder, 104*f*, 105*f*
  of shoulder arthrogram, 133*f*, 134*f*
 coronal view
  of arm, 169*f*
  of pectoral girdle and chest wall, 89*f*, 90*f*
 oblique coronal view
  of shoulder, 122*f*
  of shoulder arthrogram, 142*f*, 143*f*
 oblique sagittal view
  of shoulder, 111*f*
  of shoulder arthrogram, 137*f*, 138*f*
 sagittal view
  of arm, 164*f*, 165*f*
  of pectoral girdle and chest wall, 79*f*
Levator ani m.
 axial view
  of female pelvis CT, 582*f*, 583*f*
  of female pelvis MRI, 617*f*
  of male pelvis CT, 568*f*
  of male pelvis MRI, 599*f*
 coronal view
  of female pelvis CT, 593*f*
  of female pelvis MRI, 625*f*, 626*f*
  of hip, 398*f*
  of male pelvis CT, 577*f*, 578*f*
  of male pelvis MRI, 610*f*, 611*f*, 612*f*
 sagittal view
  of female pelvis CT, 586*f*
  of female pelvis MRI, 619*f*
  of male pelvis CT, 571*f*
  of male pelvis MRI, 603*f*, 604*f*, 605*f*
Levator costae m., coronal view, of pectoral girdle
  and chest wall, 96*f*
Levator scapulae m.
 axial view, of pectoral girdle and chest wall, 70*f*
 coronal view
  of cervical spine MRI, 294*f*, 295*f*
  of pectoral girdle and chest wall, 92*f*, 93*f*,
   94*f*, 95*f*
  of thoracic spine, 303*f*
 origin, insertion, and nerve supply of, 306*t*–308*t*
 sagittal view
  of cervical spine MRI, 291*f*
  of pectoral girdle and chest wall, 85*f*, 86*f*
Ligamentum avum, axial view, of cervical spine
  MRI, 289*f*
Ligamentum flavum
 axial view, of cervical spine MRI, 290*f*
 axial view, of lumbar spine, 310*f*, 314*f*
 sagittal view
  of cervical spine MRI, 293*f*
  of lumbar spine, 316*f*
  of thoracic spine, 301*f*
Ligamentum teres
 coronal view, of abdomen CT, 338*f*
 fissure
  axial view
   of abdomen CT, 327*f*, 328*f*
   of abdomen MRI, 349*f*
  coronal view, of abdomen MRI, 362*f*, 363*f*
  sagittal view, of abdomen MRI, 360*f*
 sagittal view, of abdomen CT, 336*f*

Ligamentum teres femoris
   axial view, of hip arthrogram, 404f, 405f, 406f
   coronal view, of hip arthrogram, 415f, 416f, 417f
   sagittal view, of hip arthrogram, 412f, 413f
Ligamentum venosum
   axial view, of abdomen MRI, 347f
   coronal view, of abdomen CT, 341f
   fissure
      axial view, of abdomen CT, 327f
      sagittal view, of abdomen MRI, 360f
   sagittal view, of abdomen CT, 334f
Linea alba
   axial view
      of abdomen CT, 328f
      of abdomen MRI, 352f, 353f
      of female pelvis CT, 580f, 581f, 582f
      of male pelvis CT, 564f, 565f, 566f
      of male pelvis MRI, 595f, 596f, 597f
   sagittal view, of abdomen MRI, 357f, 358f
Linea aspera, axial view, of thigh, 423f
Linea semilunaris, axial view
   of female pelvis CT, 580f, 581f
   of male pelvis CT, 565f, 566f
   of male pelvis MRI, 596f
Liver
   axial view
      of abdomen CT, 327f, 328f, 329f, 330f
      of abdomen MRI, 346f, 347f, 348f, 349f, 350f, 351f, 352f, 353f
      of heart MRI, 57f
      of thorax CT, 41f, 42f
   coronal view
      of abdomen CT, 338f, 339f, 340f, 341f, 342f, 343f
      of abdomen MRI, 362f, 363f, 364f, 365f, 366f, 368f, 369f
      of heart MRI, 61f, 62f
      of thoracic spine, 302f
      of thorax CT, 47f, 49f, 51f
   sagittal view
      of abdomen CT, 332f, 333f, 334f, 335f, 336f, 337f
      of abdomen MRI, 355f, 356f, 357f, 358f, 359f, 360f, 361f
      of heart MRI, 58f, 60f
      of thorax CT, 44f, 45f, 46f
Longissimus capitis m.
   axial view
      of brain CT, 9f
      of cervical spine MRI, 288f
   origin, insertion, and nerve supply of, 306t–308t
Longissimus cervicis m., origin, insertion, and nerve supply of, 306t–308t
Longissimus dorsi m.
   axial view
      of abdomen CT, 326f, 328f, 330f, 331f
      of male pelvis CT, 564f
   coronal view
      of abdomen CT, 343f
      of female pelvis CT, 593f
      of male pelvis CT, 577f, 578f
   sagittal view
      of abdomen CT, 332f, 333f, 334f, 335f, 336f, 337f
      of male pelvis CT, 571f
Longissimus thoracis m.
   axial view
      of abdomen MRI, 346f, 347f, 348f, 349f, 350f, 351f, 352f, 353f
      of thoracic spine, 297f, 298f
   coronal view
      of abdomen MRI, 369f
      of thoracic spine, 304f
   origin, insertion, and nerve supply of, 306t–308t
   sagittal view
      of abdomen MRI, 356f
      of lumbar spine, 314f, 315f
Longitudinal lig., anterior, sagittal view
   of lumbar spine, 316f
   of thoracic spine, 301f
Longitudinal lig., posterior, sagittal view
   of lumbar spine, 316f
   of thoracic spine, 301f

Longus capitis m.
   axial view
      of brain CT, 9f
      of brain MRI, 24f
      of cervical spine MRI, 288f, 289f
   coronal view, of brain CT, 15f
   sagittal view, of cervical spine MRI, 292f
Longus colli m.
   axial view, of cervical spine MRI, 289f, 290f
   axial view, of pectoral girdle and chest wall, 70f
   sagittal view, of cervical spine MRI, 292f
Lumbar a.
   axial view, of lumbar spine, 310f
   coronal view, of lumbar spine, 317f
Lumbar plexus, coronal view, of female pelvis CT, 592f
Lumbar spine, coronal view, of abdomen MRI, 365f, 366f, 367f
Lumbar triangle
   inferior, axial view, of abdomen CT, 331f
   superior, axial view, of abdomen CT, 330f
Lumbar v.
   axial view
      of abdomen CT, 328f, 329f
      of lumbar spine, 310f
   coronal view, of lumbar spine, 317f
   sagittal view, of abdomen CT, 333f
Lumbar vertebral a., coronal view, of lumbar spine, 318f
Lumbar vertebral v., coronal view, of lumbar spine, 318f
Lumbar vertebral vessels, coronal view, of lumbar spine, 319f
Lumbar vessels, sagittal view, of abdomen CT, 335f
Lumbosacral fascia, dorsal, axial view, of lumbar spine, 313f
Lumbosacral trunk
   axial view, of lumbar spine, 311f, 313f
   coronal view, of lumbar spine, 319f, 320f
   sagittal view, of lumbar spine, 315f
Lumbrical m.
   1st
      axial view, of hand, 266f, 267f
      sagittal view, of hand, 272f, 273f
   2nd
      axial view, of hand, 266f, 267f
      sagittal view, of hand, 273f
   3rd
      axial view, of hand, 266f
      sagittal view, of hand, 274f, 275f
   4th, sagittal view, of hand, 276f
   axial view, of hand, 275f
   coronal view, of hand, 279f, 280f
   origin, insertion, and nerve supply of, 284t
Lumbrical t., axial view, of hand, 268f
Lunate, coronal view, of hand, 280f, 281f, 282f
Lung
   left
      axial view
         of abdomen CT, 326f
         of abdomen MRI, 346f
         of heart MRI, 54f, 56f, 57f
      coronal view
         of abdomen CT, 343f
         of abdomen MRI, 364f, 365f, 366f, 367f, 368f, 369f
         of heart MRI, 61f, 62f, 63f
      sagittal view
         of abdomen CT, 332f, 333f
         of abdomen MRI, 354f, 355f, 356f
         of heart MRI, 58f
         of thoracic spine, 299f, 300f
   right
      axial view
         of abdomen CT, 326f
         of abdomen MRI, 346f
         of heart MRI, 54f, 56f, 57f
         of pectoral girdle and chest wall, 71f, 72f, 73f, 74f
      coronal view
         of abdomen CT, 343f
         of abdomen MRI, 364f, 365f, 366f, 367f, 368f, 369f
         of heart MRI, 61f, 62f, 63f

Lung (Continued)
      of pectoral girdle and chest wall, 89f, 90f, 91f, 92f, 93f, 94f
   sagittal view
      of abdomen CT, 335f, 337f
      of abdomen MRI, 360f, 361f
      of heart MRI, 60f
      of pectoral girdle and chest wall, 83f, 84f, 85f
Lung apex, coronal view, 294f, 295f
Lymph node
   axial view
      of abdomen MRI, 353f
      of hip, 377f, 379f, 380f, 381f
      of male pelvis MRI, 598f, 599f, 600f
      of shoulder, 105f, 106f
   coronal view, of hip, 393f
   oblique coronal view
      of elbow, 203f
      of shoulder, 121f
   oblique sagittal view
      of shoulder, 118f
      of shoulder arthrogram, 140f
   sagittal view
      of hip, 389f, 390f
      of knee, 458f
      of male pelvis MRI, 601f, 602f
      of thigh, 433f

M
Malleolus, lateral
   axial view, of ankle, 504f, 505f, 506f
   coronal view
      of ankle, 528f, 529f, 530f
      of leg, 492f, 493f
   oblique axial view, of ankle, 512f, 513f
   sagittal view
      of ankle, 517f, 518f
      of leg, 485f, 486f
Malleolus, medial
   axial view, of ankle, 504f
   coronal view
      of ankle, 526f, 527f, 528f
      of leg, 492f
   oblique axial view, of ankle, 512f, 513f
   sagittal view
      of ankle, 522f, 523f
      of leg, 489f
Malleolus, posterior, axial view, of ankle, 504f
Mammary a., internal
   axial view, of heart MRI, 54f, 55f, 56f
   sagittal view, of abdomen CT, 336f
Mammary v., internal, axial view, of heart MRI, 54f, 55f, 56f
Mammary vessels, internal, coronal view
   of heart MRI, 61f
   of pectoral girdle and chest wall, 88f
Mammillary body
   axial view, of brain MRI, 22f
   sagittal view, of brain MRI, 25f
Mandible
   axial view
      of brain CT, 9f
      of brain MRI, 24f
      of cervical spine MRI, 288f
   coronal view, of brain CT, 15f
   sagittal view
      of brain CT, 12f
      of brain MRI, 26f, 27f, 29f
Mandibular condyle, axial view
   of brain CT, 8f
   of brain MRI, 23f
Manubrium
   axial view, of thorax CT, 37f
   coronal view, of pectoral girdle and chest wall, 88f, 89f
   sagittal view
      of pectoral girdle and chest wall, 87f
      of thorax CT, 45f, 46f
Masseter m.
   axial view
      of brain CT, 8f
      of brain MRI, 23f, 24f
   coronal view, of brain CT, 15f
   of heart MRI, 61f, 62f, 63f

Masseter m. *(Continued)*
  sagittal view, of brain MRI, 29*f*
Mastoid air cells
  axial view
    of brain CT, 7*f*, 8*f*
    of brain MRI, 23*f*
  coronal view, of brain CT, 16*f*
  sagittal view, of brain CT, 12*f*
Maxillary bone
  axial view, of brain MRI, 24*f*
  sagittal view, of brain MRI, 28*f*
Maxillary bone, axial view, of brain CT, 8*f*, 9*f*
Maxillary sinus
  axial view
    of brain CT, 8*f*, 9*f*
    of brain MRI, 23*f*, 24*f*
  coronal view
    of brain CT, 13*f*, 14*f*
  sagittal view
    of brain CT, 11*f*
    of brain MRI, 26*f*, 28*f*
Meckel cave, axial view, of brain CT, 7*f*
Medial cutaneous n., of forearm, axial view, of
    arm, 156*f*, 157*f*, 159*f*
Medial meniscus
  anterior horn
    coronal view, of knee, 466*f*
    sagittal view, of knee, 460*f*, 461*f*
  body, coronal view, of knee, 467*f*, 468*f*, 469*f*
  posterior horn
    coronal view, of knee, 469*f*
    sagittal view, of knee, 460*f*, 461*f*
  sagittal view, of knee, 462*f*
Medial rectus m.
  axial view
    of brain CT, 8*f*
    of brain MRI, 22*f*
  coronal view, of brain CT, 13*f*, 14*f*
  sagittal view, of brain MRI, 28*f*, 29*f*
Median basilic v.
  axial view
    of elbow, 183*f*, 184*f*, 185*f*, 186*f*, 187*f*, 188*f*,
      189*f*
    of forearm, 209*f*, 210*f*, 211*f*, 212*f*, 213*f*, 214*f*,
      215*f*, 216*f*
  coronal view, of forearm, 225*f*
  oblique coronal, of elbow, 199*f*, 200*f*
  oblique sagittal view, of elbow, 196*f*
Median cubital v.
  axial view, of elbow, 179*f*, 180*f*, 181*f*, 182*f*
  oblique coronal, of elbow, 199*f*, 200*f*, 201*f*, 202*f*
  oblique sagittal view, of elbow, 195*f*, 196*f*
  sagittal view, of forearm, 219*f*
Median n.
  axial view
    of arm, 155*f*, 156*f*, 157*f*, 158*f*, 159*f*, 160*f*
    of elbow, 181*f*, 182*f*, 183*f*, 184*f*, 185*f*, 186*f*,
      187*f*, 188*f*, 189*f*, 190*f*
    of forearm, 209*f*, 210*f*, 211*f*, 212*f*, 213*f*, 214*f*,
      215*f*, 216*f*, 217*f*, 218*f*
    of hand, 262*f*, 263*f*, 264*f*, 265*f*, 266*f*
  coronal view
    of forearm, 227*f*
    of hand, 279*f*
  oblique coronal, of elbow, 192*f*, 193*f*
  oblique sagittal view, of elbow, 195*f*, 196*f*
  sagittal view
    of arm, 165*f*
    of forearm, 220*f*, 221*f*
Median raphe, coronal view, of leg, 496*f*, 497*f*
Median v.
  axial view, of elbow, 179*f*, 180*f*, 181*f*, 182*f*
  sagittal view, of forearm, 219*f*
Medulla
  axial view
    of brain CT, 8*f*
    of brain MRI, 23*f*, 24*f*
  coronal view, of brain CT, 16*f*
  sagittal view
    of brain CT, 10*f*
    of brain MRI, 25*f*, 31*f*
    of cervical spine MRI, 293*f*
Meniscal lig., transverse
  axial view, of knee, 451*f*
  coronal view, of knee, 465*f*

Meniscal lig., transverse *(Continued)*
  sagittal view, of knee, 458*f*
Meniscofemoral (Humphrey's) lig.
  axial view, of knee, 450*f*
  coronal view, of knee, 469*f*
  sagittal view, of knee, 459*f*
Meniscus homologue, coronal view,
    of hand, 281*f*
Mesenteric a., inferior
  axial view
    of abdomen CT, 331*f*
    of male pelvis CT, 564*f*
  coronal view
    of abdomen CT, 339*f*
    of female pelvis CT, 590*f*
    of male pelvis CT, 575*f*
  sagittal view, of abdomen CT, 334*f*
Mesenteric a., superior
  axial view
    of abdomen CT, 328*f*, 329*f*, 330*f*
    of abdomen MRI, 350*f*, 351*f*, 352*f*, 353*f*
  coronal view
    of abdomen CT, 339*f*, 340*f*, 341*f*
    of abdomen MRI, 364*f*, 365*f*, 366*f*
    of female pelvis CT, 589*f*
    of male pelvis CT, 574*f*
    of thorax CT, 47*f*, 48*f*, 49*f*
  sagittal view
    of abdomen CT, 334*f*
    of abdomen MRI, 357*f*, 358*f*
    of female pelvis CT, 586*f*
    of thorax CT, 44*f*
Mesenteric v., inferior
  coronal view
    of abdomen CT, 339*f*, 340*f*, 341*f*
    of male pelvis CT, 574*f*
  sagittal view, of abdomen CT, 333*f*
Mesenteric v., superior
  axial view
    of abdomen CT, 329*f*, 330*f*
    of abdomen MRI, 351*f*, 352*f*, 353*f*
  coronal view
    of abdomen CT, 339*f*
    of abdomen MRI, 364*f*
    of female pelvis CT, 589*f*
  sagittal view
    of abdomen CT, 334*f*
    of female pelvis CT, 586*f*
Mesenteric vessels
  axial view
    of abdomen CT, 330*f*, 331*f*
    of male pelvis CT, 564*f*
  sagittal view
    of abdomen CT, 332*f*, 334*f*
    of abdomen MRI, 355*f*, 356*f*, 357*f*
Mesentery
  axial view
    of abdomen CT, 330*f*, 331*f*
    of male pelvis CT, 564*f*
  coronal view
    of abdomen CT, 338*f*
    of female pelvis CT, 589*f*
  sagittal view, of abdomen CT, 332*f*, 334*f*
Mesocolon, sigmoid
  axial view, of male pelvis CT, 566*f*
  sagittal view, of abdomen CT, 334*f*
Metacarpal
  1st
    axial view, of hand, 262*f*, 263*f*, 264*f*, 265*f*
    coronal view, of hand, 280*f*
    sagittal view, of hand, 269*f*, 270*f*, 271*f*
  2nd
    axial view, of hand, 262*f*, 263*f*, 264*f*, 265*f*
    sagittal view, of hand, 271*f*, 272*f*, 273*f*, 274*f*
  3rd
    axial view, of hand, 262*f*, 263*f*
    sagittal view, of hand, 273*f*, 274*f*
  4th
    axial view, of hand, 262*f*, 263*f*
    sagittal view, of hand, 274*f*
  5th
    axial view, of hand, 262*f*, 263*f*
    sagittal view, of hand, 275*f*, 276*f*, 277*f*
Metacarpal a., palmar, axial view, of hand, 263*f*,
    264*f*, 265*f*

Metacarpal base
  1st, coronal view, of hand, 279*f*
  2nd, coronal view, of hand, 281*f*, 282*f*
  3rd, coronal view, of hand, 281*f*, 282*f*
  4th, coronal view, of hand, 281*f*, 282*f*
  5th, coronal view, of hand, 281*f*
Metacarpal head
  2nd, axial view, of hand, 268*f*
  3rd
    axial view, of hand, 268*f*
    sagittal view, of hand, 275*f*
  4th, sagittal view, of hand, 275*f*, 276*f*
  5th
    coronal view, of hand, 281*f*
    sagittal view, of hand, 276*f*, 277*f*
Metacarpophalangeal joint
  axial view, of hand, 265*f*
  sagittal view, of hand, 270*f*, 272*f*, 274*f*, 276*f*,
    277*f*
Metatarsal
  1st
    axial view, of foot, 535*f*, 536*f*, 537*f*, 538*f*
    coronal view, of foot, 545*f*, 546*f*
    sagittal view, of foot, 550*f*, 551*f*
  2nd
    axial view, of foot, 535*f*, 536*f*, 537*f*
    coronal view, of foot, 544*f*, 545*f*, 546*f*
    sagittal view, of foot, 550*f*, 551*f*
  3rd
    axial view, of foot, 537*f*, 538*f*
    coronal view, of foot, 551*f*, 552*f*, 553*f*, 554*f*,
      555*f*
    sagittal view, of foot, 543*f*
  4th
    axial view, of foot, 538*f*
    coronal view, of foot, 551*f*, 552*f*, 553*f*, 554*f*,
      555*f*
    sagittal view, of foot, 542*f*
  5th
    axial view
      of ankle, 508*f*, 509*f*
      of foot, 539*f*
    coronal view, of foot, 551*f*, 552*f*, 553*f*, 554*f*,
      555*f*
    sagittal view, of foot, 541*f*
Metatarsal base
  1st
    axial view, of foot, 535*f*, 537*f*
    sagittal view, of foot, 545*f*, 546*f*
  2nd
    axial view, of foot, 535*f*
    sagittal view, of foot, 544*f*
  3rd
    axial view, of foot, 536*f*
    sagittal view
      of ankle, 521*f*
      of foot, 542*f*, 543*f*, 544*f*
  4th
    axial view, of foot, 537*f*, 538*f*
    sagittal view
      of ankle, 519*f*, 520*f*, 521*f*
      of foot, 541*f*, 542*f*, 543*f*
  5th
    axial view
      of ankle, 509*f*, 510*f*
      of foot, 538*f*, 540*f*
    coronal view, of foot, 556*f*
    sagittal view
      of ankle, 519*f*, 520*f*
      of foot, 541*f*
Metatarsal head
  1st
    axial view, of foot, 538*f*, 539*f*
    coronal view, of foot, 550*f*
    sagittal view, of foot, 547*f*, 548*f*
  2nd
    axial view, of foot, 538*f*, 539*f*
    coronal view, of foot, 550*f*
    sagittal view, of foot, 545*f*, 546*f*
  3rd
    axial view, of foot, 538*f*, 539*f*
    coronal view, of foot, 550*f*
    sagittal view, of foot, 544*f*
  4th
    axial view, of foot, 538*f*, 539*f*

Metatarsal head *(Continued)*
  coronal view, of foot, 550*f*
  sagittal view, of foot, 543*f*
  5th
    axial view, of foot, 540*f*
    coronal view, of foot, 550*f*, 551*f*
    sagittal view, of foot, 541*f*
Metatarsophalangeal joint
  1st, coronal view, of foot, 549*f*, 550*f*
  2nd, coronal view, of foot, 549*f*
  3rd, coronal view, of foot, 549*f*
  4th, coronal view, of foot, 550*f*
Midbrain
  axial view
    of brain CT, 6*f*, 7*f*
    of brain MRI, 22*f*
  coronal view, of brain CT, 15*f*, 16*f*
  sagittal view
    of brain CT, 10*f*
    of brain MRI, 25*f*, 31*f*
Middle cerebellar peduncle
  axial view, of brain MRI, 23*f*
  sagittal view, of brain MRI, 25*f*
Middle cerebral a.
  axial view, of brain CT, 7*f*
  coronal view, of brain CT, 15*f*
Middle frontal gyrus, of brain MRI, 19*f*
Middle nasal conchae
  coronal view, of brain CT, 13*f*
  sagittal view, of brain MRI, 28*f*, 29*f*
Middle phalanx
  index finger, sagittal view, 271*f*
  long finger
    coronal view, 280*f*
    sagittal view, 273*f*, 274*f*
  ring finger
    coronal view, 280*f*
    sagittal view, 276*f*
  small finger
    coronal view, 280*f*, 281*f*
    sagittal view, 277*f*, 278*f*
Middle scalene m., coronal view, of cervical spine
    MRI, 294*f*
Mitral valve, axial view, of heart MRI, 56*f*
Mitral valve plana
  axial view, of thorax CT, 40*f*
  coronal view, of thorax CT, 49*f*
Moderator band, axial view, of thorax CT, 40*f*
Mons pubis
  axial view, of female pelvis CT, 588*f*
  coronal view
    of female pelvis CT, 588*f*
    of female pelvis MRI, 622*f*
Multifidus and rotatores mm., axial view, of
    cervical spine MRI, 290*f*
Multifidus m.
  axial view
    of abdomen CT, 326*f*, 328*f*, 331*f*
    of abdomen MRI, 346*f*, 347*f*, 348*f*, 349*f*, 350*f*,
      351*f*, 352*f*, 353*f*
    of cervical spine MRI, 289*f*
    of lumbar spine, 310*f*, 311*f*, 312*f*, 313*f*
    of pectoral girdle and chest wall, 68*f*, 69*f*
    of thoracic spine, 297*f*
  coronal view
    of abdomen CT, 343*f*
    of abdomen MRI, 369*f*
    of female pelvis CT, 593*f*
    of lumbar spine, 321*f*, 322*f*
    of male pelvis CT, 577*f*, 578*f*
    of male pelvis MRI, 611*f*
    origin, insertion, and nerve supply of,
      306*t*–308*t*
    of pectoral girdle and chest wall, 92*f*, 94*f*
  sagittal view
    of abdomen CT, 335*f*
    of abdomen MRI, 357*f*, 358*f*
    of female pelvis CT, 586*f*, 587*f*
    of lumbar spine, 314*f*, 315*f*, 316*f*
Musculocutaneous n., axial view
  of arm, 156*f*
  of elbow, 179*f*, 180*f*, 181*f*
Myometrium
  junctional zone
    axial view, of female pelvis MRI, 615*f*

Myometrium *(Continued)*
    coronal view, of female pelvis MRI, 623*f*, 624*f*
    sagittal view, of female pelvis MRI, 621*f*
  peripheral zone
    axial view, of female pelvis MRI, 615*f*
    coronal view, of female pelvis MRI, 623*f*, 624*f*
    sagittal view, of female pelvis MRI, 621*f*

N
Nail, sagittal view, of hand, 275*f*
Nasal bone, axial view, of brain CT, 8*f*, 9*f*
Nasal cavity
  axial view, of brain MRI, 23*f*, 24*f*
  coronal view, of brain CT, 13*f*, 14*f*
  sagittal view, of brain MRI, 28*f*
Nasal septum, axial view, of brain CT, 8*f*, 9*f*
Nasolacrimal canal, axial view, of brain CT, 8*f*
Nasopharyn, axial view, of brain CT, 9*f*
Navicular
  axial view
    of ankle, 505*f*, 506*f*
    of foot, 535*f*, 536*f*
  coronal view
    of ankle, 524*f*, 525*f*
    of foot, 557*f*
  oblique axial view, of ankle, 515*f*
  sagittal view
    of ankle, 520*f*, 521*f*, 522*f*, 523*f*
    of foot, 544*f*, 545*f*, 546*f*, 547*f*
Navicular tuberosity, sagittal view, of foot, 547*f*
Nerve root, coronal view, of thorax CT, 52*f*
Neural foramina
  coronal view, of thorax CT, 52*f*
  sagittal view, of abdomen MRI, 357*f*
Neuroforamen, lateral, sagittal view, of thoracic
      spine, 300*f*, 301*f*
Neurovascular bundle
  axial view, of pectoral girdle and chest wall, 76*f*
  sagittal view, of pectoral girdle and chest wall,
      81*f*
Nuchal lig
  axial view, of cervical spine MRI, 288*f*
  sagittal view, of cervical spine MRI, 293*f*
Nutrient a., axial view, of thigh, 423*f*

O
Oblique m., external
  axial view
    of abdomen CT, 328*f*, 329*f*, 331*f*
    of abdomen MRI, 350*f*, 351*f*
    of male pelvis CT, 564*f*, 565*f*
    of male pelvis MRI, 595*f*
  coronal view
    of abdomen CT, 338*f*, 340*f*, 341*f*, 343*f*
    of abdomen MRI, 363*f*, 364*f*, 365*f*, 366*f*
    of female pelvis CT, 589*f*, 590*f*
    of male pelvis CT, 573*f*, 574*f*, 575*f*, 576*f*
    origin, insertion, and nerve supply of, 344*t*
Oblique m., internal
  axial view
    of abdomen CT, 329*f*, 331*f*
    of hip, 374*f*
    of male pelvis CT, 564*f*, 565*f*
    of male pelvis MRI, 595*f*
  coronal view
    of abdomen CT, 338*f*, 340*f*, 341*f*
    of abdomen MRI, 363*f*, 364*f*, 365*f*, 366*f*, 367*f*
    of female pelvis CT, 589*f*, 590*f*
    of female pelvis MRI, 622*f*
    of hip, 393*f*
    of male pelvis CT, 573*f*, 574*f*, 575*f*, 576*f*
    origin, insertion, and nerve supply of, 344*t*
  sagittal view, of abdomen CT, 332*f*
Obturator a.
  axial view, of male pelvis CT, 567*f*
  coronal view, of male pelvis CT, 576*f*
  sagittal view, of hip, 392*f*
Obturator externus m.
  axial view
    of female pelvis CT, 583*f*, 584*f*
    of female pelvis MRI, 617*f*
    of hip, 378*f*, 379*f*
    of male pelvis CT, 568*f*, 569*f*

Obturator externus m. *(Continued)*
    of male pelvis MRI, 599*f*
  coronal view
    of female pelvis CT, 590*f*, 591*f*, 592*f*
    of female pelvis MRI, 623*f*, 624*f*
    of hip, 394*f*, 395*f*, 396*f*, 397*f*
    of male pelvis CT, 575*f*, 576*f*, 577*f*
    of male pelvis MRI, 608*f*, 609*f*, 610*f*
    origin, insertion, and nerve supply of, 400*t*–401*t*
  sagittal view
    of female pelvis CT, 585*f*, 586*f*
    of female pelvis MRI, 618*f*, 619*f*
    of hip, 389*f*, 390*f*, 391*f*, 392*f*
    of male pelvis CT, 570*f*, 571*f*
    of male pelvis MRI, 601*f*, 602*f*, 603*f*, 604*f*
    of thigh, 433*f*, 434*f*, 435*f*, 436*f*
Obturator externus t.
  axial view
    of hip, 378*f*
    of hip arthrogram, 405*f*
  coronal view
    of hip, 396*f*, 397*f*
    of hip arthrogram, 418*f*
  sagittal view, of hip, 386*f*, 387*f*
Obturator foramen, sagittal view
  of hip, 392*f*
  of male pelvis MRI, 602*f*
Obturator internus m.
  axial view
    of female pelvis CT, 582*f*, 583*f*
    of female pelvis MRI, 615*f*, 616*f*, 617*f*
    of hip, 375*f*, 376*f*, 377*f*, 378*f*, 379*f*
    of male pelvis CT, 566*f*, 567*f*, 568*f*
    of male pelvis MRI, 597*f*, 598*f*, 599*f*
  coronal view
    of female pelvis CT, 590*f*, 591*f*, 592*f*, 593*f*
    of female pelvis MRI, 623*f*, 624*f*, 625*f*
    of hip, 395*f*, 396*f*, 397*f*
    of male pelvis CT, 575*f*, 576*f*, 577*f*
    of male pelvis MRI, 609*f*
    origin, insertion, and nerve supply of, 400*t*–401*t*
  sagittal view
    of female pelvis CT, 585*f*, 586*f*
    of female pelvis MRI, 618*f*, 619*f*
    of hip, 386*f*, 387*f*, 388*f*, 389*f*, 390*f*, 391*f*, 392*f*
    of male pelvis CT, 570*f*, 571*f*
    of male pelvis MRI, 602*f*, 603*f*, 604*f*
    of thigh, 436*f*.
Obturator internus t.
  axial view
    of female pelvis CT, 582*f*
    of hip, 377*f*, 378*f*
    of hip arthrogram, 406*f*
    of male pelvis CT, 568*f*
    of male pelvis MRI, 598*f*
  coronal view
    of female pelvis CT, 592*f*
    of female pelvis MRI, 625*f*
    of hip arthrogram, 418*f*
    of male pelvis CT, 577*f*
    of male pelvis MRI, 611*f*
  sagittal view
    of hip, 387*f*
    of hip arthrogram, 409*f*, 410*f*, 411*f*, 412*f*,
      413*f*
Obturator n.
  axial view
    of female pelvis CT, 583*f*
    of female pelvis MRI, 616*f*
    of lumbar spine, 313*f*
    of male pelvis CT, 568*f*
  coronal view
    of lumbar spine, 318*f*
    of male pelvis CT, 575*f*
  sagittal view
    of female pelvis MRI, 618*f*
    of hip, 392*f*
    of male pelvis CT, 570*f*
Obturator v.
  axial view, of male pelvis CT, 567*f*
  coronal view, of male pelvis CT, 576*f*
  sagittal view, of hip, 392*f*
Obturator vessels
  axial view
    of female pelvis CT, 583*f*

Obturator vessels (Continued)
 of female pelvis MRI, 616f
 of male pelvis CT, 568f
 sagittal view, of female pelvis MRI, 618f
Occipital bone
 coronal view, of cervical spine MRI, 294f
 sagittal view, of cervical spine MRI, 291f, 292f, 293f
Occipital condyle
 coronal view
  of brain CT, 16f
  of cervical spine MRI, 294f
 sagittal view
  of brain MRI, 31f
  of cervical spine MRI, 292f
Occipital lobe
 axial view
  of brain CT, 5f, 6f
  of brain MRI, 20f, 21f, 22f
 coronal view, of brain CT, 16f, 17f
 sagittal view
  of brain CT, 10f, 11f, 12f
  of brain MRI, 25f, 26f, 27f, 31f, 32f
  of cervical spine MRI, 291f, 292f
Occiput, axial view, of brain MRI, 24f
Olecranon
 axial view, of elbow, 180f, 181f, 182f, 183f, 184f
 coronal view, of arm, 171f, 172f
 oblique coronal view, of elbow, 205f, 206f, 207f
 oblique sagittal view, of elbow, 194f, 195f, 196f
 sagittal view, of arm, 164f, 165f
Olecranon fossa
 axial view, of elbow, 180f, 181f, 183f
 coronal view, of arm, 171f
 oblique coronal, of elbow, 205f
 oblique sagittal view, of elbow, 195f
 sagittal view, of arm, 164f, 165f
Omental vessels
 coronal view, of abdomen CT, 338f
 sagittal view, of abdomen CT, 334f, 335f
Omentum
 coronal view, of abdomen CT, 338f
 sagittal view, of abdomen CT, 334f, 335f
Omohyoid m., inferior
 axial view, of shoulder, 101f
 coronal view, of pectoral girdle and chest wall, 90f, 91f
 oblique coronal view, of shoulder, 119f, 120f
 sagittal view, of pectoral girdle and chest wall, 83f, 84f
Omohyoid t., inferior
 axial view, of shoulder, 101f, 102f
 coronal view, of pectoral girdle and chest wall, 91f
 oblique coronal view, of shoulder, 120f
 sagittal view, of pectoral girdle and chest wall, 83f, 84f
Opponens digiti minimi m.
 axial view, of hand, 262f, 263f, 264f, 265f
 coronal view
  of foot, 552f, 555f
  of hand, 279f, 280f, 281f
 origin, insertion, and nerve supply of, 284t, 558t–560t
 sagittal view, of hand, 274f, 275f, 276f, 277f
Opponens pollicis brevis m., axial view, of hand, 262f, 263f, 264f
Opponens pollicis m.
 coronal view, of hand, 279f
 origin, insertion, and nerve supply of, 284t
 sagittal view, of hand, 271f, 272f, 273f
Optic chiasm
 axial view
  of brain CT, 7f
  of brain MRI, 22f
 sagittal view
  of brain CT, 10f
  of brain MRI, 25f
Optic nerve
 axial view
  of brain CT, 8f
  of brain MRI, 22f
 coronal view, of brain CT, 14f
 sagittal view
  of brain CT, 11f

Optic nerve (Continued)
 of brain MRI, 26f, 28f, 29f
Optic tract, of brain MRI, 30f
Os, internal, axial view, of female pelvis MRI, 615f
Ovary
 axial view
  of female pelvis CT, 580f, 581f
  of female pelvis MRI, 615f
 coronal view
  of female pelvis CT, 591f, 592f
  of female pelvis MRI, 624f
 sagittal view
  of female pelvis CT, 585f, 586f
  of female pelvis MRI, 618f

P
Palmar aponeurosis
 axial view
  of hand, 262f, 263f, 264f, 265f
  of wrist, 244f
 coronal view, of hand, 279f
 sagittal view
  of hand, 273f, 274f
  of wrist, 248f, 249f
Palmar arch, deep
 axial view
  of hand, 262f, 263f
  of wrist, 244f
 coronal view, of hand, 280f, 281f
 sagittal view, of wrist, 245f, 246f, 247f, 248f, 249f, 250f
Palmar arch, sagittal view, of wrist, 246f, 249f, 250f
Palmar arch, superficial
 axial view, of hand, 262f, 263f
 coronal view, of hand, 279f
 sagittal view, of wrist, 246f, 249f, 250f
Palmar digital a., common, sagittal view of, 246f, 257f
Palmar v., sagittal view, of wrist, 248f
Palmaris brevis m.
 axial view, of hand, 262f, 263f
 coronal view
  of hand, 279f
  of wrist, 254f
 origin, insertion, and nerve supply of, 284t
 sagittal view, of wrist, 250f, 251f, 252f
Palmaris longus m.
 axial view
  of elbow, 183f, 184f, 185f, 186f, 187f, 188f, 189f
  of forearm, 209f, 210f, 211f, 212f, 213f
 coronal view, of forearm, 225f
 oblique coronal, of elbow, 200f, 201f, 202f
 oblique sagittal view, of elbow, 197f, 198f
 origin, insertion, and nerve supply of, 233t–234t
 sagittal view, of forearm, 222f, 223f
Palmaris longus t.
 axial view
  of forearm, 214f, 215f, 216f, 217f, 218f
  of wrist, 236f, 237f, 238f, 239f, 240f, 241f, 242f, 243f
 coronal view
  of forearm, 225f, 226f, 227f
  of hand, 279f
  of wrist, 254f
 sagittal view, of wrist, 248f, 249f
Pancreas
 axial view
  of abdomen CT, 328f, 329f
  of abdomen MRI, 348f
 body
  axial view
   of abdomen CT, 329f
   of abdomen MRI, 348f, 349f, 350f
  coronal view
   of abdomen CT, 339f, 340f, 341f
   of abdomen MRI, 364f, 365f, 366f
  sagittal view
   of abdomen CT, 333f, 334f
   of abdomen MRI, 356f, 357f, 358f
 head
  axial view
   of abdomen CT, 329f

Pancreas (Continued)
 of abdomen MRI, 350f, 351f, 352f, 353f
 coronal view
  of abdomen CT, 339f, 340f
  of abdomen MRI, 364f, 365f, 366f
  of thorax CT, 47f
 sagittal view
  of abdomen CT, 335f, 336f
  of abdomen MRI, 359f, 360f, 361f
 neck
  axial view, of abdomen CT, 328f
  coronal view, of abdomen CT, 339f
  sagittal view, of abdomen CT, 334f
 tail
  axial view
   of abdomen CT, 329f
   of abdomen MRI, 349f, 350f
  coronal view
   of abdomen CT, 341f, 342f, 343f
   of abdomen MRI, 366f, 367f, 368f
  sagittal view
   of abdomen CT, 332f
   of abdomen MRI, 354f, 355f
Pancreatic duct
 axial view, of abdomen CT, 329f
 coronal view
  of abdomen CT, 340f
  of abdomen MRI, 364f
Pancreaticoduodenal v., superior, sagittal view, of abdomen CT, 335f
Papillary m., anterior
 axial view, of thorax CT, 40f
 coronal view, of thorax CT, 47f
Papillary m., left ventricular, coronal view, of thorax CT, 48f
Papillary m., posterior
 axial view, of thorax CT, 41f
 sagittal view, of thorax CT, 43f
Parametrium, sagittal view
 of female pelvis CT, 586f
 of female pelvis MRI, 619f, 620f
Parietal lobe
 axial view
  of brain CT, 4f, 5f, 6f
  of brain MRI, 19f, 20f, 21f
 coronal view, of brain CT, 15f, 16f, 17f
 sagittal view
  of brain CT, 10f, 11f, 12f
  of brain MRI, 25f, 26f, 27f, 30f, 31f, 32f
Parotid gland
 axial view
  of brain CT, 9f
  of cervical spine MRI, 288f
 coronal view, of cervical spine MRI, 294f
 sagittal view
  of brain MRI, 30f
  of cervical spine MRI, 291f
Patella
 axial view, of knee, 449f, 450f
 coronal view, of knee, 463f
 sagittal view, of knee, 455f, 456f, 457f, 458f, 459f
 upper pole, axial view, of knee, 448f
Patellar facet
 lateral, axial view, of knee, 449f
 medial, axial view, of knee, 449f
Patellar lig., sagittal view, of leg, 486f, 487f, 488f
Patellar retinaculum
 coronal view, of knee, 463f
 lateral
  axial view, of knee, 448f, 449f, 451f
  coronal view, of knee, 463f, 464f, 465f
 medial
  axial view, of knee, 448f, 449f, 450f
  coronal view, of knee, 463f, 464f, 465f, 466f
 sagittal view, of knee, 460f
Patellar t., axial view, of knee, 450f, 451f, 452f, 453f
Pectineus m.
 axial view
  of female pelvis CT, 583f, 584f
  of female pelvis MRI, 617f
  of hip, 377f, 378f, 379f, 380f
  of male pelvis CT, 568f, 569f

Pectineus m. *(Continued)*
  of male pelvis MRI, 598*f*, 599*f*, 600*f*
  of thigh, 420*f*
  coronal view
    of female pelvis CT, 589*f*, 590*f*, 591*f*
    of female pelvis MRI, 622*f*, 623*f*
    of hip, 394*f*, 395*f*
    of male pelvis CT, 574*f*, 575*f*, 576*f*
    of male pelvis MRI, 608*f*, 609*f*
  origin, insertion, and nerve supply of, 445*t*
  sagittal view
    of female pelvis CT, 585*f*, 586*f*
    of female pelvis MRI, 618*f*
    of hip, 388*f*, 389*f*, 390*f*, 391*f*, 392*f*
    of male pelvis CT, 570*f*
    of male pelvis MRI, 601*f*, 602*f*, 603*f*
    of thigh, 433*f*, 434*f*, 435*f*, 436*f*
Pectoralis major m.
  ABER view, of shoulder arthrogram, 148*f*, 149*f*,
    150*f*
  axial view
    of heart MRI, 54*f*
    of shoulder, 103*f*, 104*f*, 105*f*, 106*f*, 107*f*, 108*f*
  coronal view
    of arm, 168*f*
    of pectoral girdle and chest wall, 90*f*
  oblique coronal view, of shoulder, 119*f*, 120*f*
  oblique sagittal view, of shoulder, 112*f*, 113*f*,
    114*f*, 115*f*, 116*f*, 117*f*, 118*f*
  origin, insertion, and nerve supply of, 129*t*
  sagittal view
    of arm, 167*f*
    of pectoral girdle and chest wall, 80*f*, 82*f*,
      83*f*, 84*f*
Pectoralis major m., clavicular head
  axial view, of pectoral girdle and chest wall,
    71*f*, 72*f*, 73*f*
  coronal view, of pectoral girdle and chest wall,
    88*f*, 89*f*
  sagittal view, of pectoral girdle and chest wall,
    81*f*, 82*f*, 84*f*, 85*f*, 86*f*
Pectoralis major m. costosternal head
  axial view, of pectoral girdle and chest wall,
    74*f*, 75*f*, 76*f*
  sagittal view, of pectoral girdle and chest wall,
    87*f*
Pectoralis major m., sternoclavicular head
  axial view, of pectoral girdle and chest wall, 73*f*
Pectoralis major m., sternocostal head
  axial view, of pectoral girdle and chest wall, 74*f*
  coronal view, of pectoral girdle and chest wall,
    88*f*, 89*f*
  sagittal view, of pectoral girdle and chest wall,
    81*f*, 82*f*, 84*f*, 85*f*, 86*f*
Pectoralis major t.
  axial view, of pectoral girdle and chest wall,
    74*f*, 75*f*
  oblique coronal view, of shoulder, 120*f*
  sagittal view
    of arm, 164*f*, 166*f*
    of pectoral girdle and chest wall, 79*f*
Pectoralis minor m.
  axial view
    of heart MRI, 54*f*
    of pectoral girdle and chest wall, 72*f*, 73*f*,
      74*f*, 75*f*, 76*f*, 77*f*
    of shoulder, 104*f*, 105*f*, 106*f*, 107*f*, 108*f*
  coronal view, of pectoral girdle and chest wall,
    90*f*
  oblique sagittal view, of shoulder, 116*f*, 117*f*,
    118*f*
  origin, insertion, and nerve supply of, 129*t*
  sagittal view, of pectoral girdle and chest wall,
    82*f*, 83*f*, 84*f*
Pectoralis minor t.
  axial view
    of pectoral girdle and chest wall, 71*f*
    of shoulder arthrogram, 133*f*, 134*f*
  long head, axial view, of shoulder, 104*f*
  oblique coronal view, of shoulder, 119*f*
  oblique sagittal view, of shoulder, 115*f*, 116*f*
Pedicle
  axial view, of lumbar spine, 310*f*
  coronal view, of thorax CT, 52*f*
  sagittal view, of abdomen MRI, 357*f*

Penis
  axial view
    of male pelvis CT, 568*f*, 569*f*
    of male pelvis MRI, 600*f*
  bulb, axial view, of male pelvis CT, 569*f*
  coronal view
    of male pelvis CT, 573*f*, 574*f*, 575*f*, 576*f*
    of male pelvis MRI, 607*f*, 608*f*, 609*f*
  coronal view, of male pelvis CT, 576*f*, 577*f*
  sagittal view
    of male pelvis CT, 571*f*, 572*f*
    of male pelvis MRI, 604*f*, 605*f*, 606*f*
Pericardial fat, sagittal view, of abdomen CT, 332*f*
Pericardium
  axial view, of thorax CT, 39*f*, 40*f*, 41*f*, 42*f*
  sagittal view, of abdomen CT, 332*f*
Periprostatic venous plexus, sagittal view, of male
    pelvis CT, 571*f*
Perirenal fascia, coronal view, of abdomen CT,
    342*f*
Perivesical venous plexus, sagittal view, of male
    pelvis CT, 571*f*
Peroneal a.
  axial view, of ankle, 501*f*
  oblique axial view, of ankle, 512*f*
Peroneal n., common
  axial view
    of knee, 447*f*, 448*f*, 449*f*, 450*f*, 451*f*, 452*f*,
      453*f*
    of leg, 474*f*
    of thigh, 426*f*, 427*f*
  coronal view, of knee, 470*f*, 471*f*, 472*f*
  sagittal view
    of knee, 454*f*, 455*f*, 456*f*
    of leg, 484*f*
Peroneal n., communicating, axial view, of knee,
    448*f*, 449*f*, 450*f*
Peroneal n., deep
  axial view
    of ankle, 501*f*, 502*f*
    of leg, 475*f*
  coronal view, of leg, 493*f*
  oblique axial view, of ankle, 512*f*, 513*f*, 514*f*
Peroneal n., superficial
  axial view, of leg, 475*f*, 476*f*
  oblique axial view, of ankle, 512*f*
Peroneal retinaculum
  inferior
    axial view, of ankle, 506*f*
    coronal view, of ankle, 528*f*, 529*f*
  oblique axial view, of ankle, 513*f*
  superior, axial view, of ankle, 503*f*, 504*f*, 505*f*
Peroneal sulcus, sagittal view, of foot, 541*f*, 542*f*
Peroneal tubercle
  axial view, of ankle, 508*f*
  coronal view, of ankle, 528*f*, 529*f*
Peroneal v.
  axial view, of ankle, 501*f*
  oblique axial view, of ankle, 512*f*
Peroneal vessels, axial view, of leg, 475*f*, 476*f*,
    477*f*, 478*f*, 479*f*, 480*f*, 481*f*, 483*f*
Peroneus brevis m.
  axial view
    of ankle, 501*f*, 502*f*, 503*f*, 504*f*, 505*f*
    of leg, 476*f*, 477*f*, 478*f*, 479*f*, 480*f*, 481*f*, 482*f*,
      483*f*
  coronal view
    of ankle, 530*f*, 531*f*
    of leg, 494*f*
  oblique axial view, of ankle, 511*f*, 512*f*
  origin, insertion, and nerve supply of,
    498*t*–499*t*
  sagittal view
    of ankle, 517*f*, 518*f*
    of leg, 484*f*, 485*f*
Peroneus brevis t.
  axial view
    of ankle, 501*f*, 502*f*, 503*f*, 504*f*, 505*f*, 506*f*,
      507*f*, 508*f*, 509*f*
    of foot, 538*f*, 539*f*
    of leg, 477*f*, 478*f*, 479*f*, 480*f*, 481*f*, 482*f*, 483*f*
  coronal view
    of ankle, 524*f*, 525*f*, 526*f*, 527*f*, 528*f*, 529*f*,
      530*f*, 531*f*
    of foot, 557*f*

Peroneus brevis t. *(Continued)*
  oblique axial view, of ankle, 511*f*, 512*f*, 513*f*,
    514*f*, 515*f*, 516*f*
  sagittal view
    of ankle, 517*f*, 518*f*
    of foot, 541*f*
    of leg, 484*f*, 485*f*
Peroneus longus m.
  axial view
    of knee, 453*f*
    of leg, 474*f*, 475*f*, 476*f*, 477*f*, 478*f*, 479*f*, 480*f*,
      481*f*, 482*f*, 483*f*
  coronal view
    of knee, 469*f*, 470*f*, 471*f*, 472*f*
    of leg, 494*f*, 495*f*
  origin, insertion, and nerve supply of, 498*t*–499*t*
  sagittal view
    of knee, 454*f*, 455*f*
    of leg, 484*f*, 485*f*, 486*f*
Peroneus longus t.
  axial view
    of ankle, 501*f*, 502*f*, 503*f*, 504*f*, 505*f*, 506*f*,
      507*f*, 508*f*, 509*f*
    of foot, 537*f*, 538*f*, 539*f*
    of leg, 477*f*, 478*f*, 479*f*, 480*f*, 481*f*, 482*f*, 483*f*
  coronal view
    of ankle, 524*f*, 525*f*, 526*f*, 527*f*, 528*f*, 529*f*,
      530*f*, 531*f*
    of foot, 555*f*, 556*f*, 557*f*
    of leg, 494*f*, 495*f*
  oblique axial view, of ankle, 511*f*, 512*f*, 513*f*,
    514*f*, 515*f*, 516*f*
  sagittal view
    of ankle, 517*f*, 518*f*, 519*f*, 520*f*
    of foot, 541*f*, 542*f*, 543*f*
    of leg, 484*f*, 486*f*
Peroneus quartus m.
  axial view, of ankle, 504*f*, 505*f*, 506*f*
  coronal view, of ankle, 530*f*, 531*f*
  sagittal view, of ankle, 518*f*
Peroneus quartus t.
  axial view, of ankle, 507*f*
  coronal view, of ankle, 530*f*
Peroneus tertius m.
  oblique axial view, of ankle, 512*f*, 513*f*
  origin, insertion, and nerve supply of, 498*t*–499*t*
Peroneus tertius t., oblique axial view, of ankle,
    515*f*, 516*f*
Pes anserinus
  axial view, of knee, 453*f*
  coronal view, of knee, 467*f*
  sagittal view, of knee, 462*f*
Petrous apex of temporal bone, axial view, of
    brain CT, 8*f*
Pharynx
  axial view, of cervical spine MRI, 288*f*, 289*f*
  sagittal view
    of brain MRI, 30*f*
    of cervical spine MRI, 292*f*, 293*f*
Pineal gland
  axial view
    of brain CT, 6*f*
    of brain MRI, 21*f*
  coronal view, of brain CT, 16*f*
  sagittal view
    of brain CT, 10*f*
    of brain MRI, 25*f*, 31*f*
Piriformis m.
  axial view
    of female pelvis CT, 580*f*, 581*f*
    of female pelvis MRI, 614*f*, 615*f*
    of hip, 374*f*, 375*f*, 376*f*
    of male pelvis CT, 565*f*, 566*f*
    of male pelvis MRI, 596*f*, 597*f*
  coronal view
    of female pelvis CT, 593*f*
    of female pelvis MRI, 625*f*, 626*f*
    of hip, 398*f*, 399*f*
    of lumbar spine, 321*f*
    of male pelvis CT, 578*f*
    of male pelvis MRI, 611*f*, 612*f*
  origin, insertion, and nerve supply of, 400*t*–401*t*
  sagittal view
    of female pelvis CT, 585*f*, 586*f*
    of female pelvis MRI, 618*f*, 619*f*

Piriformis m. (Continued)
  of hip, 387f, 388f, 389f, 390f, 391f, 392f
  of lumbar spine, 315f
  of male pelvis CT, 570f, 571f
  of male pelvis MRI, 601f, 602f, 603f, 604f
Piriformis t.
  axial view, of hip, 376f, 377f
  coronal view, of male pelvis MRI, 610f
  sagittal view, of hip, 387f
Pisiform
  coronal view, of hand, 279f, 280f
  sagittal view, of hand, 275f
Pisohamate lig., coronal view, of hand, 280f
Pituitary gland
  axial view
    of brain CT, 7f
    of brain MRI, 22f
  sagittal view
    of brain CT, 10f
    of brain MRI, 25f, 30f
    of cervical spine MRI, 293f
Plantar a., lateral, coronal view
  of ankle, 525f
  of foot, 554f, 555f
Plantar a., medial
  coronal view
    of ankle, 524f, 525f, 526f
    of foot, 554f, 556f, 557f
  sagittal view, of ankle, 521f
Plantar aponeurosis
  coronal view, of ankle, 524f, 525f, 529f, 530f, 531f
  oblique axial view, of ankle, 514f
Plantar aponeurosis, lateral
  axial view, of ankle, 510f
  coronal view
    of ankle, 527f, 528f, 529f
    of foot, 557f
  oblique axial view, of ankle, 516f
Plantar aponeurosis, medial
  coronal view
    of ankle, 526f, 527f, 528f, 529f
    of foot, 553f, 554f, 555f, 557f
  oblique axial view, of ankle, 516f
Plantar fascia, lateral, sagittal view, of ankle, 519f, 520f
Plantar fascia, medial, sagittal view
  of ankle, 520f, 521f, 522f, 523f
  of foot, 544f
Plantar fascia, sagittal view, of foot, 544f
Plantar lig., long
  coronal view, of ankle, 527f, 528f
  sagittal view, of ankle, 520f
Plantar n., lateral
  axial view, of ankle, 508f, 509f
  coronal view
    of ankle, 525f, 527f, 528f
    of foot, 554f, 555f
Plantar n., medial
  axial view
    of ankle, 508f, 509f
    of foot, 538f, 539f
  coronal view
    of ankle, 524f, 525f, 526f
    of foot, 554f, 556f, 557f
  sagittal view
    of ankle, 522f, 523f
    of foot, 546f
Plantar vessels, lateral
  axial view, of ankle, 508f, 509f
  oblique axial view, of ankle, 513f, 514f, 515f, 516f
  sagittal view, of ankle, 522f
Plantar vessels, medial
  axial view
    of ankle, 508f, 509f
    of foot, 538f, 539f
  oblique axial view, of ankle, 513f, 514f, 515f, 516f
  sagittal view
    of ankle, 522f, 523f
    of foot, 546f
Plantaris m.
  axial view, of knee, 449f, 450f, 451f, 452f
  coronal view, of knee, 469f, 470f

Plantaris m. (Continued)
  origin, insertion, and nerve supply of, 498t–499t
  sagittal view, of knee, 455f, 456f, 457f, 458f
Plantaris t.
  axial view
    of ankle, 504f, 505f, 506f, 507f
    of knee, 453f
    of leg, 474f, 475f, 481f, 483f
  sagittal view, of knee, 459f, 460f
Platysma m., axial view, of pectoral girdle and chest wall, 68f
Pons
  axial view
    of brain CT, 7f
    of brain MRI, 23f
  coronal view, of brain CT, 16f
  sagittal view
    of brain CT, 10f
    of brain MRI, 25f, 31f
Popliteal a.
  axial view
    of knee, 447f, 448f
    of leg, 474f
    of thigh, 426f, 427f
  coronal view, of leg, 494f
  sagittal view, of leg, 487f
Popliteal v.
  axial view
    of knee, 447f, 448f
    of leg, 474f
    of thigh, 426f, 427f
  coronal view, of thigh, 440f
Popliteal vessels
  axial view, of knee, 448f, 449f, 450f, 451f, 452f
  coronal view
    of knee, 469f, 470f, 471f, 472f
    of leg, 495f
    of thigh, 440f, 441f
  sagittal view
    of leg, 488f
    of thigh, 429f, 431f
Popliteus m.
  axial view
    of knee, 451f, 452f, 453f
    of leg, 474f, 475f, 476f
  coronal view
    of knee, 470f, 471f
    of leg, 494f
  origin, insertion, and nerve supply of, 498t–499t
  sagittal view
    of knee, 456f, 457f, 458f, 459f, 460f
    of leg, 486f, 487f, 488f
Popliteus t.
  axial view, of knee, 451f
  coronal view, of knee, 468f, 469f
  sagittal view, of knee, 455f, 456f
Portacaval space, axial view, of abdomen CT, 328f
Portal v.
  axial view, of abdomen CT, 327f, 328f
  coronal view, of thorax CT, 48f
  left
    axial view
      of abdomen CT, 326f
      of abdomen MRI, 348f
    coronal view
      of abdomen CT, 339f, 340f
      of abdomen MRI, 363f, 364f
    sagittal view
      of abdomen CT, 335f, 336f
      of abdomen MRI, 360f
    umbilical portion
      axial view, of abdomen CT, 335f
      axial view, of abdomen MRI, 347f
      sagittal view, of abdomen CT, 335f
  main
    axial view
      of abdomen CT, 327f
      of abdomen MRI, 348f, 349f, 350f
    coronal view
      of abdomen CT, 340f
      of abdomen MRI, 365f
    sagittal view
      of abdomen CT, 335f
      of abdomen MRI, 360f
  posterior branch

Portal v. (Continued)
  axial view, of abdomen CT, 327f, 328f
  coronal view, of abdomen CT, 342f
  sagittal view, of abdomen CT, 337f
  right
    anterior branch
      axial view, of abdomen CT, 327f, 328f
      coronal view, of abdomen CT, 340f
      sagittal view, of abdomen CT, 337f
    axial view
      of abdomen CT, 327f
      of abdomen MRI, 347f, 348f
    coronal view, of abdomen CT, 341f, 342f
    sagittal view
      of abdomen CT, 336f
      of abdomen MRI, 360f, 361f
    sagittal view, of thorax CT, 46f
Postcentral gyrus
  axial view
    of brain CT, 4f
    of brain MRI, 19f, 20f
  sagittal view
    of brain CT, 11f, 12f
    of brain MRI, 26f, 27f
Postcentral sulcus, brain MRI, 19f, 20f
Posterior bands
  axial view, of elbow, 182f
  oblique sagittal view
    of elbow, 197f
    of shoulder arthrogram, 139f
Posterior belly digastric m., axial view
  of brain CT, 9f
  of cervical spine MRI, 288f
Precentral gyrus
  axial view
    of brain CT, 4f
    of brain MRI, 19f, 20f
  sagittal view
    of brain CT, 11f, 12f
    of brain MRI, 26f, 27f
Prepontine cistern, axial view, of brain CT, 7f
Profunda brachii a.
  axial view, of arm, 155f, 156f, 157f, 158f
  sagittal view, of arm, 164f, 165f
Profunda femoris a., axial view, of male pelvis MRI, 599f, 600f
Pronator quadratus m.
  axial view, of forearm, 216f, 217f, 218f
  coronal view, of forearm, 226f, 227f, 228f
  origin, insertion, and nerve supply of, 233t–234t
  sagittal view, of forearm, 221f, 222f, 223f
Pronator teres m.
  axial view
    of elbow, 180f, 181f, 182f, 183f, 184f, 185f, 186f, 187f, 188f, 189f
    of forearm, 209f, 210f, 211f, 212f
  coronal view, of forearm, 226f, 227f, 228f, 229f, 230f
  oblique coronal, of elbow, 199f, 200f, 201f, 202f, 203f, 204f
  oblique sagittal view, of elbow, 194f, 195f, 196f, 197f, 198f
  origin, insertion, and nerve supply of, 233t–234t
  sagittal view
    of arm, 166f, 167f
    of forearm, 221f
Pronator teres m., deep head
  axial view
    of elbow, 185f, 186f, 187f, 188f
    of forearm, 209f
  oblique coronal, of elbow, 203f, 204f
  oblique sagittal view, of elbow, 195f, 196f
Pronator teres t.
  axial view
    of elbow, 188f, 189f
    of forearm, 209f, 210f, 211f
  coronal view, of forearm, 229f, 230f
  oblique sagittal view, of elbow, 197f, 198f
Prostate gland
  axial view
    of male pelvis CT, 567f, 568f
    of male pelvis MRI, 599f
  coronal view
    of male pelvis CT, 576f
    of male pelvis MRI, 609f, 610f

Prostate gland (Continued)
  sagittal view
    of male pelvis CT, 572f
    of male pelvis MRI, 605f, 606f
Proximal phalanx
  2nd toe
    coronal view, 549f
    sagittal view, 545f, 546f, 548f
  3rd toe
    axial view, 539f
    coronal view, 549f
    sagittal view, 544f
  4th toe
    axial view, 539f
    coronal view, 549f
    sagittal view, 542f
  5th toe
    axial view, 538f, 539f
    coronal view, 549f
    sagittal view, 541f
  axial view, of hand, 268f
  great toe
    axial view, 538f, 539f
    coronal view, 549f
    sagittal view, 547f
  index finger
    coronal view, 281f, 282f
    sagittal view, 271f, 272f, 273f
  little toe, coronal view, 550f
  long finger
    coronal view, 281f, 282f
    sagittal view, 273f, 274f, 275f
  ring finger
    coronal view, 281f, 282f
    sagittal view, 275f, 276f
  small finger
    coronal view, 280f, 281f
    sagittal view, 277f, 278f
  thumb
    axial view, 266f, 267f
    coronal view, 281f
    sagittal view, 269f, 270f
Psoas m.
  axial view
    of abdomen CT, 330f, 331f
    of abdomen MRI, 353f
    of female pelvis CT, 580f
    of female pelvis MRI, 614f
    of lumbar spine, 310f, 311f, 312f, 313f, 314f
    of male pelvis CT, 564f, 565f
    of male pelvis MRI, 595f, 596f
  coronal view
    of abdomen CT, 340f, 341f, 342f
    of abdomen MRI, 365f, 366f, 367f, 368f
    of female pelvis CT, 589f, 590f, 592f, 593f
    of female pelvis MRI, 623f, 624f
    of hip, 395f
    of lumbar spine, 310f, 311f, 312f, 313f, 314f
    of male pelvis CT, 574f, 575f, 576f
    of male pelvis MRI, 608f, 609f, 610f
  sagittal view
    of abdomen CT, 332f, 333f, 336f, 337f
    of abdomen MRI, 355f, 356f, 360f, 361f
    of female pelvis CT, 585f, 586f
    of female pelvis MRI, 618f, 619f
    of lumbar spine, 315f
    of male pelvis CT, 570f
    of male pelvis MRI, 602f, 603f, 604f
Psoas major m., origin, insertion, and nerve supply of, 400t–401t
Pterygoid mm.
  brain CT, 8f, 9f
  brain MRI, 24f
Pterygoid process, axial view, of brain CT, 8f, 9f
Pubic bone
  axial view
    of female pelvis CT, 583f
    of male pelvis CT, 568f
  coronal view, of male pelvis CT, 574f
  sagittal view
    of male pelvis CT, 571f
    of male pelvis MRI, 604f
Pubic ramus
  axial view
    of female pelvis CT, 584f

Pubic ramus (Continued)
  of male pelvis CT, 569f
  sagittal view, of female pelvis MRI, 619f
Pubic ramus, inferior
  axial view
    of female pelvis MRI, 617f
    of hip, 379f, 380f
  coronal view
    of female pelvis CT, 591f, 592f
    of hip, 396f
    of male pelvis CT, 575f, 576f
  sagittal view, of female pelvis CT, 586f
Pubic ramus, superior
  axial view
    of female pelvis CT, 583f
    of hip, 377f, 378f
  coronal view
    of female pelvis CT, 588f, 589f, 590f
    of female pelvis MRI, 622f, 623f
    of hip, 394f, 395f
    of hip arthrogram, 414f
    of male pelvis CT, 574f, 575f
    of male pelvis MRI, 608f
    of thigh, 439f
  sagittal view
    of female pelvis CT, 585f
    of female pelvis MRI, 618f
    of hip, 392f
    of male pelvis CT, 570f, 571f
    of male pelvis MRI, 602f, 603f, 604f
Pubic symphysis
  axial view
    of female pelvis CT, 583f
    of male pelvis MRI, 599f
  coronal view
    of female pelvis CT, 589f
    of female pelvis MRI, 623f
    of male pelvis MRI, 607f, 608f
    of thigh, 439f
  sagittal view
    of female pelvis CT, 587f
    of female pelvis MRI, 621f
    of male pelvis MRI, 606f
Pubis
  axial view, of male pelvis MRI, 599f
  coronal view, of hip, 395f
  sagittal view
    of female pelvis CT, 586f
    of female pelvis MRI, 620f
    of male pelvis MRI, 605f, 606f
    of thigh, 435f, 436f
Puborectalis m., axial view, of female pelvis CT, 584f
Pulmonary a.
  coronal view
    of heart MRI, 61f
    of thorax CT, 47f, 49f
  left
    axial view
      of heart MRI, 55f
      of thorax CT, 38f
    coronal view, of thorax CT, 51f
    sagittal view
      of heart MRI, 58f
      of thorax CT, 43f
  main
    axial view
      of heart MRI, 55f
      of pectoral girdle and chest wall, 75f
      of thorax CT, 38f, 39f
    coronal view
      of heart MRI, 62f
      of thorax CT, 47f, 48f, 50f
    sagittal view
      of heart MRI, 58f
      of thorax CT, 44f
  right
    axial view
      of heart MRI, 55f
      of pectoral girdle and chest wall, 75f
      of thorax CT, 38f
    coronal view
      of heart MRI, 62f
      of thorax CT, 49f
    sagittal view

Pulmonary a. (Continued)
  of heart MRI, 59f
  of thorax CT, 43f, 44f, 45f, 47f
Pulmonary outflow tract
  axial view
    of heart MRI, 56f
    of thorax CT, 40f
  coronal view
    of heart MRI, 61f
    of thorax CT, 47f
  sagittal view
    of heart MRI, 58f, 59f
    of thorax CT, 43f, 44f
Pulmonary trunk, axial view, of thorax CT, 39f
Pulmonary v.
  left
    axial view
      of heart MRI, 55f, 56f
      of thorax CT, 39f
    coronal view
      of heart MRI, 62f
      of thorax CT, 48f, 50f
    sagittal view
      of heart MRI, 58f
      of thorax CT, 43f, 44f
  middle, axial view, of heart MRI, 56f
  right
    axial view, of heart MRI, 56f
    coronal view, of thorax CT, 48f, 51f
    sagittal view
      of heart MRI, 60f
      of thorax CT, 46f
  sagittal view, of heart MRI, 60f
  segmental, sagittal view, of thorax CT, 43f
Pulmonic valve, axial view, of heart MRI, 55f
Putamen
  axial view
    of brain CT, 6f
    of brain MRI, 21f
  coronal view, of brain CT, 14f
  sagittal view
    of brain CT, 11f
    of brain MRI, 26f, 29f, 30f

Q
Quadrangular space
  axial view, of pectoral girdle and chest wall, 72f, 73f
  coronal view, of pectoral girdle and chest wall, 92f, 93f
  oblique coronal view, of shoulder, 125f, 126f
  sagittal view, of arm, 164f
Quadratus femoris m.
  axial view
    of female pelvis CT, 583f
    of female pelvis MRI, 617f
    of hip, 379f, 380f, 381f
    of male pelvis CT, 564f, 569f
    of male pelvis MRI, 599f, 600f
  coronal view
    of female pelvis CT, 592f, 593f
    of female pelvis MRI, 624f
    of hip, 396f, 397f
    of male pelvis CT, 577f
    of male pelvis MRI, 611f
    of thigh, 442f
  origin, insertion, and nerve supply of, 400t–401t
  sagittal view
    of hip, 387f, 388f, 389f
    of male pelvis CT, 570f
    of thigh, 430f, 431f, 432f, 433f
Quadratus lumborum m.
  axial view
    of abdomen CT, 329f, 330f, 331f
    of abdomen MRI, 353f
    of lumbar spine, 310f, 312f
    of male pelvis CT, 564f
  coronal view
    of abdomen CT, 342f, 343f
    of abdomen MRI, 367f, 368f
    of female pelvis CT, 593f
    of female pelvis MRI, 625f
    of lumbar spine, 314f, 319f, 320f
    of male pelvis CT, 576f, 577f

Quadratus lumborum m. *(Continued)*
  sagittal view
    of abdomen CT, 332f, 337f
    of abdomen MRI, 354f, 355f
    of lumbar spine, 314f
    of male pelvis CT, 570f
Quadratus lumborum t., axial view, of lumbar
    spine, 311f
Quadratus plantae m.
  axial view
    of ankle, 507f, 508f, 509f
    of foot, 538f, 539f
  coronal view
    of ankle, 524f, 525f, 526f, 527f, 528f, 529f,
        530f, 531f
    of foot, 555f, 556f, 557f
  oblique axial view, of ankle, 513f, 514f, 515f,
      516f
  origin, insertion, and nerve supply of, 558t–560t
  sagittal view
    of ankle, 520f, 521f
    of foot, 543f, 544f, 545f
Quadriceps t.
  axial view, of knee, 447f, 448f
  coronal view
    of knee, 463f
    of thigh, 438f
  sagittal view
    of knee, 456f, 457f, 458f, 459f
    of thigh, 432f
Quadrilateral plate
  axial view, of female pelvis CT, 582f
  coronal view, of hip, 396f
  sagittal view, of hip, 391f

R
Radial a.
  axial view
    of elbow, 184f, 185f, 186f, 187f, 188f, 189f
    of forearm, 209f, 210f, 211f, 212f, 213f, 214f
    of hand, 262f
  coronal view
    of forearm, 227f, 228f, 229f
    of hand, 280f, 281f
  oblique coronal, of elbow, 199f, 200f, 201f
  oblique sagittal view, of elbow, 194f
  sagittal view, of forearm, 219f, 220f
Radial collateral lig.
  axial view
    of elbow, 182f, 183f, 184f
    of hand, 268f
  coronal view, of hand, 281f, 282f
  oblique coronal, of elbow, 203f, 204f
  oblique sagittal view, of elbow, 191f
  sagittal view, of hand, 270f
Radial fossa
  oblique sagittal view, of elbow, 193f
  sagittal view, of arm, 163f
Radial head
  axial view, of elbow, 184f, 185f
  coronal view, of arm, 169f, 170f
  oblique coronal, of elbow, 203f, 204f
  oblique sagittal view, of elbow, 191f, 192f,
      193f, 194f
  sagittal view, of arm, 162f, 163f
Radial n.
  axial view
    of arm, 155f, 158f
    of elbow, 179f
    of pectoral girdle and chest wall, 75f, 76f, 77f
  coronal view
    of arm, 172f
    of pectoral girdle and chest wall, 93f, 94f, 95f
  oblique coronal view
    of elbow, 203f, 204f
    of shoulder, 125f
  oblique sagittal view
    of elbow, 191f, 192f
    of shoulder, 115f
  sagittal view
    of arm, 163f, 164f, 165f
    of pectoral girdle and chest wall, 80f
Radial n., deep
  axial view

Radial n., deep *(Continued)*
    of elbow, 180f, 181f, 182f, 183f, 184f, 185f,
        186f, 187f, 188f, 189f
    of forearm, 209f, 210f
  oblique coronal, of elbow, 201f, 202f, 203f,
      204f, 205f
  oblique sagittal view, of elbow, 192f, 193f
  sagittal view, of forearm, 220f, 221f
Radial n., superficial
  axial view
    of elbow, 180f, 181f, 182f, 183f, 184f, 185f,
        186f, 187f, 188f, 189f
    of forearm, 209f, 210f, 211f, 212f, 213f, 214f,
        215f, 216f, 217f, 218f
  coronal view, of forearm, 228f, 229f, 230f
  oblique coronal, of elbow, 201f
  oblique sagittal view, of elbow, 193f
Radial neck
  axial view, of elbow, 185f, 186f
  oblique coronal, of elbow, 204f
  sagittal view, of forearm, 221f
Radial notch of ulna, axial view, of elbow, 184f
Radial recurrent a.
  axial view, of elbow, 184f, 185f
  oblique coronal view, of elbow, 205f
Radial sesamoid
  axial view, of hand, 265f
  sagittal view, of hand, 271f
Radial styloid, coronal view, of hand, 281f
Radial tuberosity
  axial view, of elbow, 186f
  coronal view, of forearm, 229f
  oblique coronal, of elbow, 203f, 204f
  oblique sagittal view, of elbow, 193f, 194f
  sagittal view, of forearm, 221f
Radioscaphocapitate lig., coronal view, of hand,
    280f
Radioulnar joint, proximal, axial view, of elbow,
    184f
Radioulnar lig., palmar
  coronal view, of wrist, 256f
  sagittal view, of wrist, 251f
Radius
  axial view, of elbow, 187f, 188f, 189f
  coronal view
    of forearm, 221f, 222f, 228f, 229f
    of hand, 280f, 281f, 282f, 283f
  oblique coronal, of elbow, 201f, 202f, 203f
  oblique sagittal view, of elbow, 193f, 194f
  sagittal view, of forearm, 220f, 221f, 222f
Rectosigmoid junction, axial view, of male pelvis
    CT, 566f
Rectovesical fossa, sagittal view, of male pelvis
    CT, 572f
Rectum
  axial view
    of female pelvis CT, 581f, 582f, 583f
    of female pelvis MRI, 614f, 615f, 616f, 617f
    of hip, 374f, 376f, 377f, 378f
    of male pelvis CT, 566f, 567f, 568f
    of male pelvis MRI, 597f, 598f, 599f
  coronal view
    of female pelvis CT, 593f
    of hip, 398f
    of male pelvis CT, 577f, 578f
    of male pelvis MRI, 610f, 611f, 612f
  sagittal view
    of female pelvis CT, 586f, 587f
    of female pelvis MRI, 620f
    of male pelvis CT, 572f
    of male pelvis MRI, 604f, 605f, 606f
Rectus abdominis m.
  axial view
    of abdomen CT, 326f, 328f, 329f, 331f
    of abdomen MRI, 350f, 351f
    of female pelvis CT, 580f, 581f, 582f, 583f
    of female pelvis MRI, 615f, 616f
    of hip, 374f, 375f, 376f
    of male pelvis CT, 564f, 565f, 566f, 567f, 568f
    of male pelvis MRI, 595f, 596f, 597f, 598f,
        599f
  coronal view
    of abdomen MRI, 363f
    of female pelvis MRI, 622f
    of hip, 393f

Rectus abdominis m. *(Continued)*
    of male pelvis CT, 573f
    of male pelvis MRI, 607f
  origin, insertion, and nerve supply of, 344t
  sagittal view
    of abdomen CT, 332f, 333f, 335f, 336f, 337f
    of abdomen MRI, 354f, 355f, 356f, 359f, 360f,
        361f
    of female pelvis CT, 585f, 586f, 587f
    of female pelvis MRI, 618f, 619f, 620f, 621f
    of hip, 391f
    of male pelvis CT, 570f, 572f
    of male pelvis MRI, 603f, 604f, 605f, 606f
  tendinous intersection
    coronal view, of abdomen MRI, 363f
    sagittal view, of abdomen MRI, 354f, 355f,
        359f, 360f
Rectus abdominis t., axial view, of male pelvis
    MRI, 599f
Rectus capitis posterior major m.
  axial view
    of brain CT, 8f
    of cervical spine MRI, 288f
  sagittal view
    of brain MRI, 32f
    of cervical spine MRI, 291f, 292f
Rectus femoris m.
  axial view
    of female pelvis CT, 582f, 583f, 584f
    of female pelvis MRI, 617f
    of hip, 376f, 377f, 378f, 379f, 380f, 381f, 382f
    of male pelvis CT, 567f, 568f, 569f
    of male pelvis MRI, 598f, 599f, 600f
    of thigh, 420f, 421f, 422f, 423f, 424f, 425f,
        426f
  coronal view
    of female pelvis CT, 588f, 589f
    of female pelvis MRI, 622f
    of hip, 393f, 394f
    of male pelvis CT, 573f, 574f, 575f
    of male pelvis MRI, 607f, 608f
    of thigh, 437f, 438f
  origin, insertion, and nerve supply of, 445t
  sagittal view
    of hip, 383f, 384f, 385f, 386f, 387f
    of thigh, 430f, 431f, 432f, 433f, 434f
Rectus femoris t.
  axial view
    of hip, 376f, 377f, 378f, 379f
    of hip arthrogram, 403f, 404f, 405f, 406f,
        407f, 408f
    of thigh, 422f, 427f
  coronal view
    of hip, 393f
    of thigh, 437f, 438f
  sagittal view, of hip, 387f
Rectus femoris t., reflected head
  axial view
    of hip, 375f
    of male pelvis CT, 567f
    of male pelvis MRI, 598f
  coronal view
    of female pelvis MRI, 623f
    of hip, 395f
    of male pelvis MRI, 608f
  sagittal view, of hip, 387f
Rectus femoris t., straight head
  axial view
    of hip, 375f
    of male pelvis CT, 567f
  coronal view
    of female pelvis MRI, 623f
    of hip, 394f
    of male pelvis MRI, 608f
Renal a.
  left
    axial view
      of abdomen CT, 329f
      of abdomen MRI, 352f
    coronal view
      of abdomen CT, 341f
      of abdomen MRI, 366f, 367f
      of lumbar spine, 317f
    sagittal view
      of abdomen CT, 333f

Renal a. (*Continued*)
    of abdomen MRI, 355*f*, 356*f*
    right
        axial view, of abdomen MRI, 351*f*
        coronal view
            of abdomen CT, 341*f*
            of abdomen MRI, 366*f*, 367*f*
            of lumbar spine, 317*f*
        sagittal view
            of abdomen CT, 335*f*, 336*f*
            of abdomen MRI, 358*f*, 359*f*, 360*f*
            of lumbar spine, 316*f*
    sagittal view, of abdomen CT, 332*f*
Renal cortex
    axial view, of abdomen CT, 329*f*
    coronal view, of abdomen CT, 343*f*
    sagittal view, of abdomen CT, 337*f*
Renal hilum, sagittal view, of abdomen CT, 332*f*
Renal medulla
    axial view, of abdomen CT, 329*f*
    coronal view, of abdomen CT, 343*f*
    sagittal view, of abdomen CT, 337*f*
Renal pelvis
    axial view
        of abdomen CT, 329*f*, 330*f*
        of abdomen MRI, 352*f*
    coronal view
        of abdomen CT, 342*f*
        of abdomen MRI, 368*f*
    sagittal view
        of abdomen CT, 336*f*
        of abdomen MRI, 355*f*, 360*f*
Renal sinus
    axial view, of abdomen MRI, 349*f*, 350*f*
    sagittal view, of abdomen MRI, 361*f*
Renal v.
    left
        axial view
            of abdomen CT, 329*f*, 330*f*
            of abdomen MRI, 350*f*, 351*f*, 352*f*
        coronal view
            of abdomen CT, 340*f*, 341*f*
            of abdomen MRI, 365*f*, 366*f*, 367*f*
            of lumbar spine, 317*f*
        sagittal view
            of abdomen CT, 333*f*, 334*f*
            of abdomen MRI, 355*f*, 356*f*, 357*f*, 358*f*
    right
        axial view
            of abdomen CT, 329*f*
            of abdomen MRI, 351*f*, 352*f*, 367*f*
            of thorax CT, 49*f*
        coronal view, of abdomen CT, 341*f*
        sagittal view
            of abdomen CT, 336*f*
            of abdomen MRI, 360*f*
    sagittal view, of abdomen CT, 332*f*
Retrobursal fat, coronal view, of knee, 463*f*
Retropubic space of Retzius, axial view
    of female pelvis CT, 583*f*
    of male pelvis CT, 568*f*
Retrotrochlear eminence
    axial view, of ankle, 507*f*, 508*f*
    coronal view, of ankle, 530*f*
Rhomboid m., axial view, of cervical spine MRI, 290*f*
Rhomboid major m.
    axial view
        of pectoral girdle and chest wall, 71*f*, 72*f*, 73*f*, 74*f*, 75*f*, 76*f*
        of thoracic spine, 297*f*
    coronal view
        of pectoral girdle and chest wall, 96*f*, 97*f*
        of thoracic spine, 304*f*
    origin, insertion, and nerve supply of, 306*t*–308*t*
    sagittal view
        of pectoral girdle and chest wall, 84*f*, 85*f*, 86*f*, 87*f*
        of thoracic spine, 299*f*
Rhomboid minor m.
    axial view, of pectoral girdle and chest wall, 71*f*
    coronal view, of pectoral girdle and chest wall, 96*f*
    origin, insertion, and nerve supply of, 306*t*–308*t*
    sagittal view

Rhomboid minor m. (*Continued*)
        of pectoral girdle and chest wall, 85*f*, 86*f*
        of thoracic spine, 299*f*
Rib
    1st, sagittal view, of thorax CT, 43*f*
    3rd, sagittal view, of pectoral girdle and chest wall, 87*f*
    6th, axial view, of thoracic spine, 297*f*
    9th, axial view, of thoracic spine, 298*f*
    10th, axial view, of thoracic spine, 298*f*
    11th, sagittal view, of lumbar spine, 314*f*, 315*f*
    12th
        coronal view
            of abdomen CT, 343*f*
            of lumbar spine, 321*f*, 322*f*
        sagittal view, of lumbar spine, 314*f*, 315*f*
    angle, sagittal view, of thoracic spine, 299*f*
    axial view
        of abdomen CT, 326*f*
        of abdomen MRI, 346*f*
        of pectoral girdle and chest wall, 70*f*, 72*f*, 73*f*, 74*f*, 75*f*, 77*f*
    coronal view
        of pectoral girdle and chest wall, 91*f*, 92*f*, 94*f*, 95*f*, 97*f*
        of thoracic spine, 303*f*, 304*f*
        of thorax CT, 51*f*
    head
        coronal view, of thorax CT, 52*f*
        sagittal view, of thoracic spine, 300*f*
    neck, sagittal view, of thoracic spine, 300*f*
    oblique coronal view, of shoulder, 119*f*, 120*f*, 121*f*
    oblique sagittal view, of shoulder, 118*f*
    posterior
        coronal view, of pectoral girdle and chest wall, 96*f*
        sagittal view
            of pectoral girdle and chest wall, 84*f*, 85*f*, 86*f*, 87*f*
            of thoracic spine, 299*f*
    sagittal view
        of abdomen CT, 332*f*
        of pectoral girdle and chest wall, 82*f*, 83*f*, 84*f*
    tubercle
        coronal view, of thoracic spine, 303*f*
        sagittal view, of thoracic spine, 300*f*
Right vertebral a.
    axial view, of cervical spine MRI, 288*f*, 289*f*, 290*f*
    coronal view, of cervical spine MRI, 294*f*
    sagittal view, of brain MRI, 31*f*
Rotator cuff interval
    oblique coronal view, of shoulder arthrogram, 142*f*
    oblique sagittal view
        of shoulder, 111*f*, 112*f*
        of shoulder arthrogram, 137*f*, 138*f*, 139*f*
Rotatores mm., origin, insertion, and nerve supply of, 306*t*–308*t*
Rotatores thoracis mm., coronal view, of pectoral girdle and chest wall, 94*f*
Round lig., axial view, of female pelvis CT, 581*f*

S
S1
    foramen, 316*f*
    nerve, 320*f*, 321*f*
    nerve root, 312*f*
        axial view, 565*f*, 596*f*
        coronal view, 577*f*, 593*f*, 626*f*
        sagittal view, 316*f*, 571*f*, 605*f*
    vertebra, 313*f*, 318*f*, 319*f*
    vertebral body, 316*f*
S2
    foramen, 316*f*
    nerve, 322*f*
    nerve root, 313*f*, 316*f*, 571*f*
Sacral ala
    axial view
        of lumbar spine, 313*f*
        of male pelvis MRI, 596*f*
    coronal view, of lumbar spine, 322*f*
Sacral crest, lateral, coronal view, of hip, 399*f*

Sacral foramen
    coronal view, of male pelvis CT, 577*f*
    sagittal view
        of male pelvis CT, 571*f*
        of male pelvis MRI, 605*f*
Sacral promontory, coronal view, of lumbar spine, 321*f*
Sacroiliac joint
    axial view
        of female pelvis CT, 580*f*
        of female pelvis MRI, 614*f*
        of lumbar spine, 313*f*
        of male pelvis CT, 565*f*
        of male pelvis MRI, 596*f*
    coronal view
        of female pelvis CT, 592*f*, 593*f*
        of female pelvis MRI, 625*f*
        of hip, 397*f*, 398*f*
        of lumbar spine, 319*f*, 320*f*, 321*f*
        of male pelvis CT, 577*f*, 578*f*
        of male pelvis MRI, 611*f*, 612*f*
    sagittal view
        of male pelvis CT, 570*f*
        of male pelvis MRI, 602*f*
Sacroiliac lig.
    anterior, axial view, of lumbar spine, 312*f*
    axial view, of lumbar spine, 313*f*
    posterior
        axial view, of lumbar spine, 313*f*
        coronal view, of lumbar spine, 320*f*, 321*f*, 322*f*
Sacrospinous lig., axial view, of hip, 377*f*
Sacrotuberous lig.
    axial view, of hip, 377*f*, 378*f*
    sagittal view, of hip, 391*f*
Sacrum
    axial view
        of female pelvis CT, 580*f*, 581*f*
        of female pelvis MRI, 614*f*
        of hip, 374*f*, 375*f*, 376*f*
        of lumbar spine, 313*f*
        of male pelvis CT, 565*f*
        of male pelvis MRI, 596*f*, 597*f*
    coronal view
        of abdomen MRI, 368*f*
        of female pelvis CT, 593*f*
        of female pelvis MRI, 624*f*, 625*f*, 626*f*
        of hip, 397*f*, 398*f*, 399*f*
        of lumbar spine, 320*f*
        of male pelvis CT, 576*f*, 577*f*
        of male pelvis MRI, 611*f*, 612*f*
    sagittal view
        of abdomen MRI, 358*f*, 359*f*, 360*f*
        of female pelvis CT, 585*f*, 586*f*, 587*f*
        of female pelvis MRI, 618*f*, 619*f*, 620*f*, 621*f*
        of hip, 392*f*
        of lumbar spine, 314*f*, 315*f*
        of male pelvis CT, 571*f*, 572*f*
        of male pelvis MRI, 602*f*, 603*f*, 604*f*, 605*f*, 606*f*
Sagittal band, axial view, of hand, 268*f*
Sartorius, coronal view, of male pelvis CT, 573*f*
Sartorius m.
    axial view
        of female pelvis CT, 581*f*, 582*f*, 583*f*, 584*f*
        of female pelvis MRI, 615*f*, 616*f*, 617*f*
        of hip, 374*f*, 375*f*, 376*f*, 377*f*, 378*f*, 379*f*, 380*f*, 381*f*, 382*f*
        of knee, 447*f*, 448*f*, 449*f*, 450*f*, 451*f*
        of male pelvis CT, 566*f*, 567*f*, 568*f*
        of male pelvis MRI, 597*f*, 598*f*, 599*f*, 600*f*
        of thigh, 420*f*, 421*f*, 422*f*, 423*f*, 424*f*, 425*f*, 426*f*, 427*f*
    coronal view
        of female pelvis CT, 588*f*
        of female pelvis MRI, 622*f*
        of hip, 393*f*
        of knee, 469*f*, 470*f*, 471*f*
        of leg, 495*f*
        of male pelvis MRI, 607*f*
        of thigh, 437*f*, 438*f*, 439*f*, 440*f*, 441*f*, 442*f*
    origin, insertion, and nerve supply of, 445*t*
    sagittal view
        of hip, 385*f*, 386*f*, 387*f*, 388*f*, 389*f*
        of knee, 461*f*, 462*f*

Sartorius m. (Continued)
  of thigh, 432f, 433f, 434f, 435f
Sartorius t.
  axial view
    of hip arthrogram, 406f
    of knee, 452f
  coronal view, of knee, 469f, 470f
Scalene m., anterior
  axial view, of pectoral girdle and chest wall,
    70f, 71f
  coronal view, of pectoral girdle and chest wall,
    91f
  sagittal view
    of pectoral girdle and chest wall, 85f, 86f
    of thoracic spine, 299f
Scalene m., middle
  axial view, of pectoral girdle and chest wall, 70f
  coronal view, of pectoral girdle and chest wall,
    91f, 92f
  sagittal view
    of pectoral girdle and chest wall, 85f, 86f
    of thoracic spine, 299f
Scalene m., posterior
  axial view, of pectoral girdle and chest wall,
    68f, 69f
  coronal view, of pectoral girdle and chest wall,
    92f
  sagittal view, of pectoral girdle and chest wall,
    85f, 86f
Scalene mm., axial view, of cervical spine MRI,
    290f
Scaphoid
  coronal view, of hand, 280f, 281f, 282f
  sagittal view, of hand, 264f, 265f
Scaphoid tuberosity, coronal view, of hand, 279f,
    280f
Scapholunate lig., coronal view, of hand, 280f,
    281f
Scaphotriquetral lig., palmar
  axial view, of wrist, 241f
  coronal view, of wrist, 256f
  sagittal view, of wrist, 247f, 248f, 249f, 250f,
    251f
Scapula
  ABER view, of shoulder arthrogram, 149f
  axial view
    of pectoral girdle and chest wall, 74f
    of shoulder, 104f, 108f
    of thorax CT, 36f, 38f
  body
    ABER view, of shoulder arthrogram, 151f,
      152f
    axial view
      of pectoral girdle and chest wall, 71f, 72f,
        73f
      of shoulder, 104f, 105f, 106f, 107f, 108f
      of shoulder arthrogram, 132f, 133f, 134f
    coronal view, of pectoral girdle and chest
      wall, 94f, 95f, 96f
    oblique coronal view
      of shoulder, 125f
      of shoulder arthrogram, 145f
    oblique sagittal view, of shoulder, 117f, 118f
    sagittal view, of pectoral girdle and chest
      wall, 84f
  coronal view
    of thoracic spine, 303f
    of thorax CT, 51f
  inferior
    axial view, of pectoral girdle and chest wall,
      74f, 75f, 76f
    coronal view, of pectoral girdle and chest
      wall, 96f, 97f
    sagittal view, of pectoral girdle and chest
      wall, 83f, 84f
  medial
    axial view, of pectoral girdle and chest wall,
      76f
    coronal view, of pectoral girdle and chest
      wall, 96f
    sagittal view, of pectoral girdle and chest
      wall, 84f
  neck
    axial view, of shoulder, 106f
    oblique sagittal view, of shoulder, 116f

Scapula (Continued)
  oblique coronal view
    of shoulder, 123f, 125f
    of shoulder arthrogram, 143f
  sagittal view
    of pectoral girdle and chest wall, 81f, 82f, 83f
    of thorax CT, 43f
  superior, coronal view, of pectoral girdle and
    chest wall, 94f
Scapular a., dorsal, coronal view, of pectoral
    girdle and chest wall, 92f, 93f
Scapular circumflex a.
  coronal view, of arm, 172f
  oblique coronal view, of shoulder, 122f, 123f,
    124f, 125f, 126f, 127f
  oblique sagittal view, of shoulder, 116f
  sagittal view, of arm, 167f
Scapular lig., superior transverse
  axial view, of shoulder, 103f
  oblique coronal view, of shoulder, 124f
Scapular notch, coronal view, of pectoral girdle
    and chest wall, 92f
Scapular spine
  ABER view, of shoulder arthrogram, 149f, 150f
  axial view
    of pectoral girdle and chest wall, 70f
    of shoulder, 100f, 101f, 102f, 103f
    of shoulder arthrogram, 131f, 132f
  coronal view
    of arm, 174f
    of pectoral girdle and chest wall, 93f, 94f, 95f
    of thoracic spine, 303f, 304f, 305f
  oblique coronal view
    of shoulder, 124f, 125f
    of shoulder arthrogram, 144f, 145f, 146f
  oblique sagittal view, of shoulder, 117f, 118f
  sagittal view, of pectoral girdle and chest wall,
    81f, 82f, 83f
Schmorl node, coronal view, of lumbar spine, 319f
Sciatic n.
  axial view
    of female pelvis CT, 582f, 583f, 584f
    of female pelvis MRI, 615f, 616f, 617f
    of hip, 375f, 376f, 377f, 378f, 379f, 380f, 381f,
      382f
    of male pelvis CT, 567f
    of male pelvis MRI, 596f, 598f, 599f, 600f
    of thigh, 420f, 421f, 422f, 423f, 424f, 425f
  coronal view
    of female pelvis MRI, 625f
    of hip, 397f
    of lumbar spine, 320f
    of male pelvis CT, 577f
    of thigh, 442f
  sagittal view
    of hip, 387f, 388f, 391f
    of male pelvis MRI, 601f, 602f
    of thigh, 430f, 431f
Semimembranosus m.
  axial view
    of knee, 447f, 448f
    of thigh, 420f, 421f, 422f, 423f, 424f, 425f,
      426f, 427f
  coronal view
    of knee, 471f, 472f
    of leg, 495f
    of male pelvis MRI, 611f, 612f
    of thigh, 441f, 442f, 443f, 444f
  origin, insertion, and nerve supply of, 400t–401t
  sagittal view
    of knee, 458f, 459f, 460f
    of thigh, 430f, 431f, 432f, 433f
Semimembranosus t.
  axial view
    of female pelvis MRI, 617f
    of hip, 380f, 381f, 382f
    of knee, 448f, 449f, 450f, 451f
    of male pelvis MRI, 600f
    of thigh, 420f, 421f, 422f, 423f, 424f
  coronal view
    of female pelvis MRI, 625f
    of knee, 470f, 471f, 472f
    of leg, 495f
    of male pelvis CT, 578f
    of thigh, 442f

Semimembranosus t. (Continued)
  sagittal view
    of hip, 389f
    of hip arthrogram, 411f
    of knee, 460f, 461f
    of leg, 489f, 490f
    of male pelvis CT, 570f
    of male pelvis MRI, 601f
    of thigh, 431f, 432f, 433f
Seminal vesicle
  axial view
    of male pelvis CT, 567f
    of male pelvis MRI, 598f
  coronal view
    of male pelvis CT, 576f, 577f
    of male pelvis MRI, 610f, 611f
  sagittal view
    of male pelvis CT, 571f
    of male pelvis MRI, 603f, 604f, 605f, 606f
Semispinalis, axial view, of thoracic spine, 297f
Semispinalis capitis m.
  axial view
    of brain CT, 7f, 8f, 9f
    of cervical spine MRI, 288f, 289f, 290f
  axial view, of pectoral girdle and chest wall, 70f
  coronal view
    of brain CT, 17f
    of cervical spine MRI, 295f
  coronal view, of pectoral girdle and chest wall,
    92f, 93f, 94f, 95f
  origin, insertion, and nerve supply of, 306t–308t
  sagittal view
    of brain MRI, 32f
    of cervical spine MRI, 291f, 292f
    of pectoral girdle and chest wall, 87f
Semispinalis cervicis m.
  axial view
    of cervical spine MRI, 289f, 290f
    of pectoral girdle and chest wall, 68f
  coronal view
    of cervical spine MRI, 295f
    of pectoral girdle and chest wall, 93f
  origin, insertion, and nerve supply of, 306t–308t
Semispinalis thoracis m.
  axial view, of pectoral girdle and chest wall,
    71f, 72f, 74f, 75f, 76f
  coronal view, of pectoral girdle and chest wall,
    95f, 97f
  origin, insertion, and nerve supply of, 306t–308t
Semitendinosus m.
  axial view
    of hip, 380f, 381f, 382f
    of knee, 447f
    of male pelvis MRI, 600f
    of thigh, 420f, 423f, 424f, 425f, 426f, 427f
  coronal view
    of female pelvis MRI, 625f
    of hip, 397f, 398f
    of male pelvis MRI, 611f, 612f
    of thigh, 442f, 443f, 444f
  origin, insertion, and nerve supply of, 400t–401t
  sagittal view
    of hip, 387f, 388f, 389f, 390f
    of male pelvis MRI, 601f
    of thigh, 430f, 431f, 432f, 433f
Semitendinosus t.
  axial view
    of hip, 382f
    of knee, 447f, 449f, 450f, 451f, 452f
    of thigh, 420f, 423f
  coronal view
    of hip, 397f
    of knee, 469f, 470f, 471f, 472f
    of male pelvis MRI, 611f
  sagittal view
    of hip, 388f, 389f
    of hip arthrogram, 411f
    of knee, 460f, 461f, 462f
    of leg, 490f
Septum pellucidum, axial view, of brain CT, 5f, 6f
Septum pellucidum, brain MRI
  axial view, 20f, 21f
  sagittal view, 29f, 30f
Serratus anterior m.
  axial view

Serratus anterior m. *(Continued)*
    of abdomen CT, 326*f*
    of abdomen MRI, 346*f*, 347*f*, 348*f*, 349*f*
    of pectoral girdle and chest wall, 70*f*, 71*f*,
        72*f*, 73*f*, 74*f*, 75*f*, 76*f*, 77*f*
    of shoulder, 102*f*
    coronal view
        of abdomen MRI, 368*f*, 369*f*
        of pectoral girdle and chest wall, 91*f*, 92*f*,
            93*f*, 94*f*, 95*f*, 96*f*, 97*f*
        of thoracic spine, 302*f*, 303*f*, 304*f*
    oblique coronal view, of shoulder, 119*f*, 120*f*
    origin, insertion, and nerve supply of, 306*t*–308*t*
    sagittal view, of pectoral girdle and chest wall,
        82*f*, 83*f*, 84*f*, 85*f*
Serratus posterior m.
    axial view
        of pectoral girdle and chest wall, 69*f*
        of thoracic spine, 298*f*
    sagittal view, of pectoral girdle and chest wall,
        85*f*
Serratus posterior m., inferior
    coronal view, of thoracic spine, 304*f*
    origin, insertion, and nerve supply of, 306*t*–308*t*
    sagittal view, of pectoral girdle and chest wall,
        85*f*, 86*f*
Serratus posterior m., superior
    coronal view
        of pectoral girdle and chest wall, 95*f*
        of thoracic spine, 303*f*, 304*f*, 305*f*
    origin, insertion, and nerve supply of, 306*t*–308*t*
    sagittal view, of pectoral girdle and chest wall,
        85*f*, 86*f*
Sesamoid
    lateral
        axial view, of foot, 539*f*
        coronal view, of foot, 550*f*, 551*f*
        sagittal view, of foot, 547*f*
    medial
        axial view, of foot, 539*f*
        coronal view, of foot, 550*f*, 551*f*
        sagittal view, of foot, 548*f*
    radial
        axial view, of hand, 265*f*
        sagittal view, of hand, 271*f*
    ulnar
        axial view, of hand, 265*f*
        sagittal view, of hand, 271*f*
    volar plate
        axial view, of hand, 268*f*
        coronal view, of hand, 280*f*
        sagittal view, of hand, 271*f*, 272*f*
Sigmoid venous sinus
    axial view, of brain CT, 7*f*
    coronal view, of brain CT, 16*f*
    sagittal view
        of brain CT, 12*f*
        of brain MRI, 27*f*, 31*f*
Sinuses of Valsalva, sagittal view, of heart MRI,
    59*f*
Small bowel
    axial view
        of abdomen CT, 329*f*, 330*f*, 331*f*
        of female pelvis CT, 580*f*
        of male pelvis CT, 564*f*
        of male pelvis MRI, 595*f*, 596*f*, 597*f*
    coronal view
        of abdomen CT, 338*f*, 339*f*, 340*f*, 341*f*, 342*f*
        of abdomen MRI, 363*f*
        of female pelvis CT, 588*f*, 589*f*, 590*f*
        of female pelvis MRI, 623*f*, 624*f*, 625*f*
        of male pelvis CT, 573*f*, 574*f*
        of male pelvis MRI, 607*f*
    loops, axial view
        of female pelvis MRI, 614*f*
        of male pelvis CT, 564*f*
    sagittal view
        of abdomen CT, 332*f*, 334*f*, 335*f*, 336*f*, 337*f*
        of abdomen MRI, 354*f*, 355*f*, 356*f*, 357*f*, 358*f*,
            359*f*, 360*f*, 361*f*
        of female pelvis CT, 585*f*, 586*f*, 587*f*
        of female pelvis MRI, 618*f*, 619*f*
        of male pelvis CT, 570*f*, 571*f*, 572*f*
        of male pelvis MRI, 601*f*, 602*f*, 603*f*, 604*f*,
            605*f*, 606*f*

Small bowel *(Continued)*
    sagittal view, of female pelvis MRI, 618*f*, 619*f*,
        620*f*
Soleus m.
    axial view
        of ankle, 501*f*, 502*f*, 503*f*, 504*f*
        of knee, 452*f*, 453*f*
        of leg, 474*f*, 475*f*, 476*f*, 477*f*, 478*f*, 479*f*, 480*f*,
            481*f*, 482*f*, 483*f*
    coronal view
        of ankle, 532*f*
        of knee, 471*f*, 472*f*
        of leg, 492*f*, 493*f*, 494*f*, 495*f*, 496*f*
    origin, insertion, and nerve supply of, 498*t*–499*t*
    sagittal view
        of ankle, 519*f*, 520*f*
        of knee, 454*f*, 455*f*, 457*f*, 458*f*, 459*f*, 460*f*
        of leg, 484*f*, 485*f*, 486*f*, 487*f*, 488*f*, 489*f*, 490*f*
Soleus t., axial view, of leg, 474*f*, 480*f*, 481*f*, 482*f*
Spermatic cord
    axial view
        of hip, 378*f*
        of male pelvis CT, 568*f*, 569*f*
        of male pelvis MRI, 599*f*, 600*f*
    coronal view
        of hip, 393*f*
        of male pelvis CT, 573*f*
        of male pelvis MRI, 607*f*
    sagittal view
        of male pelvis CT, 571*f*
        of male pelvis MRI, 603*f*, 604*f*
Sphenoid sinus
    axial view, of brain CT, 7*f*, 8*f*
    sagittal view, of brain CT, 10*f*
Spinal canal
    axial view, of abdomen MRI, 346*f*
    coronal view, of abdomen MRI, 367*f*, 368*f*, 369*f*
    sagittal view
        of abdomen MRI, 357*f*, 358*f*
        of female pelvis MRI, 620*f*
Spinal cord
    axial view
        of abdomen MRI, 346*f*, 347*f*
        of thoracic spine, 298*f*
    coronal view
        of abdomen MRI, 369*f*
        of brain CT, 16*f*
        of pectoral girdle and chest wall, 95*f*
        of thoracic spine, 302*f*
        of thorax CT, 51*f*, 52*f*
    sagittal view
        of abdomen MRI, 357*f*, 358*f*
        of brain MRI, 31*f*
        of thoracic spine, 301*f*
        of thorax CT, 45*f*
Spinal n., sagittal view, of thoracic spine, 300*f*
Spinalis capitis m., origin, insertion, and nerve
    supply of, 306*t*–308*t*
Spinalis cervicis m., origin, insertion, and nerve
    supply of, 306*t*–308*t*
Spinalis thoracis m.
    axial view, of thoracic spine, 297*f*
    coronal view
        of pectoral girdle and chest wall, 95*f*
        of thoracic spine, 304*f*
    origin, insertion, and nerve supply of, 306*t*–308*t*
    sagittal view, of thoracic spine, 301*f*
Spinoglenoid notch
    axial view
        of shoulder, 103*f*
        of shoulder arthrogram, 131*f*, 132*f*
    coronal view, of pectoral girdle and chest wall,
        93*f*
    oblique coronal view, of shoulder arthrogram,
        144*f*
    oblique sagittal view, of shoulder, 116*f*
Spinolaminal junction, sagittal view, of lumbar
    spine, 316*f*
Spinous process
    axial view
        of cervical spine MRI, 289*f*
        of lumbar spine, 310*f*
        of male pelvis MRI, 595*f*
    coronal view
        of abdomen CT, 343*f*

Spinous process *(Continued)*
    of abdomen MRI, 369*f*
    of cervical spine MRI, 295*f*
    of male pelvis CT, 578*f*
    of pectoral girdle and chest wall, 97*f*
    of thoracic spine, 303*f*, 304*f*
    sagittal view
        of abdomen MRI, 358*f*
        of thoracic spine, 301*f*
Spleen
    axial view
        of abdomen CT, 326*f*, 327*f*, 328*f*, 329*f*, 330*f*
        of abdomen MRI, 346*f*, 347*f*, 348*f*, 349*f*, 350*f*,
            351*f*, 352*f*
    coronal view
        of abdomen CT, 342*f*, 343*f*
        of abdomen MRI, 364*f*, 365*f*, 366*f*, 367*f*, 368*f*,
            369*f*
        of lumbar spine, 321*f*
        of thoracic spine, 302*f*
        of thorax CT, 51*f*
    sagittal view
        of abdomen CT, 332*f*, 333*f*
        of abdomen MRI, 354*f*, 355*f*
        of thoracic spine, 299*f*
        of thorax CT, 43*f*
Splenic a.
    axial view, of abdomen MRI, 349*f*
    coronal view
        of abdomen CT, 339*f*, 340*f*, 341*f*, 342*f*
        of abdomen MRI, 366*f*, 367*f*
        of thorax CT, 48*f*
    sagittal view
        of abdomen CT, 332*f*, 333*f*, 334*f*
        of abdomen MRI, 355*f*, 356*f*, 357*f*
Splenic hilum, sagittal view, of abdomen CT, 332*f*
Splenic v.
    axial view
        of abdomen CT, 327*f*, 328*f*, 329*f*
        of abdomen MRI, 350*f*
    coronal view
        of abdomen CT, 340*f*, 341*f*, 342*f*, 343*f*
        of thorax CT, 48*f*
    sagittal view
        of abdomen CT, 332*f*, 333*f*, 334*f*
        of abdomen MRI, 355*f*, 356*f*, 357*f*, 358*f*
Splenic vessels
    axial view, of abdomen MRI, 347*f*, 348*f*
    coronal view, of abdomen MRI, 367*f*
    sagittal view, of abdomen MRI, 354*f*
Splenium of corpus callosum
    axial view
        of brain CT, 5*f*
        of brain MRI, 20*f*, 21*f*
    coronal view, brain CT, 16*f*
    sagittal view
        of brain CT, 10*f*
        of brain MRI, 25*f*, 31*f*
Splenius capitis m.
    axial view, of pectoral girdle and
        chest wall, 70*f*, 71*f*, 72*f*
    coronal view, of pectoral girdle and
        chest wall, 93*f*, 94*f*, 95*f*, 96*f*
    origin, insertion, and nerve supply
        of, 306*t*–308*t*
    sagittal view, of pectoral girdle and
        chest wall, 86*f*, 87*f*
Splenius mm.
    axial view
        of brain CT, 9*f*
        of cervical spine MRI, 288*f*, 289*f*, 290*f*
    coronal view
        of brain CT, 17*f*
        of cervical spine MRI, 295*f*
    sagittal view, of cervical spine MRI, 291*f*
Splenoportal confluence
    axial view, of abdomen CT, 329*f*
    coronal view, of abdomen CT, 339*f*
    sagittal view, of abdomen CT, 334*f*
Sternoclavicular joint
    axial view, of pectoral girdle and chest wall, 72*f*
    coronal view, of pectoral girdle and chest wall,
        88*f*, 89*f*
    sagittal view, of pectoral girdle and chest wall,
        87*f*

Sternocleidomastoid m.
  axial view
    of brain CT, 9f
    of cervical spine MRI, 288f, 289f, 290f
    of pectoral girdle and chest wall, 70f
  clavicular head
    axial view, of pectoral girdle and chest wall, 70f
    sagittal view, of pectoral girdle and chest wall, 85f, 86f, 87f
  coronal view
    of brain CT, 16f
    of cervical spine MRI, 294f, 295f
    of pectoral girdle and chest wall, 89f, 90f, 91f
  sagittal view
    of brain MRI, 31f
    of cervical spine MRI, 291f
    of pectoral girdle and chest wall, 87f
  sternal head
    axial view, of pectoral girdle and chest wall, 70f, 71f, 72f
    coronal view, of pectoral girdle and chest wall, 89f
Sternohyoid m.
  axial view, of pectoral girdle and chest wall, 70f, 71f, 72f
  sagittal view, of pectoral girdle and chest wall, 86f, 87f
Sternothyroid m., axial view, of pectoral girdle and chest wall, 71f, 72f
Sternum
  axial view
    of abdomen MRI, 346f
    of heart MRI, 54f
    of pectoral girdle and chest wall, 73f, 74f, 75f, 76f, 77f
    of thorax CT, 38f, 40f
  coronal view
    of abdomen CT, 338f
    of abdomen MRI, 362f
    of heart MRI, 61f
    of pectoral girdle and chest wall, 88f
  sagittal view
    of abdomen CT, 334f
    of abdomen MRI, 358f
    of heart MRI, 59f
    of thorax CT, 45f
Stomach
  antrum
    axial view
      of abdomen CT, 329f, 330f
      of abdomen MRI, 350f, 351f, 352f
    coronal view
      of abdomen CT, 338f
      of abdomen MRI, 363f
    sagittal view
      of abdomen CT, 333f, 334f
      of abdomen MRI, 360f
  axial view, of abdomen CT, 326f, 327f, 328f, 329f, 330f
  body
    axial view
      of abdomen CT, 328f, 329f, 330f
      of abdomen MRI, 348f, 349f, 350f
    coronal view
      of abdomen CT, 338f
      of abdomen MRI, 362f, 363f
    sagittal view
      of abdomen CT, 332f
      of abdomen MRI, 356f, 357f, 358f, 359f
  coronal view
    of abdomen CT, 339f, 340f
    of thorax CT, 47f
  fundus
    axial view
      of abdomen CT, 328f
      of abdomen MRI, 346f, 347f
    coronal view
      of abdomen CT, 342f, 343f
      of abdomen MRI, 363f, 364f, 365f, 366f, 367f
    sagittal view
      of abdomen CT, 332f
      of abdomen MRI, 355f, 356f

Stomach (Continued)
  pylorus ring, coronal view, of abdomen MRI, 364f
  sagittal view
    of abdomen CT, 332f, 333f, 334f
    of thorax CT, 43f
Straight venous sinus, coronal view, of brain CT, 17f
Styloid process, axial view, of brain CT, 9f
Subarachnoid space, sagittal view, of thoracic spine, 301f
Subclavian a.
  axial view
    of pectoral girdle and chest wall, 70f
    of thorax CT, 36f, 37f
  coronal view
    of heart MRI, 62f
    of pectoral girdle and chest wall, 91f
    of thorax CT, 48f, 49f
  sagittal view
    of cervical spine MRI, 291f, 292f
    of pectoral girdle and chest wall, 85f, 86f
    of thorax CT, 43f, 44f
Subclavian v.
  axial view
    of pectoral girdle and chest wall, 71f
    of thorax CT, 36f
  coronal view
    of pectoral girdle and chest wall, 89f, 90f, 91f
    of thorax CT, 47f, 48f, 49f
  sagittal view
    of pectoral girdle and chest wall, 85f, 86f
    of thorax CT, 43f, 46f
Subclavius m.
  axial view
    of pectoral girdle and chest wall, 71f
    of shoulder, 101f, 102f, 103f
  coronal view, of pectoral girdle and chest wall, 89f, 90f
  oblique coronal view, of shoulder, 119f
  oblique sagittal view, of shoulder, 118f
  origin, insertion, and nerve supply of, 129t
  sagittal view, of pectoral girdle and chest wall, 82f, 83f, 84f, 85f
Subcutaneous fat, coronal view, of abdomen MRI, 362f, 369f
Subcutaneous vessels, coronal view, of abdomen MRI, 362f
Sublabral sulcus, oblique coronal view, of shoulder, 122f
Sublime process
  axial view, of elbow, 184f, 185f
  oblique coronal, of elbow, 204f
Submandibular gland, sagittal view, brain MRI, 30f
Subscapular a.
  axial view
    of pectoral girdle and chest wall, 73f
    of shoulder, 107f, 108f
  coronal view, of pectoral girdle and chest wall, 92f
  oblique coronal view, of shoulder, 121f
  oblique sagittal view, of shoulder, 116f, 117f
Subscapular recess
  oblique coronal view, of shoulder arthrogram, 142f, 143f
  oblique sagittal view, of shoulder arthrogram, 141f
  superior
    axial view, of shoulder arthrogram, 133f
    oblique coronal view, of shoulder arthrogram, 142f
    oblique sagittal view, of shoulder arthrogram, 140f, 141f
Subscapularis m.
  ABER view, of shoulder arthrogram, 149f, 150f, 151f, 152f, 153f
  axial view
    of heart MRI, 54f
    of pectoral girdle and chest wall, 70f, 71f, 72f, 73f, 74f, 75f
    of shoulder, 102f, 103f, 104f, 105f, 106f, 107f, 108f
    of shoulder arthrogram, 131f, 132f, 133f, 134f
  coronal view

Subscapularis m. (Continued)
    of arm, 170f, 171f, 172f, 173f
    of pectoral girdle and chest wall, 90f, 91f, 92f, 93f, 94f, 95f, 96f
    of thoracic spine, 303f, 304f, 305f
  oblique coronal view
    of shoulder, 119f, 120f, 121f, 122f, 123f
    of shoulder arthrogram, 142f, 143f, 144f, 145f
  oblique sagittal view
    of shoulder, 114f, 115f, 116f, 117f, 118f
    of shoulder arthrogram, 140f, 141f
  origin, insertion, and nerve supply of, 129t
  sagittal view
    of arm, 166f
    of pectoral girdle and chest wall, 80f, 81f, 82f, 83f
Subscapularis t.
  ABER view, of shoulder arthrogram, 148f, 149f
  axial view
    of shoulder, 103f, 104f, 105f
    of shoulder arthrogram, 132f, 133f, 134f
  coronal view, of arm, 169f
  oblique coronal view
    of shoulder, 121f
    of shoulder arthrogram, 142f
  oblique sagittal view
    of shoulder, 111f, 112f, 113f, 114f
    of shoulder arthrogram, 136f, 137f, 138f, 139f, 140f, 141f
  sagittal view, of pectoral girdle and chest wall, 79f
Subtalar joint, anterior
  coronal view, of ankle, 525f, 526f
  sagittal view, of ankle, 520f, 521f
Subtalar joint, middle
  coronal view, of ankle, 527f
  oblique axial view, of ankle, 514f
  sagittal view
    of ankle, 521f, 522f
    of foot, 545f
Subtalar joint, posterior
  coronal view, of ankle, 528f, 529f, 530f
  oblique axial view, of ankle, 513f
  sagittal view, of ankle, 518f, 519f, 520f, 521f
Subtrapezial plexus, coronal view, of thoracic spine, 304f
Sulcus, posterior, axial view, of ankle, 506f
Superior frontal gyrus, brain MRI, 19f
Superior rectus m., brain CT
  axial view, 7f
  coronal view, 13f, 14f
  sagittal view, 29f
Superior rectus m., brain MRI
  axial view, 22f
  sagittal view, 28f
Superior sagittal sinus, sagittal view, of brain CT, 10f
Superior sagittal venous sinus
  axial view
    of brain CT, 4f, 5f
    of brain MRI, 19f, 20f
  coronal view, brain CT, 13f, 15f, 16f, 17f
  sagittal view, brain MRI, 28f, 32f
Superior vena cava
  axial view
    of heart MRI, 54f, 55f, 56f
    of pectoral girdle and chest wall, 73f, 74f, 75f
    of thorax CT, 38f, 39f
  coronal view
    of pectoral girdle and chest wall, 90f, 91f
    of thorax CT, 48f, 49f
  sagittal view, of thorax CT, 45f
Supinator m.
  axial view
    of elbow, 185f, 186f, 187f, 188f, 189f
    of forearm, 209f, 210f, 211f
  coronal view
    of forearm, 227f, 228f, 229f, 230f, 231f
  oblique coronal
    of elbow, 201f, 202f, 203f, 204f, 205f
  oblique sagittal view
    of elbow, 191f, 192f, 193f, 194f
  origin, insertion, and nerve supply of, 233t–234t
  sagittal view, of forearm, 220f, 221f, 222f
Supinator ridge, axial view, of elbow, 186f

Supracondylar crest, lateral
  axial view, of arm, 158f, 159f, 160f
  sagittal view, of arm, 162f, 163f
Supraglenoid tubercle
  axial view, of shoulder, 131f
  oblique sagittal view, of shoulder, 115f, 140f
Suprascapular a.
  axial view
    of pectoral girdle and chest wall, 71f
    of shoulder, 101f, 102f, 103f, 104f
  coronal view, of pectoral girdle and chest wall,
    92f, 93f
  oblique coronal view
    of shoulder, 119f, 120f, 121f, 122f, 123f, 124f
    of shoulder arthrogram, 143f, 144f
  oblique sagittal view, of shoulder, 116f
Suprascapular n.
  axial view
    of pectoral girdle and chest wall, 71f
    of shoulder, 102f, 103f, 104f
  coronal view, of pectoral girdle and chest wall,
    92f, 93f
  oblique coronal view
    of shoulder, 119f, 122f, 123f, 124f
    of shoulder arthrogram, 143f, 144f
Suprascapular neurovascular bundle
  axial view, of pectoral girdle and chest
    wall, 71f
  sagittal view, of pectoral girdle and chest wall,
    81f
Suprascapular notch
  axial view, of pectoral girdle and chest wall, 71f
  oblique coronal view
    of shoulder, 123f, 124f
    of shoulder arthrogram, 143f
Suprascapular v., axial view, of shoulder, 102f
Suprasellar cistern, axial view, of brain CT, 7f
Supraspinatus lig.
  axial view, of thoracic spine, 297f, 298f
  coronal view, of thoracic spine, 305f
Supraspinatus m.
  ABER view, of shoulder arthrogram, 148f, 149f
  axial view
    of pectoral girdle and chest wall, 70f
    of shoulder, 100f, 101f, 102f
  coronal view
    of arm, 172f, 173f
    of pectoral girdle and chest wall, 91f, 92f,
      93f, 94f
    of thoracic spine, 302f, 303f, 304f
  oblique coronal view
    of shoulder, 121f, 122f, 123f, 124f
    of shoulder arthrogram, 142f, 143f, 144f
  oblique sagittal view
    of shoulder, 112f, 113f, 114f, 115f, 116f, 117f,
      118f
    of shoulder arthrogram, 139f, 140f, 141f
  origin, insertion, and nerve supply of, 129t,
    306t–308t
  sagittal view
    of arm, 163f, 164f, 166f, 167f
    of pectoral girdle and chest wall, 80f, 81f,
      82f, 83f, 84f
Supraspinatus t.
  ABER view, of shoulder arthrogram, 149f
  axial view
    of pectoral girdle and chest wall, 70f
    of shoulder, 101f, 102f
    of shoulder arthrogram, 131f, 132f
  coronal view
    of arm, 171f, 172f
    of pectoral girdle and chest wall, 90f, 91f
  oblique coronal view
    of shoulder, 123f, 124f
    of shoulder arthrogram, 142f, 143f, 144f
  oblique sagittal view
    of shoulder, 110f, 111f, 112f, 113f
    of shoulder arthrogram, 136f, 137f, 138f,
      139f, 140f, 141f
  sagittal view
    of arm, 166f
    of pectoral girdle and chest wall, 80f
Supraspinous lig., sagittal view
  of lumbar spine, 316f
  of thoracic spine, 301f

Supraspinous lig., sagittal view, of cervical spine
  MRI, 293f
Sural cutaneous n., medial, axial view, of leg, 477f
Sural n.
  axial view, of ankle, 501f, 502f
  medial, axial view, of leg, 474f, 475f, 476f, 479f
Suspensory lig., coronal view, of male pelvis MRI,
    607f
Sustentaculum tali
  axial view, of ankle, 507f
  coronal view, of ankle, 527f, 528f
  oblique axial view, of ankle, 513f, 514f
  sagittal view
    of ankle, 521f, 522f
    of foot, 545f, 546f
Sylvian fissure
  axial view
    of brain CT, 6f, 7f
    of brain MRI, 21f, 22f
  coronal view, of brain CT, 14f, 15f
  sagittal view
    of brain CT, 11f, 12f
    of brain MRI, 27f, 29f, 30f
Sympathetic trunk, axial view, of lumbar spine,
    312f
Symphysis pubis
  axial view, of male pelvis CT, 568f
  coronal view
    of female pelvis CT, 588f
    of male pelvis CT, 574f
Synovial space
  axial view, of knee, 449f
  sagittal view, of knee, 456f, 457f, 458f, 459f

T
T5
  spinous process, 297f
T6
  lamina, 297f
  vertebra, 297f
T7
  inferior facet, 297f
  superior facet, 297f
T9
  pedicle, 298f
  vertebra, 298f
T10
  pedicle, 298f
  vertebra, 298f
T12 vertebra, 320f
T12 vertebral a. and v., sagittal view, of lumbar
    spine, 316f
T12–L1
  annulus fibrosus, 320f
  nucleus pulposus, 320f
Talar dome
  coronal view, of ankle, 527f, 528f
  oblique axial view, of ankle, 504f, 512f
  sagittal view, of ankle, 518f, 519f, 520f, 521f
Talocalcaneal joint, posterior facet, axial view, of
    ankle, 506f
Talocalcaneal lig.
  coronal view, of ankle, 526f, 527f
  sagittal view, of ankle, 518f, 519f, 520f
Talofibular lig., anterior
  axial view, of ankle, 505f
  coronal view, of ankle, 528f
Talofibular lig., posterior
  axial view, of ankle, 506f
  coronal view, of ankle, 529f, 530f
  oblique axial view, of ankle, 512f
  sagittal view, of ankle, 517f, 518f, 519f
Talonavicular joint
  axial view, of ankle, 505f, 506f
  coronal view, of ankle, 524f
  sagittal view, of ankle, 521f
Talonavicular lig., oblique axial view, of ankle,
    514f
Talus
  axial view
    of ankle, 506f
    of foot, 536f
  body
    axial view, of ankle, 505f

Talus (Continued)
  coronal view, of ankle, 527f, 528f
  sagittal view, of ankle, 519f, 520f, 521f
  coronal view
    of ankle, 525f, 526f, 529f, 530f
    of leg, 492f
  head
    axial view
      of ankle, 505f, 506f
      of foot, 535f
    coronal view, of ankle, 524f, 525f
    sagittal view
      of ankle, 520f, 521f
      of foot, 544f, 545f
  lateral process
    coronal view, of ankle, 528f, 529f
    sagittal view, of ankle, 518f, 519f
  neck
    axial view, of ankle, 505f
    sagittal view, of foot, 544f
  oblique axial view, of ankle, 513f, 514f
  posterior process
    axial view, of ankle, 506f
    oblique axial view, of ankle, 512f
    sagittal view, of ankle, 520f
  sagittal view
    of ankle, 522f
    of foot, 543f, 546f
Tarsal sinus
  axial view, of ankle, 506f
  coronal view, of ankle, 526f
  sagittal view, of ankle, 520f
Tarsometatarsal joint, 5th, axial view, of ankle,
    508f
Tectal plate
  axial view
    of brain CT, 6f
    of brain MRI, 22f
  sagittal view
    of brain CT, 10f
    of brain MRI, 25f
Temporal lobe
  axial view
    of brain CT, 6f, 7f, 8f
    of brain MRI, 21f, 22f
  coronal view
    of brain CT, 14f, 15f, 16f
  sagittal view
    of brain CT, 11f, 12f
    of brain MRI, 26f, 27f, 29f, 30f
    of cervical spine MRI, 291f, 292f
Temporalis m.
  axial view
    of brain CT, 5f, 6f, 7f, 8f
    of brain MRI, 20f, 21f, 22f, 23f, 24f
  coronal view, brain CT, 14f
  sagittal view, brain MRI, 29f
Tensor fasciae latae m.
  axial view
    of female pelvis CT, 582f, 583f, 584f
    of female pelvis MRI, 616f, 617f
    of hip, 374f, 375f, 376f, 377f, 378f, 379f,
      380f, 381f
    of male pelvis CT, 566f, 567f, 568f, 569f
    of male pelvis MRI, 598f, 599f, 600f
    of thigh, 420f, 421f
  coronal view
    of female pelvis CT, 588f, 589f, 590f
    of female pelvis MRI, 622f, 623f
    of hip, 394f, 395f
    of male pelvis CT, 573f, 574f, 575f
    of male pelvis MRI, 607f, 608f
    of thigh, 437f, 438f, 439f
  origin, insertion, and nerve supply of,
    400t–401t
  sagittal view
    of hip, 383f, 384f, 385f
    of thigh, 428f, 429f, 430f
Tentorium cerebelli
  coronal view, of brain CT, 16f, 17f
  sagittal view
    of brain CT, 10f, 11f, 12f
    of brain MRI, 25f, 26f, 32f
Teres major m.
  axial view

Teres major m. *(Continued)*
    of pectoral girdle and chest wall, 73f, 74f,
        75f, 76f
    of shoulder, 108f
    coronal view
        of arm, 172f, 173f, 174f, 176f
        of pectoral girdle and chest wall, 92f, 93f,
            94f, 95f, 96f, 97f
        of thoracic spine, 303f, 304f, 305f
    oblique coronal view, of shoulder, 124f, 125f,
        126f, 127f
    oblique sagittal view
        of shoulder, 113f, 114f, 115f, 116f, 117f, 118f
        of shoulder arthrogram, 141f
    origin, insertion, and nerve supply of, 129t,
        306t–308t
    sagittal view
        of arm, 164f, 166f, 167f
        of pectoral girdle and chest wall, 79f, 80f,
            81f, 82f, 83f
Teres major t.
    axial view
        of pectoral girdle and chest wall, 74f
        of shoulder, 107f, 108f
    coronal view
        of arm, 171f
        of pectoral girdle and chest wall, 92f
    oblique sagittal view, of shoulder, 112f, 113f,
        114f
Teres minor m.
    axial view
        of pectoral girdle and chest wall, 72f, 73f, 74f
        of shoulder, 105f, 106f, 107f, 108f
        of shoulder arthrogram, 134f, 135f, 152f
    coronal view
        of arm, 172f, 173f, 174f, 175f, 176f
        of pectoral girdle and chest wall, 93f, 94f,
            95f, 96f
        of thoracic spine, 303f, 304f
    oblique coronal view
        of shoulder, 125f, 126f, 127f
        of shoulder arthrogram, 147f
    oblique sagittal view
        of shoulder, 112f, 113f, 114f, 115f, 116f, 117f,
            118f
        of shoulder arthrogram, 139f, 140f, 141f
    origin, insertion, and nerve supply of, 129t,
        306t–308t
    sagittal view
        of arm, 163f, 164f, 165f, 166f, 167f
        of pectoral girdle and chest wall, 79f, 80f, 81f
Teres minor t.
    ABER view, of shoulder arthrogram, 151f, 152f,
        153f
    axial view, of shoulder arthrogram, 136f
    oblique coronal view
        of shoulder, 127f
        of shoulder arthrogram, 147f
    oblique sagittal view
        of shoulder, 111f, 112f, 113f
        of shoulder arthrogram, 136f, 137f, 138f,
            139f, 140f
    sagittal view
        of arm, 165f
        of pectoral girdle and chest wall, 79f
Testis
    axial view, of male pelvis MRI, 600f
    coronal view, of male pelvis MRI, 607f
    sagittal view, of male pelvis MRI, 603f, 604f,
        605f, 606f
Thalamus
    axial view
        of brain CT, 6f
        of brain MRI, 21f
    coronal view, of brain CT, 15f, 16f
    sagittal view
        of brain CT, 10f
        of brain MRI, 25f, 30f, 31f
Thecal sac
    axial view
        of cervical spine MRI, 288f
        of lumbar spine, 310f, 311f, 312f, 313f
        of male pelvis CT, 565f
        of male pelvis MRI, 595f, 596f
    coronal view

Thecal sac *(Continued)*
        of female pelvis CT, 593f
        of female pelvis MRI, 625f
        of lumbar spine, 320f
        of male pelvis CT, 577f
        of thoracic spine, 302f
    sagittal view
        of female pelvis CT, 586f, 587f
        of lumbar spine, 316f
        of male pelvis MRI, 606f
Thoracic a.
    lateral, oblique sagittal view, of shoulder, 118f
    segmental, coronal view, of thoracic spine, 302f
Thoracic a., internal
    axial view
        of pectoral girdle and chest wall, 74f, 75f,
            76f, 77f
        of thorax CT, 37f, 38f
    coronal view, of pectoral girdle and chest wall,
        88f, 89f
Thoracic duct, axial view, of thoracic spine, 298f
Thoracic lamina, coronal view, of thoracic spine,
    303f
Thoracic n., lateral, oblique sagittal view, of
    shoulder, 118f
Thoracic neurovascular bundle
    lateral, coronal view, of pectoral girdle and
        chest wall, 95f
    long, coronal view, of pectoral girdle and chest
        wall, 95f
Thoracic pars interarticularis, sagittal view, of
    thoracic spine, 301f
Thoracic pedicle
    coronal view, of thoracic spine, 302f
    sagittal view, of thoracic spine, 301f
Thoracic spinal cord, coronal view, of cervical
    spine MRI, 295f
Thoracic spinal n.
    coronal view, of thoracic spine, 302f
    sagittal view, of thoracic spine, 301f
Thoracic v., internal
    axial view
        of pectoral girdle and chest wall, 74f, 75f,
            76f, 77f
        of thorax CT, 38f
    coronal view, of pectoral girdle and chest wall,
        88f, 89f
Thoracic v., segmental, coronal view, of thoracic
    spine, 302f
Thoracic vertebra
    coronal view, of pectoral girdle and chest wall,
        92f
    sagittal view, of thoracic spine, 301f
Thoracic vertebral body
    axial view
        of heart MRI, 54f
        of pectoral girdle and chest wall, 73f
    coronal view, of pectoral girdle and chest wall,
        93f, 94f
Thoracic vertebral vessels
    axial view, of thoracic spine, 297f
    sagittal view, of thoracic spine, 300f
Thoracoacromial a.
    axial view, of pectoral girdle and chest wall, 71f
    oblique coronal view, of shoulder, 119f
Thoracoacromial a., acromial branch
    axial view
        of pectoral girdle and chest wall, 70f
        of shoulder, 101f
Thoracoacromial a., deltoid branch, axial view, of
    shoulder, 104f
Thoracoacromial v., acromial branch, axial view,
    of shoulder, 101f
Thoracolumbar fascia
    axial view
        of lumbar spine, 312f
            posterior part, 310f, 311f, 312f, 313f
        of thoracic spine, posterior part, 298f
    sagittal view
        of lumbar spine, 315f, 316f
            posterior part, 314f, 315f
        of thoracic spine, 300f
Thumb
    distal phalanx
        coronal view, 281f

Thumb *(Continued)*
        sagittal view, 269f, 270f
    interphalangeal joint, coronal view, 282f
    proximal phalanx
        axial view, 266f
        coronal view, 281f
        sagittal view, 269f, 270f
Thyrocervical trunk, coronal view, of pectoral
    girdle and chest wall, 91f
Thyroid
    axial view
        of pectoral girdle and chest wall, 69f
        of thorax CT, 41f
    coronal view, of thorax CT, 36f
Thyroid cartilage
    axial view, of pectoral girdle and chest wall, 68f
    coronal view, of pectoral girdle and chest wall,
        89f
Thyroid gland, axial view, of cervical spine MRI,
    290f
Tibia
    axial view
        of ankle, 501f, 502f, 503f, 504f
        of knee, 452f, 453f
        of leg, 474f, 475f, 476f, 478f, 479f, 481f, 483f
    coronal view
        of ankle, 526f, 527f, 528f, 529f, 530f
        of knee, 466f, 467f, 468f, 469f, 470f
        of leg, 492f, 493f, 494f
    distal, sagittal view, of leg, 486f, 488f
    oblique axial view, of ankle, 511f, 512f, 513f
    sagittal view
        of ankle, 518f, 519f, 520f, 521f, 523f
        of knee, 455f, 456f, 457f, 458f, 459f, 461f,
            462f
        of leg, 487f, 488f, 489f
Tibial a., posterior, coronal view, of leg, 494f
Tibial (medial) collateral lig.
    axial view, of knee, 450f, 451f
    coronal view
        of knee, 467f, 468f
        of leg, 493f
Tibial condyle, medial, axial view, of knee, 452f
Tibial cortex, coronal view, of leg, 492f, 493f
Tibial eminence, coronal view
    of knee, 468f, 469f
    of leg, 487f
Tibial n.
    axial view
        of ankle, 501f, 502f, 503f, 504f, 505f
        of knee, 447f, 448f, 449f, 450f, 451f, 452f,
            453f
        of leg, 474f, 475f, 476f, 477f, 478f, 479f, 480f,
            481f, 482f, 483f
        of thigh, 426f, 427f
    coronal view
        of ankle, 530f, 531f
        of knee, 469f, 470f, 471f, 472f
        of leg, 494f
        of thigh, 441f
    oblique axial view, of ankle, 511f
    sagittal view
        of ankle, 521f, 522f
        of knee, 457f
Tibial plafond
    coronal view, of ankle, 526f, 527f, 528f, 529f
    sagittal view
        of ankle, 518f, 519f, 520f, 521f
        of leg, 487f
Tibial plateau, lateral
    axial view, of knee, 451f
    coronal view
        of knee, 466f, 467f, 470f, 471f
        of leg, 493f, 494f
    sagittal view
        of knee, 454f, 455f, 456f
        of leg, 485f, 486f, 487f
Tibial plateau, medial
    axial view, of knee, 451f
    coronal view
        of knee, 465f, 470f
        of leg, 493f, 494f
    sagittal view
        of knee, 460f, 461f
        of leg, 489f, 490f

Tibial tubercle
  axial view
    of ankle, 503f
    of knee, 452f, 453f
    of leg, 474f
  sagittal view, of leg, 486f
Tibial tuberosity
  coronal view, of knee, 465f
  sagittal view, of knee, 458f
Tibialis anterior a.
  axial view
    of ankle, 501f, 502f, 503f
    of leg, 475f
  coronal view, of leg, 493f, 494f
  oblique axial view, of ankle, 512f, 513f, 514f
Tibialis anterior m.
  axial view
    of knee, 452f, 453f
    of leg, 474f, 475f, 476f, 477f, 478f, 479f, 480f, 481f, 482f, 483f
  coronal view
    of knee, 466f, 467f, 468f
    of leg, 492f, 493f
  oblique axial view, of ankle, 511f
  origin, insertion, and nerve supply of, 498t–499t
  sagittal view
    of knee, 455f, 456f
    of leg, 484f, 485f, 486f
Tibialis anterior t.
  axial view
    of ankle, 501f, 502f, 503f, 504f, 505f
    of foot, 535f, 536f
    of leg, 477f, 478f, 479f, 480f, 481f, 482f, 483f
  coronal view
    of ankle, 524f, 525f
    of foot, 555f, 556f, 557f
    of leg, 492f, 493f
  oblique axial view, of ankle, 511f, 512f, 513f, 514f, 515f, 516f
  sagittal view
    of ankle, 521f, 522f
    of foot, 546f, 547f
    of leg, 486f, 487f
Tibialis anterior vessels
  axial view, of leg, 474f, 476f, 477f, 479f, 480f, 481f, 483f
  coronal view, of ankle, 525f, 526f
  sagittal view
    of ankle, 519f, 520f
    of leg, 488f
Tibialis posterior a.
  axial view, of ankle, 501f, 502f, 503f, 504f, 505f
  coronal view, of ankle, 531f
  oblique axial view, of ankle, 513f
Tibialis posterior m.
  axial view
    of knee, 453f
    of leg, 474f, 475f, 476f, 477f, 478f, 479f, 480f, 481f, 482f, 483f
  coronal view
    of knee, 468f, 469f, 470f
    of leg, 493f, 494f
  origin, insertion, and nerve supply of, 498t–499t
  sagittal view
    of knee, 456f
    of leg, 486f, 487f, 488f
Tibialis posterior t.
  additional slip
    coronal view, of foot, 556f, 557f
    oblique axial view, of ankle, 514f, 515f, 516f
  axial view
    of ankle, 501f, 502f, 503f, 504f, 505f, 506f, 507f
    of foot, 536f
    of leg, 475f, 478f, 479f, 480f, 481f, 482f, 483f
  coronal view
    of ankle, 524f, 525f, 526f, 527f, 528f, 529f
    of foot, 557f
    of leg, 493f, 494f
  cuneiform slip
    axial view
      of ankle, 507f
      of foot, 536f, 537f
    sagittal view
      of ankle, 523f

Tibialis posterior t. (Continued)
    of foot, 546f
  oblique axial view, of ankle, 511f, 512f, 513f, 514f, 515f
  sagittal view
    of ankle, 522f, 523f
    of foot, 546f, 547f
    of leg, 487f, 488f, 489f
Tibialis posterior v., axial view, of ankle, 501f, 502f, 503f, 504f, 505f
Tibialis posterior vessels
  axial view
    of ankle, 506f, 507f, 508f
    of leg, 474f, 475f, 476f, 477f, 478f, 479f, 480f, 481f, 482f, 483f
  coronal view
    of ankle, 529f
    of knee, 471f
  oblique axial view, of ankle, 511f, 512f
Tibiocalcaneal lig., sagittal view, of ankle, 522f
Tibiofibular joint, proximal, sagittal view
    of knee, 455f
    of leg, 485f, 486f
Tibiofibular lig., anterior inferior
  axial view, of ankle, 504f
  oblique axial view, of ankle, 512f
  sagittal view, of ankle, 517f, 518f
Tibiofibular lig., posterior inferior
  axial view, of ankle, 504f
  coronal view, of ankle, 530f
  oblique axial view, of ankle, 512f
Tibiotalar joint, axial view, of ankle, 504f
Tibiotalar lig.
  anterior, sagittal view, of ankle, 522f
  posterior, sagittal view, of ankle, 522f
Toe, 1st (great), proximal phalanx
  axial view, 538f, 539f
  coronal view, 549f
  sagittal view, 547f, 548f
Toe, 2nd
  extensor t., sagittal view, 545f
  proximal phalanx
    coronal view, 549f
    sagittal view, 545f, 546f
Toe, 3rd, proximal phalanx
  axial view, 539f
  coronal view, 549f
  sagittal view, 544f
Toe, 4th
  proximal phalanx
    axial view, 539f
    coronal view, 549f
    sagittal view, 542f
Tongue, brain MRI, 29f
Trachea
  axial view
    of cervical spine MRI, 290f
    of heart MRI, 54f
    of pectoral girdle and chest wall, 71f, 72f, 73f
    of thorax CT, 36f, 37f
  coronal view
    of heart MRI, 62f
    of pectoral girdle and chest wall, 88f, 90f, 91f
    of thorax CT, 48f, 49f, 50f
  sagittal view
    of heart MRI, 59f
    of thorax CT, 45f
Tracheal carina
  axial view, of thorax CT, 38f
  coronal view, of thorax CT, 50f
Transverse acetabular lig.
  axial view, of hip arthrogram, 406f
  coronal view, of hip arthrogram, 414f, 415f, 416f, 417f
  sagittal view, of hip arthrogram, 412f, 413f
Transverse cervical vessels
  axial view, of pectoral girdle and chest wall, 69f
  coronal view, of pectoral girdle and chest wall, 92f, 93f
Transverse humeral lig., axial view, of shoulder, 105f, 106f
Transverse lig
  axial view, of cervical spine MRI, 288f
  sagittal view, of cervical spine MRI, 293f

Transverse meniscal lig
  coronal view, of knee, 465f
  sagittal view, of knee, 458f
Transverse process
  axial view
    of lumbar spine, 310f
    of thoracic spine, 298f
  coronal view, of thoracic spine, 303f
Transverse sinus, sagittal view, of brain CT, 10f, 11f, 12f
Transverse venous sinus
  axial view, of brain CT, 6f
  coronal view, of brain CT, 17f
Transversospinalis m.
  axial view, of thoracic spine, 297f, 298f
  coronal view, of thoracic spine, 303f
  sagittal view, of thoracic spine, 300f
Transversus abdominis m
  axial view
    of abdomen CT, 329f, 331f
    of abdomen MRI, 350f, 351f
    of hip, 374f
    of male pelvis CT, 564f, 565f
    of male pelvis MRI, 595f
  coronal view
    of abdomen CT, 338f, 340f, 341f
    of female pelvis CT, 589f, 590f
    of male pelvis CT, 573f, 574f, 575f, 576f
  origin, insertion, and nerve supply of, 344t
  sagittal view, of abdomen CT, 332f, 337f
Trapezium
  coronal view, of hand, 279f, 280f, 281f
  sagittal view, of hand, 271f, 272f
Trapezius m.
  axial view, 99f, 100f
    of cervical spine MRI, 288f, 289f, 290f
    of heart MRI, 54f
    of pectoral girdle and chest wall, 70f, 71f, 72f, 73f, 74f
    of shoulder, 99f, 100f
    of thoracic spine, 297f, 298f
  coronal view
    of cervical spine MRI, 295f
    of pectoral girdle and chest wall, 91f, 92f, 93f, 94f, 95f, 96f, 97f
    of thoracic spine, 302f, 303f, 304f, 305f
  oblique coronal view, of shoulder, 119f, 120f, 121f, 122f, 123f, 124f
  oblique sagittal view
    of shoulder, 116f, 117f, 118f
    of shoulder arthrogram, 140f, 141f
  origin, insertion, and nerve supply of, 306t–308t
  sagittal view
    of brain MRI, 32f
    of cervical spine MRI, 291f, 292f
    of pectoral girdle and chest wall, 81f, 82f, 83f, 84f, 85f, 86f, 87f
    of thoracic spine, 299f, 300f, 301f
Trapezoid
  coronal view, of hand, 280f, 281f, 282f
  sagittal view, of hand, 272f, 273f
Trapezoid lig., coracoclavicular portion, coronal view, of pectoral girdle and chest wall, 90f, 91f
Trapezotriquetral lig., dorsal, coronal view, of hand, 281f, 282f
Triangular fibrocartilage, coronal view, of hand, 280f, 281f, 282f
Triangular space
  coronal view
    of arm, 173f
    of pectoral girdle and chest wall, 93f
  oblique coronal view, of shoulder, 125f
Triceps brachii m.
  axial view
    of arm, 158f, 159f, 160f
    of elbow, 180f
  coronal view
    of arm, 172f, 173f
    of pectoral girdle and chest wall, 94f, 95f, 96f, 97f
  oblique coronal, of elbow, 203f, 204f
  origin, insertion, and nerve supply of, 177t
  sagittal view
    of arm, 162f, 163f, 164f

Triceps brachii m. (Continued)
    of pectoral girdle and chest wall, 79f
Triceps brachii m., lateral head
    axial view
        of arm, 155f, 156f, 157f
        of elbow, 179f, 180f
        of pectoral girdle and chest wall, 74f, 75f, 76f
        of shoulder, 108f
    coronal view
        of arm, 172f, 173f, 174f, 175f
        of pectoral girdle and chest wall, 94f, 95f
    oblique coronal view
        of elbow, 206f, 207f
        of shoulder, 126f, 127f
    oblique sagittal view
        of elbow, 190f, 191f, 192f, 197f
        of shoulder, 112f, 113f
    sagittal view
        of arm, 161f, 162f, 163f, 164f
        of pectoral girdle and chest wall, 78f, 79f
Triceps brachii m., long head
    axial view
        of arm, 155f, 156f, 157f
        of elbow, 179f, 180f
        of pectoral girdle and chest wall, 72f, 73f,
            74f, 75f, 76f, 77f
        of shoulder, 107f, 108f
        of shoulder arthrogram, 135f
    coronal view
        of arm, 173f, 174f, 175f
        of pectoral girdle and chest wall, 94f, 95f,
            96f, 97f
    oblique coronal view, of elbow, 204f, 205f, 206f
    oblique sagittal view
        of elbow, 195f, 196f, 197f
        of shoulder, 112f, 113f, 114f, 115f, 116f, 117f
    sagittal view
        of arm, 162f, 163f, 164f, 165f, 166f
        of pectoral girdle and chest wall, 78f, 79f
        of shoulder, 125f, 126f, 127f, 128f
Triceps brachii m., medial head
    axial view
        of arm, 155f, 156f, 157f
        of elbow, 179f, 180f
        of pectoral girdle and chest wall, 76f, 77f
    coronal view
        of arm, 171f, 172f
        of pectoral girdle and chest wall, 94f, 95f
    oblique coronal, of elbow, 204f, 205f, 206f, 207f
    oblique sagittal view, of elbow, 192f, 193f, 194f
    sagittal view
        of arm, 164f, 165f, 166f, 167f
        of pectoral girdle and chest wall, 79f
Triceps brachii musculotendinous unit, coronal
        view, of arm, 172f
Triceps brachii t.
    axial view
        of arm, 158f, 159f, 160f
        of elbow, 179f, 180f, 181f
    coronal view, of arm, 172f, 173f
    oblique coronal, of elbow, 206f, 207f
    oblique sagittal view, of elbow, 191f, 192f,
        194f, 195f, 196f
    sagittal view, of arm, 164f, 165f
Triceps brachii t., long head
    ABER view, of shoulder arthrogram, 153f
    axial view, of shoulder, 107f, 108f
    coronal view
        of arm, 173f
        of pectoral girdle and chest wall, 93f
    oblique sagittal view
        of shoulder, 114f
        of shoulder arthrogram, 140f, 141f
Triceps m., lateral head, axial view, of pectoral
        girdle and chest wall, 73f
Tricipital aponeurosis, axial view, of elbow, 180f,
    181f
Tricuspid plane, axial view, of heart MRI, 57f
Trigeminal nerve
    axial view, brain MRI, 23f
    sagittal view, brain MRI, 30f
Trigone of lateral ventricle, axial view, of brain
    CT, 5f
Triquetrum
    coronal view, of hand, 280f, 281f, 282f

Triquetrum (Continued)
    sagittal view
        of hand, 275f
        of wrist, 275f
Trochlea
    axial view, of elbow, 181f, 182f, 183f
    femoral
        axial view, of knee, 449f, 450f
        coronal view, of knee, 463f
    oblique coronal, of elbow, 203f, 204f
    oblique sagittal view, of elbow, 195f, 196f, 197f
    sagittal view, of arm, 163f, 164f, 165f, 166f
Trochlear notch
    oblique sagittal view, of elbow, 195f, 196f
    sagittal view, of arm, 164f, 165f
Trunk of corpus callosum
    coronal view, of brain CT, 14f, 15f
    sagittal view
        of brain CT, 10f
        of brain MRI, 29f, 30f
Tunica albuginea, axial view, of male pelvis MRI,
    600f

U
Ulna
    axial view, of elbow, 184f, 185f, 186f, 187f,
        188f, 189f
    coronal view
        of forearm, 226f, 227f, 228f, 229f, 230f
        of hand, 281f, 282f, 283f
    oblique coronal, of elbow, 204f, 205f
    oblique sagittal view, of elbow, 193f, 194f, 195f
    radial notch, axial view, of elbow, 184f
    sagittal view, of forearm, 222f, 223f, 224f
Ulnar a.
    axial view
        of elbow, 184f, 185f, 186f, 187f, 188f, 189f
        of forearm, 209f, 210f, 211f, 212f, 213f, 214f,
            215f, 216f, 217f, 218f
    coronal view
        of forearm, 225f, 226f, 227f, 228f
        of hand, 279f, 280f
    oblique coronal, of elbow, 201f, 202f, 203f
    oblique sagittal view, of elbow, 194f, 195f
    sagittal view, of forearm, 221f, 222f
Ulnar a., deep
    axial view, of hand, 262f
    coronal view, of hand, 280f
Ulnar a., superficial, axial view, of hand, 262f,
    263f
Ulnar collateral a., inferior, axial view, of arm,
    159f, 160f
Ulnar collateral a., superior, axial view
    of arm, 156f, 157f, 158f, 159f
    of elbow, 182f, 183f, 184f, 185f, 186f, 187f
Ulnar collateral lig.
    accessory, coronal view, of hand, 281f
    axial view
        of elbow, 182f, 183f
        of hand, 268f
    coronal view
        of arm, 170f
        of hand, 281f, 282f
    lateral
        axial view, of elbow, 183f, 184f, 185f, 186f,
            187f
        oblique coronal, of elbow, 204f, 205f
        oblique sagittal view, of elbow, 191f, 192f,
            193f
    oblique coronal, of elbow, 204f
    oblique sagittal view, of elbow, 197f
    sagittal view, of hand, 270f
Ulnar head
    axial view, of elbow, 187f, 188f
    oblique sagittal view, of elbow, 197f, 198f
Ulnar n.
    axial view
        of arm, 155f, 157f, 158f, 159f
        of elbow, 179f, 180f, 181f, 182f, 183f, 184f,
            185f, 186f, 187f, 188f, 189f
        of forearm, 209f, 210f, 211f, 212f, 213f, 214f,
            215f, 216f, 217f, 218f
    coronal view
        of forearm, 225f, 226f

Ulnar n. (Continued)
    of hand, 279f, 280f
    oblique coronal, of elbow, 203f, 204f, 205f,
        206f
    oblique sagittal view, of elbow, 196f, 197f
    sagittal view
        of forearm, 222f, 223f
        of hand, 275f
Ulnar recurrent a., oblique coronal, of elbow, 203f
Ulnar sesamoid
    axial view, of hand, 265f
    sagittal view, of hand, 271f
Ulnar styloid, coronal view, of hand, 281f, 282f
Ulnar tuberosity, oblique sagittal view, of elbow,
    195f
Ulnotriquetral lig., palmar, sagittal view, of wrist,
    252f
Umbilical a., obliterated, axial view, of male pelvis
    MRI, 597f
Umbilicus
    axial view
        of abdomen CT, 331f
        of male pelvis MRI, 595f
    coronal view
        of abdomen MRI, 362f
        of female pelvis MRI, 622f
    sagittal view
        of abdomen CT, 334f
        of abdomen MRI, 358f
Uncinate process
    axial view
        of abdomen CT, 330f
        of abdomen MRI, 351f, 352f
    coronal view, of abdomen CT, 339f
    sagittal view, of abdomen CT, 335f
Uncus
    axial view, brain MRI, 23f
    sagittal view, brain MRI, 30f
Ureter
    axial view
        of abdomen MRI, 353f
        of male pelvis CT, 564f, 565f, 566f
    coronal view
        of abdomen MRI, 367f
        of female pelvis CT, 590f
        of male pelvis CT, 574f
    sagittal view, of male pelvis CT, 571f
Ureterovesicular junction, axial view, of male
    pelvis CT, 567f
Urethra
    axial view
        of female pelvis CT, 583f, 584f
        of female pelvis MRI, 617f
        of male pelvis CT, 568f
    coronal view
        of female pelvis CT, 591f
        of female pelvis MRI, 624f
        of male pelvis MRI, 607f
    membranous, axial view, of male pelvis CT, 569f
    prostatic segment, axial view, of male pelvis
        MRI, 599f
    sagittal view
        of female pelvis CT, 587f
        of female pelvis MRI, 620f
    spongiose segment, axial view, of male pelvis
        CT, 569f
Urinary bladder
    axial view
        of female pelvis CT, 582f, 583f
        of female pelvis MRI, 616f, 617f
        of hip, 378f
        of male pelvis CT, 567f, 568f
        of male pelvis MRI, 598f
    coronal view
        of female pelvis CT, 588f, 589f, 590f, 591f,
            592f
        of female pelvis MRI, 623f, 624f
        of hip, 394f, 395f
        of male pelvis CT, 574f, 575f, 576f
        of male pelvis MRI, 608f, 609f
    sagittal view
        of female pelvis CT, 585f, 586f, 587f
        of female pelvis MRI, 618f, 619f, 620f, 621f
        of male pelvis CT, 571f, 572f
        of male pelvis MRI, 603f, 604f, 605f, 606f

Urogenital diaphragm
  coronal view, of female pelvis CT, 592*f*
  sagittal view, of male pelvis CT, 571*f*
Uterine a.
  axial view, of female pelvis CT, 582*f*
  coronal view, of female pelvis CT, 592*f*
Uterine body
  coronal view, of female pelvis CT, 593*f*
  sagittal view, of female pelvis CT, 586*f*, 587*f*
Uterine cervix
  axial view, of female pelvis CT, 582*f*
  coronal view
    of female pelvis CT, 593*f*
    of female pelvis MRI, 624*f*, 625*f*
  sagittal view
    of female pelvis CT, 586*f*, 587*f*
    of female pelvis MRI, 620*f*, 621*f*
Uterine corpus, sagittal view, of female pelvis MRI, 620*f*
Uterine fundus
  axial view, of female pelvis MRI, 615*f*
  sagittal view, of female pelvis CT, 587*f*
Uterine v.
  axial view, of female pelvis CT, 582*f*
  coronal view, of female pelvis CT, 592*f*
Uterosacral lig., axial view, of female pelvis CT, 582*f*
Uterus
  axial view, of female pelvis CT, 580*f*, 581*f*, 582*f*
  coronal view, of female pelvis CT, 592*f*
  sagittal view, of female pelvis MRI, 621*f*

V

Vagina
  axial view
    of female pelvis CT, 583*f*, 584*f*
    of female pelvis MRI, 616*f*, 617*f*
  coronal view
    of female pelvis CT, 591*f*, 592*f*, 593*f*
    of female pelvis MRI, 624*f*, 625*f*
    posterior fornix, sagittal view, of female pelvis MRI, 621*f*
  sagittal view
    of female pelvis CT, 586*f*, 587*f*
    of female pelvis MRI, 620*f*, 621*f*
Vagus n., axial view, of thorax CT, 36*f*
Valsalva, sinuses of, sagittal view, of heart MRI, 59*f*
Vas deferens
  axial view, of male pelvis MRI, 597*f*
  coronal view, of male pelvis MRI, 610*f*, 611*f*
Vastus intermedius m.
  axial view
    of female pelvis CT, 584*f*
    of hip, 380*f*, 381*f*, 382*f*
    of male pelvis CT, 569*f*
    of male pelvis MRI, 600*f*
    of thigh, 420*f*, 423*f*, 424*f*, 425*f*, 426*f*, 427*f*
  coronal view
    of female pelvis CT, 590*f*, 591*f*
    of female pelvis MRI, 623*f*, 624*f*
    of hip, 394*f*, 395*f*
    of male pelvis CT, 577*f*
    of male pelvis MRI, 608*f*, 609*f*
    of thigh, 439*f*, 440*f*
  origin, insertion, and nerve supply of, 445*t*
  sagittal view
    of hip, 384*f*, 385*f*, 386*f*, 387*f*
    of thigh, 428*f*, 429*f*, 430*f*, 431*f*, 432*f*

Vastus intermedius t., axial view, of thigh, 426*f*, 427*f*
Vastus lateralis m.
  axial view
    of female pelvis CT, 584*f*
    of female pelvis MRI, 617*f*
    of hip, 378*f*, 379*f*, 380*f*, 381*f*, 382*f*
    of knee, 447*f*, 448*f*
    of male pelvis CT, 568*f*, 569*f*
    of male pelvis MRI, 599*f*, 600*f*
    of thigh, 420*f*, 421*f*, 422*f*, 423*f*, 424*f*, 425*f*, 426*f*, 427*f*
  coronal view
    of female pelvis CT, 590*f*, 591*f*, 592*f*
    of female pelvis MRI, 623*f*, 624*f*
    of hip, 394*f*, 395*f*, 396*f*
    of knee, 465*f*, 466*f*, 467*f*
    of male pelvis CT, 576*f*, 577*f*
    of male pelvis MRI, 608*f*, 609*f*, 610*f*, 611*f*
    of thigh, 437*f*, 438*f*, 440*f*, 441*f*, 442*f*
  origin, insertion, and nerve supply of, 445*t*
  sagittal view
    of hip, 383*f*, 384*f*, 385*f*
    of knee, 454*f*
    of thigh, 428*f*, 429*f*, 430*f*, 431*f*
Vastus medialis m.
  axial view
    of knee, 447*f*, 448*f*
    of thigh, 424*f*, 425*f*, 426*f*, 427*f*
  coronal view
    of knee, 463*f*, 464*f*, 465*f*, 466*f*, 467*f*, 468*f*
    of thigh, 439*f*, 440*f*, 441*f*
  origin, insertion, and nerve supply of, 445*t*
  sagittal view
    of knee, 459*f*, 460*f*, 461*f*, 462*f*
    of thigh, 432*f*, 433*f*, 434*f*
Ventricle
  coronal view
    of abdomen CT, 338*f*, 339*f*, 341*f*
    of heart MRI, 61*f*, 62*f*
    of thorax CT, 47*f*
  left
    axial view
      of heart MRI, 56*f*, 57*f*
      of thorax CT, 40*f*, 41*f*
    coronal view
      of abdomen CT, 339*f*, 341*f*
      of abdomen MRI, 364*f*
      of heart MRI, 61*f*, 62*f*
      of thorax CT, 47*f*, 49*f*
    sagittal view
      of abdomen CT, 332*f*, 333*f*, 334*f*
      of heart MRI, 58*f*
      of thorax CT, 43*f*, 44*f*, 45*f*
  right
    axial view
      of heart MRI, 56*f*, 57*f*
      of thorax CT, 40*f*, 41*f*, 42*f*
    sagittal view
      of abdomen CT, 332*f*, 333*f*
      of heart MRI, 58*f*, 60*f*
      of thorax CT, 43*f*, 44*f*, 45*f*
Ventricular cavity
  left
    coronal view, of heart MRI, 62*f*
    sagittal view, of heart MRI, 58*f*
  right, sagittal view, of heart MRI, 59*f*
Ventricular myocardium, left
  coronal view, of heart MRI, 62*f*
  sagittal view, of heart MRI, 58*f*

Ventricular outflow tract, right, sagittal view, of heart MRI, 58*f*
Ventricular papillary m., left, coronal view, of thorax CT, 48*f*
Vertebra, thoracic
  coronal view, of pectoral girdle and chest wall, 92*f*
  sagittal view, of thoracic spine, 301*f*
Vertebral a.
  axial view
    of pectoral girdle and chest wall, 68*f*
    of thorax CT, 36*f*
  sagittal view
    of brain MRI, 25*f*
    of cervical spine MRI, 291*f*, 292*f*
    of lumbar spine, 316*f*
Vertebral body
  axial view
    of heart MRI, 54*f*
    of pectoral girdle and chest wall, 73*f*, 74*f*, 75*f*, 77*f*
  coronal view
    of abdomen MRI, 365*f*, 366*f*, 367*f*
    of heart MRI, 62*f*
    of pectoral girdle and chest wall, 93*f*, 94*f*
    of thorax CT, 51*f*
  sagittal view, of abdomen MRI, 357*f*, 358*f*, 359*f*
Vertebral v.
  axial view, of thorax CT, 36*f*
  sagittal view, of lumbar spine, 316*f*
Vertebral vessels, thoracic
  axial view, of thoracic spine, 297*f*
  sagittal view, of thoracic spine, 300*f*
Vestibule, axial view, of female pelvis CT, 584*f*
Volar plate
  axial view, of hand, 266*f*, 268*f*
  coronal view, of hand, 279*f*, 280*f*, 281*f*
  sagittal view, of hand, 272*f*, 274*f*, 275*f*, 276*f*, 277*f*, 278*f*

X

Xiphoid process
  axial view
    of abdomen MRI, 348*f*
    of thorax CT, 40*f*, 41*f*
  coronal view
    of abdomen CT, 338*f*
    of abdomen MRI, 362*f*
    of heart MRI, 61*f*
  sagittal view, of thorax CT, 45*f*

Z

Zona articularis, coronal view, of hip arthrogram, 418*f*
Zona orbicularis
  axial view, of hip arthrogram, 405*f*, 406*f*, 407*f*, 408*f*
  coronal view, of hip arthrogram, 415*f*, 416*f*, 417*f*, 418*f*
  sagittal view, of hip arthrogram, 409*f*, 410*f*
Zygapophyseal (facet) joint, sagittal view, of thoracic spine, 300*f*, 301*f*
Zygomatic arch
  axial view, of brain CT, 8*f*
  coronal view, of brain CT, 14*f*
  sagittal view, of brain CT, 12*f*
Zygomatic bone, axial view, of brain CT, 7*f*